Neurodevelopment and Schizophrenia

Since the early 1990s, developmental neurobiology has made important strides towards eluci-dating the pathophysiology of psychiatric disorders. Nowhere has this link between basic science and clinical insights become more evident than in the field of schizophrenia research. In this volume, the editors bring together some of the most active investigators in this field. Each con-tributor provides an up-to-date overview of the relevant research, including directions for further investigation.

The book begins with a section on advances in developmental neurobiology. This is followed by sections on etiological and pathophysiological developments, and models that integrate this knowledge. The final section addresses the clinical insights that emerge from the developmental models and sets the scene for future efforts at early detection and prevention of schizophrenia.

This book will be valuable to researchers in psychiatry and neurobiology, students in medicine and psychology, and all mental health practitioners.

Neurodevelopment and Schizophrenia

Edited by

Matcheri S. Keshavan

University of Pittsburgh and Western Psychiatric Institute and Clinic,
Pittsburgh, PA and Wayne State University, Detroit, MI, USA

James L. Kennedy

University of Toronto Centre for Mental Health and Addiction,
Toronto, Canada

and

Robin M. Murray

King's College London and Institute of Psychiatry, London, UK

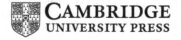

CAMBRIDGE
UNIVERSITY PRESS

CAMBRIDGE UNIVERSITY PRESS
Cambridge, New York, Melbourne, Madrid, Cape Town, Singapore,
São Paulo, Delhi, Dubai, Tokyo

Cambridge University Press
The Edinburgh Building, Cambridge CB2 8RU, UK

Published in the United States of America by Cambridge University Press, New York

www.cambridge.org
Information on this title: www.cambridge.org/9780521126595

First published 2004
This digitally printed version 2009

A catalogue record for this publication is available from the British Library

Library of Congress Cataloguing in Publication data
Neurodevelopment and schizophrenia / [edited by] Matcheri S. Keshavan,
James L. Kennedy, Robin M. Murray.
       p.   cm.
Includes bibliographical references and index.
ISBN 0 521 82331 5 (hardback)
1. Schizophrenia – Etiology.   2. Schizophrenia – Pathophysiology.   3. Developmental neurobiology.
4. Brain – Growth.   I. Keshavan, Matcheri S., 1953–   II. Kennedy, James L.   III. Murray, Robin, M.
[DNLM: 1. Brain – growth & development.   2. Schizophrenia – etiology.   3. Brain – abnormalities.
4. Models, neurological.   5. Neurobiology – methods.   WM 203 N49318   2004]
RC514.N4433   2004
616.89′8071 – dc22   2004045710

ISBN 978-0-521-82331-9 Hardback
ISBN 978-0-521-12659-5 Paperback

Additional resources for this publication at www.cambridge.org/9780521126595

Contents

Part III   Pathophysiology

Contributors

Matthew Allin
Institute of Psychiatry at The Maudsley and
Department of Psychiatry, King's College
London, De Crespigny Park, London
SE5 8AF, UK

Vicki Anderson
Department of Psychology, University
of Melbourne and the Murdoch
Children's Research Institute, Royal
Children's Hospital, Melbourne,
Australia

Francine M. Benes
Program in Structural and Molecular
Neuroscience, McLean Hospital, Belmont
and Program in Neuroscience and
Department of Psychiatry, Harvard
Medical School, Boston, MA,
USA

Jonathan D. Blumenthal
Child Psychiatry Branch, National Institute
of Mental Health, National
Institutes of Health, Bethesda,
MD 20892, USA

Jane Boydell
Institute of Psychiatry at The Maudsley and
Department of Psychiatry, King's College
London, De Crespigny Park, London
SE5 8AF, UK

Mary Cannon
Division of Psychological Medicine,
Institute of Psychiatry, De Crespigny
Park, Denmark Hill, London
SE5 8AF, UK

Chih-Ken Chen
Department of Psychiatry, Chang Gung
Memorial Hospital, 222 Mai-Chin Road,
Keelung, Taiwan

Liv S. Clasen
Child Psychiatry Branch, National Institute
of Mental Health, National Institutes of
Health, Bethesda, MD 20892,
USA

Barbara A. Cornblatt
Recognition and Prevention (RAP)
Program, 444 Lakeville Road, Lake Success,
NY 11042, USA

David Cotter
Division of Psychological Medicine,
Institute of Psychiatry, De Crespigny Park,
Denmark Hill, London SE5 8AF, UK

Michael Craig
Division of Psychological Medicine,
Institute of Psychiatry, De Crespigny Park,
Denmark Hill, London
SE5 8AF, UK

William Cutter
Division of Psychological Medicine,
Institute of Psychiatry, De Crespigny Park,
Denmark Hill, London
SE5 8AF, UK

Paola Dazzan
Division of Psychological Medicine,
Institute of Psychiatry, De Crespigny
Park, Denmark Hill, London
SE5 8AF, UK

Kimberlie Dean
Division of Psychological Medicine,
Institute of Psychiatry, De Crespigny Park,
Denmark Hill, London SE5 8AF, UK

Cinzia R. De Luca
Departments of Psychology and Psychiatry,
University of Melbourne and Melbourne
Neuropsychiatry Centre, Sunshine
Hospital, Melbourne,
Australia

Richard R. Dopp
Child Psychiatry Branch, National
Institute of Mental Health, National
Institutes of Health, Bethesda, MD 20892,
USA

Stephan Eliez
Division of Child and Adolescent
Psychiatry, University of Geneva School of
Medicine, 41 Chemin Crts-de-Champel,
1206 Geneva, Switzerland

Paul Fearon
Division of Psychological Medicine,
Institute of Psychiatry at the
Maudsley NHS Trust, De Crespigny Park,
Denmark Hill, London SE5 8AF,
UK

Carl Feinstein
Stanford University School of Medicine,
401 Quarry Road, Stanford, CA
94305–5719, USA

Daniel J. Fridberg
Child Psychiatry Branch, National
Institute of Mental Health, National
Institutes of Health, Bethesda, MD 20892,
USA

Jay N. Giedd
Child Psychiatry Branch, National
Institute of Mental Health, National
Institutes of Health, Bethesda, MD 20892,
USA

John H. Gilmore
Department of Psychiatry, UNC Conte
Center for Neuroscience of Mental
Disorders, University of North Carolina
School of Medicine, Chapel Hill, NC 27599,
USA

Nitin Gogtay
Child Psychiatry Branch, National Institute
of Mental Health, National Institutes of
Health, Bethesda, MD 20892,
USA

Anthony A. Grace
Department of Neuroscience,
458 Crawford Hall, University of
Pittsburgh, Pittsburgh, PA 15206,
USA

L. Fredrik Jarskog
Department of Psychiatry, UNC Conte
Center for Neuroscience of Mental
Disorders, University of North Carolina
School of Medicine, Chapel Hill, NC 27599,
USA

Peter B. Jones
Department of Psychiatry, University of
Cambridge, Addenbrooke's Hospital,
Cambridge CB2 2QQ, UK

James L. Kennedy
Centre for Addiction and Mental Health,
University of Toronto, 250 College St,
Toronto, ON M5T1R8, Canada

Matcheri S. Keshavan
University of Pittsburgh School of
Medicine, Department of Psychiatry and
Western Psychiatric Institute and Clinic,
Pittsburgh and the Department of
Psychiatry and Behavioral Neurosciences,
Wayne State University School of Medicine,
4201 St Antoine Boulevard,
Detroit, MI 48201,
USA

Timothy A. Klempan
Centre for Addiction and Mental Health,
University of Toronto, 250 College St,
Toronto, ON M5T1R8,
Canada

Eugenia Kravariti
Division of Psychological Medicine,
Institute of Psychiatry, De Crespigny Park,
Denmark Hill, London SE5 8AF, UK

Christian W. Kreipke
Cellular and Clinical Neurobiology,
Department of Psychiatry and Behavioral
Neurosciences, Wayne State University
School of Medicine, 540 E. Canfield,
Detroit, MI 48201, USA

Stephen M. Lawrie
Division of Psychiatry, Royal Edinburgh
Hospital, Edinburgh EH10 5HF, UK

Pat Levitt
Kennedy Center, Vanderbilt University,
Nashville, TN 37235, USA

David A. Lewis
Departments of Psychiatry and
Neuroscience, University of Pittsburgh,
Pittsburgh, PA 15213, USA

Jeffrey A. Lieberman
Department of Psychiatry, UNC Conte
Center for Neuroscience of Mental
Disorders, University of North Carolina
School of Medicine, Chapel Hill,
NC 27599, USA

Beatriz Luna
Laboratory of Neurocognitive
Development, Western Psychiatric
Institute and Clinic, University of
Pittsburgh Medical Center, 3501 Forbes
Ave, Pittsburgh, PA 15213,
USA

Sahebarao P. Mahadik
Department of Psychiatry and Health
Behavior, Medical College of Georgia and
Medical Research Service, VA Medical
Center, 1 Freedom Way, Augusta,
GA 30904, USA

Colm McDonald
Division of Psychological Medicine,
Institute of Psychiatry, De Crespigny Park,
Denmark Hill, London SE5 8AF, UK

Darlene S. Melchitzky
Department of Psychiatry, University of
Pittsburgh, Pittsburgh, PA 15213 and
Department of Biology, Mercyhurst
College, Erie, PA 16546,
USA

Karoly Mirnics
Departments of Psychiatry and
Neurobiology, University of Pittsburgh,
Pittsburgh, PA 15213, USA

Elizabeth Molloy
Child Psychiatry Branch, National Institute of Mental Health, National Institutes of Health, Bethesda, MD 20892, USA

Pierandrea Muglia
Centre for Addiction and Mental Health, University of Toronto, 250 College St, Toronto, ON M5T1R8, Canada

Declan Murphy
Division of Psychological Medicine, Institute of Psychiatry, De Crespigny Park, Denmark Hill, London SE5 8AF, UK

Robin M. Murray
Institute of Psychiatry at The Maudsley and Department of Psychiatry, King's College London, De Crespigny Park, London SE5 8AF, UK

Ray Norbury
Division of Psychological Medicine, Institute of Psychiatry, De Crespigny Park, Denmark Hill, London SE5 8AF, UK

Chiara Nosarti
Institute of Psychiatry at The Maudsley and Department of Psychiatry, King's College London, De Crespigny Park, London SE5 8AF, UK

Christos Pantelis
Melbourne Neurospychiatry Centre Department of Psychiatry, University of Melbourne and Sunshine Hospital, Melbourne, Australia

Carmine M. Pariante
Division of Psychological Medicine, Institute of Psychiatry, De Crespigny Park, Denmark Hill, London SE5 8AF, UK

Arturas Petronis
The Krembil Family Epigenetics Laboratory, Centre for Addiction and Mental Health, 250 College St, Toronto, ON M5T1R8, Canada

Larry Rifkin
Institute of Psychiatry at The Maudsley and Department of Psychiatry, King's College London, De Crespigny Park, London SE5 8AF, UK

A. Blythe Rose
Child Psychiatry Branch, National Institute of Mental Health, National Institutes of Health, Bethesda, MD 20892, USA

David R. Rosenberg
Department of Psychiatry and Behavioral Neurosciences, Wayne State University School of Medicine, 4201 St Antoine Boulevard, Detroit, MI 48201, USA

Michael A. Rosenthal
Child Psychiatry Branch, National Institute of Mental Health, National Institutes of Health, Bethesda, MD 20892, USA

John A. Sweeney
Department of Psychiatry, University of Illinois at Chicago, The Psychiatric Institute, 1601 W. Taylor St, Chicago, IL 60612, USA

Jim van Os
Maastricht University, PO Box 616, 6200 MD Maastricht, the Netherlands

Stephen J. Wood
Melbourne Neuropsychiatry Centre and Department of Psychiatry, University of Melbourne and Sunshine Hospital and The Brain Research Institute, Melbourne, Australia

Foreword

Although both Kraepelin and Bleuler noted that premorbid abnormalities in childhood could be present many years before a schizophrenic psychosis developed (Marenco and Weinberger, 2000), until the late 1980s and 1990s, most people viewed schizophrenia as an adult-onset mental illness. As a result, most biological studies focused on a search for possible neurodegenerative changes that might account for the onset of the condition. During the 1960s and 1970s (see Garmezy, 1974; Offord and Cross, 1969), evidence began to accumulate from developmentally oriented follow-up and follow-back studies that abnormalities in interpersonal relationships, neurodevelopmental immaturities, and attentional deficits in childhood all predicted the later onset of schizophrenia (see Rutter and Garmezy, 1983). However, it was not until 1987 (Murray and Lewis, 1987; Weinberger, 1987) that psychiatrists concerned with adult patients firmly took on board the notion that schizophrenia might be a neurodevelopmental disorder. Since then, there has been a veritable explosion of research tackling this proposition using a variety of research strategies. In parallel, there has been an upsurge in studies of brain development and function, giving rise to a much better understanding of brain plasticity and of the role of neurotransmitters in both normal functioning and disease states. Clearly, the time is ripe for a book that brings together the findings and concepts deriving from both basic and clinic neuroscience, in order to examine the neurodevelopmental hypothesis in a critical but constructive fashion and then to consider the implications for clinical practice. This book does just that, and does it extremely well.

There is abundant consistent evidence that there are strong genetic influences on the underlying liability to develop schizophrenia. Accordingly, one key challenge for the neurodevelopmental hypothesis is to make explicit how neurodevelopmental risk factors relate to genetic risk for schizophrenia. It is appropriate, therefore, that the book begins with an account of what is known about genetic influences on brain development, followed by reviews of what has been learned about normal brain development from structural and functional magnetic resonance imaging studies. Contrary to some people's view that brain development is confined to infancy, it is evident that there are important neural changes that extend into late adolescence and early adult life. It remains the case that we have much to learn still about how these changes relate to both normal and abnormal development, but they provide a possible basis for the transition from the premorbid features of childhood to the overt psychosis seen in adult life. This transition is also discussed with respect to the evidence that there may be new abnormal brain changes that occur at this time.

The velo-cardio-facial syndrome is put forward as a possible model for the interplay between genes, brain, behavior, and cognition, and it is also suggested that structural magnetic resonance imaging could provide a useful endophenotype for genetic studies. This reflects the growing awareness that susceptibility genes probably do not act directly on mental disorders and that, therefore, it may be useful to examine genetic effects on neurobiological abnormalities representing more proximal effects of genes.

The neurodevelopmental hypothesis has been accompanied by indications of the possible contributory causal role of epigenetic factors, malnutrition, pre- and perinatal risk factors (including infection), minor physical anomalies, and adverse rearing environment. The evidence on all of these is succinctly reviewed, with the conclusion that the risk effects are probably real even though their effect size is small.

Initially, with the advent of persuasive findings in genetics and in biological psychiatry more generally, it became unfashionable to consider either social risk factors or the effects of drug abuse: both of which had constituted a major focus of interest in the 1960s and 1970s. However, animal studies and migration studies of humans have shown that there is now reasonable evidence that social factors are influential, even though we do not understand how they operate. What is quite different from the 1960s and 1970s is the appreciation that it is necessary to understand how social factors may impact on brain development and that there may well be a synergistic interplay between environmental risk and genetic vulnerability, with the risks largely dependent on the presence of genetic susceptibility. Much the same message derives from the study of recreational drugs, with the specific suggestion that the drug effects associated with heavy early usage affect neurotransmitters in ways that may precipitate the onset of psychosis when combined with genetic susceptibility.

Further chapters provide a more detailed consideration of the possible role of the dopamine system, of mis-wired limbic lobe or thalamocortical circuitry, of estrogen and X-chromosome effects on brain development, of premorbid structural brain abnormalities, and of neurodegenerative models.

From a clinical perspective, it is crucial to know whether the neurodevelopmental features are specific to schizophrenia or apply to a broader range of psychiatric conditions. In frustrating fashion, the evidence suggests both substantial commonalities and important specificities. A key chapter considers whether the extensive evidence of premorbid abnormalities means that it should now be possible to identify children who are likely to develop schizophrenia. It is concluded that this is not yet possible, yet combining risk factors from different functional domains can usefully enhance the accuracy of predictive models. The final chapter discusses how it may be possible for the pathophysiology to be explained by an integrative neurochemical model and how there is now the beginning of a basis for possible preventive interventions.

The book provides a rich intellectual meal of great interest and importance. Nevertheless, we have to ask where all these creative ideas and empirical findings get us. The book has two main achievements. First, it provides an excellent compilation of what is known about the neurodevelopmental origins of schizophrenia, what the findings explain, and what research challenges remain (together with invaluable suggestions on how these challenges might be met). The evidence is compelling that, in crucial ways, schizophrenia is a neurodevelopmental disorder and that research using this concept has been immensely productive. There is the promise of a better understanding of how neurodevelopmental features relate to genetic risk, but that understanding has not yet been achieved. Similarly, although the onset in late adolescence/adult life, long after premorbid manifestations have been evident in childhood, is no longer quite the mystery that it was, the causal pathways have still to be delineated. Nevertheless, the book clearly documents that neurodevelopmental approaches are now mainstream in the study of schizophrenia and that much has been learned in the last decade or so.

The second achievement is that the consideration of neurodevelopmental origins of schizophrenia has thrown invaluable light on the broader issues involved in normal and abnormal brain development. This gives the book an interest that extends well beyond the world of schizophrenia clinicians and researchers. It is not light bedtime reading, but the book does provide an engrossing read that is richly rewarding.

Michael Rutter

REFERENCES

Garmezy, N. (1974). Children at risk: the search for the antecedents to schizophrenia. *Schizophr Bull* **8**: 14–55; **9**: 90–125.

Marenco, S., Weinberger, D. R. (2000). The neurodevelopmental hypothesis of schizophrenia: following a trail of evidence from cradle to grave. *Dev Psychopath* **12**: 501–527.

Murray, R. M., Lewis, S. W. (1987). Is schizophrenia a neurodevelopmental disorder? *Br Med J* **295**: 681–682.

Offord, D. R., Cross, L. A. (1969). Behavioral anticedents of adult schizophrenia. *Arch Gen Psychiatry* **21**: 267–283.

Rutter, M., Garmezy, N. (1983). Developmental psychopathology. In *Mussen's Handbook of Child Psychology*, 4th edn, Vol. 4: *Socialization, Personality, and Child Development*, ed. M. Hetherington, New York Wiley, pp. 775–911.

Weinberger, D. R. (1987). Implications of normal brain development for the pathogenesis of schizophrenia. *Arch Gen Psychiatry* **44**: 660–669.

Preface

This volume arises out of a widely perceived need to take stock of our new knowledge about the developmental pathophysiology of schizophrenia. In 1997, we published our first book on this topic, entitled *Neurodevelopment and Psychopathology*. That volume, which was surprisingly well received, covered neurodevelopmental approaches to adult psychopathology, though many of the chapters concerned schizophrenia. The enormous progress made in the subsequent years, particularly on schizophrenia, has led us to focus the current volume exclusively on this disorder, arguably the most debilitating of all psychiatric illnesses.

Since the early 1990s, our understanding of the developmental origins of schizophrenia has *"come of age,"* with impressive advances emerging from both the basic sciences and clinical studies. In retrospect, it is clear that the early neurodevelopmental models that emerged in the mid-1980s were extremely simplistic and too often relied on speculations about cellular and molecular mechanisms that were not subsequently confirmed. Furthermore, to a large extent, they ignored the contribution of psychology and certainly they included no mention of the role of the social environment. We believe that the recent explosion of knowledge in both neuroscience and cognitive science, as well as in imaging and epidemiology, has allowed us to begin to remedy such deficiencies. Therefore, this new book brings together many of the most productive and admired investigators in those areas of research, individuals who we believe have contributed most to contemporary developmental models of schizophrenia. Each of the chapters provides a state-of-the-art overview of the authors' area of expertise, including directions for the future.

We start with a section on recent advances in developmental neurobiology. The current state of our knowledge of genetics is reviewed, including the recent identification and apparent replication of susceptibility genes for schizophrenia (Ch. 1). The latter is no small cause for rejoicing as claims for the identification of genes had previously materialized and dematerialized with disturbing regularity, rather like the sightings of alien spacecraft. Then, progress in our understanding of the normal development of the human brain and its structural (Ch. 2), functional (Ch. 3), and cognitive (Ch. 4) properties is successively outlined. Such a perspective is vital since schizophrenia researchers have all too often attempted to outline the abnormal psychology and physiology underlying the condition before the normal had been charted. The important field of brain plasticity and its limits is then discussed in Ch. 5 with its implications for long-term functioning and psychopathology.

The next section contains overviews of pathophysiology and etiology of schizophrenia. The lessons for schizophrenia from the study of unusual genetic disorders such as the velo-cardio-facial syndrome are discussed, as is the impact of genetic loading for schizophrenia on brain structure (Chs. 7 and 8). The important and now well-documented effects of early environmental factors such as perinatal complications (Ch. 11) and nutritional anomalies (Ch. 9) on risk of schizophrenia are reviewed. Then the newer field of the effects of risk factors nearer to the onset of psychosis is considered, such as psychosocial adversity (Ch. 13) and drug abuse (Ch. 14) in pathogenetics, their epigenetic interaction (Ch. 10), and their impact on gene expression (Ch. 12). Chapter 6 outlines a novel theory on the etiological role of stress on schizophrenia and how its effects may be mediated by glucocorticoids. At a pathophysiological level, the developmental dysregulation of the neurotransmitter systems such as dopamine (Ch. 15), and the limbic (Ch. 16) and thalamocortical (Ch. 17) circuitry are critically reviewed. The important role of X chromosome and estrogens in brain development and its relevance for schizophrenia are discussed in Ch. 18. The possible premorbid neurodegenerative changes in the schizophrenic illness (Ch. 20) and the commonalities versus differences between developmental/degenerative changes in common neuropsychiatric disorders beginning in childhood/adolescence (Ch. 21) are discussed.

In the final section, some of the important clinical questions that drive pathophysiological research are considered. Can we identify preschizophrenia children? What do studies of those at high genetic risk of the disorder teach us? Does understanding of pathophysiology lead to specific predictions for preventive and therapeutic approaches?

For too long, the origins of schizophrenia have been considered to be shrouded in mystery. However, the exciting advances that have been made in schizophrenia research in the past decades, captured in this volume, have made the disease more comprehensible, even though the puzzle continues to unravel. We also hope that this volume will be of value for both researchers and practicing clinicians. Throughout this volume, the implications of research findings for clinical practice are discussed. The book will have served its purpose if the topics discussed herein provided stimulation and new learning for a new generation of researchers and clinicians in their efforts to inch toward better scientific knowledge and therapeutic possibilities as applied to the patient with schizophrenia.

We wish to express our sincere gratitude to Drs Vaibhav Diwadkar, Debra Montrose, Raj Rajarethinam, and Vandana Shashi for providing peer reviews of the chapters in this book. We are in particular grateful to Karol L. Rosengarth for her painstaking efforts in formatting and proofreading this work.

Part I

Basic aspects

Genes and brain development

Timothy A. Klempan, Pierandrea Muglia, and James L. Kennedy

Centre for Addiction and Mental Health, University of Toronto, Toronto, Canada

The mechanisms underlying development of the mammalian central nervous system (CNS) are of fundamental importance for research into psychiatric disorders. The processes of neurulation, patterning, neuronal specification, and synaptogenesis, as well as the functional dynamics of neurotransmission, are governed by the coordinated actions of products from a wide array of genes. Our knowledge of the expression and complex interactions between the products controlling these processes has been broadened by developmental studies using animal models (primarily fruit fly and nematode but increasingly in the mouse); biochemical, histochemical, and imaging studies; and analysis using high-throughput, non-selective techniques such as microarray hybridization. Undoubtedly, the identification of novel brain-expressed transcripts through the Human Genome Project has also provided a solid framework for investigation of CNS function.

A neurodevelopmental etiology of schizophrenia is suggested by neuroimaging and postmortem studies revealing significant and replicated lateral ventricular enlargement, hippocampal and gray matter deficits, and cellular disarray, independent of duration of illness and antipsychotic treatment. As these features remain some of the best non-behavioral correlates of schizophrenia, the genetic investigation of neurodevelopmental candidate genes, especially those with well-characterized neural function and within chromosomal regions demonstrating prior linkage or association with schizophrenia, is an important research focus.

This chapter will provide an overview of the major mechanisms involved in the development of the mammalian CNS, with specific reference to the identity and patterning of genes that are known to regulate these developmental phases (Table 1.1). This pattern of gene expression will be related to the etiology of schizophrenia through evidence provided by genetic, postmortem, imaging, electrophysiological, and behavioral investigations of the disorder. In this fashion, a set of possible determinants of both aberrant neurodevelopment and psychosis will be suggested.

Neurodevelopment and Schizophrenia, ed. Matcheri S. Keshavan *et al.* Published by Cambridge University Press. © Cambridge University Press 2004.

Table 1.1. Neurodevelopmental genes and reports of expression-based and genetic analysis in schizophrenia

Gene	Function	Locus of interest	Genetic and expression-based analysis
Mash1	Neurulation -		
Notch		NOTCH4 (6p21.3)	(Wei & Hemmings, 2000 and see text)
Delta		DLL1 (6q27)	
Neurogenin		NGN1 (5q23-q31)	
NeuroD		NEUROD (2q32)	
Sonic Hedgehog		SHH (7q36)	
Wnt		WNT1 (12q12-q13)	(Cotter *et al.*, 1998; Miyaoka *et al.*, 1999)
Krox20	Patterning	EGR2 (10q21.1-q22.1)	
Hox		HOXB (17q21.3)	(Kennedy and Kidd, unpublished)
Dlx		DLX1 (2q32)	
Emx		EMX2 (10q26.1)	
Gbx		GBX2 (2q36-q37)	
Nkx		TITF1 (14q13)	
Otx		OTX2 (14q21-q22)	
Pax		PAX6 (11p13)	(Stober *et al.*, 1999)
POU		POU3F3 (3p14.2)	
NCAM	Cell migration/ neurite extension	NCAM1 (11q23.1)	(Vicente *et al.*, 1997; Doherty *et al.*, 1990)
L1CAM			
N-Cadherin		NCAD (18q11.2)	
Reelin		RELN (7q22)	(Fatemi *et al.*, 2000; Guidotti *et al.*, 2000)
NGF	Neuronal	NGFB (1p13.1)	
BDNF	Survival	BDNF (11p13)	(Muglia *et al.*, 2003)
NT-3		NTF3 (12p13)	(Nanko *et al.*, 1994 and see text)
NT-4/5		NTF5 (19q13.3)	
GDNF		GDNF (5p13.1-p12)	(Lee *et al.*, 2001)
CNTF		CNTF (11q12.2)	(Thome *et al.*, 1996 and see text)
SNAP25	Presynaptic/ exocytosis	SNAP25 (20p11.2-p12)	(Tachikawa *et al.*, 2001; Wong *et al.*, 2003)
Syntaxin		STX1A (7q11.23)	(A. Wong *et al.*, unpublished data)
Synaptobrevin		VAMP1 (12p)	
Synapsin		SYN3 (22q12.3)	(Ohmori *et al.*, 2000) and see text
Complexin		CPLX2 (5q35.3)	(Harrison and Eastwood, 1998 and see text)
Synaptophysin		SYP (Xp11.23-p11.22)	
Synaptotagmin		SYT1 (12cen-q21)	

Neurulation

The coordinated development of the human brain, from a single cell to some 10^{12} neurons with a possible 1000 connections between each, is a feat of unimaginable intricacy. The function of individual groups of neurons within this framework in the control of essential processes such as learning and memory, perception, mood, and motor activity adds a further level of complexity. While the differentiative pathways followed by neurons are topologically similar to those in other cell types, one unique aspect of nervous system morphogenesis is the essential connectivity of its units through axonal and dendritic outgrowth, allowing for interactions in a highly plastic system. Despite the apparent difficulties of dissecting such a detailed system, the changes involved in neuronal specification and overall CNS development are becoming increasingly well understood. Much of our present state of awareness in the field has been gathered through research using simple organisms such as sea slug, squid and nematode, while recombinant DNA technology has allowed generalization to vertebrates through investigations in mice. The cascade of events proceeding from early gastrulation of the embryo to maturation can now be adequately described.

The events leading to formation of the neural tube are known collectively as neurulation. Two distinct developmental programs may be used: primary neurulation, during which the chordamesoderm instructs the overlying ectoderm to divide, invaginate, and separate from the surface to form the neural tube, and secondary neurulation, during which a cylindrical zone of cells descends into the embryo and hollows to form the tube. In mammals, this appears to occur in regionally differentiated processes, with primary neurulation in the anterior region and secondary neurulation posterior to somite 35.

The first signals responsible for the determination of anterior/posterior identity in the ectoderm during gastrulation emanate from Hensen's node, a small group of cells at the anterior end of the primitive streak. The neural ectoderm is induced through vertical signals from the mesodermal tissues beneath and adjacent to it. The neural ectoderm gives rise to the neural plate, which is polarized through the dorsal–ventral and anterior–posterior axes. The edges of the plate fold upwards to join at the dorsal midline, producing the neural tube. Cells overlying the dorsal midline of the neural tube form neural crest cells and migrate to form the brain and spinal cord from the anterior and posterior portions, respectively. A commitment to cell fates is revealed with the closure of the tube, with ventricular CNS generated from the interior of the tube and epithelial cells at the interior periphery eventually forming neurons and glia.

The brain becomes further divided through a series of constrictions into the forebrain (prosencephalon), midbrain (mesencephalon), and hindbrain (rhombencephalon). Further compartmentalization results in regions within these vesicles known as neuromeres, where mixing of cells becomes restricted to others within the same region (as within rhombomeres of the hindbrain), laying the ground plan for specification of neurogenesis. The forebrain gives rise to the telencephalon (forming the olfactory lobes, hippocampus, basal ganglia, and cerebral cortex in the adult brain following proliferation and folding) and the diencephalon (forming the thalamus, epithalamus, hypothalamus, and the retina). The midbrain forms the mesencephalon (including regions of connectivity between rostral and caudal brain, the optic lobes, and tectum), while the hindbrain develops into the metencephalon (producing the cerebellum and pons) and myelencephalon (forming the medulla).

The localization and development of these highly specialized regions of the brain is regulated principally through the actions of transcription factors: DNA-binding proteins that direct the expression of specific genes. The phenotype of all neurons is dictated by the precise set of genes expressed within the cell, allowing for functional specialization. While the initial effect of transcription factors on the cell may be brief, the influence of individual factors may be carried through numerous cell divisions and persist beyond migration and diversification of a specific cell lineage. The coordinated boundaries of expression of these factors serve to delineate clearly morphological boundaries and to impart organization to the adult CNS. Much of the information that we now possess regarding the determination of neural cell fate and patterning in the early embryo has been made possible through research conducted in *Drosophila*, *Xenopus*, and mice, where factors such as single neuroblast ablation, ease of manipulation, and the ability to knock out specific genes are advantageous. The extrapolation of findings from these organisms to humans is facilitated by the remarkable degree of conservation of the factors controlling neural fate across species.

The selection of distinct areas within the ectoderm to form neural precursor cells is regulated through the expression of proneural genes, encoding transcription factors of the basic helix-loop-helix (bHLH) class. The expression of these genes provides the potential for the cell to become neural. Proneural genes are typified by *Mash1*, encoding a factor in the central and peripheral nervous systems that selects for neural fate and acts in subsequent differentiation. Knockout analysis of *Mash1* reveals its role in neurogenesis within the ventral telencephalon (Casarosa *et al.*, 1999). Overexpression of the *Xash3*, the homologue of *Mash1* in *Xenopus*, leads to selection of neural over epidermal cell fate and ectopic neuronal differentiation (Ferreiro *et al.*, 1994). Lateral specification within the cluster of proneural cells then allows specific cells within the equivalent group to become neural. The transmembrane proteins encoded by the neurogenic genes *Notch* and *Delta* permit the division between neuronal and epidermal cell fates to become established in a mechanism incorporating cell-to-cell signaling and an amplified feedback loop. Neural precursors express the Delta ligand, which, on binding to the Notch receptor, represses further proneural gene expression and downregulates the expression of Delta. When *Notch* transcription is absent from the embryo, all ectodermal cells develop into neural precursors in *Drosophila* (Artavanis-Tsakonis *et al.*, 1983), while markers of neurogenesis are markedly increased in the absence of *Notch1* transcription in mouse (de la Pompa *et al.*, 1997).

Neurogenins are proneural bHLH proteins that function as transcriptional activators of neuronal differentiation genes. The neurogenin Ngn1, for instance, promotes neurogenesis and inhibits differentiation of neural stem cells into astrocytes (Sun *et al.*, 2001). Another neurogenin, Ngn2, restricts cell migration from the cortex to the striatum (Chapouton *et al.*, 2001) and is expressed in dorsal telencephalic cells, defining a boundary through repression by Mash1, which defines the ventral telencephalon (Parras *et al.*, 2002). A regulator of differentiation known as NeuroD is directly regulated by the neurogenins in many regions of the brain and maintains expression in fully differentiated neurons (Lee, 1997). The overexpression of NeuroD in *Xenopus* will direct the development of non-neural ectoderm into neurons and accelerate the differentiation of neural precursors (Lee *et al.*, 1995). A host of additional factors act to convey positional information to groups of cells, instruct the development of specific phenotypes through cascades of gene expression and repression, and preserve the differentiated states of various cell lineages in the CNS.

Sonic hedgehog (*Shh*), a member of a vertebrate gene family corresponding to the *Drosophila* gene *hedgehog*, is a secreted factor that acts in a concentration-dependent fashion to induce cells of the floor plate and neural tube (Ericson *et al.*, 1995), in addition to its role in axial specification over various regions of the body. Regionalization within the developing telencephalon is controlled by the ventralizing properties of *Shh* expression (Kohtz *et al.*, 1998) and distinct dopaminergic and serotonergic neuronal subpopulations are induced along the anterior–posterior axis at different times by Shh signaling (Hynes and Rosenthal, 1999). Signaling mediated by the Wnt family of glycoproteins is tightly connected to those controlled through the *hedgehog* family. The expression of *wnt1* (and the gene for fibroblast growth factor 8) is coordinated with establishment of the mesencephalon–metencephalon boundary; and mice lacking Wnt1 fail to develop midbrain structures and cerebellum (McMahon and Bradley, 1990).

The recent description of a strong association between a promoter base-pair substitution and the exon 1 $(CTG)_n$ repeat of *NOTCH4* with schizophrenia (Wei and Hemmings, 2000) in a region (6p21.3) previously associated with the disease (Schwab *et al.*, 1995; Straub *et al.*, 1995) has ignited interest in this candidate gene. Of six *NOTCH* homologues identified in vertebrates, *NOTCH4* is the most divergent phylogenetically (Kortschak *et al.*, 2001) and shows a pattern of expression that is primarily endothelial and myocardial (Li *et al.*, 1998) with minimal expression in brain. A number of follow-up reports on *NOTCH4* have failed to replicate the original finding for both individual markers and haplotypes using case–control and family-based association approaches (Fan *et al.*, 2002; Imai *et al.*, 2001b; Klempan *et al.*, 2001; McGinnis *et al.*, 2001; Sklar *et al.*, 2001; Swift-Scanlan *et al.*, 2002; Ujike *et al.*, 2001). The extreme biases in transmission of *NOTCH4* alleles witnessed in the first study now appear more likely to be a false-positive association, although an unusual population specific effect cannot be excluded since differences between the African-American and European populations have been noted at the *NOTCH4* locus (Luo *et al.*, 2004).

Abnormalities of the Wnt signaling pathway have been suggested by several recent studies which have described reductions of β-catenin and γ-catenin staining in the CA3 and CA4 hippocampal subregions and increases in Wnt1 staining in these regions of schizophrenic brains relative to controls (Cotter *et al.*, 1998; Miyaoka *et al.*, 1999). Furthermore, levels of glycogen synthase kinase-3β (GSK-3β) are significantly reduced in the prefrontal cortex of schizophrenia patients and Wnt is known to act as a repressor of GSK-3β (Beasley *et al.*, 2001). GSK-3β also participates in apoptosis, a form of programmed cell death, and, therefore, aberrant GSK-3β expression may provide a rationale for observations of irregular neuronal distributions found in schizophrenia (Kozlovsky *et al.*, 2002). Many of the signaling components of the Wnt pathway have been localized and some of these map within susceptibility regions for psychosis (Rhoads *et al.*, 1999).

Segmentation

Patterning of the specialized cell groups that will eventually specify distinct regions of the CNS is carried out by other groups of transcription factors, whose expression is confined to discrete segments of the developing embryo. The compartmentalization granted by division of regions of the brain into segments (prosomeres in the forebrain and rhombomeres in the hindbrain) prevents the mixing of various lineages of cells and the activity of expressed genes and restricts the targets and navigational properties of axons within these segments.

One gene, for example, that is known to be critical in the establishment of neural tube boundaries is the zinc-finger transcription factor Krox20. *Krox20* is expressed in the neural plate in alternating segments (rhombomeres r3 and r5) prior to distinct rhombomere formation, as revealed by lineage tracing studies in the chick. Mice that are null for *Krox20* display a disruption of segmental identity with a fused r2/r4/r6 region (Schneider-Manoury *et al.*, 1997). The function of *Krox20* is considered comparable to that of the *Drosophila* pair-rule genes, which translate information from previously expressed genes into periodic stripes of further expression. At the early stages of segmental specification, however, there is very little conservation of specific genes between flies and vertebrates.

One family of genes that is critical in the determination of regional identity along the anterior–posterior axis is known as the homeobox (*Hox*) family. Based upon homeotic genes in *Drosophila*, these master regulatory factors are strongly conserved from fly to mammals. Homeobox proteins are characterized by a 60 amino acid residue motif (the homeodomain), which binds to specific sequences of DNA. The *Hox* genes show colinearity with positions of genes within clusters along the chromosome corresponding to their domains of expression along the embryo. Those genes located further 3' within the cluster are expressed both earlier during development and in a more anterior location. The limits of rostral expression of the *Hox* genes are strongly coordinated with the divisions between rhombomeres, suggesting that they may be involved in the specification and/or maintenance of segment identity (Krumlauf, 1994). The influence of specific *Hox* members on actual segment phenotype is illustrated by *Hoxb1*. The expression of *Hoxb1* is particularly strong in rhombomere r4 and loss of Hoxb1 in mutant mice transforms r4 to an r2 phenotype (Studer *et al.*, 1996), while ectopic *Hoxb1* expression in chick produces the opposite result (Bell *et al.*, 1999).

In addition to the *Hox* family of transcription factors, a number of other homeodomain-containing proteins impart positional information to the developing brain. Mice lacking both *Dlx1* and *Dlx2*, for instance, do not demonstrate proper migration of cortical cells from subcortical regions and show disrupted cell migration within the striatum (Anderson *et al.*, 1997). In the absence of functional Emx1 protein, the corpus callosum fails to develop, while *Emx2* mutants lack hippocampal dentate gyrus and Cajal–Retzius cells of the neocortex. These *Emx2* mutants are also similar to the reeler mouse, with disturbances of lamination and neuronal migration (Mallamaci *et al.*, 2000). The expression of *Gbx2*, required in rostral hindbrain differentiation (Wassarman *et al.*, 1997), acts in concert with Otx2 to establish the isthmic signaling region (Broccoli *et al.*, 1999). The function of Otx2 is perhaps even more critical in neural induction, as targeted mutations of *Otx2* result in absence of rostral brain areas.

Another family of transcriptional regulatory factors expressed in the mammalian forebrain with persistence into adulthood is known as the POU domain family. Members of this group contain a POU homeodomain and a POU specific domain and are generally expressed in restricted regions late in forebrain development. The severe defects produced by mutations in many early patterning genes (such as *Hox*) make these unlikely candidates for the subtle structural alterations witnessed in schizophrenia; however, many members of the POU class of factors are expressed specifically in frontal cortical and hippocampal areas implicated in disease processes (Turner *et al.*, 1997). The POU-III subclass of factors includes Brn-1, Brn-2, and SCIP (among others), which have been extensively studied in null mutant mice. *Brn-1* null mice show cellular disorganization of the hippocampus and transitional cortex and disorganized cortical lamination, while *Brn-2* mutants are defective in hypothalamic development (Schonemann *et al.*, 1995). Brn-1 and Brn-2, coexpressed in layer II–V cortical neurons, have roles in the initiation of radial migration (McEvilly *et al.*, 2002). Reelin, also involved in radial migration of cortical neurons, is reduced in a subpopulation of cortical plate neurons normally colocalizing with Brn-1 expression in *Brn-1* mutants, suggesting cross-regulation between these pathways.

Transcriptional regulatory molecules can act in a hierarchical fashion to enhance or inhibit the expression of downstream targets and sometimes may compensate for others in their absence. The roles played by these factors can be diverse, acting in neuroepithelial patterning, differentiation, and survival through cues given at different times throughout embryogenesis. Numerous genes have been identified as targets for these molecules, as seen in the enhancement of neuronal cell adhesion molecule (NCAM) expression by Otx2 (Nguyen Ba-Charvet *et al.*, 1999) and the regulation of the *SNAP25* promoter by Brn-3 POU transcription factors (Morris *et al.*, 1997). The cascade of gene expression induced by these factors would classify them as interesting targets for investigation in schizophrenia, yet few studies have been undertaken, perhaps because it is felt that the consequences of their misregulation would be dire. One report has shown a mild association between a high-activity variant of a *Pax6* (paired-box family transcription factor) polymorphism, and paranoid schizophrenia (Stober *et al.*, 1999), while others have suggested that Pax6 may contribute to schizophrenia through disrupted retinoic acid signaling (LaMantia, 1999).

Cell adhesion

In the developing brain, once a neuron has become committed to its phenotype it must migrate to its proper layer of the maturing brain (Ruiz i Altaba, 1994). Cell adhesion molecules (CAMs) are cell membrane proteins that mediate adhesion between neural cells, exerting a key role in the morphogenesis, differentiation, and migration of neurons as well as in the guidance of outgrowing axons in the developing brain (see Fig. 1.1). CAMs can be classified functionally into calcium-dependent and calcium-independent groups. The calcium-dependent category contains at least 80 proteins belonging to the cadherin superfamily, while the Ca^{2+}-independent CAMs comprise the immunoglobulin (Ig) superfamily (IgSF). Most of the cadherin

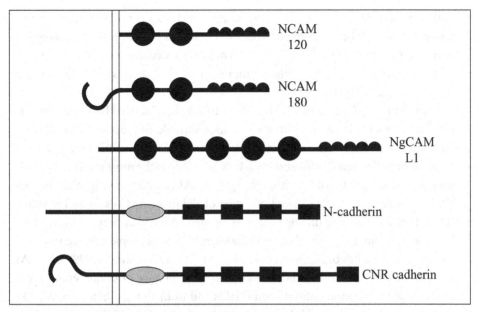

NCAM
120

NCAM
180

NgCAM
L1

N-cadherin

CNR cadherin

Fig. 1.1.   Members of the cadherin and immunoglobulin superfamilies of cell adhesion molecules. Several prominent members of these transmembrane protein families are depicted, with known roles in neurite outgrowth and morphogenesis. CNR, cadherin neuronal-related receptor; NCAM, neuronal cell adhesion molecule; Ng CAM, neurogenin cell adhesion molecule.

superfamily genes are expressed in the brain, and the protein structure is character-ized by a unique domain named the cadherin motif, which is involved in calcium binding (Takeichi, 1990). The cadherin motif (also called the EF motif) is repeated a variable number of times in the different members of the superfamily (Yagi and Takeichi, 2000). In addition to the classic cadherins, other members of the pro-tocadherins superfamily are cadherin neuronal-related receptors (CNRs) and the so-called seven-pass transmembrane cadherins. The seven-pass transmembrane cadherins have a transmembrane structure similar to G-protein-coupled recep-tors and appear to be involved in polarity orientation of the developing neuron, as shown in *Drosophila* (Usui *et al.*, 1999). The CNRs are coded by a cluster of 13 genes that map to 5q31.1 in humans and play a role in both the formation of neuronal circuits at the synaptic level and the strengthening of the synapse during long-term potentiation (LTP) (Yagi and Takeichi, 2000). It is interesting to note that a significant linkage region for schizophrenia, derived from meta-analysis of data from 20 genome scans, is located in a 30 cM stretch across 5q23–34 (Lewis *et al.*, 2003), which includes the CNR gene cluster. CNRs are distinguished from the other cadherins that exhibit homophilic interactions since they show etherophilic inter-actions. They have been observed to bind to the Reelin protein and to the integrins (Karecla *et al.*, 1996; Senzaki *et al.*, 1999). The genetic structure of the CNRs resem-ble the organization of genes of the immunologic system, such as the T cell receptor genes (Wu and Maniatis, 1999).

The calcium-independent CAMs (the IgSF) are characterized by a large amino-terminal extracellular domain that contains a variable number of Ig motifs and fibronectin repeats, which characterize the various members of the family sharing a similar organization (Fields and Itoh, 1996). NCAM is the most extensively stud-ied and characterized protein within the IgSF. NCAM contains five Ig folds and two fibronectin repeats in the extracellular part of the protein (Crossin and Krushel, 2000). Further to its role during CNS development, NCAM appears to be involved in the remodeling, regeneration, and maintenance of neuronal connections and pathways in the adult brain (Kiss *et al.*, 2001; Murase and Schuman, 1999). NCAM also plays a role in learning and memory, and in guidance of brain development in response to environmental stimuli (Fields and Itoh, 1996). Changes in NCAM expression are also observed during synaptic remodeling and LTP in the rat hip-pocampus (Fields and Itoh, 1996). NCAM is encoded by a single gene (*NCAM1*) consisting of 26 exons located at 11q23.1 (Bello *et al.*, 1989), which undergoes alternative splicing generating at least 30 different forms with different spatial and temporal patterns of expression in vertebrates (Akbarian *et al.*, 1996). Three NCAM isoforms (NCAM 180, NCAM 140 and NCAM 120) represent the most common variants. NCAM 180 knockout mice have minor brain development abnormal-ities, such as decreased size of the olfactory bulb, anterior ventricle enlargement, and hippocampal dentate gyrus thinning (Andrews and Wood, 1986; Treloar *et al.*, 1997). In addition, the NCAM 180 knockouts exhibit behavioural deficits during learning tasks and in the prepulse inhibition of startle (Wood *et al.*, 1998). Both Hox and Pax transcription factors appear to have a regulatory role on NCAM transcrip-tion (Jones *et al.*, 1993). NCAM functions as a cell–cell and cell–matrix homophilic and heterophilic adhesion receptor; however, the mechanisms of interaction are not completely understood. The binding of NCAM activates transmembrane-signaling reactions and contributes to the initiation of cellular responses implicated in synap-tic plasticity. The signaling downstream of neural NCAM not only impacts on morphological changes but also can affect transcription factor activation and gene induction (Krushel *et al.*, 1999). Two main pathways are activated in response to NCAM-mediated interactions, represented by the mitogen-activated protein kinase and phospholipase C cascades (Crossin and Krushel, 2000). Other pathways involve the interaction of the NCAM molecule with tyrosine kinase-linked recep-tors (Beggs *et al.*, 1997). The function of NCAM is also regulated by the molecule's content of polysialic acid (Fields and Itoh, 1996). The PSA residue makes the NCAM less adhesive, thereby facilitating neuronal movement (Cunningham, 1995; Gower *et al.*, 1988). The addition of the PSA to NCAM is made possible by two sialyltrans-ferases and their activity in directing polysialylated NCAM synthesis is controlled at the mRNA level (Eckhardt *et al.*, 1995; Nakayama *et al.*, 1995). New interac-tions and mechanisms are emerging from the study of NCAM. For example, it is likely that NCAM binds to the brain-derived neurotrophic factor (BDNF) receptor TrkB at the synapse level, since the deficient LTP observed in NCAM knockout mice is recovered by addition of BDNF (Muller *et al.*, 2000). It is also likely that polysialylated NCAM can sensitize pyramidal cells to the action of BDNF as NCAM knockout mice exhibit blunted activation of Trk B in response to BDNF (Muller *et al.*, 2000).

The role of NCAM in the schizophrenic brain has been investigated through expression studies as well as molecular genetic association and linkage studies. One study found a decreased number of neurons expressing the polysialylated form of NCAM in the hippocampus of brains from individuals with schizophrenia (Doherty *et al.*, 1990). The abnormal levels of polysialylated NCAM in the brain of schizophrenics might be responsible for the commonly observed abnormalities of migration. This finding stimulated one group (Vicente *et al.*, 1997) to investigate whether variants in the *NCAM* gene were associated with susceptibility to develop schizophrenia. Linkage analysis in five multiplex families was performed and an association analysis was conducted in 71 nuclear families with one affected off-spring. Linkage analysis of the polymorphic dinucleotide (CA) repeat in the region of the *NCAM* gene, considering the disease as either autosomal dominant or reces-sive, found no evidence of linkage. The association studies in the nuclear families also did not find association between another (CA) repeat found at the *NCAM* locus and schizophrenia. Subsequent to the initial report, a number of studies have revealed NCAM alterations in schizophrenia, including decreased polysialy-lated NCAM in the hippocampus (Barbeau *et al.*, 1995), increased NCAM in the prefrontal cortex and hippocampus (Honer *et al.*, 1997), and increased NCAM in cerebrospinal fluid (van Kammen *et al.*, 1998). Several lines of evidence have shown that other CAMs such as L1, fibroblast growth factor receptor, laminin, and integrins interact with NCAM (Doherty and Walsh, 1996; Kristiansen *et al.*, 1999; Takei *et al.*, 1999).

A major role in the layering of neurons into their specific target area of the CNS once their migration is completed in several brain areas, including the hippocam-pus, is ascribed to Reelin (Rice and Curran, 2001). The spontaneous mutation occurring in the gene *reelin* in mice bred at the Institute of Animal Genetics in Edinburgh (Falconer, 1951) has initiated five decades of research into *reelin* func-tion and its involvement in brain development. The *reeler* mouse displays impaired motor coordination, ataxia, and tremor evident since day 12 after birth. The *reeler* mutation is also associated with severe cerebellar hypoplasia, disorganization of cerebral and cerebellar cortices, and disruption of other structures such as the hippocampus (Rakic and Caviness, 1995). In spite of the altered neuronal positioning, most neuronal fibers make appropriate connections in the *reeler* brain although with longer and more intricate paths (Steindler and Colwell, 1976). Yet, connections are aberrant in cerebellar neurons. Several known alleles in *reelin* determine very similar phenotypes in the mouse (D'Arcangelo and Curran, 1998).

Reelin is a large protein coded by the *reelin* gene (*Reln*), located on chromosome 5 in the mouse (Goffinet and Dernoncourt, 1991). In humans, the gene (*RELN*) maps to 7q22 (DeSilva *et al.*, 1997). It contains 65 exons and encodes a mRNA of approximately 12 kb, which translates into a 3461 amino acid residue protein with 94% homology to the murine amino acid sequence. Reelin is abundantly synthesized and secreted in the extracellular matrix during early stages of brain development by the Cajal–Retzius neurons located in the marginal zone. It has been shown in both rodents and primates that, once the Cajal–Retzius cells disappear, a few months before gestation in primates (Rodriguez *et al.*, 2000), Reelin is synthesized throughout life by a select population of interneurons utilizing gamma-aminobutyric acid (GABA) including cells within layers I and II of various cortical areas (Rodriguez *et al.*, 2000).

In the search for etiological factors underlying the neurodevelopmental anomalies described in schizophrenia brains, the expression pattern of Reelin has been investigated. According to two independent findings (Fatemi *et al.*, 2000; Guidotti *et al.*, 2000), schizophrenia brains show a 30 to 60% reduction of *RELN* expression in the prefrontal cortex and in the hippocampus. Patients with bipolar disorder and associated psychotic features also show a reduction in *RELN* expression (Guidotti *et al.*, 2000). Several polymorphisms have been described for *RELN* including a trinucleotide repeat in the 5′ untranslated region (UTR) region of the gene. One study has found an association between this polymorphism and autism in a family-based association study (Persico *et al.*, 2001); however, at present, few studies (Akatone *et al.*, 2002) have investigated the possible role of *RELN* sequence variants in schizophrenia.

Neuronal survival

With the development of the nervous system, as axons innervate their appropriate target regions and connections become established, a naturally occurring cell death takes place to refine the complex network of connections. This process serves to establish a balance between the requirements of the target tissue and the characteristics of the innervating neuronal population (Purves, 1988). The primary molecules involved in this target-derived regulation of neuronal survival and differentiation

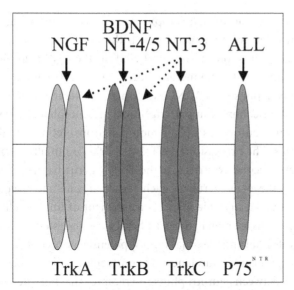

Fig. 1.2.   Specificity of neurotrophic factor binding to tyrosine kinase receptors. All factors activate receptors of the trk class. While neurotrophin 3 acts weakly through TrkA and TrkB in addition to TrkC, all factors can act through the low-affinity receptor p75NTR. BDNF, brain-derived neurotrophic factor; NGF, nerve growth factor; NT, neurotrophin.

are the neurotrophins (see Fig. 1.2). The neurotrophin family of growth factors display functional similarity through the promotion of neuronal survival, as first seen with nerve growth factor (NGF) (Levi-Montalcini, 1987) and later for BDNF (Leibrock *et al.*, 1989). Neurotrophins now also include neurotrophin 3 (NT-3) (Ernfors *et al.*, 1990; Hohn *et al.*, 1990), neurotrophin 4/5 (NT-4/5) (Berkmeier *et al.*, 1991; Ip *et al.*, 1992), and neurotrophin 6 (NT-6) (Gotz *et al.*, 1994), all cloned through homology to NGF and BDNF. These also play key roles in neuronal differentiation, cell body growth, promotion of neurite sprouting/extension, and, in the mature CNS, the control of short-term synaptic transmission and LTP, considered a mechanism for the processes of memory and learning (Thoenen, 1995).

Neurotrophin signaling is thought to occur primarily through the Trk family of tyrosine kinase receptors. Binding of neurotrophin ligand induces transphosphorylation of Trk receptors, initiating signal transduction through phosphorylation of further intracellular proteins. Specificity is exhibited in the binding of neurotrophins for individual Trk receptors: TrkA is a receptor for NGF, TrkB is a receptor for BDNF and NT-4/5, and TrkC is a receptor for NT-3. A further receptor known as p75NTR binds all neurotrophins with low affinity and acts selectively to increase or decrease the response to different neurotrophins in neurons expressing Trk receptors. In the absence of Trk receptors, p75NTR controls an apoptotic response to both NGF and BDNF in some neurons.

The domains of expression of neurotrophins and their cognate high-affinity receptors have been extensively mapped in both the peripheral and the central nervous systems. The expression of TrkA and NGF in the CNS is localized primarily to basal forebrain, striatal cholinergic neurons, and cerebellar Purkinje cells. Neuronal populations responsive to BDNF and, to a lesser extent, NT-4/5 comprise basal forebrain cholinergic, hippocampal, trigeminal mesencephalic, and substantia nigra dopaminergic neurons, as well as motor neurons, retinal ganglion and cerebellar granule cells. The expression of NT-3 and TrkC is initially strong in the hippocampus and later becomes restricted to the dentate gyrus, basal forebrain, and adrenergic neurons of the locus coeruleus. Each of these ligands and receptors have also been knocked out in transgenic mice for assessment of functionality. While profound losses of neurons are seen in the peripheral nervous system, deficits in the CNS are generally quite mild and the situation is apparently more complex. It is currently believed that significant redundancy in neurotrophin activity occurs within the CNS, as cross-talk between neurotrophins and receptors has been described and receptor knockouts are generally more severe than their ligand counterparts (Snider, 1994). The neurotrophins play vital roles in cell survival and differentiation in all regions of the brain and may be associated with reductions in cortical and whole brain volume (Lawrie and Abukmeil, 1998) and with the high neuronal density (Selemon *et al.*, 1995) seen in morphometric analyses of the schizophrenic brain.

Significant alterations of BDNF protein levels have been seen in postmortem studies of schizophrenia patients compared with normal controls, specifically increases in cortical regions and decreases in the hippocampus (Brouha *et al.*, 1996; Durany *et al.*, 2001), although others have seen the opposite effect in hippocampus (Takahashi *et al.*, 2000). It has also been observed that treatment with haloperidol and risperidone decreases the expression of BDNF in frontal cortex, occipital cortex, and hippocampus of rat brain (Angelucci *et al.*, 2000; Takahashi *et al.*, 2000) and alters the level of TrkB expression in similar regions. These findings complicate the interpretation of human expression studies, suggesting that results in the hippocampus may be a confound of neuroleptic exposure, and further indicating that these antipsychotic medications may be unlikely to have an effect through mediation of neurotrophin levels. Nevertheless, the reductions in BDNF-deficient mice of immunoreactivity for neuropeptide Y, the calcium-binding proteins calbindin and parvalbumin, somatostatin, and cholecystokinin indicate that neuronal maturation and calcium trafficking is perturbed. Research using rat brain striatal slices in vitro shows that BDNF induces release of GABA, dopamine, and serotonin (Goggi *et al.*, 2002). A direct induction of dopamine D_3 receptor expression by BDNF has also been described during early development and adulthood (Guillin *et al.*, 2001), linking molecular findings between two factors of potential etiological significance in schizophrenia.

Genetic investigation of the gene *BDNF* in schizophrenia was initiated following discovery of a dinucleotide repeat polymorphism located within what was initially recognized as the promoter (now determined as intronic) region of the gene (Proschel *et al.*, 1992). The first published reports included a Japanese case–control study (Sasaki *et al.*, 1997a) and an Irish study using over 200 cases and controls for association analysis and 250 families for linkage disequilibrium analysis (Hawi *et al.*, 1998); both reports were negative for this polymorphism. While the small sample size of the first study may limit any conclusions, the high power of the sample from the second report discredits a role for *BDNF* (although variations in allele frequencies and population effects for this microsatellite may contribute to these findings). Recently, additional studies have also been negative for association of *BDNF* with schizophrenia; however, these have provided support for an effect of *BDNF* alleles on parietal lobe volume (Wassink *et al.*, 1999) and shown increased dinucleotide repeat marker length with treatment-responsive schizophrenia (Krebs *et al.*, 2000). The results of transmission disequilibrium test-based analysis of a schizophrenia sample of Italian and Canadian families (Muglia *et al.*, 2003) have shown increased transmission of the 170 bp allele and reduced transmission of the 174 bp allele to probands. Of further interest, a recent study (Egan *et al.*, 2003) has shown that the Val66Met polymorphism of BDNF influences intracellular distribution of the precursor protein, alters hippocampal activity as measured by functional magnetic resonance imaging (FMRI), and affects performance on episodic memory tasks. The availability of extensive sequence data for the *BDNF* gene should facilitate its further examination as a putative schizophrenia susceptibility factor.

The *NT-3* gene, with significant hippocampal expression (Maisonpierre *et al.*, 1990), has been extensively examined following a positive association between a highly polymorphic dinucleotide repeat polymorphism of *NT-3* and schizophrenia in a Japanese study (Nanko *et al.*, 1994). This group also identified a missense mutation in the *NT-3* gene that was associated with severe schizophrenia (Hattori and Nanko, 1995). Subsequent investigations of *NT-3* have failed to replicate these findings (Arinami *et al.*, 1996; Jonsson *et al.*, 1997; Nimgaonkar *et al.*, 1995; Thome *et al.*, 1997a). One study has replicated the original finding, but only in male schizophrenics (Dawson *et al.*, 1995). Recent reports have shown an association of illness with *NT-3* in female probands (Virgos *et al.*, 2001) and a reduction of *NT-3* expression in frontal and parietal cortical regions using enzyme-linked immunosorbant assays (Durany *et al.*, 2001). These diverse results are difficult to reconcile, although heterogeneity of samples and methods is a likely contributor to the inconsistency.

Two additional molecules not structurally related to the neurotrophins that serve to promote survival of neurons during development are glial cell-derived neurotrophic factor (GDNF) and ciliary neurotrophic factor (CNTF). GDNF is related to transforming growth factor-β, which initiates induction of mesoderm and is a trophic factor for midbrain dopaminergic (Lin *et al.*, 1993), cholinergic (Ha *et al.*, 1996), and noradrenergic (Arenas *et al.*, 1995) neurons. The role of GDNF in differentiation of dopaminergic neurons has prompted its study as a putative susceptibility locus for schizophrenia; however, negative results were obtained for a polymorphic trinucleotide repeat marker of *GDNF* in a recent association study (Lee *et al.*, 2001). CNTF is a cytokine that promotes the survival of various populations of neurons during development (Sendtner *et al.*, 1994) through activation of multiple signaling pathways. While the presence of a *CNTF* null mutation initially appeared to associate with schizophrenia in one sample studied (Thome *et al.*, 1996), further investigation by other groups has been predominantly negative (Arinami and Toru, 1996; Gelernter *et al.*, 1997; Sakai *et al.*, 1997b; Thome *et al.*, 1997a; Virgos *et al.*, 2001). Some associations, however, have been made to schizoaffective disorder (Tanaka *et al.*, 1998) and other schizophrenia subtypes (Thome *et al.*, 1997b).

Neurotransmission

The process of neurotransmission at its most fundamental level involves regulated exocytosis through recruitment of synaptic vesicles, fusion to the plasma membrane and neurotransmitter release, and eventual re-establishment of the vesicle pool through endocytosis. The processes and molecules associated with vesicular trafficking are also critical for cell division, fertilization, and secretion of hormones and other proteins, and they are strongly conserved from yeast to human. Exocytosis is regulated most centrally by a group of proteins known as soluble *N*-ethylmaleimide-sensitive attachment factor protein receptors (SNAREs), which are small (18–42 kDa) integral (or anchored) membrane proteins that interact with each other through amphipathic helical domains known as SNARE motifs. The three core SNARE proteins can be categorized into target-SNAREs (t-SNAREs) such as SNAP-25 (synaptosomal-associated protein of 25 kDa) and the syntaxins, and vesicle-SNAREs (v-SNAREs) such as the synaptobrevins (or VAMPs). While this core complex of SNARE proteins is known to regulate vesicular fusion (Hodel, 1998), the cyclical and quantal aspects of neurotransmitter release are facilitated through a host of synaptic protein interactions, which are seen to be quite strongly location-specific among regions of the brain (Bark and Wilson, 1994). The array of synaptic terminal proteins involved in generalized neurotransmission includes the core complex and interactors, which are either soluble or bound to the synaptic vesicle or plasma membrane, such as soluble SNAPs, *N*-ethylmaleimide sensitive

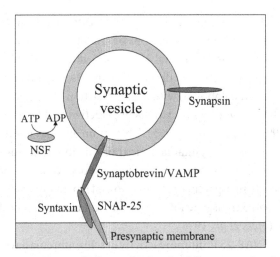

Fig. 1.3.   Synaptic terminal proteins involved in exocytosis. The core complex required for vesicle fusion to the presynaptic membrane includes synaptosomal associated protein of 25 kDa (SNAP-25), syntaxins, and synaptobrevins (or VAMP). Proteins such as *N*-ethylmaleimide-sensitive factor (NSF), which recycle this complex, and synapsins, which interact between the vesicle and the cytoskeleton, are also involved, as well as numerous others.

factor (NSF), synapsins, synaptophysins, synaptogyrins, synaptotagmin, dynamin, and complexins, among others (see Fig. 1.3).

Vesicles are recruited in a calcium-dependent process to active zones on the presynaptic membrane. It has been suggested that vesicle-bound synapsins contribute during the recruitment phase by releasing actin following phosphorylation by calmodulin-dependent protein kinase II, permitting vesicles to untether from the cytoskeleton. Vesicle docking at appropriate sites on the plasma membrane is regulated through a strong connection between vesicle and membrane-bound SNAREs. A slow, ATP-driven priming event then occurs, driven by interaction of the ATPase NSF with the primary SNAREs through soluble α-SNAPs, forming a stable 20S complex. A number of accessory proteins are capable of binding to individual SNARE members, including munc-18, syntaphilin, and CDCrel-1, which bind to syntaxin; synaptophysin, which binds to VAMP; and synaptotagmin, which binds to SNAP-25. Changes in the degree of expression or interaction of specific presynaptic proteins are likely to constitute a major element in the determination of brain structure and function, and the genes encoding these proteins are becoming a topic of investigation in schizophrenia research.

SNAP-25, a t-SNARE that binds to the plasma membrane on palmitoylation, shows a pattern of expression coinciding with synaptogenesis during early embryonic differentiation (Catsicas *et al.*, 1991; Lou and Bixby, 1995). SNAP-25 is most strongly expressed in neurons of neocortex, hippocampus, anterior thalamic and pontine nuclei, and cerebellar granule cells (also pancreatic β-cells and adrenal chromaffin cells), and it is associated with regions of synaptic plasticity. Antisense oligonucleotides to SNAP-25 inhibit axonal elongation in rat cortical neurons, specifically preventing complete terminal differentiation (Osen-Sand et al., 1993). A strain of mouse designated coloboma, with a 2 cM deletion of a region of chromosome 2 containing the Snap-25 gene, exhibits hyperactivity and delayed development (Hess et al., 1996; Heyser et al., 1995). This strain also has abnormalities in dopaminergic, serotonergic, and glutamatergic transmission in dorsal striatum (Raber et al., 1997). This suggests that it may act as a model of attention-deficit hyperactivity disorder and other psychiatric conditions. Hyperactivity is corrected on introduction of a Snap-25 transgene into the strain, indicating the specificity of this feature to the gene (Hess et al., 1996).

Postmortem assays of SNAP-25 immunoreactivity in schizophrenia have revealed changes in the inferior temporal and prefrontal association cortices (Thompson et al., 1998), with decreased expression in Brodmann areas 10 and 20 and increased expression in area 9. A study of hippocampal connectivity found reduced cortical SNAP-25 protein, most notably in the terminal fields of entorhinal cortex projections of schizophrenics (Young et al., 1998). More recently, decreased SNAP-25 expression has been seen in the cerebellum of schizophrenics (Mukaetova-Ladinska et al., 2002), further implicating this molecule in the etiology of the disease. Altered levels of SNAP-25 have also been witnessed in cerebral spinal fluid by quantitative dot blotting (Thompson et al., 1999), with significant elevation of SNAP-25 over that in control subjects and those with headaches. A further study was able to confirm the original SNAP-25 findings in area 10 (along with reduced synaptophysin expression) yet showed no alteration in SNAP-25 mRNA expression (Karson et al., 1999). Enhanced cortical expression of SNAP-25 has been identified through subtraction suppression polymerase chain reaction (PCR) in several rodent models of schizophrenia, including haloperidol-treated versus control and Fischer 344 versus Lewis rats (Wong et al., 2003).

The human SNAP-25 gene has been localized to 20p11.2-12 (Maglott et al., 1996), near a region identified in a multi-center schizophrenia genome scan (Moises et al., 1995). Three single nucleotide polymorphisms have been identified (Barr et al., 2000) in the 3′ untranslated region of SNAP-25, and the transmission of alleles of these polymorphisms have been evaluated in 200 small, nuclear schizophrenia families. Preliminary results indicate unbiased transmission of SNAP-25 alleles and haplotypes within these families (Wong et al., 2003). A polymorphic tetranucleotide repeat identified in the SNAP-25 promoter region also shows no association with affection, subtypes, or family history in a recent case–control study (Tachikawa et al., 2001); consequently, further investigation of additional markers and sample groups is warranted.

The synapsins comprise a family of phosphoproteins localized to the cytoplasmic surface of synaptic vesicles. Until recently, two differentially spliced synapsin genes (*synapsin I* at Xp11.23 and *synapsin II* at 3p25) have been identified, with well-characterized roles in synaptic vesicle release (Jovanovic *et al.*, 2000; Rosahl *et al.*, 1995) and efficiency of neurotransmission (Greengard *et al.*, 1993). A third member of this family, synapsin III, with neuron-specific expression and extensive structural similarity to other members, was recently described (Kao *et al.*, 1998) and localized to chromosome 22q12-13, distal to the psychosis-associated deletion region responsible for DiGeorge and velo-cardio-facial syndrome. A role of synapsins in development of the presynaptic terminal is indicated by studies in rat neuroblastoma cells, which showed that overexpression of synapsin IIb produces an increase in the number of varicosities and the synaptic vesicle content of the varicosities (Han *et al.*, 1991).

Decreased expression of synapsin I protein, as determined through quantitative Western blotting, has been observed in the hippocampus of postmortem brains from individuals with schizophrenia (Browning *et al.*, 1993). Further research shows age-related abnormalities in expression of synapsin Ia and Ib, suggested by data showing that mRNA expression of these isoforms in schizophrenics under age 75 is approximately twofold higher in the left middle and superior temporal gyrus than in age-matched controls, while normalizing in individuals above this age (Tcherepanov and Sokolov, 1997). A preliminary investigation into the possible role of *synapsin I* variants in schizophrenia has given negative results for one microsatellite polymorphism in over 100 families using both linkage- and linkage disequilibrium-based approaches (A. M. Vicente and J. L. Kennedy, unpublished data).

Reduced transcripts for synapsin II (among others, including NSF, synaptotagmin 5, and synaptojanin I) were noted during microarray expression profiling of schizophrenic versus matched control prefrontal cortical brain tissue (Mirnics *et al.*, 2000). This study demonstrated highly significant changes in expression of the presynaptic gene group, among 250 other groups examined, which were verified using *in situ* hyridization and a second cohort for confirmation. These changes were quite consistent in the sample studied (nine of ten and ten of ten pairs showed reduction of synapsin II and NSF, respectively) and appeared unrelated to administration of antipsychotic medication based on patient history and comparison of arrays between haloperidol-treated and control monkeys. The report suggests the presence of global rather than individual modifiers of presynaptic gene expression, as potentially dictated by pre-existing changes in developmental molecules, aberrant cytoarchitecture, or survival/connectivity in the prefrontal cortex. It can be suggested that schizophrenia is, in fact, a disease of the synapse, of polygenic inheritance, and determined by alterations in genes related to trafficking and regulated neurotransmission or their antecedents, with onset related to maturational processes occurring in puberty (Mirnics et al., 2001). Combined with this finding, an early study of synapsin II detected increased numbers of molecular weight variants of the protein in postmortem brain tissue of schizophrenic and alcoholic individuals in comparison with controls (Grebb and Greengard, 1990). A recent attempt to confirm the observations of the Mirnics study on NSF and synapsin II expression using immunoblotting and real-time PCR has been negative (Imai et al., 2001a), raising doubts as to the generalizability of the findings.

The localization of the *synapsin III* gene to a segment of chromosome 22q, associated with a 25-fold elevation in rates of psychiatric disorders and elevated numbers of deletions in individuals with schizophrenia (Murphy et al., 1999), has made this synaptic candidate gene a promising area of study. However, to date, at least six studies (Imai et al., 2001c; Klempan et al., 2002; Ohmori et al., 2000; Ohtsuki et al., 2000; Stober et al., 2000; Tsai et al., 2002) using both linkage and family-based association analysis of eight separate polymorphisms in schizophrenia families have been resoundingly negative.

Complexins are SNARE accessory proteins that bind to syntaxin and limit its interaction with other SNARE proteins. Complexin I is a marker of inhibitory synapses while complexin II occurs in synapses that are primarily excitatory. Investigation of complexin expression identified a reduction in complexin protein and mRNA in medial temporal lobe structures of schizophrenia patients (Harrison and Eastwood, 1998). This was later confirmed specifically in the hippocampus and found to be unaffected by antipsychotic treatment in rats (Eastwood and Harrison, 2000), although complexin mRNA is altered in other regions of the rat forebrain by antipsychotics (Eastwood et al., 2000). Changes in cytoarchitecture and protein expression in the anterior cingulate cortex prompted the examination of this region for levels of complexins (Eastwood and Harrison, 2001); however, no changes were observed in schizophrenia, although they were for mood disorders. This group also identified reduced complexin II expression in the cerebellum (Eastwood et al., 2001). A selective and progressive loss of complexin II and other SNARE proteins in the striatum (and enrichment in the hippocampus) of patients with Huntington's disease has been observed, with possible functional consequences for this disorder (Morton et al., 2001). No genetic investigations of the complexins as candidate genes for schizophrenia have yet been reported in the literature.

A number of additional studies have revealed expression-based changes of synaptic terminal molecules in schizophrenia. Increases in levels of syntaxin within the cingulate cortex have been detected in several studies (Gabriel et al., 1997; Honer et al., 1997), along with changes in the anterior prefrontal cortex (Honer et al., 2002). A negative correlation between age of individuals with schizophrenia and expression of many presynaptic proteins in the temporal cortex (Sokolov et al., 2000) highlights the relative non-specificity of this process and suggests that changes may arise from an abnormality of synaptic connectivity determined much earlier in life. These quantifiable changes in protein levels reflect actual biochemical changes at the presynaptic terminal, potentially leading to synaptic dysfunction, as loss of neuropil is not evident in these regions. An imbalance in stoichiometry between critical regulatory elements may have severe consequences for both response capacity following calcium influx and rates of vesicle fusion and recycling, leading to an increase or deficit in neurotransmission at the synapse. These changes in neuronal phenotype or maturational state may account for the disorganization and volume loss witnessed in various brain regions.

Apart from the recent microarray-based analysis described (Mirnics *et al.*, 2000; also see Ch. 12), other reports are providing increasing evidence for cortical presynaptic dysfunction in schizophrenia, including findings of synaptic vesicle clustering (Soustek, 1989) and alterations of many presynaptic protein and mRNA levels. In addition to a fundamental role in neurotransmission, these molecules are critical during early embryonic development, influence neurite outgrowth and growth cone maturation, and regulate morphological plasticity (Hepp and Langley, 2001). These changes in presynaptic protein expression are also affected by neurotrophic factors such as BDNF (Tartaglia *et al.*, 2001), thus pointing to the need for further elaboration of epistasis in these pathways when examining genetic variants.

Conclusions

While a staggering number of genes are involved in the patterning and function of the human brain, the rapid pace of human genome sequence analysis has facilitated the isolation and further characterization of brain-expressed sequences. Many of the proteins encoded by these genes will participate in complex biological activities integral to the establishment and maintenance of proper neuronal connectivity, which, in turn, provides a template for higher-order cognitive function. It is natural to consider, therefore, given the demonstrated genetic liability for schizophrenia, that a number of these loci are likely to be involved as either direct etiological determinants or phenotypic modifiers of the disease. As most researchers would now agree that schizophrenia is inherited in a decidedly non-Mendelian fashion, the best question that we can ask at present would be what set of DNA alterations are consistently linked to a particular phenotype of schizophrenia? Possible modifiers of cognitive abilities are beginning to be found through assessment of candidate gene influence on neuropsychological tests (Bilder *et al.*, 2002; Egan *et al.*, 2003) and further genetic determinants of individual disease components will likely be identified as the complexities of the human genome are unraveled.

This chapter has outlined the role played in the developing brain by various genes within broad functional categories. A myriad of other factors (both genetic and environmental) await investigation, and the final understanding of schizophrenia etiology may only be known with improvements in methodologies for detection of gene–gene and gene–environment interaction. Until fairly recently, the relative permanency of individual cells and populations/networks within the brain was undisputed; however, we now know that the CNS is highly plastic and responsive, with the capacity for neurogenesis throughout life from discrete sets of neural stem cells (Eriksson *et al.*, 1998). We should perhaps not be surprised, therefore, to learn that the complex set of phenotypes collectively known as schizophrenia is anticipated by an equally complex set of genetic alterations, from which only particular combinations may be identified within any given individual at risk for the disorder. Of particular interest in this regard is the recent description of epistasis between alleles of the *G72* and D-amino acid oxidase (*DAOO*) genes in conferring risk for schizophrenia (Chumakov *et al.*, 2002). Together with *neuregulin 1* and *dysbindin*, these genes may induce schizophrenia susceptibility through a common *N*-methyl-D-aspartate receptor pathway (Cloninger, 2002), a pathway that could alter the neurodevelopmental trajectory of the brain. If replicated, the finding of Chumakov and colleagues would constitute the first significant observation of gene–gene interaction in the etiology of schizophrenia, with likely expansion as the interactions between various susceptibility factors are uncovered in the years to come.

Acknowledgements

We thank the Canadian Institutes of Health Research for grant support and Mary Smirniw for her assistance with this manuscript.

REFERENCES

Akatone, A., Kunugi, H., Tanaka, H., Nanko, S. (2002). Association analysis of polymorphic CGG repeat in 5′ UTR of the *reelin* and *VLDLR* genes with schizophrenia, *Schizophr Res* **58**: 37–41.

Akbarian, S., Kim, J. J., Potkin, S. G., *et al.* (1996). Maldistribution of interstitial neurons in prefrontal white matter of the brains of schizophrenic patients. *Arch Gen Psychiatry* **53**: 425–436.

Anderson, S. A., Eisenstat, D. D., Shi, L., Rubenstein, J. L. R. (1997). Interneuron migration from basal forebrain to neocortex: dependence on *Dlx* genes. *Science* **278**: 474–476.

Andrews, P. L., Wood, K. L. (1986). Systemic baclofen stimulates gastric motility and secretion via a central action in the rat. *Br J Pharmacol* **89**: 461–467.

Angelucci, F., Mathe, A. A., Aloe, L. (2000). Brain-derived neurotrophic factor and tyrosine kinase receptor TrκB in rat brain are significantly altered after haloperidol and risperidone administration. *J Neurosci Res* **60**: 783–794.

Arenas, E., Trupp, M., Akerud, P., Ibanez, C. F. (1995). GDNF prevents degeneration and promotes the phenotype of brain noradrenergic neurons in vivo. *Neuron* **15**: 1465–1473.

Arinami, T., Toru, M. (1996). No evidence for association between CNTF null mutant allele and schizophrenia. *Br J Psychiatry* **169**: 253.

Arinami, T., Takekoshi, K., Itokawa, M., Hamaguchi, H., Toru, M. (1996). Failure to find associations of the CA repeat polymorphism in the first intron and the Gly-63/Glu-63 polymorphism of the neurotrophin-3 gene with schizophrenia. *Psychiatry Genet* **6**: 13–15.

Artavanis-Tsakonis, S., Muskavitch, M. A., Yedvobnick, Y. (1983). Molecular cloning of *Notch*, a locus affecting neurogenesis in *Drosophila melanogaster*. *Proc Natl Acad Sci* USA **80**: 1977–1981.

Barbeau, D., Liang, J. J., Robitalille, Y., Quirion, R., Srivastava, L. K. (1995). Decreased expression of the embryonic form of the neural cell adhesion molecule in schizophrenic brains. *Proc Natl Acad Sci* USA **92**: 2785–2789.

Bark, I. C., Wilson, M. C. (1994). Regulated vesicular fusion in neurons: snapping together the details. *Proc Natl Acad Sci USA* **91**: 4621–4624.

Barr, C. L., Feng, Y., Wigg, K., *et al.* (2000). Identification of DNA variants in the SNAP-25 gene and linkage study of these polymorphisms and attention-deficit hyperactivity disorder. *Mol Psychiatry* **5**: 405–409.

Beasley, C., Cotter, D., Khan, N., *et al.* (2001). Glycogen synthase kinase-3beta immunoreactivity is reduced in the prefrontal cortex in schizophrenia. *Neurosci Lett* **302**: 117–120.

Beggs, H. E., Baragona, S. C., Hemperly, J. J., Maness, P. F. (1997). NCAM140 interacts with the focal adhesion kinase p125(fak) and the SRC-related tyrosine kinase p59(fyn). *J Biol Chem* **272**: 8310–8319.

Bell, E., Wingate, R. J. T., Lumsden, A. (1999). Homeotic transformation of rhombomere identity after localized *Hoxb1* misexpression. *Science* **284**: 2168–2171.

Bello, M. J., Salagnon, N., Rey, J. A., *et al.* (1989). Precise *in situ* localization of NCAM, ETS1, and D11S29 on human meiotic chromosomes. *Cytogenet Cell Genet* **52**: 7–10.

Berkmeier, L. R., Winslow, J. W., Kaplan, D. R., *et al.* (1991). Neurotrophin-5: a novel neurotrophic factor that activates *trk* and *trkB*. *Neuron* **4**: 189–201.

Bilder, R. M., Volavka, J., Czobor, P., *et al.* (2002). Neurocognitive correlates of the COMT Val(158)Met polymorphism in chronic schizophrenia. *Biol Psychiatry* **52**: 701–707.

Broccoli, V., Boncinelli, E., Wurst, W. (1999). The caudal limit of *Otx2* expression positions the isthmic organizer. *Nature* **401**: 164–168.

Brouha, A. K., Weickert, C. S., Hyde, T. M., *et al.* (1996). Reductions in brain derived neurotrophic factor mRNA in the hippocampus of patients with schizophrenia. In *Proceedings of the Society for Neuroscience*. Washington, DC: Society for Neuroscience, pp. 1680.

Browning, M. D., Dudek, E. M., Rapier, J. L., Leonard, S., Freedman, R. (1993). Significant reductions in synapsin but not synaptophysin specific activity in the brains of some schizophrenics. *Biol Psychiatry* **34**: 529–535.

Casarosa, S., Fode, C., Guillemot, F. (1999). *Mash1* regulates neurogenesis in the ventral telencephalon. *Development* **126**: 525–534.

Catsicas, S., Larhammar, D., Blomqvist, A., *et al.* (1991). Expression of a conserved cell-type-specific protein in nerve terminals coincides with synaptogenesis. *Proc Natl Acad Sci USA* **88**: 785–789.

Chapouton, P., Schuurmans, C., Guillemot, F., Gotz, M. (2001). The transcription factor neurogenin 2 restricts cell migration from the cortex to the striatum. *Development* **128**: 5149–5159.

Chumakov, I., Blumenfeld, M., Guerassimenko, O., *et al.* (2002). Genetic and physiological data implicating the new human gene *G72* and the gene for D-amino acid oxidase in schizophrenia. *Proc Natl Acad Sci* USA **99**: 13675–13680.

Cloninger, C. R. (2002). The discovery of susceptibility genes for mental disorders. *Proc Natl Acad Sci* USA **99**: 13365–13367.

Cotter, D., Kerwin, R., al-Sarraji, S., *et al.* (1998). Abnormalities of Wnt signalling in schizophrenia: evidence for neurodevelopmental abnormality. *Neuroreport* **9**: 1379–1383.

Crossin, K. L., Krushel, L. A. (2000). Cellular signaling by neural cell adhesion molecules of the immunoglobulin superfamily. *Dev Dyn* **218**: 260–279.

Cunningham, B. A. (1995). Cell adhesion molecules as morphoregulators. *Curr Opin Cell Biol* **7**: 628–633.

D'Arcangelo, G., Curran, T. (1998). Reeler: new tales on an old mutant mouse. *Bioessays* **20**: 235–244.

Dawson, E., Powell, J. F., Sham P. C., *et al.* (1995). An association study of a neurotrophin-3 (NT-3) gene polymorphism with schizophrenia. *Acta Psychiatr Scand* **92**: 425–428.

de la Pompa, J. L., Wakeham, A., Correia, K. M., *et al.* (1997). Conservation of the Notch signalling pathway in mammalian neurogenesis. *Development* **124**: 1139–1148.

DeSilva, U., D'Arcangelo, G., Braden, V. V., *et al.* (1997). The human reelin gene: isolation, sequencing, and mapping on chromosome 7. *Genome Res* **7**: 157–164.

Doherty, P., Walsh, F. S. (1996). CAM–FGF receptor interactions: a model for axonal growth. *Mol Cell Neurosci* **8**: 99–111.

Doherty, P., Fruns, M., Seaton, P., *et al.* (1990). A threshold effect of the major isoforms of NCAM on neurite outgrowth. *Nature* **343**: 464–466.

Durany, N., Michel, T., Zochling, R., *et al.* (2001). Brain-derived neurotrophic factor and neurotrophin 3 in schizophrenic psychoses. *Schizophr Res* **52**: 79–86.

Eastwood, S. L., Harrison, P. J. (2000). Hippocampal synaptic pathology in schizophrenia, bipolar disorder and major depression: a study of complexin mRNAs. *Mol Psychiatry* **5**: 425–432.

(2001). Synaptic pathology in the anterior cingulate cortex in schizophrenia and mood disorders. A review and a Western blot study of synaptophysin, GAP-43 and the complexins. *Brain Res Bull* **55**: 569–578.

Eastwood, S. L., Burnet, P. W., Harrison, P. J. (2000). Expression of complexin I and II mRNAs and their regulation by antipsychotic drugs in the rat forebrain. *Synapse* **36**: 167–177.

Eastwood, S. L., Cotter, D., Harrison, P. J. (2001). Cerebellar synaptic protein expression in schizophrenia. *Neuroscience* **105**: 219–229.

Eckhardt, M., Muhlenhoff, M., Bethe, A., *et al.* (1995). Molecular characterization of eukaryotic polysialyltransferase-1. *Nature* **373**: 715–718.

Egan, M. F., Kojima, M., Callicott, J. H., *et al.* (2003). The BDNF val66met polymorphism affects activity-dependent secretion of BDNF and human memory and hippocampal function. *Cell* **112**: 257–269.

Ericson, J., Murh, J., Placzek, M., *et al.* (1995). Sonic hedgehog induces the differentiation of ventral forebrain neurons: a common signal for ventral patterning within the neural tube. *Cell* **81**: 747–756.

Eriksson, P. S., Perfilieva, E., Bjork-Eriksson, T., *et al.* (1998). Neurogenesis in the adult human hippocampus. *Nat Med* **4**: 1313–1317.

Ernfors, P., Ibanez, C. F., Ebendal, T., Olson, L., Persson, H. (1990). Molecular cloning and neurotrophic activities of a protein with structural similarities to nerve growth factor: developmental and topographical expression in brain. *Proc Natl Acad Sci USA* **87**: 5454–5458.

Falconer, D. S. (1951). Two new mutants *trembler* and *reeler*, with neurological actions in the house mouse. *J Genet* **50**: 192–201.

Fan, J. B., Tang, J. X., Gu, N. F., *et al.* (2002). A family-based and case–control association study of the NOTCH4 gene and schizophrenia. *Mol Psychiatry* **7**: 100–103.

Fatemi, S. H., Earle, J. A., McMenomy, T. (2000). Reduction in Reelin immunoreactivity in hippocampus of subjects with schizophrenia, bipolar disorder and major depression. *Mol Psychiatry* **5**: 654–663, 571.

Ferreiro, B., Kintner, C., Zimmerman, K., Anderson, D. J., Harris, W. (1994). *XASH1* genes promote neurogenesis in *Xenopus* embryos. *Development* **120**: 3649–3655.

Fields, R. D., Itoh, K. (1996). Neural cell adhesion molecules in activity-dependent development and synaptic plasticity. *Trends Neurosci* **19**: 473–480.

Gabriel, S. M., Haroutunian, V., Powchik, P., *et al.* (1997). Increased concentrations of presynaptic proteins in the cingulate cortex of subjects with schizophrenia. *Arch Gen Psychiatry* **54**: 559–566.

Gelernter, J., Van Dyck, C., van Kammen, D. P., *et al.* (1997). Ciliary neurotrophic factor null allele frequencies in schizophrenia, affective disorders, and Alzheimer's disease. *Am J Med Genet* **74**: 497–500.

Goffinet, A. M., Dernoncourt, C. (1991). Localization of the reeler gene relative to flanking loci on mouse chromosome 5. *Mamm Genome* **1**: 100–103.

Goggi, J., Pullar, I. A., Carney, S. L., Bradford, H. F. (2002). Modulation of neurotransmitter release induced by brain-derived neurotrophic factor in rat brain striatal slices in vitro. *Brain Res* **941**: 34–42.

Gotz, R., Koster, R., Winkler, C., *et al.* (1994). Neurotrophin-6 is a new member of the nerve growth factor family. *Nature* **372**: 266–269.

Gower, H. J., Barton, C. H., Elsom, V. L., *et al.* (1988). Alternative splicing generates a secreted form of N-CAM in muscle and brain. *Cell* **55**: 955–964.

Grebb, J. A., Greengard, P. (1990). An analysis of synapsin II, a neuronal phosphoprotein, in postmortem brain tissue from alcoholic and neuropsychiatrically ill adults and medically ill children and young adults. *Arch Gen Psychiatry* **47**: 1149–1156.

Greengard, P., Valtorta, F., Czernik, A. J., Benfenati, F. (1993). Synaptic vesicle phosphoproteins and regulation of synaptic function. *Science* **259**: 780–785.

Guidotti, A., Auta, J., Davis, J. M., *et al.* (2000). Decrease in reelin and glutamic acid decarboxylase67 (GAD67) expression in schizophrenia and bipolar disorder: a postmortem brain study. *Arch Gen Psychiatry* **57**: 1061–1069.

Guillin, O., Diaz, J., Carroll, P., *et al.* (2001). BDNF controls dopamine D3 receptor expression and triggers behavioural sensitization. *Nature* **411**: 86–89.

Ha, D. H., Robertson, R. T., Ribak, C. E., Weiss, J. H. (1996). Cultured basal forebrain cholinergic neurons in contact with cortical cells display synapses, enhanced morphological features, and decreased dependence on nerve growth factor. *J Comp Neurol* **373**: 451–465.

Han, H. Q., Bahler, M., Greengard, P., Nichols, R. A., Rubin, M. R. (1991). Induction of formation of presynaptic terminals in neuroblastoma cells by synapsin IIb. *Nature* **349**: 697–700.

Harrison, P. J., Eastwood, S. L. (1998). Preferential involvement of excitatory neurons in medial temporal lobe in schizophrenia. *Lancet* **352**: 1669–1673.

Hattori, M., Nanko, S. (1995). Association of neurotrophin-3 gene variant with severe forms of schizophrenia. *Biochem Biophys Res Commun* **209**: 513–518.

Hawi, Z., Straub, R. E., O'Neill, A., *et al.* (1998). No linkage or linkage disequilibrium between brain-derived neurotrophic factor (BDNF) dinucleotide repeat polymorphism and schizophrenia in Irish families. *Psychiatry Res* **81**: 111–116.

Hepp, R., Langley, K. (2001). SNAREs during development. *Cell Tissue Res* **305**: 247–253.

Hess, E. J., Collins, K. A., Wilson, M. C. (1996). Mouse model of hyperkinesis implicates SNAP-25 in behavioral regulation. *J Neurosci* **16**: 3104–3111.

Heyser, C. J., Wilson, M. C., Gold, L. H. (1995). Coloboma hyperactive mutant exhibits delayed neurobehavioral developmental milestones. *Brain Res Dev Brain Res* **89**: 264–269.

Hodel, A. (1998). Snap-25. *Int J Biochem Cell Biol* **30**: 1069–1073.

Hohn, A., Leibrock, J., Bailey, K., Barde, Y. A. (1990). Identification and characterization of a novel member of the nerve growth factor/brain-derived neurotrophic factor family. *Nature* **344**: 339–341.

Honer, W. G., Falkai, P., Young, C., *et al.* (1997). Cingulate cortex synaptic terminal proteins and neural cell adhesion molecule in schizophrenia. *Neuroscience* **78**: 99–110.

Honer, W. G., Falkai, P., Bayer, T. A., *et al.* (2002). Abnormalities of SNARE mechanism proteins in anterior frontal cortex in severe mental illness. *Cereb Cortex* **12**: 349–356.

Hynes, M., Rosenthal, A. (1999). Specification of dopaminergic and serotonergic neurons in the vertebrate CNS. *Curr Opin Neurobiol* **9**: 26–36.

Imai, C., Sugai, T., Iritani, S., *et al.* (2001a). A quantitative study on the expression of synapsin II and *N*-ethylmaleimide-sensitive fusion protein in schizophrenic patients. *Neurosci Lett* **305**: 185–188.

Imai, K., Harada, S., Kawanishi, Y., *et al.* (2001b). The $(CTG)_n$ polymorphism in the *NOTCH4* gene is not associated with schizophrenia in Japanese individuals. *BMC Psychiatry* **1**: 1.

(2001c). Polymorphisms in the promoter and coding regions of the synapsin III gene. A lack of association with schizophrenia. *Neuropsychobiology* **43**: 237–241.

Ip, N. Y., Ibanez, C. F., Nye, S. H., *et al.* (1992). Mammalian neurotrophin-4: structure, chromosomal localization, tissue distribution, and receptor specificity. *Proc Natl Acad Sci USA* **89**: 3060–3064.

Jones, F. S., Holst, B. D., Minowa, O., De Robertis, E. M., Edelman, G. M. (1993). Binding and transcriptional activation of the promoter for the neural cell adhesion molecule by HoxC6 (Hox-3.3). *Proc Natl Acad Sci USA* **90**: 6557–6561.

Jonsson, E., Brene, S., Zhang, X. R., *et al.* (1997). Schizophrenia and neurotrophin-3 alleles. *Acta Psychiatr Scand* **95**: 414–419.

Jovanovic, J. N., Czernik, A. J., Fienberg, A. A., Greengard, P., Sihra, T. S. (2000). Synapsins as mediators of BDNF-enhanced neurotransmitter release. *Nat Neurosci* **3**: 323–329.

Kao, H. T., Porton, B., Czernik, A. J., *et al.* (1998). A third member of the synapsin gene family. *Proc Natl Acad Sci USA* **95**: 4667–4672.

Karecla, P. I., Green, S. J., Bowden, S. J., Coadwell, J., Kilshaw, P. J. (1996). Identification of a binding site for integrin alphaEbeta7 in the N-terminal domain of E-cadherin. *J Biol Chem* **271**: 30909–30915.

Karson, C. N., Mrak, R. E., Schluterman, K. O., *et al.* (1999). Alterations in synaptic proteins and their encoding mRNAs in prefrontal cortex in schizophrenia: a possible neurochemical basis for "hypofrontality". *Mol Psychiatry* **4**: 39–45.

Kiss, J. Z., Troncoso, E., Djebbara, Z., Vutskits, L., Muller, D. (2001). The role of neural cell adhesion molecules in plasticity and repair. *Brain Res Brain Res Rev* **36**: 175–184.

Klempan, T. A., Trakalo, J. M., Pato, C. N., *et al.* (2001). Polymorphisms of the *NOTCH4* gene and schizophrenia. *Am J Hum Genet* **69** (Suppl. 4): 567.

Klempan, T. A., Trakalo, J., King, N., *et al.* (2002). Transmission of SYNAPSIN3 gene variants in schizophrenia families. In *Proceeding of the 52nd Annual Meeting of the American Society for Human Genetics*. Bethesda, MD: American Society for Human Genetics, p. 489.

Kohtz, J. D., Baker D. P., Corte, G., Fishell, G. (1998). Regionalization within the mammalian telencephalon is mediated by changes in responsiveness to Sonic hedgehog. *Development* **125**: 5079–5089.

Kortschak, R. D., Tamme, R., Lardelli, M. (2001). Evolutionary analysis of vertebrate *Notch* genes. *Dev Genes Evol* **211**: 350–354.

Kozlovsky, N., Belmaker, R. H., Agam, G. (2002). GSK-3 and the neurodevelopmental hypothesis of schizophrenia. *Eur Neuropsychopharmacol* **12**: 13–25.

Krebs, M. O., Guillin, O., Bourdell, M. C., *et al.* (2000). Brain derived neurotrophic factor (BDNF) gene variants association with age at onset and therapeutic response in schizophrenia. *Mol Psychiatry* **5**: 558–562.

Kristiansen, L. V., Marques F. A., Soroka, V., *et al.* (1999). Homophilic NCAM interactions interfere with L1 stimulated neurite outgrowth. *FEBS Lett* **464**: 30–34.

Krumlauf, R. (1994). *Hox* genes in vertebrate development. *Cell* **78**: 191–201.

Krushel, L. A., Cunningham, B. A., Edelman, G. M., Crossin, K. L. (1999). NF-kappaB activity is induced by neural cell adhesion molecule binding to neurons and astrocytes. *J Biol Chem* **274**: 2432–2439.

LaMantia, A. S. (1999). Forebrain induction, retinoic acid, and vulnerability to schizophrenia: insights from molecular and genetic analysis in developing mice. *Biol Psychiatry* **46**: 19–30.

Lawrie, S. M., Abukmeil, S. S. (1998). Brain abnormality in schizophrenia. A systematic and quantitative review of volumetric magnetic resonance imaging studies. *Br J Psychiatry* **172**: 110–120.

Lee, J. E. (1997). Basic helix–loop–helix genes in neural development. *Curr Opin Neurobiol* **7**: 13–20.

Lee, J. E., Hollenberg, S. M., Lipnick, N., *et al.* (1995). Conversion of *Xenopus* ectoderm into neurons by NeuroD, a basic helix–loop–helix protein. *Science* **268**: 836–844.

Lee, K., Kunugi, H., Nanko, S. (2001). Glial cell line-derived neurotrophic factor (GDNF) gene and schizophrenia: polymorphism screening and association analysis. *Psychiatry Res* **104**: 11–17.

Leibrock, J., Lottspeich, F., Hohn, A., *et al.* (1989). Molecular cloning and expression of brain-derived neurotrophic factor. *Nature* **341**: 149–152.

Levi-Montalcini, R. (1987). The nerve growth factor 35 years later. *Science* **237**: 1154–1162.

Lewis, C. M., Levinson, D. F., Wise, L. H., *et al.* (2003). Genome scan meta-analysis of schizophrenia and bipolar disorder, part II: schizophrenia. *Am J Hum Genet* **73**: 34–48.

Li, L., Huang, G. M., Banta, A. B., *et al.* (1998). Cloning, characterization, and the complete 56.8-kilobase DNA sequence of the human *NOTCH4* gene. *Genomics* **51**: 45–58.

Lin, L. H., Doherty, D. H., Lile, J. D., Bektesh, S., Collins, F. (1993). GDNF: a glial cell-derived neurotrophic factor for midbrain dopaminergic neurons. *Science* **260**: 1130–1132.

Lou, X. J., Bixby, J. L. (1995). Patterns of presynaptic gene expression define two stages of synaptic differentiation. *Mol Cell Neurosci* **6**: 252–262.

Luo, X. J., Klempan, T. A., Lappalainen, J., *et al.* (2004). *NOTCH4* gene haplotype is associated with schizophrenia in African-Americans. *Biol Psychiatry* **55**: 112–117.

Maglott, D. R., Feldblyum, T. V., Durkin, A. S., Nierman, W. C. (1996). Radiation hybrid mapping of SNAP, PCSK2, and THBD (human chromosome 20p). *Mamm Genome* **7**: 400–401.

Maisonpierre, P., Belluscio, L., Friedman, B., *et al.* (1990). NT-3, BDNF, and NGF in the developing rat nervous system: parallel as well as reciprocal patterns of expression. *Neuron* **5**: 501–509

Mallamaci, A., Mercurio, S., Muzio, L., *et al.* (2000). The lack of Emx2 causes impairment of Reelin signaling and defects of neuronal migration in the developing cerebral cortex. *J Neurosci* **20**: 1109–1118.

McEvilly, R. J., de Diaz, M. O., Schonemann, M. D., Hooshmand, F., Rosenfeld, M. G. (2002). Transcriptional regulation of cortical neuron migration by POU domain factors. *Science* **295**: 1528–1532.

McGinnis, R. E., Fox, H., Yates, P., *et al.* (2001). Failure to confirm NOTCH4 association with schizophrenia in a large population-based sample from Scotland. *Nat Genet* **28**: 128–129.

McMahon, A. P., Bradley, A. (1990). The *Wnt-1* (*int-1*) proto-oncogene is required for the development of a large region of the mouse brain. *Cell* **62**: 1073–1085.

Mirnics, K., Middleton, F. A., Marquez, A., Lewis, D. A., Levitt, P. (2000). Molecular characterization of schizophrenia viewed by microarray analysis of gene expression in prefrontal cortex. *Neuron* **28**: 53–67.

Mirnics, K., Middleton, F. A., Lewis D. A., Levitt, P. (2001). Analysis of complex brain disorders with gene expression microarrays: schizophrenia as a disease of the synapse. *Trends Neurosci* **24**: 479–486.

Miyaoka, T., Seno, H., Ishino, H. (1999). Increased expression of Wnt-1 in schizophrenic brains. *Schizophr Res* **38**: 1–6.

Moises, H. W., Kristbjarnarson, H., Wiese, C., *et al.* (1995). An international two-stage genome-wide search for schizophrenia susceptibility genes. *Nat Genet* **11**: 321–324.

Morris, P. J., Dawson, S. J., Wilson, M. C., Latchman, D. S. (1997). A single residue within the homeodomain of the Brn-3 POU family transcription factors determines whether they activate or repress the SNAP-25 promoter. *Neuroreport* **8**: 2041–2045.

Morton, A. J., Faull, R. L. M., Edwardson, J. M. (2001). Abnormalities in the synaptic vesicle fusion machinery in Huntington's disease. *Brain Res Bull* **56**: 111–117.

Muglia, P., Vicente, A. M., Verga, M., *et al.* (2003). Association between the BDNF gene and schizophrenia. *Mol Psychiatry* **8**: 147–148.

Mukaetova-Ladinska, E. B., Hurt, J., Honer, W. G., Harrington, C. R., Wischik, C. M. (2002). Loss of synaptic but not cytoskeletal proteins in the cerebellum of chronic schizophrenics. *Neurosci Lett* **317**: 161–165.

Muller, D., Djebbara-Hannas, Z., Jourdain, P., *et al.* (2000). Brain-derived neurotrophic factor restores long-term potentiation in polysialic acid-neural cell adhesion molecule-deficient hippocampus. *Proc Natl Acad Sci USA* **97**: 4315–4320.

Murase, S., Schuman, E. M. (1999). The role of cell adhesion molecules in synaptic plasticity and memory. *Curr Opin Cell Biol* **11**: 549–553.

Murphy, K. C., Jones, L. A., Owen, M. J. (1999). High rates of schizophrenia in adults with velo-cardio-facial syndrome. *Arch Gen Psychiatry* **56**: 940–945.

Nakayama, J., Fukuda, M. N., Fredette, B., Ranscht, B., Fukuda, M. (1995). Expression cloning of a human polysialyltransferase that forms the polysialylated neural cell adhesion molecule present in embryonic brain. *Proc Natl Acad Sci USA* **92**: 7031–7035.

Nanko, S., Hattori, M., Kuwata, S., *et al.* (1994). Neurotrophin-3 gene polymorphism associated with schizophrenia. *Acta Psychiatr Scand* **89**: 390–392.

Nguyen Ba-Charvet, K. T., von Boxberg, Y., Godement, P. (1999). The mouse homeodomain protein OTX2 regulates NCAM promoter activity. *Brain Res Mol Brain Res* **67**: 292–295.

Nimgaonkar, V. L., Zhang, X. R., Brar, J. S., DeLeo, M., Ganguli, R. (1995). Lack of association of schizophrenia with the neurotrophin-3 gene locus. *Acta Psychiatr Scand* **92**: 464–466.

Ohmori, O., Shinkai, T., Hori, H., Kojima, H., Nakamura, J. (2000). Synapsin III gene polymorphisms and schizophrenia. *Neurosci Lett* **279**: 125–127.

Ohtsuki, T., Ichiki, R., Toru, M., Arinami, T. (2000). Mutational analysis of the synapsin III gene on chromosome 22q12-q13 in schizophrenia. *Psychiatry Res* **94**: 1–7.

Osen-Sand, A., Catsicas, M., Staple, J. K., *et al.* (1993). Inhibition of axonal growth by SNAP-25 antisense oligonucleotides in vitro and in vivo. *Nature* **364**: 445–448.

Parras, C. M., Schuurmans, C., Scardigli, R., *et al.* (2002). Divergent functions of the proneural genes *Mash1* and *Ngn2* in the specification of neuronal subtype identity. *Genes Dev* **16**: 324–338.

Persico, A. M., D'Agruma, L., Maiorano, N., *et al.* (2001). Reelin gene alleles and haplotypes as a factor predisposing to autistic disorder. *Mol Psychiatry* **6**: 150–159.

Proschel, M., Saunders, A., Roses, A. D., Muller, C. R. (1992). Dinucleotide repeat polymorphism at the human gene for the brain-derived neurotrophic factor (BDNF). *Hum Mol Genet* **1**: 353.

Purves, D. (1988) *Body and Brain: A Trophic Theory of Neural Connections*. Cambridge, MA: Harvard University Press.

Raber, J., Mehta, P. P., Kreifeldt, M., *et al.* (1997). Coloboma hyperactive mutant mice exhibit regional and transmitter-specific deficits in neurotransmission. *J Neurochem* **68**: 176–186.

Rakic, P., Caviness, V. S., *Jr.* (1995). Cortical development: view from neurological mutants two decades later. *Neuron* **14**: 1101–1104.

Rhoads, A. R., Karkera, J. D., Detera-Wadleigh, S. D. (1999). Radiation hybrid mapping of genes in the lithium-sensitive wnt signaling pathway. *Mol Psychiatry* **4**: 437–442.

Rice, D. S., Curran, T. (2001). Role of the reelin signaling pathway in central nervous system development. *Annu Rev Neurosci* **24**: 1005–1039.

Rodriguez, M. A., Pesold, C., Liu, W. S., et al. (2000). Colocalization of integrin receptors and Reelin in dendritic spine postsynaptic densities of adult nonhuman primate cortex. *Proc Natl Acad Sci USA* **97**: 3550–3555.

Rosahl, T. W., Spillane, D., Missler, M., et al. (1995). Essential functions of synapsins I and II in synaptic vesicle regulation. *Nature* **375**: 488–493.

Ruiz i Altaba, A. (1994). Pattern formation in the vertebrate neural plate. *Trends Neurosci* **17**: 233–243.

Sasaki, T., Dai, X. Y., Kuwata, S., et al. (1997a). Brain-derived neurotrophic factor gene and schizophrenia in Japanese subjects. *Am J Med Genet* **74**: 443–444.

Sakai, T., Sasaki, T., Tatsumi, M., et al. (1997b). Schizophrenia and the ciliary neurotrophic factor (CNTF) gene: no evidence for association. *Psychiatry Res* **71**: 7–10.

Schneider-Manoury, S., Seitanidou, T., Charnay, P., Lumsden, A. (1997). Segmental and neuronal architecture of the hindbrain of *Krox-20* mouse mutants. *Development* **124**: 1215–1226.

Schonemann, M. D., Ryan A. K., McEvilly, R. J., et al. (1995). Development and survival of the endocrine hypothalamus and posterior pituitary gland requires the neuronal POU domain factor Brn-2. *Genes Dev* **9**: 3122–3135.

Schwab, S. G., Albus, M., Hallmayer, J., et al. (1995). Evaluation of a susceptibility gene for schizophrenia on chromosome 6p by multipoint affected sib-pair linkage analysis. *Nat Genet* **11**: 325–327.

Selemon, L. D., Rajkowska, G., Goldman-Rakic, P. S. (1995). Abnormally high neuronal density in the schizophrenic cortex. A morphometric analysis of prefrontal area 9 and occipital area 17. *Arch Gen Psychiatry* **52**: 805–818.

Sendtner, M., Carroll, P., Holtmann, B., Hughes, R., Thoenen, H. (1994). Ciliary neurotrophic factor. *J Neurobiol* **25**: 1436–1453.

Senzaki, K., Ogawa, M., Yagi, T. (1999). Proteins of the CNR family are multiple receptors for Reelin. *Cell* **99**: 635–647.

Sklar, P., Schwab, S. G., Williams, N. M., et al. (2001). Association analysis of *NOTCH4* loci in schizophrenia using family and population-based controls. *Nat Genet* **28**: 126–128.

Snider, W. (1994). Functions of the neurotrophins during nervous system development: what the knockouts are teaching us. *Cell* **77**: 627–638.

Sokolov, B. P., Tcherepanov, A. A., Haroutunian, V., Davis, K. L. (2000). Levels of mRNAs encoding synaptic vesicle and synaptic plasma membrane proteins in the temporal cortex of elderly schizophrenic patients. *Biol Psychiatry* **48**: 184–196.

Soustek, Z. (1989). Ultrastructure of cortical synapses in the brain of schizophrenics. *Zentralbl Allg Pathol* **135**: 25–32.

Steindler, D. A., Colwell, S. A. (1976). Reeler mutant mouse: maintenance of appropriate and reciprocal connections in the cerebral cortex and thalamus. *Brain Res* **113**: 386–393.

Stober, G., Syagailo, Y. V., Okladnova, O., et al. (1999). Functional *PAX*-6 gene-linked polymorphic region: potential association with paranoid schizophrenia. *Biol Psychiatry* **45**: 1585–1591.

Stober, G., Meyer, J., Nanda, I., et al. (2000). Linkage and family-based association study of schizophrenia and the synapsin III locus that maps to chromosome 22q13. *Am J Med Genet* **96**: 392–397.

Straub, R. E., MacLean, C. J., O'Neill, F. A., *et al.* (1995). A potential vulnerability locus for schizophrenia on chromosome 6p24–22: evidence for genetic heterogeneity. *Nat Genet* **11**: 287–293.

Studer, M., Lumsden, A., Ariza-McNaughton, L., Bradley, A., Krumlauf, R. (1996). Altered segmental identity and abnormal migration of motor neurons in mice lacking *Hoxb1*. *Nature* **384**: 630–634.

Sun, Y., Nadal-Vicens, M., Misono, S., *et al.* (2001). Neurogenin promotes neurogenesis and inhibits glial differentiation by independent mechanisms. *Cell* **104**: 365–376.

Swift-Scanlan, T., Lan, T. H., Fallin, M. D., *et al.* (2002). Genetic analysis of the $(CTG)_n$ NOTCH4 polymorphism in 65 multiplex bipolar pedigrees. *Psychiatr Genet* **12**: 43–47.

Tachikawa, H., Harada, S., Kawanishi, Y., Okubo, T., Suzuki, T. (2001). Polymorphism of the 5′-upstream region of the human SNAP-25 gene: an association analysis with schizophrenia. *Neuropsychobiology* **43**: 131–133.

Takahashi, M., Shirakawa, O., Toyooka, K., *et al.* (2000). Abnormal expression of brain-derived neurotrophic factor and its receptor in the corticolimbic system of schizophrenic patients. *Mol Psychiatry* **5**: 293–300.

Takei, K., Chan, T. A., Wang, F. S., Deng, H., Rutishauser, U., Jay, D. G. (1999). The neural cell adhesion molecules L1 and NCAM-180 act in different steps of neurite outgrowth. *J Neurosci* **19**: 9469–9479.

Takeichi, M. (1990). Cadherins: a molecular family important in selective cell–cell adhesion. *Annu Rev Biochem* **59**: 237–252.

Tanaka, Y., Ujike, H., Fujiwara, Y., *et al.* (1998). Schizophrenic psychoses and the CNTF null mutation. *Neuroreport* **9**: 981–983.

Tartaglia, N., Du, J., Tyler, W. J., *et al.* (2001). Protein synthesis-dependent and -independent regulation of hippocampal synapses by brain-derived neurotrophic factor. *J Biol Chem* **276**: 37585–37593.

Tcherepanov, A. A., Sokolov, B. P. (1997). Age-related abnormalities in expression of mRNAs encoding synapsin 1A, synapsin 1B, and synaptophysin in the temporal cortex of schizophrenics. *J Neurosci Res* **49**: 639–644.

Thoenen, H. (1995) Neurotrophins and neuronal plasticity. *Science* **270**: 593–598.

Thome, J., Durany, N., Harsanyi, A., *et al.* (1996). A null mutation allele in the CNTF gene and schizophrenic psychoses. *Neuroreport* **7**: 1413–1416.

Thome, J., Durany, N., Palomo, A., *et al.* (1997a). Variants in neurotrophic factor genes and schizophrenic psychoses: no associations in a Spanish population. *Psychiatry Res* **71**: 1–5.

Thome, J., Jonsson, E., Foley, P., *et al.* (1997b). Ciliary neurotrophic factor null mutation and schizophrenia in a Swedish population. *Psychiatr Genet* **7**: 79–82.

Thompson, P. M., Sower, A. C., Perrone-Bizzozero, N. I. (1998). Altered levels of the synaptosomal associated protein SNAP-25 in schizophrenia. *Biol Psychiatry* **43**: 239–243.

Thompson, P. M., Rosenberger, C., Qualls, C. (1999). CSF SNAP-25 in schizophrenia and bipolar illness. A pilot study. *Neuropsychopharmacology* **21**: 717–722.

Treloar, H., Tomasiewicz, H., Magnuson, T., Key, B. (1997). The central pathway of primary olfactory axons is abnormal in mice lacking the N-CAM-180 isoform. *J Neurobiol* **32**: 643–658.

Tsai, M. T., Hung, C. C., Tsai, C. Y., *et al.* (2002). Mutation analysis of synapsin III gene in schizophrenia. *Am J Med Genet* **114**: 79–83.

Turner, E. E., Fedtsova, N., Jeste, D. V. (1997). Cellular and molecular neuropathology of schizophrenia: new directions from developmental neurobiology. *Schizophr Res* **27**: 169–180.

Ujike, H., Takehisa, Y., Takaki, M., *et al.* (2001). *NOTCH4* gene polymorphism and susceptibility to schizophrenia and schizoaffective disorder. *Neurosci Lett* **301**: 41–44.

Usui, T., Shima, Y., Shimada, Y., *et al.* (1999). Flamingo, a seven-pass transmembrane cadherin, regulates planar cell polarity under the control of Frizzled. *Cell* **98**: 585–595.

van Kammen, D. P., Poltorak, M., Kelley, M. E., *et al.* (1998). Further studies of elevated cerebrospinal fluid neuronal cell adhesion molecule in schizophrenia. *Biol Psychiatry* **43**: 680–686.

Vicente, A. M., Macciardi, F., Verga, M., *et al.* (1997). NCAM and schizophrenia: genetic studies. *Mol Psychiatry* **2**: 65–69.

Virgos, C., Martorell, L., Valero, J., *et al.* (2001). Association study of schizophrenia with polymorphisms at six candidate genes. *Schizophr Res* **49**: 65–71.

Wassarman, K. M., Lewandoski, M., Campbell, K., *et al.* (1997). Specification of the anterior hindbrain and establishment of a normal mid/hindbrain organizer is dependent on Gbx2 gene function. *Dev Suppl* **124**: 2923–2934.

Wassink, T. H., Nelson J. J., Crowe, R. R., Andreasen, N. C. (1999). Heritability of BDNF alleles and their effect on brain morphology in schizophrenia. *Am J Med Genet* **88**: 724–728.

Wei, J., Hemmings, G. P. (2000). The *NOTCH4* locus is associated with susceptibility to schizophrenia. *Nat Genet* **25**: 376–377.

Wong, A., Macciardi, F., Klempan, T., *et al.* (2003). Identification of candidate genes for psychosis in rat models, and possible association between schizophrenia and the *14-3-3η* gene. *Mol Psychiatry* **8**: 156–166.

Wood, G. K., Tomasiewicz, H., Rutishauser, U., *et al.* (1998). NCAM-180 knockout mice display increased lateral ventricle size and reduced prepulse inhibition of startle. *Neuroreport* **9**: 461–466.

Wu, Q., Maniatis, T. (1999). A striking organization of a large family of human neural cadherin-like cell adhesion genes. *Cell* **97**: 779–790.

Yagi, T., Takeichi, M. (2000). Cadherin superfamily genes: functions, genomic organization, and neurologic diversity. *Genes Dev* **14**: 1169–1180.

Young, C. E., Arima, K., Xie, J., *et al.* (1998). SNAP-25 deficit and hippocampal connectivity in schizophrenia. *Cereb Cortex* **8**: 261–268.

2

Brain development in healthy children and adolescents: magnetic resonance imaging studies

Jay N. Giedd, Michael A. Rosenthal, A. Blythe Rose, Jonathan D. Blumenthal, Elizabeth Molloy, Richard R. Dopp, Liv S. Clasen, Daniel J. Fridberg, and Nitin Gogtay

Child Psychiatry Branch, National Institute of Mental Health, Bethesda, USA

Any parent of a teenager can tell you that the brain of a 13 year old is different than the brain of an 8 year old; yet, actually pinning down the neuroanatomical substrates of those differences has proved elusive. Nature has gone through a great deal of trouble to protect the brain. It is wrapped in a tough leathery membrane, surrounded by a protective moat of fluid, and completely encased in bone. This has shielded the brain from falls or attacks from predators, but it has also shielded the brain from scientists.

Magnetic resonance imaging (MRI) has changed that. It allows for the acquisition of exquisitely accurate pictures of the living growing human brain and it does so without the use of ionizing radiation. This has opened the door not only for scanning healthy children but also for acquiring repeated scans throughout development.

Using MRI, the team at the Child Psychiatry Branch of the National Institute of Mental Health has been collecting brain MRI scans on healthy children and adolescents since 1989. As of 2003, we have acquired over 300 scans from 150 healthy subjects. The data presented in this chapter will be largely drawn from this cohort unless otherwise stated.

Total brain size

The relationship between brain size and function is complex. Evidence for the relative unimportance of brain size within a broad range of extremes is demonstrated by observations that (a) healthy children with similar intelligence quotients (IQs)

Neurodevelopment and Schizophrenia, ed. Matcheri S. Keshavan *et al.* Published by Cambridge University Press. © Cambridge University Press 2004.

can have a 50% difference in brain volume, (b) there are robust differences in brain sizes between males and females with similar functional capacity, and (c) there is a paucity of established correlations between the size of any given brain structure and a specific cognitive ability. However, from a computational science perspective it seems likely that the number of neuronal connections in a structure reflects its information processing capacity.

Also, modest positive correlation between IQ and total cerebral volume and a possible relationship between hippocampal size and memory recall have been reported. The intricacy of various neurochemical systems and the diversity of afferent and efferent connections to the many distinct nuclei of most brain structures make straightforward relationships between volumes of a single structure and performance on a particular cognitive task uncommon. This supports the concept of *distributed neural systems*, whereby functional attributes are not thought to lie so much within a single structure as within a network of structures. Across species there is a strong correlation between body size and brain size (Jerison, 1991), and animals with large brains such as elephants and dolphins demonstrate greater behavioral complexity.

Total brain volume is approximately 90% of its adult size by age six years. Data of total brain size, as is the case for data of the subcomponents of the brain, is characterized by a high degree of variability (Fig. 2.1). This large variability necessitates large sample sizes to detect group differences (Lange *et al.*, 1997).

MRI is adept at discerning gray matter, white matter, and fluid on brain images. These boundaries are used to define the size and shape of a variety of brain structures or regions.

White matter

White matter consists of myelinated axons (Fig. 2.2). The amount of white matter in the brain increases throughout childhood and adolescence. Myelination greatly speeds up transmission between neurons, up to 100 times the speed in unmyelinated fibers. The greater speed of neuronal processing may facilitate cognitive complexity. The myelinated axons comprising white matter can be projectional, connecting the brain to the brainstem or spinal cord; associational, connecting one type of brain part to another; or commissural, connecting like parts of the brain in the left and right hemispheres. Diffusion tensor imaging, a structural brain imaging technique, may help to discern these different types of white matter connection although our group has not yet acquired diffusion tensor imaging scans on pediatric populations (see Ch. 3 for a discussion of this approach).

The most conspicuous white matter component of the brain is the corpus callosum (CC). It is the main connection between the left and right hemispheres and

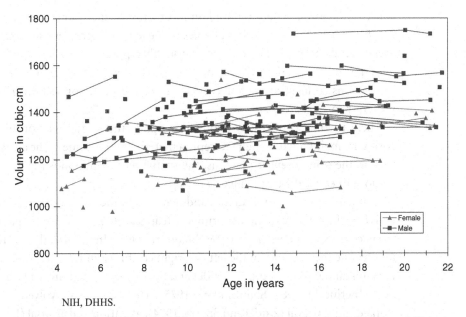

NIH, DHHS.

Fig. 2.1.   Total cerebral volume for 145 children and adolescents (ages 4–22) based on 243 brain magnetic resonance imaging scans. (Jay N. Giedd, Child Psychiatry Branch, NIMH, NIH, DHHS.)

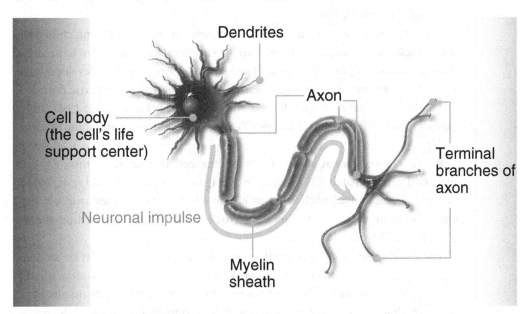

Fig. 2.2.   The neuron. (Donald Bliss, NIH Medical Arts and Photography Branch for Jay N. Giedd, Child Psychiatry Branch, NIMH, NIH, DHHS.)
For a colour version of this figure, see www.cambridge.org/9780521126595.

consists of approximately 180 million mostly myelinated axons (Tomasch, 1954). The fibers usually connect similar areas in the left and right hemispheres. Because they generally take the shortest route, a roughly topographic pattern is maintained, with the anterior sections consisting of fibers connecting frontal brain areas, middle sections connecting middle cortical areas, and posterior sections connecting posterior cortical areas.

There is some controversy about how tightly the spatial relationships of the cortex are maintained in their CC representation, but for some of the areas studied, such as the somatosensory regions, the spatial representation is highly preserved (Innocenti *et al.*, 1974; Spidalieri *et al.*, 1985).

Although absent in monotrenes and marsupials, the CC is present in most animals from insectivores to higher primates. It appears to have evolved in parallel with the neocortex (Kappers *et al.*, 1936; Rapoport, 1990). In general, the CC functions to integrate the activities of the left and right cerebral hemispheres, such as organizing bimanual motor output (Zaidel and Sperry, 1977) and unifying the sensory fields (Berlucchi, 1981; Shanks *et al.*, 1975). The CC is also involved in memory storage and retrieval (Zaidel and Sperry, 1974), attention and arousal (Levy, 1985), language and auditory functions (Cook, 1986), and possibly in the perception of consciousness (Joseph, 1980). Creativity and intelligence are linked to interhemispheric integration (Bogen and Bogen, 1969) and the more difficult the cognitive task the more critical interhemispheric integration becomes (Hellige *et al.*, 1979; Levy and Trevarthen, 1981).

These functions subserved by the CC continue to improve during childhood and adolescence, highlighting interest in the structural changes shown to progress during that developmental period (Giedd *et al.*, 1996). Further developmental interest stems from CC anomalies reported for several neuropsychiatric disorders of childhood (Bigelow *et al.*, 1983; Giedd *et al.*, 1994; Hynd *et al.*, 1990, 1991; Njiokiktjien, 1991; Parashos *et al.*, 1995; Peterson *et al.*, 1994; Rosenthal and Bigelow, 1972).

In our cross-sectional study of 114 healthy pediatric subjects, total CC size increased approximately 2% per year on average for the group (Giedd *et al.*, 1996). However, when individual children are followed longitudinally, the changes in specific subcomponents of the CC are shown to be occurring much more dramatically (Thompson, 2000).

The CC changes occur in a front-to-back direction, with the anterior sections reaching adult sizes sooner than the posterior sections. This was somewhat surprising because, in general, frontal regions of the brain are thought to mature later. Another white matter area that has particularly strong age effects is the left arcuate fasciculus. This tract connects Wernicke's area, involved in the reception of speech, with Broca's area, involved in the production of speech (Paus *et al.*, 1999).

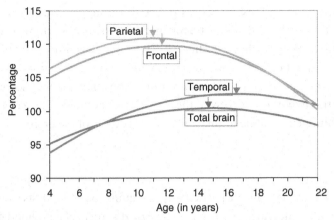

Fig. 2.3.   Standardized regional brain development for 145 children and adolescents (ages 4–22) based on 243 brain magnetic resonance imaging scans. (Jay N. Giedd, Child Psychiatry Branch, NIMH, NIH, DHHS.)

Gray matter

Gray matter consists largely of cell bodies and is home to the nucleus and the dendrites, the antennae-like connections that receive input from other cells (Fig. 2.2). Gray matter comprises the cortex (Latin for "bark"), the outermost layer of the brain, and certain subcortical structures such as the basal ganglia and the thalamus.

Initial cross-sectional studies showed a general decrease in the amount of cortical gray matter during childhood, beginning at the earliest ages of the study design, which was often around age 5 years (Jernigan *et al.*, 1991; Pfefferbaum *et al.*, 1994; Sowell *et al.*, 2002; Steen *et al.*, 1997). However, when scans were acquired in the same individuals at approximately two year intervals, cortical gray matter was shown to follow an inverted U-type pattern (Fig. 2.3). In the frontal lobes, involved in planning, organizing, strategizing, and other "executive" functions, the cortical gray matter reaches its maximal thickness at 11.0 years in girls and 12.1 years in boys (Giedd *et al.*, 1997, 1999). Temporal lobe cortical gray matter peaks at 16.7 years in girls and 16.2 years in boys. Parietal lobe cortical gray matter peaks at 10.2 years in girls and 11.8 years in boys.

The thickening and thinning of gray matter is thought to reflect changes in the size and complexity of neurons, not a change in the actual number. The increasing size may reflect a process called arborization, as the cells grow extra branches, twigs, and roots, thus growing "bushier" and making a greater number of connections to other cells. The decreasing amount of gray matter may reflect the process of pruning where certain connections are eliminated.

The forces guiding these processes of arborization and pruning are not well understood. Genetics, nutrition, toxins, bacteria, viruses, hormones, and many other factors have been shown to have an effect. One hypothesis for the pruning phase is the "use it or lose it" principle, in which those connections that are used well survive and flourish whereas those connections that are not used will wither and die. If this hypothesis is correct, the activities of the child or teenager may have a powerful influence on the ultimate physical structure of the brain.

Sex differences

Sex differences in the brain are particularly intriguing to psychiatrists studying children and adolescents since nearly all psychiatric disorders of childhood onset have different ages of onset, prevalence, and symptomatology between boys and girls. Whether environmental or other genetic factors interact with normal differences between boy and girl brains to account for some of these clinical differences is a topic of active research (see Ch. 18 for a review of this topic).

In an analysis of 71 male and 50 female healthy subjects between the ages of 4 and 18 years, males had a 9% larger cerebral volume. This difference was consistent across the entire age range of 4 to 18 years and is similar to that found in adult postmortem brain (Dekaban and Sadowsky, 1978; Ho *et al.*, 1980) and in vivo imaging studies (Flaum *et al.*, 1995).

Given the myriad of factors that determine brain structure size, and findings of enlarged brains in patient groups such as those with fragile X syndrome (Reiss *et al.*, 1994) and autism (Piven *et al.*, 1995), size difference should not be interpreted as imparting any sort of functional advantage or disadvantage. The fact that gross structural size may be insensitive to sexual differences in receptor density or connectivity between different neurons further emphasizes the complexity of interpreting the implications of size differences in brain structures.

Other structures examined in that study included the lateral ventricles, caudate, putamen, globus pallidus temporal lobe, amygdala, and hippocampus. Of these structures, when adjusted for total cerebral volume difference by analysis of covariance, only the basal ganglia demonstrated sex differences in mean volume, with the caudate being relatively larger in females and the globus pallidus being relatively larger in males.

The sexual dimorphism of the basal ganglia is interesting in light of the frequent implication of basal ganglia involvement in neuropsychiatric disorders such as attention-deficit hyperactivity disorder (Castellanos *et al.*, 1994; Hynd *et al.*, 1991) and Tourette's syndrome (Hyde *et al.*, 1995; Peterson *et al.*, 1993; Singer, 1993), which have a higher incidence in males. Obsessive–compulsive disorder, which has an approximately equal incidence for males and females in late adolescence and adulthood, may be more common in boys in early childhood (Swedo *et al.*, 1989). Also, a developmental subtype of this disorder, which demonstrates a more treatment-refractory course and neurological/basal ganglia abnormalities, is more common in young boys (Blanes and McGuire, 1997).

Amygdala and hippocampal volume increased for both sexes, but with the amygdala increasing significantly more in males than females and hippocampal volume increasing more in females. The amygdala and hippocampus findings are consistent with the preponderance of androgen receptors in the amygdala (Clark *et al.*, 1988) and of estrogen receptors in the hippocampus of rhesus monkeys (Sholl and Kim, 1989). Further evidence of a relationship between estrogen and hippocampal volume in rodents is the decreased fiber outgrowth and altered density of dendritic spines in the hippocampus of gonadectomized adult females, which is reversed with hormone replacement (Gould *et al.*, 1990; Morse *et al.*, 1986). Similarly, in humans, women with gonadal hypoplasia have been found to have smaller hippocampi than controls (Murphy *et al.*, 1993).

Conclusions

MRI has allowed for the safe acquisition of brain scans in healthy children and has helped to launch a new era of pediatric neuroscience. Characterization of normal brain development is imperative to assess the hypothesis that many of the most severe neuropsychiatric disorders of childhood onset are manifestations of deviations from that normative path. White matter volumes tend to increase in a roughly linear fashion from ages 4 to 18 years and slopes do not differ significantly by lobe of the brain. Gray matter volumes, by comparison, tend to follow an inverted U-shaped developmental curve and differ by lobe. Sexual dimorphism in healthy brain development may lead to differential vulnerability, which would account for some of the clinical differences in childhood neuropsychiatric disorders.

REFERENCES

Berlucchi, G. (1981). Interhemispheric asymmetries in visual discrimination: a neurophysiological hypothesis. *Doc Opthal Proc Ser* **30**: 87–93.

Bigelow, L. H., Nasrallah, H. A., Rauscher, F. P. (1983). Corpus callosum thickness in chronic schizophrenia. *Br J Psychiatry* **142**: 284–287.

Blanes, T., McGuire, P. (1997). Heterogeneity within obsessive compulsive disorder: evidence for primary and neurodevelopmental subtypes. In *Neurodevelopment and Adult Psychopathology*, ed. M. S. Keshavan, R. Murray. Cambridge, UK: Cambridge University Press, pp. 206–216.

Bogen, J. E., Bogen, G. M. (1969). The other side of the brain. 3, The corpus callosum and creativity. *Bull Los Ang Neurol Soc* **34**: 191–220.

Castellanos, F. X., Giedd, J. N., Eckburg, P., *et al.* (1994). Quantitative morphology of the caudate nucleus in attention deficit hyperactivity disorder. *Am J Psychiatry* **151**: 1791–1796.

Clark, A. S., MacLusky, N. J., Goldman-Rakic, P. S. (1988). Androgen binding and metabolism in the cerebral cortex of the developing rhesus monkey. *Endocrinology* **123**: 932–940.

Cook, N. D. (1986). *The Brain Code: Mechanisms of Information Transfer and the Role of the Corpus Callosum.* London: Methuen.

Dekaban, A. S., Sadowsky, D. (1978). Changes in brain weight during the span of human life: relation of brain weights to body heights and body weights. *Ann Neur* **4**: 345–356.

Flaum, M., Swayze, V. W., O'Leary, D. S., *et al.* (1995). Brain morphology in schizophrenia: effects of diagnosis, laterality and gender. *Am J Psychiatry* **152**: 704–714.

Giedd, J. N., Castellanos, F. X., Casey, B. J., *et al.* (1994). Quantitative morphology of the corpus callosum in attention deficit hyperactivity disorder. [See comments] *Am J Psychiatry* **151**: 665–669.

Giedd, J. N., Rumsey, J. M., Castellanos, F. X., *et al.* (1996). A quantitative MRI study of the corpus callosum in children and adolescents. *Brain Res Dev Brain Res* **91**: 274–280.

Giedd, J. N., Castellanos, F. X., Rajapakse, J. C., Vaituzis, A. C., Rapoport, J. L. (1997). Sexual dimorphism of the developing human brain. *Prog Neuropsychopharmacol Biol Psychiatry* **21**: 1185–1201.

Giedd, J. N., Blumenthal, J., Jeffries, N. O., *et al.* (1999). Brain development during childhood and adolescence: a longitudinal MRI study. *Nat Neurosci* **2**: 861–863.

Gould, E., Allan, M. D., McEwen, B. S. (1990). Dendritic spine density of adult hippocampal pyramidal cells is sensitive to thyroid hormone. *Brain Res* **525**: 327–329.

Hellige, J. B., Cox, J. P., Litvac, L. (1979). Information processing in the hemispheres: selective hemisphere activation and capacity limitations. *J Exp Psychol Gen* **108**: 251–259.

Ho, K. C., Roessmann, U., Straumfjord, J. V., Monroe, G. (1980). Analysis of brain weight. I. Adult brain weight in relation to sex, age, and race. *Arch Pathol Lab Med* **104**: 635–639.

Hyde, T. M., Stacey, M. E., Coppola, R., *et al.* (1995). Cerebral morphometric abnormalities in Tourette's syndrome: a quantitative MRI study of monozygotic twins. *Neurology* **45**: 1176–1182.

Hynd, G. W., Semrud-Clikeman, M., Lorys, A. R., Novey, E. S., Eliopulos, D. (1990). Brain morphology in developmental dyslexia and attention deficit disorder/hyperactivity. *Arch Neurol* **47**: 919–926.

   (1991). Corpus callosum morphology in attention deficit–hyperactivity disorder: morphometric analysis of MRI. *J Learn Disabil* **24**: 141–146.

Innocenti, G. M., Manzoni, T., Spidalieri, G. (1974). Patterns of somesthetic messages transferred through the corpus callosum. *Exp Brain Res* **19**: 447–466.

Jerison, H. J. (1991). *Brain Size and the Evolution of Mind.* New York: American Museum of Natural History.

Jernigan, T. L., Trauner, D. A., Hesselink, J. R., Tallal, P. A. (1991). Maturation of human cerebrum observed in vivo during adolescence. *Brain* **114**: 2037–2049.

Joseph, R. (1980). Awareness, the origin of thought, and the role of conscious self-deception in resistance and repression. *Psychol Rep* **46**: 767–781.

Kappers, C. U. A., Huber, G. C., Crosby, C. C. (1936). *The Comparative Anatomy of the Nervous System of Vertebrates including Man*, Vol. 2. New York: MacMillan.

Lange, N., Giedd, J. N., Castellanos, F. X., Vaituzis, A. C., Rapoport, J. L. (1997). Variability of human brain structure size: ages 4 to 20. *Psychiatry Res Neuroimaging* **74**: 1–12.

Levy, J. (1985). Interhemispheric collaboration: single mindedness in the asymmetric brain. In *Hemisphere Function and Collaboration in the Child*, ed. C. T. Best. New York: Academic Press, pp. 11–32.

Levy, J., Trevarthen, C. (1981). Color-matching, color naming and color memory in split brain patients. *Neuropsychology* **19**: 523–541.

Morse, J. K., Scheff, S. W., DeKosky, S. T. (1986). Gonadal steroids influence axonal sprouting in the hippocampal dentate gyrus: a sexually dimorphic response. *Exp Neur* **94**: 649–658.

Murphy, D. G. M., DeCarli, C. D., Daly, E., *et al.* (1993). Effects of the X chromosome on female brain: a study of turner syndrome using quantitative magnetic resonance imaging. *Lancet* **342**: 1197–1200.

Njiokiktjien, C. (1991). *Pediatric Behavioral Neurology*, Vol. 3 *The Child's Corpus Callosum*. Amsterdam: Suyi Publications.

Parashos, I. A., Wilkinson, W. E., Coffey, C. E. (1995). Magnetic resonance imaging of the corpus callosum: predictors of size in normal adults. *J Neuropsychiatry Clin Neurosci* **7**: 35–41.

Paus, T., Zijdenbos, A., Worsley, K., *et al.* (1999). Structural maturation of neural pathways in children and adolescents: in vivo study. *Science* **283**: 1908–1911.

Peterson, B., Riddle, M. A., Cohen, D. J., *et al.* (1993). Reduced basal ganglia volumes in Tourette's syndrome using three-dimensional reconstruction techniques from magnetic resonance images. *Neurology* **43**: 941–949.

Peterson, B. S., Leckman, J. F., Duncan, J. S., Wetzles, R., Riddle, M. A. (1994). Corpus callosum morphology from magnetic resonance images in Tourette's syndrome. *Psychiatry Res Neuroimaging* **55**: 85–99.

Pfefferbaum, A., Mathalon, D. H., Sullivan, *et al.* (1994). A quantitative magnetic resonance imaging study of changes in brain morphology from infancy to late adulthood. *Arch Neurol* **51**: 874–887.

Piven, J., Arndt, S., Bailey, J., *et al.* (1995). An MRI study of brain size in autism. *Am J Psychiatry* **152**: 1145–1149.

Rapoport, S. I. (1990). Integrated phylogeny of the primate brain, with special reference to humans and their diseases. *Brain Res Rev* **15**: 267–294.

Reiss, A. L., Lee, J., Freund, L. (1994). Neuroanatomy of fragile X syndrome: the temporal lobe. *Neurology* **44**: 1317–1324.

Rosenthal, R. Bigelow, L. (1972). Quantitative brain measurements in chronic schizophrenia. *Br J Psychiatry* **121**: 259–264.

Shanks, M. F., Rockel, A. J., Powel, T. P. S. (1975). The commissural fiber connections of the primary somatic sensory cortex. *Brain Res* **98**: 166–171.

Sholl, S. A., Kim, K. L. (1989). Estrogen receptors in the rhesus monkey brain during fetal development. *Dev Brain Res* **50**: 189–196.

Singer, H., Reiss, A. L., Brown, J. E., *et al.* (1993). Volumetric MRI changes in basal ganglia of children with Tourette's syndrome. *Neurology* **43**: 950–956.

Sowell, E., Trauner, D. A., Gamst, A., Jernigan, T. L. (2002). Development of cortical and subcortical brain structures in childhood and adolescence: a structural MRI study. *Dev Med Child Neurol* **44**: 4–16.

Spidalieri, G., Franchi, G., Guandalini, P. (1985). Somatic receptive-field properties of single fibers in the rostral portion of the corpus callosum in awake cats. *Exp Brain Res* **58**: 75–81.

Steen, R. G., Ogg, R. J., Reddick, W. E., Kingsley, P. B. (1997). Age-related changes in the pediatric brain: quantitative MR evidence of maturational changes during adolescence. *Am J Neuroradiol* **18**: 819–828.

Swedo, S. E., Rapoport, J. L., Leonard, H., Lenane, M., Cheslow, D. (1989). Obsessive–compulsive disorder in children and adolescents. Clinical phenomenology of 70 consecutive cases. *Arch Gen Psychiatry* **46**: 335–341.

Thompson, P., Giedd, J. N., Blanton, R. E., *et al.* (2000). Growth patterns in the developing brain detected by using continuum mechanical tensor maps. *Nature* **404**: 190–192.

Tomasch, J. (1954). Size, distribution and number of fibers in the human corpus callosum. *Anat Rec* **119**: 119–135.

Zaidel, D., Sperry, R. W. (1974). Memory impairment after commissurotomy in man. *Brain* **97**: 263–272.

(1977). Some long-term effects of cerebral commissurotomy in man. *Neuropsychology* **15**: 193–204.

3

Cognitive development: functional magnetic resonance imaging studies

Beatriz Luna[1] and John A. Sweeney[2]

[1] Western Psychiatric Institute and Clinic, Pittsburgh, USA
[2] The Psychiatric Institute, University of Illinois, Chicago, USA

Given the developmental etiology of schizophrenia and its neurobiological profile, neurodevelopmental models promise to provide important insights into the causes of this debilitating disorder (Hyde *et al.*, 1992; Keshavan *et al.*, 1994; Waddington *et al.*, 1991; Weinberger and Lipska, 1995). The onset of schizophrenia typically presents in late adolescence or early adulthood and is marked by psychotic symptoms and cognitive impairments that are believed to have a neurodevelopmental basis (Ch. 4). Although progress has been made in characterizing structural brain impairments that may underlie these behavioral deficits, little is known about how these may play out through development and how they may affect brain function. Brain abnormalities may result in different adaptive mechanisms, especially given developmental plasticity, that could affect brain function in a manner not evident by information of the location of the structural impairment. Regions that are connected to, but distant from, the location of injury could demonstrate impaired function although the distant structure itself might not be intrinsically impaired. Pediatric neuroimaging techniques can probe the integrity of brain function and normal brain maturational processes and provide a window into possible abnormalities in neurocognitive development (Luna and Sweeney, 2001). First, however, we must characterize the development of brain function in a healthy population, especially during adolescence, in order to identify the processes that are vulnerable to impairment in schizophrenia. This is a relatively new field and work has only begun towards the understanding of developmental changes in brain function. In this chapter, we will describe the initial investigations and discuss what has been found regarding the changes in brain function that support the healthy maturation of cognitive control of behavior.

Neurodevelopment and Schizophrenia, ed. Matcheri S. Keshavan *et al.* Published by Cambridge University Press. © Cambridge University Press 2004.

Brain and cognitive maturation

Basic cognitive processes, which are evident in infancy and show dramatic changes throughout childhood (Diamond and Goldman-Rakic, 1989), continue to develop throughout adolescence. This period of late childhood and adolescent development is characterized by improvement in the capacity for abstract thought, planning, and cognitive flexibility (Levin *et al.*, 1991; Luciana and Nelson, 1998; Welsh *et al.*, 1991). As adult levels of basic cognitive processes are reached, we see improvements in executive processes, such as working memory and voluntary response suppression, that support goal-directed behavior.

Cognitive development occurs concurrently with significant changes in brain maturation. The degree of cortical folding (Armstrong *et al.*, 1995), overall size, and regional functional specialization of the brain is, for the most part, in adult form by early childhood (Caviness *et al.*, 1996). However, significant refinements of brain systems, including synaptic pruning, elaboration of dendritic arborization (Changeux and Danchin, 1976; Huttenlocher, 1990), and increased myelination (Jernigan *et al.*, 1991; Pfefferbaum *et al.*, 1994; Yakovlev and Lecours, 1967), continue into adolescence. Of special relevance to the maturation of executive abilities is the continued elimination of synapses in the prefrontal cortex (layer III of the middle frontal gyrus) throughout adolescence (Huttenlocher, 1990). The emergence of higher-order cognitive control of behavior is believed to be subserved by the integration of prefrontal cortex with other brain regions in widely distributed circuits (Chugani, 1998; Fuster, 1997; Goldman-Rakic, 1990; Thatcher, 1991). Huttenlocher's (1990) findings, indicating a late stabilization of synaptic pruning in prefrontal relative to visual cortex, have led to a traditional view that brain maturation occurs last in frontal cortex. In contrast, histological studies and recent magnetic resonance imaging (MRI) studies indicate that, similar to the non-human primate, the human cortex develops in a concurrent fashion (Giedd *et al.*, 1999; Rakic *et al.*, 1986; Yakovlev and Lecours, 1967). The effectiveness of prefrontal control of behavior however, may continue to develop as other regions become more specialized and myelination allows for the integration of function throughout the brain.

In order to understand how cognitive development is supported by brain maturation, it is crucial to investigate brain function. Changes in the microstructure of the brain during childhood, and especially adolescence, though highly significant from a functional perspective, are not readily observable in vivo with conventional anatomic neuroimaging techniques (Ch. 2). Cognitive capabilities, however, improve at a relatively dramatic pace, indicating that robust changes in brain microstructure and organization must also be occurring. Investigating brain *function* allows us to assess how brain processes develop relative to their structural capacity. Brain weight is more than 90% of the adult level by school age (Caviness *et al.*, 1996); however, myelination and synaptic pruning continue throughout this period without dramatic consequences on gross brain anatomy. Investigating brain function allows us to see the effects of these structurally subtle, but significant, processes. The elimination of redundant synaptic connections supports quicker and more efficient regional neuronal processes, allowing for more focused brain function with the increased capacity for more complicated neuronal operations. Myelination speeds up neuronal transmission and allows distant brain regions to participate more effectively in widely distributed circuitry, which, allows for top-down, prefrontal executive control of behavior.

It has only recently become feasible to use neuroimaging procedures in healthy pediatric populations. The available neuroimaging methods, such as positron emission tomography (PET) and single photon emission tomography, depend upon ionizing radiation. Consequently, these two lines of investigation, cognitive development and brain maturation, had remained separate with limited efforts at reconciling or integrating them. With the advent of functional MRI (fMRI), which allows non-invasive in vivo investigation of brain processes that underlie cognitive function, we can now study the link between these psychological and neurobiological phenomena. This technique has been used to investigate how the functional organization of brain regions contributing to cognitive abilities changes with development to support the emergence of adult-level cognition. Initial studies have provided crucial information for delineating the brain circuitry underlying healthy cognitive development.

Electroencephalography and PET were initially used to characterize developmental changes in brain function. Thatcher (1991) measured electroencephalography coherence among neocortical regions and reported an increase in coherence activity throughout adolescence, especially between frontal and other cortical areas. PET results support these findings by indicating that local cerebral resting metabolic rates decrease in frontal, parietal, and temporal regions throughout childhood and only reach adult levels in adolescence (Chugani, 1998). These are significant findings indicating a late integration of frontal regions to widely distributed brain function; however, there are limitations to these methods and findings. The electroencephalography studies lack sufficient spatial resolution to localize adequately developmental changes in specific brain regions. Because PET is invasive, it has rarely been used to study healthy pediatric populations.

Functional magnetic resonance imaging

Brain function can be imaged in vivo during cognitive activity using fMRI. Because it is non-invasive, this method permits the characterization of changes in brain activity that occur during development in pediatric populations. The minimal

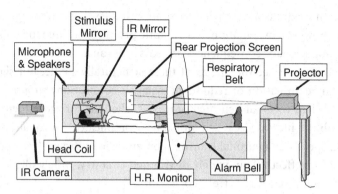

Fig. 3.1.   Schematic of the MR environment. IR, infrared; H.R., heart rate.

health risk from repeated MRI studies also permits longitudinal fMRI studies of developmental changes in brain–behavior systems. This is especially important as it provides a basis for actually following developmental trajectories in individual subjects, rather than utilizing only cross-sectional studies to investigate developmental trends. Since development often proceeds in bursts rather than in a smooth, gradual way (Thatcher, 1991), longitudinal studies provide a better way to characterize patterns of development. For these reasons, fMRI is a valuable tool for bridging cognitive and biological studies of brain development.

The principle of fMRI is that neuronal activation associated with cognitive activity results in an increased metabolic demand; that metabolic demand, in turn, brings increased blood flow to the active region. The increase in blood flow produces a change in the ratio of oxygenated to deoxygenated blood, which changes the magnetic properties of blood in a way that can be detected. Using sophisticated image reconstruction and analysis procedures, these changes in regional magnetic properties can be used to provide a detailed picture of brain regions involved in performing a particular cognitive act. The psychological tasks subjects perform in the MRI scanner need to be carefully selected to probe specific cognitive processes of interest. A diagram of the MRI environment is presented in Fig. 3.1.

There are two primary fMRI methods used for identifying brain regions underlying specific cognitive processes: *block design* and *event-related* procedures. The block design is a boxcar method used to identify the group of regions participating in a cognitive process. Blocks of experimental trials are contrasted with alternating blocks of baseline brain function; analyses identify the voxels where signal fluctuates in accordance with changing block trial types. Baseline trials can vary from eyes closed or fixation to trials identical to experimental trials except for the variable of interest. The boxcar design provides the best characterization of specific brain regions. The advantage of this method is that it is relatively easy to implement and analyze, and it generates a relatively high signal-to-noise ratio, resulting in robust brain activation. The limitation to this method is that one cannot disassociate the different cognitive processes occurring in each experimental trial since these are averaged across blocks, limiting the ability to investigate the relative contributions of each of the brain regions in a circuit. Event-related designs are used to answer this concern by acquiring brain images time-locked to the occurrence of each cognitive event in a trial. In this manner, different brain regions can be associated with specific cognitive steps in a task and regions that are primary to each cognitive process can be identified. This method, however, typically has a significantly reduced signal-to-noise ratio compared with block design studies, generating modest areas of brain activation. Because of the limitations of each method, investigators will often use both designs. A block design is used to identify all the brain regions in a circuit; event-related designs are then used to disentangle the specific contributions of each region to a cognitive process of interest.

Studies using fMRI to characterize brain function in healthy adults are relatively straightforward. However, pediatric studies necessitate the comparison of brain activation between different age groups, which requires additional methodological considerations and statistical analyses. Initial studies reported differences in brain activation determined from visual inspection between a group of children and separate, but similar, adult studies (Casey *et al.*, 1995; Hertz-Pannier *et al.*, 1997). Presently, pediatric studies study children and adult comparison groups in the same study. Testing subjects ranging in age from childhood to adulthood provides the greatest power, as regression analyses can identify brain regions that change with age.

Changes in brain function supporting cognitive development

Two higher-order cognitive abilities crucial to the voluntary control of behavior are working memory (Case, 1992; Fry and Hale, 1996) and voluntary suppression of context-inappropriate responses (Bjorklund and Harnishfeger, 1990; Case, 1992; Ridderinkhof and van der Molen, 1997; Wilson and Kipp, 1998). These processes require brain circuitry that supports online calculations for the appropriate behavioral responses to ongoing environmental demands. It is these cognitive processes that have a protracted developmental sequence into adolescence and are impaired in schizophrenia (Cohen *et al.*, 1999; Merriam *et al.*, 1999; Park and Holzman, 1992; Weinberger *et al.*, 1986).

Working memory

Working memory is the ability to maintain and manipulate information online in order to guide goal-directed behavior (Baddeley, 1983). This circuitry has been well delineated in the single-cell literature and is known to be subserved by a widely distributed circuitry in which prefrontal regions play a primary role (Fuster, 1997; Goldman-Rakic, 1992). Delay-dependent cells found in prefrontal cortex have the unique feature of responding exclusively to the maintenance of information, as distinct from sensory and motor responses. Brain regions with neurons having this property and that are part of a circuitry that supports these processes are critical for working memory.

Several pediatric studies have compared brain activation between children and adults during performance of spatial and non-spatial working memory tasks. Working memory studies require that subjects retain a spatial location or a sequence of non-spatial stimuli in memory and use this information to guide a future response. These studies have either found similar brain function in children and adults or increased activation in children relative to adults. In one spatial working memory task, six children aged 6–11 years and six adults were asked to recall the location of a visual stimulus that occurred in previous trials (Thomas *et al.*, 1999). Despite differences in performance, children demonstrated similar patterns of activation as that in adults in their prefrontal and parietal regions. They did not, however, show bilateral activation of cingulate cortex, temporal regions, and premotor regions, which are known to underlie response preparation and were recruited by adults. In another study, nine children aged 8–11 years performed a spatial working memory task where they had to press a button corresponding to the location of a previous prompt (Nelson *et al.*, 2000). The children activated the same brain regions as adults, including dorsal prefrontal, anterior cingulate, and posterior parietal cortices. These results suggest that the brain circuitry underlying working memory is mainly in place by 8–11 years of age; however, differences in the relative contribution of different regions of this circuitry may change with age. In a non-spatial working memory n-back task, six children aged 9–11 years were required to press a button when a letter was repeated with one intervening non-match letter (Casey *et al.*, 1995). Brain activation during these test trials were compared with blocks of trials where subjects pressed a button whenever the letter "X" appeared. Coronal slices focused on prefrontal regions. Results indicated a greater magnitude of activation in prefrontal cortex in children than adults. These results suggest that, while the correct circuitry is accessed by children when they maintain information in working memory, children rely on a greater contribution of prefrontal cortex than do adults. Increased activation of prefrontal cortex could indicate either an immature specialization of the underlying neuronal processes, such as synaptic pruning, or a higher reliance on prefrontal cortex during a task that is harder for children to perform. (See below for issues regarding age-related performance differences in developmental fMRI studies.) Increases in task difficulty are known to generate increases in brain activation (Szameitat *et al.*, 2002).

Other studies have found evidence for increased participation of brain regions with age during working memory tasks. Thirteen subjects aged 9–18 years performed a spatial working memory task during whole-brain imaging (Klingberg et al. 2002). Subjects were presented with stimuli that appeared sequentially in a 4 by 4 grid for three or five steps. After a 1.5 second delay, subjects had to respond if the present stimulus was in a location prompted in the previous sequence. Age-related increases in activation were found in the superior frontal sulcus and intra-parietal sulcus, which corresponded to increased working memory capacity. Similar results were found in another spatial working memory task that was used to characterize changes in brain function related to age progression in eight children, eight adolescents, and seven adults (Kwon et al., 2002). A block design compared activation during trials where subjects had to press a key if an "O" appeared in the same location as two previous trials (2-back) compared with rest trials where subjects responded when the "O" stimulus appeared at center. Reaction time decreased with age while accuracy remained stable. Multiple regression analyses were used to correlate the magnitude of brain function with age. Results showed that brain function increased with age throughout prefrontal and premotor regions as well as throughout posterior parietal regions, while no age-related decreases in activation were found. These results remained after factoring out performance differences between age groups. These two studies are unique in that they looked at age as a continuous variable from childhood to adulthood and, therefore, may be more sensitive than studies on discrete age groups in identifying brain regions that show subtle changes with age.

Taken together, these studies indicate that the basic brain circuitry underlying spatial working memory is in place by childhood; however, with increasing age, there are changes in the degree that different regions in this circuitry are recruited. The prefrontal cortex, which is known to play a primary role in mature working memory, demonstrates the most consistent change with age in these different studies.

Voluntary response suppression

The ability to choose, through response suppression and interference control, what stimulus or plan to use to guide behavior is another essential aspect of higher executive cognition (Bjorklund and Harnishfeger, 1995). This ability, though present in infancy, matures throughout adolescence, supporting increasing voluntary control of behavior (Bjorklund and Harnishfeger, 1990). This is also a cognitive process that is impaired in neurodevelopmental disorders, especially schizophrenia (Klein et al., 2000; McDowell and Clementz, 2001; Sereno and Holzman, 1995).

Initial studies established that, like in the working memory task, children and adults recruit a similar brain network during response suppression. Prefrontal cortex was imaged in nine children aged 7–12 years and nine adults while they performed a go–no-go task (Casey *et al.*, 1997). Subjects had to button press in response to a centrally presented letter (go-trials) except when the letter was an "X" (no-go trials). Children made more false-alarm errors than adults. Children activated the middle frontal gyrus (Broca's area 9, 10, 46) as adults did; however, they showed a greater volume of activation. This study, as in the working memory results, provides evidence that children rely on increased participation of prefrontal cortex during response suppression, which could be a result of changes in the underlying anatomy or of increased effort by children to complete the task.

Evidence for increasing participation of multiple brain regions with age during performance of tasks requiring voluntary response suppression has also been provided by whole-brain fMRI. In one study, 16 children aged 8–12 years and 16 adults performed a combination task with flanker and go–no-go trials (Bunge *et al.*, 2001). In the flanker trials, subjects pressed a button corresponding to the direction of a central arrow flanked on both sides by two arrows pointing in the opposite direction to the central arrow (response interference), two arrows pointing in the same direction as the central arrow (no response interference), diamond shapes (no response interference), or "X" symbols to indicate no response (no-go trials). Children made more interference and response-suppression errors than adults. Results from correct trials only indicated that children, as well as adults, recruited prefrontal cortex during successful *interference suppression*, but in the opposite hemisphere. During successful *response inhibition*, children, unlike adults, relied more heavily on posterior rather than prefrontal regions. Children did not recruit right ventrolateral prefrontal cortex as adults did during both tasks. These results indicate that, with age, there is increased participation of prefrontal regions during response-suppression tasks. A study on adolescents showed similar results. Nine subjects aged 12–19 years were compared with eight healthy adults aged 22–40 years. Dorsal cortical regions were imaged while subjects performed a stop task, where they were required to press a button only if a picture of an airplane was not followed by a picture of a bomb (Rubia *et al.*, 2000). Performance did not differ between age groups; however, adolescents demonstrated reduced activation of prefrontal regions and increased activation in caudate and inferior frontal gyrus relative to adults. Age-related increases in prefrontal function were also found during a Stroop interference task (Adleman *et al.*, 2002). Thirty subjects aged 7–22 years performed a Stroop test where subjects had to read a list of color words printed in black font, name the color of a series of "X" symbols, and say the color of the ink of color words that were discordant for color font. Dorsal cortical regions of the brain were imaged. Results indicated that parietal involvement in the Stroop task is mature by adolescence, while prefrontal activation continues to increase into adulthood. These results support findings from working memory studies indicating that specialization of prefrontal function changes with age in a way that extends or elaborates its primary role in the voluntary control of behavior.

While it is generally accepted that prefrontal cortex plays a crucial role in higher-order cognition, it is also now well established that higher-order executive cognitive functions are subserved by widely distributed and integrated brain systems rather than by the prefrontal cortex independently (Goldman-Rakic, 1988). It is possible that, in conjunction with developmental improvements in the intrinsic computational capacity of prefrontal cortex, there is increased integration with other brain regions as well. We do not yet know details about the maturation of the functional integration of widely distributed circuitry.

Our own work has focused on characterizing changes in the distribution of brain function from childhood through adolescence during the performance of a voluntary response suppression task (Luna *et al.*, 2001). We conducted an fMRI study of 36 healthy subjects ranging in age from 8 to 30 years to study developmental changes in the brain substrate of antisaccade task performance. The antisaccade task requires that the prepotent tendency to make an eye movement towards a new visual stimulus be suppressed and instead a voluntary eye movement be generated to the opposite location. Developmental studies have indicated that the number of instances of response-suppression failures significantly decreases with age through adolescence (Fischer *et al.*, 1997; Munoz *et al.*, 1998) suggesting that, the *capacity* to suppress a response is present early on (a child can perform a correct antisaccade) but *efficiency* (the ability to perform correct antisaccades consistently) continues to improve into adolescence. In our fMRI study, the subjects were instructed to look in the opposite direction of targets that appeared in the periphery when preceded by a red fixation cross-hair. These were compared with blocks of trials where a green cross-hair indicated that subjects were to look toward peripheral targets. Activation across whole brain was compared in children, adolescents, and adults. Results indicated that, across the age span, subjects recruited a widely distributed circuitry, including frontal, supplementary, and parietal eye fields; dorsolateral prefrontal cortex; thalamus; and striatum (Fig. 3.2). In contrast, adults demonstrated increased activation in regions known to play a role in the establishment of the preparatory state needed to perform antisaccades successfully including frontal and parietal eye fields as well as the superior colliculus (Everling *et al.*, 1999; Everling and Munoz, 2000). Additionally, only adults recruited regions in the lateral cerebellum that underlie cognitive processes related to timing and learning (Kim *et al.*, 1994). Adolescents demonstrated increased activation of the dorsolateral prefrontal cortex and striatum relative to children, apparently reflecting their ability to recruit frontostriatal circuitry more effectively to perform the antisaccade task. Children, compared with older subjects, relied more on posterior parietal regions, reflecting increased use of visuospatial processing. Taken together, fMRI and behavioral

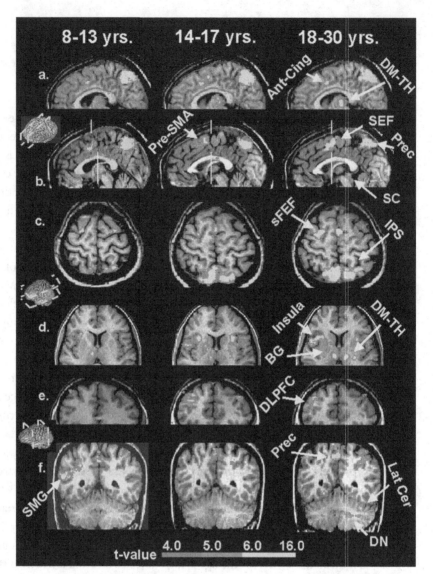

Fig. 3.2.   Group activation maps (t ≥ 4.0) during an antisaccade task relative to a visually guided prosaccade task superimposed on the structural anatomic image of a representative subject (Female aged 26 years) warped into Talairach space. Columns show the average activation for each age group. Rows depict the orientation (a,b, sagittal; d, axial; e,f, coronal) that optimally illustrate activation in brain regions of interest. Ant-Cing, anterior cingulate; DM-TH, dorsomedial thalamus; Pre-SMA, presupplementary area; SEF, supplementary eye fields; Prec, precuneus; SC, superior colliculus; sFEF, superior precentral sulcus aspect of the frontal eye field; IPS, intraparietal sulcus; BG, basal ganglia; DLPFC, dorsolateral prefrontal cortex; SMG, supramarginal sulcus; Lat Cer, lateral cerebellum; DN, dentate nucleus. (Reprinted from *NeuroImage*, Vol. 13, Luna, B., Thulborn, K. R., Munoz, D. P., Merriam, E. P., Garver, K. E., Minshew, N. J., *et al.*, "Maturation of widely distributed brain function subserves cognitive development" 786–793, Copyright 2001, with permission from Elsevier.)
For a colour version of this figure, see www.cambridge.org/9780521126595.

studies indicate that the increased integration of distant brain regions underlie improved efficiency in the voluntarily cognitive control of behavior that occurs throughout childhood and adolescence.

These results support other studies indicating that the increased participation of brain regions that underlie executive and attentional control are important in the maturation of voluntary response suppression. We extend these findings by proposing that the recruitment of regions that underlie preparatory and refined responses are also crucial to adult-level performance. Children are able to suppress prepotent responses and interference, but what improves with age is the consistency in which this behavioral state is maintained. We propose that this stage of maturation, encompassing adolescence, may be characterized by increased reliance on more widely distributed brain function that incorporates regions which are not primary in the generating of a voluntary response but, instead, improve the consistent control of behavior by a more concerted effort of the whole brain.

Developmental fMRI studies of both working memory and voluntary-response suppression indicate that brain function does change with age and with increases in performance; however, these changes are subtle and require further study. We still need to characterize the relative contributions of localized brain regions and the activities that are dependent on the integration of whole-brain processes. These initial studies do show us that there are important changes occurring during adolescence that could be vulnerable either to emergence of schizophrenia or the neurodevelopmental pathology that precedes it. With the background of methods and findings from normative psychological developmental research, we can now begin to explore possible failures in development that are associated with this disorder. The occurrence of abnormalities of prefrontal processes in schizophrenia is now widely supported by a range of histological, neuroimaging, and behavioral studies. We have seen that this region is particularly sensitive to developmental changes and may be vulnerable to impairment. Additionally, with neuroimaging techniques, we can characterize the integrity of integrated brain function and begin to understand the implications of localized impairment or failure to integrate the whole brain and the relationship these might have to neurodevelopmental psychiatric disorders (Luna and Sweeney, 1999; Luna et al., 2002). By studying at-risk populations, we can examine when the developmental dysmaturation of executive abilities begins to diverge most dramatically from normal processes (Ch. 23 reviews high-risk studies). As discussed below, we are still refining fMRI tools, especially with relevance to pediatric populations; however, well-defined developmental experiments with pediatric patient populations can begin to elucidate the nature of an impairment. In the next section, we present how pediatric fMRI studies have informed us of the development of other abilities and what they have shown us about impaired development.

Development of brain function supporting language

Pediatric fMRI studies of language development have demonstrated similar trajectories as those characterized in studies of the development of executive abilities.
Most pediatric fMRI studies have been performed to assist in the localization of
language areas to guide excision lesions to relieve epileptic seizures (Benson *et al.*,
1996; Hertz-Pannier *et al.*, 1997; Stapleton *et al.*, 1997). These studies provide further evidence of changing brain function with increasing language proficiency with
age. The integrity of temporal regions has most typically been assessed using reading
and passive language listening tasks. Results demonstrate similar language circuitry
and lateralization for children and adults (Hertz-Pannier *et al.*, 2001). Activation
of brain regions known to underlie sentence processing, including Broca's and
Wernicke's areas, as well as prefrontal and occipital cortices, was evident in children aged 8–13 years. These children also showed increases in activation of left
temporal cortex during reading, as previously shown for healthy adults (Gaillard
et al., 2001a). Children also demonstrate recruitment similar to adults of frontal,
parietal, occipital, and cingulate cortices during auditory sentence comprehension
and verb generation (Booth *et al.*, 1999). These results, like those from studies of
executive abilities, demonstrate that the basic circuitry needed for higher-order
function is in place by childhood.

Increases with age in activation within this circuitry have also been reported. Left
hemisphere lateralization of Broca's area for semantic language function during a
verb generation task was found to increase significantly with age from 7 to 18 years,
concurrent with increases in linguistic proficiency (Holland *et al.*, 2001). Evidence
from a fMRI study of 74 healthy subjects aged 7 to 17 years demonstrated no
changes in brain function with age in phonological processing, but age-related
changes in brain function in inferior frontal gyrus and precentral sulcus during
a semantic categorization task (Shaywitz *et al.*, 2002). Frontal lobe activation was
compared in 10 children aged 8–13 years and 10 healthy adults aged 19–48 years
while they performed a verbal fluency task (Gaillard *et al.*, 2000). Children were
found to activate the same frontal regions as adults including posterior inferior
frontal gyrus, dorsolateral prefrontal cortex, and cingulate cortex, but with a 60%
greater extent of activation. As mentioned above, this increase in the recruitment
of frontal regions could reflect the larger effort exerted by children to perform the
task or may be related to immature neuronal processes. Taken together, these results
confirm the primary role in the integration of frontal regions in the maturation of
higher-order cognition.

In order to delineate age changes in brain activation resulting from differences
in performance, children who performed at adult levels were compared with those
who performed worse than adults (Schlaggar *et al.*, 2002). Results indicated that age

differences detected in lateral prefrontal regions and posterior extrastriate regions were related to performance differences; however, those detected in neighboring areas in more dorsal medial prefrontal regions (absent in children) and more anterior extrastriate regions (increased activation in children) resulted only from age differences and may reflect maturational changes in the brain that affect how regions are recruited. These results show both increases and decreases in age-related activation. Greater activation in children relative to adults, as discussed above, may reflect the increased effort by children to perform at adult levels. Decreases in activation in children relative to adults may reflect decreased access to that region, immature local circuitry, or the recruitment of an alternative circuitry.

The above results support findings from fMRI studies of cognitive development showing continued changes in brain function with increases in development throughout childhood and adolescence. It is striking how, in both cognitive and language development, frontal regions appear to account for a significant number of age-related differences.

Abnormal populations

Pediatric fMRI studies have already provided insight into the possible factors underlying the etiology of developmental abnormalities such as ADHD and dyslexia.

Attention-deficit hyperactivity disorder

Attention-deficit hyperactivity disorder (ADHD) is the most prevalent childhood developmental disorder and is characterized by inattention, impulsivity, and hyperactivity. Studies using fMRI have indicated impaired function of prefrontal cortex and striatum. In one study, subjects aged 12–18 years who had been diagnosed with ADHD performed a response-suppression task, which showed decreased function in prefrontal cortex while the premotor and parietal cortices and caudate nucleus demonstrated similar activation as controls (Rubia *et al.*, 2000). In another study, 10 subjects aged 8–13 years diagnosed with ADHD were compared with six age-matched controls (Vaidya *et al.*, 1998). Subjects were tested before and after methylphenidate treatment. Subjects performed a letter go–no-go task where they refrained from responding on trials where an "X" appeared. Children with ADHD demonstrated poorer inhibitory performance and increased frontal and reduced striatal activation than controls. Methylphenidate improved performance and normalized activation in prefrontal and striatal regions in patients. These results provide evidence for frontostriatal involvement in ADHD.

Dyslexia

Dyslexia is an impairment in the ability to read that is not caused by reduced intellectual capabilities. Neuroimaging studies indicate abnormalities in the systems underlying phonological processes in dyslexic individuals, and fMRI has indicated that dyslexic children fail to recruit parietotemporal and extrastriate regions known to support orthographic processing (Temple *et al.*, 2001). Similar results were obtained when a large number (74) of dyslexic subjects aged 7–18 years were compared with 70 normal readers aged 7–17 years (Shaywitz *et al.*, 2002). Dyslexic children had reduced activation of parietotemporal and occipitotemporal regions compared with normal readers, instead relying on homologous right hemisphere regions and the anterior cingulate cortex to perform the semantic category task. These studies indicate a failure to recruit regions throughout circuits known to underlie processes crucial to reading, primarily in parietotemporal regions, in dyslexic subjects. Additionally, abnormalities in cortical visual region V5/MT have also been found during motion processing in dyslexic subjects, indicating that, in addition to abnormalities in phonological processing, impaired visual processing may also underlie this disorder (Eden *et al.*, 1996). Instead, dyslexics demonstrate increased activation of Broca's area as they struggle with phonological processing (Georgiewa *et al.*, 2002). In contrast to ADHD, these results illustrate abnormalities associated with dysfunction of posterior brain processes.

Pediatric fMRI studies of schizophrenia

Given the very low incidence of childhood schizophrenia and the additional complications making that diagnosis in young children, it is difficult to test neurodevelopmental theories of schizophrenia directly on sufficient numbers of child patients. Further, studies of affected children would make it difficult to disentangle disease effects from neurodevelopmental risk mechanisms. Pediatric offspring of a schizophrenia parent are particularly well suited to investigate the developmental nature of schizophrenia. Offspring of schizophrenia patients have a 10–16% risk of developing schizophrenia–related disorders, compared with 1% in the general population (Gottesman *et al.*, 1982). We have initiated pediatric fMRI studies in the offspring of individuals with schizophrenia (a high-risk group) to investigate brain function underlying executive function in schizophrenia (Keshavan *et al.*, 2002). Brain function during a spatial working memory task, the oculomotor delayed response task, were compared between four high-risk adolescents and four age- and sex-matched healthy controls. In this task, subjects had to generate a saccade in the absence of a visual stimulus to a location that had been previously indicated and had been retained in working memory for several seconds. In order to isolate brain function associated with working memory from oculomotor processes, the block of oculomotor delayed response trials were compared with blocks of visually guided saccade trials where subjects made similar saccadic eye movements but to visual targets appearing in the periphery. During the working memory task, the high-risk subjects had reduced prefrontal Broadmann's areas 9 and 46 and parietal activation relative to the healthy group. These results suggest that abnormalities in frontal and parietal heteromodal association cortex may precede illness onset and represent a neurodevelopmental failure that contributes to risk for the disorder, indicating that studies of the high-risk group may be valuable in testing neurodevelopmental models of schizophrenia.

Challenges to pediatric neuroimaging

Pediatric neuroimaging requires consideration of issues specific to the testing of children. Non-compliance has to be considered and methods are used to engage the child's participation while ameliorating any fears. Training with the tasks that will be presented in the scanner previous to the MRI session is often very helpful to enable the child to focus on attainable goals when testing occurs. Using stimuli and tasks that are particularly amenable to attract children's attention can also be of benefit during long tasks. The prospect of being "tested," especially inside an enclosed space such as an MR scanner, can be particularly stressful to children. In order to reduce the anxiety and acclimate subjects to this constrained environment, many laboratories now have subjects spend time inside a non-working model of a scanner previous to the testing. In our experience, children and adolescents who spend time inside a "mock" scanner prior to imaging studies have significantly reduced heart rates and self-reported distress levels during subsequent imaging studies (Rosenberg *et al.*, 1997). Children who did not spend time in a "mock" scanner had higher heart rates and self-reported distress levels in the actual scanner than did simulation-trained subjects.

Head motion is one of the most significant sources of artifact in fMRI imaging. fMRI activation maps are typically developed using more than 100 images of the brain, which are acquired over the course of a study that may last 5 to 10 minutes. Head movement during image acquisition compromises the ability to detect brain function because the brain tissue from which image data are obtained varies over the course of a study. For this reason, head motion artifact can dramatically underestimate brain function. This is particularly problematic with children and patient groups, who can have a more difficult time than adults remaining still (Logan, 1999; Poldrack *et al.*, 2002; Thomas *et al.*, 1999). Head motion is usually corrected for by algorithms that align all images to a reference image (Cox, 1996; Eddy *et al.*, 1996; Woods *et al.*, 1993). Head movement larger than the level of resolution prescribed, displacement larger than a half to two-thirds of a voxel, can often not be adequately corrected and such data cannot be included in analyses. Therefore, restraints are often used to reduce head motion. A bite bar affords an anchor that reduces head motion significantly; however, subjects, especially children and patient groups, can actually move more with such devices because they do not tolerate the discomfort. Less-restrictive systems include using pillows to pack the head into the head coil, minimizing range of movement, and visual feedback of head location to help subjects to reposition themselves to their original position (Thulborn and Shen, 1999). Training subjects to keep their heads still through sensory feedback in a mock scanner also helps to minimize head motion (Slifer, 1996). Pediatric neuroimaging studies must report the amount of head movement found in their subjects lest their results be confounded by this artifact. This is of particular concern when studies find a reduction of activation throughout the brains of children relative to adults with no regions demonstrating similar magnitude of activation.

Children have faster respiratory and heart rate cycles than adults. Respiration can lead to physiological artifact by introducing variations in the static magnetic field, which can lead to spurious and decreased activation (Kemna and Posse, 2001; Raj et al., 2001). Increased pulse rate can result in motion within the brain, affecting brainstem structures the most, but also basal ganglia and, to a lesser degree, the cortical surface (Gaillard et al., 2001b). Algorithms are being devised to remove this artifact (Frank et al., 2001) but there is still limited experience in using such approaches with pediatric samples.

A great misconception is that there are dramatic differences in the gross morphology of the child and adult brains that make any direct comparison of functional responses between age groups seriously flawed. This view implies that children's brains would be warped to a higher degree than adults when warping brain structure into a common adult brain atlas such as the Talairach atlas (Talairach and Tournoux, 1988). Studies have shown, however, that brain size and gross morphology at age 5 is not significantly different from that of adults (Caviness et al., 1996; Giedd et al., 1996; Reiss et al., 1996) and the variability in brain structure between children and adults is less than the normal variance between adult subjects. Nasal sinuses continue to form into adolescence, perhaps resulting in increasing sources of artifacts in brain regions bordering these areas. Neck length also continues to increase developmentally, raising concerns regarding the optimal placement of a child's head on a head coil designed for an adult (Gaillard et al., 2001b). This could result in children not reaching the "sweet" spot of the head coil where optimal images are obtained.

Differences in performance

A major concern of pediatric neuroimaging is understanding if age differences in brain function result from differences in performance or actually reflect differences in functional brain systems (Bookheimer, 2000). Some investigators choose to use tasks where children perform at the same levels as adults (Casey et al., 1995). The primary result in these studies, perhaps not surprisingly, has been similar activation across ages. When differences in activation are found, these may reflect underlying differences in anatomy or differences in the computational demand required to equate performance across age groups. However, age differences in brain activation where performance levels of the task differ does not exclude the possibility that adult patterns of activation would be evident in the child brain if performance was equated. These two approaches are useful in answering different questions regarding development. The former approach is needed to identify the presence of mature brain circuitry, while the latter allows the characterization of the immature aspects of the brain systems supporting a specific cognitive process. Although mature circuitry may be accessed by children given optimal conditions, it is important to characterize the brain regions that are not being accessed when performance fails.

There are methods available to gain the benefits of both approaches. One approach is to identify the brain regions that demonstrate age-related changes owing to differences in performance and those that are independent of performance differences. One study identified performance-related activity by identifying regions that had greater activation in children that performed worse than adults but not in children with equivalent performance levels as adults (Schlaggar et al., 2002). Brain regions that show age-related differences in children with both poor and equivalent performance as adults are independent from performance differences and may reflect differences in the underlying neuroanatomy. Another approach is to change task difficulty parametrically. As task difficulty increases, differences in brain activation resulting from age differences should emerge. The variables that consistently differ between ages across different task difficulties can be identified as demonstrating developmental changes. In this manner, we can identify regions that demonstrate age differences owing to performance differences and those that are independent of performance and may indicate differences in neuroanatomy (Benson et al., 1996).

Future directions

The goal of pediatric neuroimaging is to characterize the interaction between brain maturation and cognitive development. We still need to characterize how synaptic pruning and myelination processes contribute to age-related changes in the functional organization of brain systems. The next step in pediatric neuroimaging is to gain more direct characterization of brain maturation while obtaining indices of brain function.

Diffusion tensor imaging (DTI) provides an indirect measure of myelination in vivo by distinguishing the motion properties of water molecules inside axonal tracts (Basser et al., 1994; Conturo et al., 1996; Le Bihan et al., 2001). The confinement produced by myelin and tract tissue forces water molecules to diffuse rapidly in an anisotropic manner in the direction of the fibers, in contrast to non-directional isotropic diffusion outside fiber tracts (Peled and Yeshurun, 2001). Similar to fMRI, DTI is a non-invasive and relatively short procedure (about 10 minutes) and can be acquired using the same echo planar imaging sequence as fMRI, which enables the direct overlay of images, permitting high resolution for localizing regions. Initial DTI studies indicated a continued increase in frontal white matter anisotropy throughout childhood (Klingberg et al., 1999). The high resolution of DTI allows the tracking of subtle white matter differences that are not evident in white matter volume, as well as sensitivity to subtle and dynamic changes in brain disorders. Decreased anisotropy in left parietotemporal regions have been reported for adult subjects with reading disabilities, providing evidence for impaired communication between visual- and language-processing regions (Klingberg et al., 2000) and a possible mechanism for the impaired brain function demonstrated in these regions (see above). DTI has also demonstrated reduced anisotropy in schizophrenia patients, indicating a lack of connective integrity in white matter volumes throughout the neocortex (Agartz et al., 2001; Foong et al., 2000; Lim et al., 1999). Understanding the changes in myelination and other potential changes in white matter tracts that concur with cognitive development will be pivotal in characterizing possible dysmaturation in schizophrenia.

Phosphorus MR spectroscopy (^{31}P MRS) allows non-invasive in vivo investigation of phosphorus-containing metabolites, which provide an indirect measure of synaptic pruning (Keshavan et al., 1991; Stanley et al., 1996). MRS probes the integrity of cell membranes by indicating the levels of phosphomonoesters (PMEs), which are membrane phospholipid precursors, and phosphodiesters (PDEs), which are phospholipid breakdown products (Keshavan et al., 1991). This can provide an indirect measure of age-related changes in synaptic integrity. MRS has provided evidence for decreases in PMEs and increases in PDEs in prefrontal cortex in schizophrenia (Pettegrew et al., 1993). The concurrent acquisition of fMRI and MRS data could potentially reveal the contribution changes in synaptic integrity to age-related changes in brain functional organization.

Finally, in order to increase power, validity, and reliability, pediatric studies should include a larger number of subjects with equal distribution of individuals across each age group. Given the variability in rates of maturation, sources of individual difference should be reduced. Variables such as gender, intelligence quotient, and puberty would decrease intersubject variability. Control groups should be carefully characterized and be free of any neurobiological abnormalities, including metabolic and neurological disorders as well as psychiatric illness in the subject and first-degree relatives. Most importantly, longitudinal studies should be performed in a well-characterized group of healthy subjects who could be tested annually with the same cognitive tasks. In this manner, developmental trajectories can be delineated and also stage-like characterization of development can be understood. Only with carefully designed studies with a large number of subjects, as suggested, will we be able to generate normative data that is sensitive to subtle dysmaturation processes present in psychiatric disorders.

Conclusions

We have recently been able to characterize the interface between cognitive development and brain maturation using fMRI, a non-invasive neuroimaging method. This is important to the understanding of neurodevelopmental models of dysmaturation in brain disorders such as schizophrenia. Initial pediatric fMRI studies have shown that the basic circuitry supporting the *capacity* to perform a task is established by childhood. Changes in the participation of frontal cortex and the ability to recruit widely distributed brain circuitry support increases in the *efficiency* of the cognitive control of behavior with age. This pattern was observed in studies investigating the cognitive development of working memory and voluntary response suppression, and language processing in healthy individuals. Studies of abnormal pediatric populations demonstrate impairments in frontal circuitry in ADHD and parietotemporal regions in dyslexia. When using fMRI with children, special precautions must be taken to eliminate factors that have the potential to confound the results. The future direction of fMRI includes the ability to probe brain anatomical changes supporting the brain functional changes that are observed during development.

REFERENCES

Adleman, N. E., Menon, V., Blasey, C. M., *et al.* (2002). A developmental fMRI study of the Stroop color–word task. *NeuroImage* **16**: 61–75.

Agartz, I., Andersson, J. L. R., Skare, S. (2001). Abnormal brain white matter in schizophrenia: a diffusion tensor imaging study. *Neuroreport* **12**: 2251–2254.

Armstrong, E., Schleicher, A., Omran, H., Curtis, M., Zilles, K. (1995). The ontogeny of human gyrification. *Cereb Cortex* **5**: 56–63.

Baddeley, A. D. (1983). Working memory. *Philos Trans R Soc Lond B* **302**: 311–324.

Basser, P. J., Mattiello, J., Lebihan, D. (1994). Estimation of the effective self-diffusion tensor from the NMR spin echo. *J Magn Reson* **103**: 247–254.

Benson R. R., Logan W. J., Cosgrove G. R., *et al.* (1996). Functional MRI localization of language in a 9-year-old child. *Can J Neurol Sci* **23**: 213–219.

Bjorklund, D. F., Harnishfeger, K. K. (1990). The resources construct in cognitive development: diverse sources of evidence and a theory of inefficient inhibition. *Dev Rev* **10**: 48–71.

(1995). The evolution of inhibition mechanisms and their role in human cognition and behavior. In *Interference and Inhibition in Cognition*, ed. F. N. Dempster, C. J. Brainerd. San Diego, CA: Academic Press, pp. 141–173.

Bookheimer, S. Y. (2000). Methodological issues in pediatric neuroimaging. *Mental Retard Dev Disabil Res Rev* **6**: 161–165.

Booth, J. R., MacWhinney, B., Thulborn, K. R., *et al.* (1999). Functional organization of activation patterns in children: whole brain fMRI imaging during three different cognitive tasks. *Prog Neuropsychopharmacol Biol Psychiatry* **23**: 669–682.

Bunge, S. A., Dudukovic, N. M., Thomason, M. E, Vaidya, C. J., Gabrieli, J. D. E. (2001). Immature frontal lobe contributions to cognitive control in children: evidence from fMRI. *Neuron* **33**: 301–311.

Case, R. (1992). The role of the frontal lobes in the regulation of cognitive development. *Brain Cogn* **20**: 51–73.

Casey, B. J., Cohen, J. D., Jezzard, P., *et al.* (1995). Activation of prefrontal cortex in children during a nonspatial working memory task with functional MRI. *NeuroImage* **2**: 221–229.

Casey, B. J., Trainor, R. J., Orendi, J. L., *et al.* (1997). A developmental functional MRI study of prefrontal activation during performance of a go-no-go task. *J Cogn Neurosci* **9**: 835–847.

Caviness, V. S., Kennedy, D. N., Bates, J. F., Makris, N. (1996). The developing human brain: a morphometric profile. In *Developmental Neuroimaging: Mapping the Development of Brain and Behavior*, ed. R. W. Thatcher, G. Reid Lyon, J. Rumsey, N. A. Krasnegor. New York: Academic Press, pp. 3–14.

Changeux, J. P., Danchin, A. (1976). Selective stabilization of developing synapses as a mechanism for the specification of neuronal networks. *Nature* **264**: 705–712.

Chugani, H. T. (1998). A critical period of brain development: studies of cerebral glucose utilization with PET. *Prev Med* **27**: 184–188.

Cohen, J. D., Barch, D. M., Carter, C., Servan-Schreiber, D. (1999). Context-processing deficits in schizophrenia: converging evidence from three theoretically motivated cognitive tasks. *J Abnorm Psychol* **108**: 120–133.

Conturo, T. E., McKinstry, R. C., Akbudak, E., Robinson, B. H. (1996). Encoding of anisotropic diffusion with tetrahedral gradients: a general mathematical diffusion formalism and experimental results. *Magn Reson Med* **35**: 399–412.

Cox, R. W. (1996). AFNI: Software for analysis and visualization of functional magnetic resonance neuroimages. *Comput Biomed Res* **29**: 162–173.

Diamond, A., Goldman-Rakic, P. S. (1989). Comparison of human infants and rhesus monkeys on Piaget's AB task: evidence for dependence on dorsolateral prefrontal cortex. *Exp Brain Res* **74**: 24–40.

Eddy, W. F., Fitzgerald, M., Genovese, C. R., Mockus, A., Noll, D. C. (1996). Functional image analysis software: computational olio. In *Proceedings in Computational Statistics*, ed. A. Prat. Heidelberg: Physica-Verlag, pp. 39–49.

Eden, G. F., Van Meter, J. W., Rumsey, J. M., *et al.* (1996). Abnormal processing of visual motion in dyslexia revealed by functional brain imaging. [See comments] *Nature* **382**: 66–69.

Everling, S., Munoz, D. P. (2000). Neuronal correlates for preparatory set associated with prosaccades and anti-saccades in the primate frontal eye field. *J Neurosci* **20**: 387–400.

Everling, S., Dorris, M. C., Klein, R. M., Munoz, D. P. (1999). Role of primate superior colliculus in preparation and execution of anti-saccades and pro-saccades. *J Neurosci* **19**: 2740–2754.

Fischer, B., Biscaldi M, Gezeck, S. (1997). On the development of voluntary and reflexive components in human saccade generation. *Brain Res* **754**: 285–297.

Foong, J., Maier, M., Clark, C. A., *et al.* (2000). Neuropathological abnormalities of the corpus callosum in schizophrenia: a diffusion tensor imaging study. *J Neurol Neurosurg Psychiatry* **68**: 242–244.

Frank, L. R., Buxton, R. B., Wong, E. C. (2001). Estimation of respiration-induced noise fluctuations from undersampled multislice fMRI data. *Magn Reson Med* **45**: 635–644.

Fry, A. F., Hale, S. (1996). Processing speed, working memory, and fluid intelligence: evidence for a developmental cascade. *Psychol Sci* **7**: 237–241.

Fuster, J. M. (1997). *The Prefrontal Cortex.* New York: Raven Press.

Gaillard, W. D., Hertz-Pannier, L., Mott, S. H., *et al.* (2000). Functional anatomy of cognitive development: fMRI of verbal fluency in children and adults. *Neurology* **54**: 180–185.

Gaillard, W. D., Pugliese, M., Grandin, C. B., *et al.* (2001a). Cortical localization of reading in normal children: an fMRI language study. *Neurology* **57**: 47–54.

Gaillard, W. D., Grandin, C. B., Xu, B. (2001b). Developmental aspects of pediatric fMRI: considerations for image acquisition, analysis, and interpretation. *NeuroImage* **13**: 239–249.

Georgiewa, P., Rzanny, R., Gaser, C., *et al.* (2002). Phonological processing in dyslexic children: a study combining functional imaging and event related potentials. *Neurosci Lett* **318**: 5–8.

Giedd, J. N., Snell, J. W., Lange, N., *et al.* (1996). Quantitative magnetic resonance imaging of human brain development: ages 4–18. *Cereb Cortex* **6**: 551–560.

Giedd, J. N., Blumenthal, J., Jeffries, N. O., *et al.* (1999). Brain development during childhood and adolescence: a longitudinal MRI study. *Nat Neurosci* **2**: 861–863.

Goldman-Rakic, P. S. (1988). Topography of cognition: parallel distributed networks in primate association cortex. *Annu Rev Neurosci* **11**: 137–156.

(1990). Parallel systems in the cerebral cortex: the topography of cognition. In *Natural and Artificial Parallel Computation*, ed. M. A. Arbib, J. A. Robinson. New York: MIT Press, pp. 155–176.

(1992). Working memory and the mind. *Sci Am* **267**: 111–117.

Gottesman, I. I., Shields, J., Hanson, D. (1982). *Schizophrenia: The Epigenetic Puzzle.* New York: Cambridge University Press.

Hertz-Pannier, L., Gaillard, W. D., Mott, S. H., *et al.* (1997). Noninvasive assessment of language dominance in children and adolescents with functional MRI: a preliminary study. *Neurology* **48**: 1003–1012.

Hertz-Pannier, L., Chiron, C., Vera, P., van de Morteele, P. F., *et al.* (2001). Functional imaging in the work-up of childhood epilepsy. *Childs Nerv Syst* **17**: 223–228.

Holland, S. K., Plante, E., Byars, A. W., *et al.* (2001). Normal fMRI brain activation patterns in children performing a verb generation task. *NeuroImage* **14**: 837–843.

Huttenlocher, P. R. (1990). Morphometric study of human cerebral cortex development. *Neuropsychologia* **28**: 517–527.

Hyde, T. M., Ziegler, J. C., Weinberger, D. R. (1992). Psychiatric disturbances in metachromatic leukodystrophy. *Arch Neurol* **49**: 401–406.

Jernigan, T. L., Trauner, D. A., Hesselink, J. R., Tallal, P. A. (1991). Maturation of human cerebrum observed in vivo during adolescence. *Brain* 114: 2037–2049.

Kemna, L. J., Posse, S. (2001). Effect of respiratory CO_2 changes on the temporal dynamics of the hemodynamic response in functional MR imaging. *NeuroImage* 14: 642–649.

Keshavan, M. S., Kapur, S., Pettegrew, J. W. (1991). Magnetic resonance spectroscopy in psychiatry: potential, pitfalls, and promise. *Am J Psychiatry* 148: 976–985.

Keshavan, M. S., Anderson, S., Pettegrew, J. W. (1994). Is schizophrenia due to excessive synaptic pruning in the prefrontal cortex? The Feinberg hypothesis revisited. *J Psychiatr Res* 28: 239–265.

Keshavan, M., Diwadkar, V., Spencer, S. M., *et al.* (2002). A preliminary functional magnetic resonance imaging study in offspring of schizophrenic parents. *Prog Neuropsychopharmacol Biol Psychiatry* 26: 1143–1149.

Kim, S. G., Ugurbil, K., Strick, P. L. (1994). Activation of a cerebellar output nucleus during cognitive processing. *Science* 265: 949–951.

Klein, C., Heinks, T., Andresen, B., Berg, P., Moritz, S. (2000). Impaired modulation of the saccadic contingent negative variation preceding antisaccades in schizophrenia. *Biol Psychiatry* 47: 978–990.

Klingberg, T., Vaidya, C. J., Gabrieli, J. D. E., Moseley, M. E., Hedehus, M. (1999). Myelination and organization of the frontal white matter in children: a diffusion tensor MRI study. *Neuroreport* 10: 2817–2821.

Klingberg, T., Hedehus, M., Temple, E., *et al.* (2000). Microstructure of temporo-parietal white matter as a basis for reading ability: evidence from diffusion tensor magnetic resonance imaging. *Neuron* 25: 493–500.

Klingberg, T., Forssberg, H., Westerberg, H. (2002). Increased brain activity in frontal and parietal cortex underlies the development of visuospatial working memory capacity during childhood. *J Cogn Neurosci* 14: 1–10.

Kwon, H., Reiss, R. L., Menon, V. (2002). Neural basis of protracted developmental changes in visuo-spatial working memory. *Proc Natl Acad Sci USA* 99: 13336–13341.

Le Bihan, D., Mangin, J. F., Poupon, C., *et al.* (2001). Diffusion tensor imaging: concepts and applications. *J Magn Reson* 13: 534–546.

Levin, H. S., Culhane, K. A., Hartmann, J., Evankovich, K., Mattson, A. J. (1991). Developmental changes in performance on tests of purported frontal lobe functioning. *Dev Neuropsychol* 7: 377–395.

Lim, K. O., Hedehus, M., Moseley, M., *et al.* (1999). Compromised white matter tract integrity in schizophrenia inferred from diffusion tensor imaging. *Arch Gen Psychiatry* 56: 367–374.

Logan, W. J. (1999). Functional magnetic resonance imaging in children. *Semin Pediatr Neurol* 6: 78–86.

Luciana, M., Nelson, C. A. (1998). The functional emergence of prefrontally-guided working memory systems in four- to eight-year-old children. *Neuropsychologia* 36: 273–293.

Luna, B., Sweeney, J. A. (1999). Cognitive functional magnetic resonance imaging at very-high-field: eye movement control. *Top Magn Reson Imaging* 10: 3–15.

(2001). Studies of brain and cognitive maturation through childhood and adolescence: a strategy for testing neurodevelopmental hypotheses. *Schizophr Bull* 27: 443–455.

Luna, B., Thulborn, K. R., Munoz, D. P., *et al.* (2001). Maturation of widely distributed brain function subserves cognitive development. *NeuroImage* **13**: 786–793.

Luna, B., Minshew, N. J., Garver, K. E., *et al.* (2002). Neocortical system abnormalities in autism: an fMRI study of spatial working memory. *Neurology* **59**: 834–840.

McDowell, J. E., Clementz, B. A. (2001). Behavioral and brain imaging studies of saccadic performance in schizophrenia. *Biol Psychol* **57**: 5–22.

Merriam, E. P., Thase, M. E., Haas, G. L., Keshavan, M. S., Sweeney, J. A. (1999). Prefrontal cortical dysfunction in depression determined by Wisconsin Card Sorting Test performance. *Am J Psychiatry* **156**: 780–782.

Munoz, D. P., Broughton, J. R., Goldring, J. E., Armstrong, I. T. (1998). Age-related performance of human subjects on saccadic eye movement tasks. *Exp Brain Res* **217**: 1–10.

Nelson, C. A., Monk, C. S., Lin, J., *et al.* (2000). Functional neuroanatomy of spatial working memory in children. *Dev Psychol* **36**: 109–116.

Park, S., Holzman, P. S. (1992). Schizophrenics show spatial working memory deficits. *Arch Gen Psychiatry* **49**: 975–982.

Peled, S., Yeshurun, Y. (2001). Superresolution in MRI: application to human white matter fiber tract visualization by diffusion tensor imaging. *Magn Reson Med* **42**: 29–35.

Pettegrew, J. W., Keshavan, M. S., Minshew, N. J. (1993). ^{31}P nuclear magnetic resonance spectroscopy: neurodevelopment and schizophrenia. *Schizophr Bull* **19**: 35–53.

Pfefferbaum, A., Mathalon, D. H., Sullivan, E. V., *et al.* (1994). A quantitative magnetic resonance imaging study of changes in brain morphology from infancy to late adulthood. *Arch Neurol* **51**: 874–887.

Poldrack, R. A., Pare-Blagoev, E. J., Grant, P. E. (2002). Pediatric functional magnetic resonance imaging: progress and challenges. *Top Magn Reson Imaging* **13**: 61–70.

Raj, D., Anderson, A. W., Gore, J. C. (2001). Respiratory effects in human functional magnetic resonance imaging due to bulk susceptibility changes. *Phys Med Biol* **46**: 3331–3340.

Rakic, P., Bourgeois, J. P., Eckenhoff, M. F., Zecevic N, Goldman-Rakic, P. S. (1986). Concurrent overproduction of synapses in diverse regions of the primate cerebral cortex. *Science* **232**: 232–235.

Reiss, A. L., Abrams, M. T., Singer, H. S., Ross, J. L., Denckla, M. B. (1996). Brain development, gender, and IQ in children: a volumetric imaging study. *Brain* **119**: 1763–1774.

Ridderinkhof, K. R., van der Molen, M. W. (1997). Mental resources, processing speed, and inhibitory control: a developmental perspective. *Biol Psychol* **45**: 241–261.

Rosenberg, D. R., Sweeney, J. A., Gillen, J., *et al.* (1997). Magnetic resonance imaging of children without sedation: preparation with simulation. *J Am Acad Child Adolesc Psychiatry* **36**: 853–859.

Rubia, K., Overmeyer S, Taylor, E., *et al.* (2000). Functional frontalisation with age: mapping neurodevelopmental trajectories with fMRI. *Neurosci Biobehav Rev* **24**: 13–19.

Schlaggar, B. L., Brown, T. T., Lugar, H. M., *et al.* (2002). Functional neuroanatomical differences between adults and school-age children in the processing of single words. *Science* **296**: 1476–1479.

Sereno, A. B., Holzman, P. S. (1995). Antisaccades and smooth pursuit eye movements in schizophrenia. *Biol Psychiatry* **37**: 394–401.

Shaywitz, B. A., Shaywitz, S. E., Pugh, K. R., *et al.* (2002). Disruption of posterior brain systems for reading in children with developmental dyslexia. *Biol Psychiatry* **52**: 101–110.

Slifer, K. J. (1996). A video system to help children cooperate with motion control for radiation treatment without sedation. *J Pediatr Oncol Nurs* **13**: 91–97.

Stanley, J. A., Williamson, P. C., Drost, D. J., *et al.* (1996). An in vivo proton magnetic resonance spectroscopy study of schizophrenia patients. *Schizophr Bull* **22**: 597–609.

Stapleton, S. R., Kiriakopoulos, E., Mikulis, D., *et al.* (1997). Combined utility of functional MRI, cortical mapping, and frameless stereotaxy in the resection of lesions in eloquent areas of brain in children. *Pediatr Neurosurg* **26**: 68–82.

Szameitat, A. J., Schubert, T., Mueller, K., von Cramon, D. Y. (2002). Localization of executive functions in dual-task performance with fMRI. *J Cogn Neurosci* **14**: 1184–1199.

Talairach, J., Tournoux, P. (1988). *Co-Planar Stereotaxic Atlas of the Human Brain.* New York: Thieme Medical.

Temple, E., Poldrack, R. A., Salidis, J., *et al.* (2001). Disrupted neural responses to phonological and orthographic processing in dyslexic children: an fMRI study. *Neuroreport* **12**: 299–307.

Thatcher, R. W. (1991). Maturation of the human frontal lobes: physiological evidence for staging. *Dev Neuropsychol* **7**: 397–419.

Thomas, K. M., King, S. W., Franzen, P. L., *et al.* (1999). A developmental functional MRI study of spatial working memory. *NeuroImage* **10**: 327–338.

Thulborn, K. R., Shen, G. X. (1999). An integrated head immobilization system and high-performance RF coil for fMRI of visual paradigms at 1.5 T. *J Magn Reson* **139**: 26–34.

Vaidya, C. J., Austin, G., Kirkorian, G., *et al.* (1998). Selective effects of methylphenidate in attention deficit hyperactivity disorder: a functional magnetic resonance study. *Proc Natl Acad Sci USA* **95**: 14494–14499.

Waddington, J. L., Torrey, E. F., Crow, T. J., Hirsch, S. R. (1991). Schizophrenia, neurodevelopment and disease. *Arch Gen Psychiatry* **48**: 271–273.

Weinberger, D. R., Lipska, B. K. (1995). Cortical maldevelopment, anti-psychotic drugs, and schizophrenia: a search for common ground. *Schizophr Res* **16**: 87–110.

Weinberger, D. R., Berman, K. F., Zec, R. F. (1986). Physiologic dysfunction of dorsolateral prefrontal cortex in schizophrenia: I. Regional cerebral blood flow evidence. *Arch Gen Psychiatry* **43**: 114–124.

Welsh, M. C., Pennington, B. F., Groisser, D. B. (1991). A normative–developmental study of executive function: a window on prefrontal function in children. *Dev Neuropsychol* **7**: 131–149.

Wilson, S. P., Kipp, K. (1998). The development of efficient inhibition: evidence from directed-forgetting tasks. *Dev Rev* **18**: 86–123.

Woods, R. P., Mazziotta, J. C., Cherry, S. R. (1993). Automated image registration. In *Quantification of Brain Function: Tracer Kinetics and Image Analysis in Brain PET*, ed. K. Uemura, N. A. Lassen, T. Jones, *et al.* Amsterdam: Elsevier Science, pp. 391–400.

Yakovlev P. I., Lecours A. R. (1967). *Regional Development of the Brain in Early Life.* Oxford: Blackwell Scientific, pp. 3–70.

4

Cognitive development in adolescence: cerebral underpinnings, neural trajectories, and the impact of aberrations

Stephen J. Wood, Cinzia R. De Luca, Vicki Anderson, and Christos Pantelis

University of Melbourne, Melbourne, Australia

Children are not born with the full complement of cognitive skills they need for adulthood; instead, they need to develop these abilities as they grow. Initial theories about this development espoused a behaviorist idea of the child as a passive participant shaped by external forces, with more recent views considering the child as developing through invariant and universal cognitive stages in an active quest to make sense of their experience (Piaget, 1965). In this scheme, adolescence heralded the final developmental progression in cognitive development, with the transition from concrete to formal operational thought. This capacity to deal with abstract concepts, "operating on operations" rather than reality, what is now referred to as meta-cognition, or encompassed in the notion of executive functions, was considered to become available to the child around the age of 11 or 12 years (Stuss, 1992; Travis, 1998).

Much of the detail of the influential cognitive model proposed by Piaget and his proponents has now been amended and extended. Nevertheless, the notion of a sequential and gradual accumulation of cognitive processes, along with the limitations and capabilities of the child as they mature, has been invaluable to the study of child development. An understanding of the normal development of cognitive function is important in order to appreciate the pattern of impairments in children and adolescents who suffer from illnesses of putative neurodevelopmental origin. In particular, we need to know when cognitive functions are due to come "on-line" during maturation, and how this differs across cognitive domains. Information on the normal progression of skill acquisition allows for better characterization of whether the onset of behavioral disturbances or symptoms of psychiatric or other disorders reflect a deviation in functioning or a failure to make age-appropriate

Neurodevelopment and Schizophrenia, ed. Matcheri S. Keshavan *et al.* Published by Cambridge University Press. © Cambridge University Press 2004.

gains. In this regard, the observation that the acute symptoms of schizophrenia arise during this final phase of cognitive transition raises interesting questions about the etiology of the disorder and how the underlying substrates of psychosis are expressed.

Adolescence

Adolescence is a loose descriptive term referring to the period of transition from childhood to adulthood. Although it comprises the teenage years and is heralded by the onset of puberty, it is not defined by specific events. Indeed, while puberty and adolescence are often used synonymously (Petersen, 1998), the two do not necessarily co-occur (Dubas, 1991). For the purposes of this review, adolescence will be taken to cover the years from ages 12 to 20, as distinct cognitive advances in higher-order thinking are seen to occur around the age of 12, with a general stabilization of most executive processes as individuals enter their twenties.

Adolescence is a time of major upheaval in behavioral and social domains as the developing child seeks to attain the skills necessary for independence. The major changes tend to be in the areas of social interaction, risk-taking behavior, and intellectual expansion. The first two are more comprehensively reviewed by Spear (2000), while the last is covered in detail. The greater emphasis placed on exploring cognitive developments unique to adolescence derives from the belief that, ultimately, the emergence of independent thinking, social and moral awareness, impulsivity, and challenging of conceptual ideas are a reflection of the higher-order executive abilities that become available to the child during the teenage years.

Brain development during adolescence

The adolescent period, which is associated with the greatest risk for psychotic disorders, is accompanied by extensive, but localized, brain maturation, which takes the form of myelination and cortical synapse elimination (Huttenlocher, 1984). It has been suggested that as many as 30 000 synapses per second are lost during primate adolescence (Rakic et al., 1994). The vast majority of these synapses are excitatory in nature (Rakic et al., 1994), so it is unsurprising that removal of these synapses is associated with a decline in brain rates of glucose metabolism from the hypermetabolic state of childhood (Chugani et al., 1987). The elimination of excess synaptic connections through apoptotic processes results in a refinement of the neural circuitry, which is thought to strengthen the remaining functional connections and reduce competition from suboptimal associations. As a result, communication between distributed information systems is thought to be vastly improved. However, the hard-wiring of neural networks, while improving communication between distributed systems, has the added consequence of reducing the redundancy available in the brain.

Postmortem studies suggest that myelination begins during the second trimester of gestation and continues well into the third decade of life (Benes *et al.*, 1994; Yakovlev and Lecours, 1967). Importantly, these studies show that myelination does not occur concurrently in all brain regions: there is a graded progression of maturation from inferior to superior and posterior to anterior, with the cerebellum developing first and the frontal lobes last (Yakovlev and Lecours, 1967). Recent advances in brain imaging have allowed the in vivo study of these maturational changes in brain structure during adolescence, with the most consistent findings being a significant decline in global gray matter volume and a contrasting increase in global white matter volume (Giedd *et al.*, 1999; Reiss *et al.*, 1996; see also Ch. 2). Klingberg *et al.* (1999) used diffusion tensor imaging to examine axonal integrity in the frontal lobes of children and adults and found that white matter continues to increase into the second decade of life in this region. These changes appear to be regionally specific in that the white matter increase is located in the dorsal prefrontal cortex and not in the orbitofrontal region (Reiss *et al.*, 1996). However, automated voxel-based methods have suggested that white matter change during adolescence is seen most prominently in frontotemporal (specifically dorsal prefrontal–lateral temporal) and corticospinal pathways (Paus *et al.*, 1999). Of relevance, it is disruption in these frontotemporal pathways that is proposed to play a large role in the pathology of schizophrenia.

These white matter changes, particularly those identified by Paus and colleagues (1999), are consistent with reported findings of striatal gray matter volume loss over the same period. These contrasting maturational changes are thought to enhance neural transmission between the motor connections of the striatal pathway with the frontal cortex, allowing for greater top-down mediation of behavioral output (Sowell *et al.*, 1999). Refinement of gray matter structure also follows heterochronous development, occurring latest in the prefrontal and parietal lobes (Giedd *et al.*, 1999). This development is associated with "thinning" of the cortex, with reductions in gray matter most prominent in the dorsal, medial, and lateral regions of the frontal lobes during adolescence (Sowell *et al.*, 2001a, 2003). Despite the loss of tissue, net brain volume continues to increase over adolescence through a combination of regressive and progressive changes (Sowell *et al.*, 2001b). Synaptic pruning of inefficient or unused connections is thought to result in the shrinkage of gray matter, while progressive myelination of these same areas leads to enhanced communication between functionally distributed systems.

The magnitude of the maturational changes taking place during adolescence holds implications for the emergence of abnormal cognitive processing and behaviors during this time. Pruning of connections and maximal activation of frontal areas, along with their various functionally connected systems, means that aberrantly formed associations will likely come to prominence during the adolescent years. The suggestion that schizophrenia involves disruption within the frontotemporal–striatal system, with psychiatric symptoms arising late in adolescence, conforms to the notion that such behavioral abnormalities correspond to the anatomically related events that have been described above (Pantelis *et al.*, 2002). It is currently proposed that dysregulation of this developmental trajectory may actually be implicated in the emergence of symptoms, as individuals with schizophrenia fail to make age-appropriate cognitive gains (Wood and Pantelis, 2001).

Cognitive changes

Cognition generally refers to "knowing" or "thinking" and includes a broad range of abilities over and above what is thought of as intelligence. These include memory, attention, executive functions, plus less-obvious skills such as appreciating humour and perceiving another's motivation: skills that are often deficient in individuals with neurodevelopmental disorders such as schizophrenia. Basic cognitive processes are in place by early childhood, and it has been shown that certain abilities are inborn (Meltzoff and Moore, 1977). However, more complex behaviors develop at a slower rate and some functions are not mastered until late in adulthood. This holds implications for the observation of deficits in areas of higher-order functions as individuals enter the adolescent period. Studies of cognitive development tend to have proceeded with little attention to studies of brain development; however, given that the predominant brain regions developing during adolescence are the frontal lobes, it is sensible to examine the cognitive development of functions thought to be mediated by these regions. The frontal lobes have been given particular attention in the mediation of executive functions, that is, those interrelated skills required for successful independent, volitional behavior in response to novelty (Anderson, 1998). The functions subsumed under the executive umbrella include higher-order processes such as strategic planning, problem solving, inhibitory control, cognitive flexibility, abstract thinking, concept formation, working memory, and self-monitoring.

Cerebral organization and cognitive functioning models initially presented executive function as an adult capacity that reaches maturity during adolescence, approximating the stage of Piaget's predicted transition from concrete to formal operational thinking (Golden, 1981; Stuss, 1992; Travis, 1998). Research has now identified a stage-like sequence of executive function development characterized by "spurts" in executive abilities beginning from as young as 12 months of age, with the majority of functions coming "online" around the age of 8 (Ardila and Rosselli, 1994; Case, 1992; Luciana and Nelson, 1998). These higher-order processes are not homogeneous, however, and are thought to observe disparate developmental trajectories. Simple planning, attentional set-shifting and hypothesis testing are reportedly available to the child at an earlier stage than other abilities, including temporal ordering and complex strategy formation (Chelune and Baer, 1986; Espy, 1997; Luciana and Nelson, 1998; Stuss, 1992). The development of working memory capacity also follows a relatively slow but steady increase over the adolescent years and into adulthood (Luciana and Nelson, 1998). The verbal modality is thought to be slightly advanced in the amount of information it can hold online in an active buffer (Nichelli *et al.*, 2001). Cognitive theories of working memory systems propose that the ability to convert visuospatial information into phonological form actually develops during adolescence, and that this is the preferred way to encode information for temporary storage and manipulation (Hitch, 2002). As such, working memory abilities in both the verbal and the visuospatial modality are thought to develop in unison into the adult years.

A number of influential developmentally oriented studies have provided evidence to support the continuing development of executive functions into adolescence. Welsh and Pennington (1988) assessed 140 children and adults from ages 3 to 28 years on several executive tasks. The data supported sequential development of these skills over childhood and into adolescence. Performance on these tests was found to be quite independent from intelligence quotient (IQ) scores, and adult levels were reached sooner on simple planning and visual search tasks than in those measuring complex planning and verbal fluency. Levin *et al.* (1991) also administered a range of "executive" ability measures to a group of 52 normal children and adolescents. The sample was divided into three age bands: 7–8, 9–12, and 13–15 years, with gains across all tasks identified with increasing age. The improvements in performance were described as reflecting progress in concept formation, mental flexibility, and goal-setting skills through childhood. Scores on different measures also provided evidence for discrepant maturation of distinct abilities, with some skills reaching adult levels by 12 years of age, while others continued to show developmental trends into mid-adolescence. A large-scale developmental study by Anderson *et al.* (1995), involving 430 children aged 7–17 years, provided complementary findings to those presented above. The data indicated significant improvements in executive skills through middle to late childhood (7–11 years), with stabilization evident by mid-adolescence.

We have recently conducted a study (De Luca *et al.*, 2003) involving 193 individuals ranging in age from 8 to 64 years, investigating the development of executive functions across the lifespan, using the Cambridge Neuropsychological Test Automated Battery (CANTAB). In particular, we examined planning and organization, working memory and strategy formation, and attentional set-shifting. In our study, we demonstrated that performance on these tasks continues to develop throughout adolescence and is at its height between the ages of 20 and 29 years. Success on these tasks is thought to result at least in part from the achievement and maintenance of maximal short-term memory capacity in the 15–19 age range, since maturation of this "capacity resource" contributes to a greater ability to define and order a strategic plan (Hitch *et al.*, 2001). However, while increases in abilities such as memory span, inhibitory control, and speed of processing may allow for more efficient executive control, advances in the last have been dissociated from the maturation of these types of general, capacity-limited factor (Ridderinkhof and van der Molen, 1997).

In our study, attentional set-shifting ability was also tested using the intradimensional/extradimensional task from the CANTAB, which assesses the ability of an individual to establish the correct response set to positive and negative feedback, to reverse this rule, and later to shift this learning to new exemplars within a previously learned set. This measure of cognitive flexibility was found to follow a swifter maturational path, and performance on this task did not differentiate any of the groups (De Luca *et al.*, 2003), confirming documented adult levels of set-shifting competence in 8 and 10 year old children (Anderson *et al.*, 2001a; Chelune and Baer, 1986; Luciana and Nelson, 1998). This would suggest that the ability to adjust responses to feedback, and to shift them to new exemplars within a previously learned set, is an executive skill acquired early in development, indicating that the purported neural circuitry subserving this ability in the lateral and orbital prefrontal cortex is connected and activated earlier than other executive systems (Rezai *et al.*, 1993; Roberts *et al.*, 1998; Stuss and Benson, 1987). However, our use of an endpoint score for this task may have obscured subtle differences in performance. Previous research would suggest that children do in fact make a greater number of errors in learning a response set, but they do not differ in the number of trials necessary to advance at either level (Luciana and Nelson, 1998; Shanab and Yasin, 1979). Consequently, they can competently complete such tasks by responding to the absolute properties of the stimuli without relevant understanding of the underlying contingency being tested. Adolescents and adults, by comparison, are found to experience greater difficulty performing a shift in set because of their more profound understanding of the dimension characteristics of the task. Having learned the relevant dimension governing the response rule, their performance is potentially impeded as they are required to extinguish the original response set and transfer this learning to new exemplars (Owen *et al.*, 1993; Whitney and White, 1993). Indeed, patients with schizophrenia are seen to perseverate on previously learned sets and perform poorly on similar tests such as the Wisconsin Card Sorting Task. Their inability to dissociate from one paradigm and shift to a new exemplar highlights deficits in attentional control and, therefore, implicates dysfunction in the lateral and orbital frontal systems that mediate this function. It is interesting to note that this skill appears to be relatively unimpaired in first-episode schizophrenia, suggesting that these brain areas, which develop earlier in life, are in fact well connected and activated appropriately during development but may be affected later by the continued insult of acute psychotic episodes.

While the set-shifting component of the attentional system appears to develop relatively early in childhood, the literature suggests that other attentional processes, such as the ability to attend to meaningful stimuli and actively inhibit distractors, continue to improve during adolescence (Anderson et al., 2001a). Greater control in the triage of incoming information with internal needs and desires places less demand on the capacity-limited attentional system, which, in turn, results in the more efficient processing of relevant information. While attentional components are found to dissociate both anatomically and in terms of their maturational course, gradual increments in performance from 6 to 15 years of age have been found for a range of these skills across modalities (Anderson et al., 2001a).

As is the case with the development of executive abilities, the prolonged trajectory of attentional skills implies that deficits may not be obvious until later in development. Within a developmental framework, the cumulative effects of attention deficits, such as distractibility or the inability to shift-set, may have serious implications for the learning of new information and coordination of internal desires with external demands at a time when these skills appear to be critical to the success of the individual. In addition, impaired executive function will affect the adolescent's ability to plan homework or find classrooms, resulting in poorer scholastic performance over and above its effect on actual learning. These practical consequences highlight the dynamic interplay that exists between cognitive and psychological factors, and how cognitive inefficiencies that arise during adolescence, already a time of considerable emotional upheaval, feed feelings of personal inadequacy and disrupt the usual process of self-discovery. It is not surprising then that the current drive in the treatment of schizophrenia is to treat aggressively first-episode patients, both to prevent the purported neurotoxic effects of repeated acute episodes and to halt the snowballing effects of chronic illness and perceived personal failure.

Links between the emergence of cognitive skills and cerebral development

Much of the research on cognitive development and cerebral maturation fails to consider the dynamic interplay that occurs between the structural and functional advances of the developing brain. This is integral to an understanding of the normal capabilities and constraints of the individual across the lifespan, along with the consequences of aberrant development at different times along the maturational trajectory. Interesting parallels can be found in anatomical and intellectual development from childhood through to adolescence, and changes in brain structure centering on the frontal lobes have been implicated as the physiological substrate for development of executive functions during this time (Anderson, 1998; Casey *et al.*, 2000). Our findings of improved performance on tasks of working memory, strategic ability, planning, and goal setting correspond to the development of functional connections involving distributed systems of the frontal cortex. As stated above, the frontal lobes are one of the latest maturing areas of the brain, with both regressive events and myelination not fully active until the second decade of life, and continuing beyond early adulthood (Giedd *et al.*, 1999; Klingberg *et al.*, 1999; Luna and Sweeney, 2001). As such, executive skills are thought to become fully available to the individual once the anterior portions of the brain have matured, allowing for whole brain systems to be maximally activated.

Working memory, a higher-order capacity that peaks around 20–29 years of age, is one of the functions that are thought to be limited in the child as a result of the immaturity of a frontoparietal–limbic circuit. Functional imaging studies have been informative in identifying a distributed neural system involved in the ability to hold and manipulate information online in an active buffer. Several areas, including the dorsolateral and ventrolateral prefrontal cortex, premotor cortex, and the posterior parietal cortex, show increased activation on working memory tasks (Kwon *et al.*, 2002). The cingulate cortex and occipital areas are also considered to form part of the visuospatial working memory circuitry (Klingberg *et al.*, 2002; Rubia *et al.*, 2000). This distributed system is activated in both children and adults; however, research looking at the development of visuospatial working memory capacity have reported positive correlations between age and working memory-related brain activity in several frontal and parietal areas into adulthood (Klingberg *et al.*, 2002; Kwon *et al.*, 2002). In fact, Kwon *et al.* (2002) showed activation in areas correlating to a left-hemisphere phonological rehearsal system and a right-hemisphere-based visuospatial attentional system, suggesting concurrent development of verbal and visual-based working memory modalities. These findings correspond to Baddeley's behavioral findings, which led to the development of his influential cognitive model of working memory (Baddeley, 1998). Progression in functional capacities and activation of neural systems are thought to correspond to the physiological changes of synaptic pruning and myelination of frontal and parietal areas, as discussed above, which continue into the second decade of life and beyond (Giedd *et al.*, 1999; Paus *et al.*, 1999; Sowell *et al.*, 1999).

Similar correlations in the development of attentional processes and the circuitry purported to mediate these functions are found in the literature. Attentional processes are thought to be controlled by an anatomically distributed system primarily involving the prefrontal cortex, cingulate gyrus, and posterior parietal cortex (Heilman *et al.*, 1997; Koski and Petrides, 2002). Areas such as the thalamus and reticular activating system also form part of this system, although they are more involved with the arousal/motivation aspects of attention. Improvements in the volitionally driven skills of divided attention and inhibitory control during the adolescent period are thought to reflect maturation of the connections in this functional system. Myelination of the cingulate gyrus and prefrontal cortex does not fully occur until at least the second decade of life (Giedd *et al.*, 1999), and these are key areas involved in the integration of emotional/biological information with intentional, cognitively driven plans (Benes, 1989; Paus *et al.*, 2001). Conversely, reductions in the gray matter of the parietal and frontal cortices during late adolescence are considered a marker of the refinement of these anterior–posterior connections (Giedd *et al.*, 1999; Sowell *et al.*, 1999).

Functional magnetic resonance imaging (fMRI) studies looking at development of selective attention and response inhibition skills have reported variable findings, with both hypo- and hyperactivation found in these brain regions in children and adolescents compared with adults (see Ch. 3). A steady increase in activation of frontal, parietal, cingulate, striatal, and thalamic areas has been shown from childhood to adulthood for tasks assessing response inhibition (Luna and Sweeney, 2001). These studies suggested that the power of activation corresponds to the extent of functional maturation and, therefore, voluntary control over one's actions (Kwon *et al.*, 2002; Rubia *et al.*, 2000). In contrast, other fMRI studies have indicated that essentially the same circuits are activated in children and adults, although the activation is greater in children, both for the volume of cortex engaged to perform the task and the percentage signal change (Casey *et al.*, 2000). These authors argue that, taken together, the decrease in structural and functional areas mediating attentional processes suggests that improvements in these skills during adolescence correspond to anatomical maturation of frontal and parietal areas. These physiological processes are thought to strengthen and enhance stable connections, leading to a decrease in the brain tissue required to perform a task and removal of competing inputs that interfere with direct communication between these interconnected regions (Klingberg *et al.*, 2002). It is specifically these later maturing systems that are found to be dysfunctional in both first-episode and chronic schizophrenia; they will be discussed in greater detail in the section below dealing with schizophrenia.

Aberrations in development that impact on adolescence

The developing brain provides a model for the study of the impact of aberrations on normal development. A unique aspect of the immature brain is the state of flux of the young system, and its lack of fixed functional connections. Lesions of developmental origin, therefore, have a dynamic impact on further maturation, rather than the expected static losses that are seen with injury during adulthood. Proponents of the vulnerability theories of childhood insult hold that children present a greater risk for cognitive impairment as they can fail to acquire the skills necessary for new learning and the organization of information. In other words, early disruption to the brain impacts most significantly on the development of higher-order functions that rely on the intact primary processing of information and the integration of this knowledge through robust associations between distributed functional systems. This corresponds closely to the current models of schizophrenia, which hold that a developmental lesion that disrupts the initial formation of system connections is necessary to explain the myriad of deficits found in psychotic individuals.

Childhood injury is also distinct from similar lesions in adulthood in the observation of emerging deficits with age, or the notion of the child "growing into deficits." This extends from the fact that not all intellectual functions are fully mature in the child, such as executive functions, which follow a prolonged maturational trajectory into young adulthood (Anderson et al., 2001a; De Luca et al., 2003; Luciana and Nelson, 1998). Therefore, aberrations involving the anterior regions, which mediate these executive and other skills, will not be immediately visible following injury, as they are not yet available to the child. When these functions are due to come "online" later during adolescence, dysfunction in various systems arise, and this is observed as a widening gap in the performance of brain-damaged children compared with their peers (Anderson et al., 2001b).

Developmental lesions

Research on the impact of developmental lesions supports the protracted and distinct consequences of disruption to the developing neural system. Of the limited studies examining the outcome of frontal lesions in the young child, pervasive behavioral and social deficits have been reported that are of a similar nature to those seen in patients with schizophrenia. In line with the developmental perspective of frontal maturation, these deficits do not arise immediately following damage in all cases but become progressively more evident as the child ages (Eslinger et al., 1992; Marlowe, 1992). Many of the features are comparable to those described in adult patients, such as a lack of initiative, disorganization, irritability, emotional lability, and disinhibited behavior (Anderson et al., 1999; Eslinger and Damasio, 1985; Eslinger et al., 1992; Leduc et al., 1999). However, the severity of impairment appears to be greater in individuals who acquired lesions in childhood, and a distinct antisocial presentation is reported in studies with adult follow-up (Price et al., 1990). This is demonstrated as a failure to learn from experience, unresponsiveness to punishment, increasing disruptive and demanding behavior, a lack of expressed guilt and remorse, with some displaying verbal and physically abusive tendencies (Eslinger and Damasio, 1985; Eslinger et al., 1992; Marlowe, 1992). The distinctive feature that sets these individuals apart from sociopaths is their rather impulsive and child-like performance of morally sanctioned acts, and the transparency with which they attempt to cover up their indiscretions (Anderson et al., 1999). This is interpreted as a reflection of the lack of insight and immature development of executive skills in these individuals. It appears that damage to the anterior lobes early in life disrupts the application of socially appropriate skills in real-life situations and compromises the establishment of adaptive behavior, the acquisition of socially relevant knowledge, and the development of moral sensibilities (Anderson *et al.*, 1999; Eslinger *et al.*, 1992).

Studies addressing the cognitive development of children with early lesions support the notion that these individuals experience more global deficits because they fail to develop in a normal manner. In one of the first studies to look specifically at cognitive outcomes of children with early brain insult, Mateer (1990) found evidence of cognitive dysfunction, alongside intact or mildly depressed intellectual ability, consistent with adult patterns of impairment. A number of more recent studies have revealed a similar pattern of poor problem-solving skills, reduced planning and strategy use, and low self-monitoring in the adult survivors of early frontal lobe damage (Anderson, 1988; Anderson and Jacobs, 2004; Anderson *et al.*, 1999, 2000; Eslinger *et al.*, 1992, 1997, 1999; Marlowe, 1992). Eslinger and colleagues (1992) reported a pattern of delayed onset of impairments, with increasing difficulties identified as executive skills failed to "come online" and mature at critical stages throughout development. The progressive emergence of deficits as the child reaches adolescence is believed to result from the combined effects of the failure to make age-appropriate gains and the increasingly complex environmental demands placed on the individual approaching adulthood. Interestingly, similar impairments in both behavioral and cognitive domains have been described in many purported neurodevelopmental and acquired pediatric conditions, including autism (Happe and Frith, 1996), schizophrenia (Pantelis *et al.*, 2002), attention-deficit hyperactivity disorder (Barkley, 1996), head injury (Pentland *et al.*, 1998), and epilepsy (Anderson *et al.*, 2001b).

Schizophrenia

Schizophrenia is a mental illness of putative neurodevelopmental origin (Murray and Lewis, 1987; Weinberger, 1987) that represents an example of aberrant development in the regions underpinning executive function. Because of this, we can use it as a model to look at changes in cognitive performance over childhood/adolescence to help to understand the neural development of brain regions mediating these skills. One example of this is the retrospective study of Walker and colleagues (1994), who used family home movies to study the neurodevelopment of children who later developed schizophrenia. Although these movies demonstrated subtle abnormalities in motor function in early life, by the time of illness onset they were much less prominent; instead these young people displayed disturbances of behavior and cognitive function. This led the authors to propose a modular developmental trajectory for schizophrenia, in which neuromotor dysfunction is most pronounced in early childhood and late in life, whereas psychotic symptomatology is most pronounced in late adolescence and early adulthood. This hypothesis was based on the literature on normal brain development suggesting that different circuits within the brain are differentially activated at various points in the life course. During infant life, the fiber tracts between motor cortex and subcortical structures are highly myelinated and the regions they connect are more metabolically active than either frontal or limbic cortices. In contrast, during late adolescence and early adulthood, the motor cortex becomes less metabolically active relative to other cortical regions, in particular limbic and frontal regions. During this period, the frontal and limbic regions are the most active, and myelination of neural pathways linking limbic regions is completed. It is hypothesized that during this period of late adolescence/early adulthood the abnormalities of limbic interconnectivity are primarily expressed behaviorally in psychotic symptoms. This would also be consistent with the abnormalities in neuropsychological function, particularly those affecting executive functions.

However, what is also apparent and not fully explained by this model is that the early abnormalities are subtler than the later manifestations and are also less-prominent features of the disorder. We propose that brain plasticity and the normal maturational trajectory of various functions define the nature and extent of their impairment over the course of the disorder. In particular, we propose that functions that normally come online early in life (i.e. during infancy) such as sensory, motor, and basic memory functions, when the brain is more adaptable, show fewer deficits at illness onset than functions normally coming online in adolescence, such as attention, working memory, and executive functions (Pantelis et al., 2001, 2003; Wood and Pantelis, 2001).

Support for this model comes from our own work on the normal development of executive function, presented above. We have found that attentional set-shifting ability is fairly well established early in development but working memory skills are not fully developed until at least the age of 20 (Fig. 4.1) (De Luca et al., 2003; Manly et al., 2001; McKay et al., 1994; Rebok et al., 1997). Our model would suggest that those cognitive functions which emerge earlier (attentional set-shifting in this example) should be less compromised in schizophrenia than those that emerge later (such as working memory). Indeed, this is consistent with the available evidence. Using the set-shifting task from the CANTAB, Hutton et al. (1998) found that first-episode patients were relatively unimpaired in set-shifting ability, while Elliott and Sahakian (1995) found that patients with moderately severe schizophrenia showed a specific deficit in set-shifting ability because of a tendency to perseverate. Further, Pantelis and colleagues (1999) showed that a group of patients with very long-standing schizophrenia performed even more poorly; these chronic schizophrenia patients manifested perseverative responding and also had difficulty in generalizing

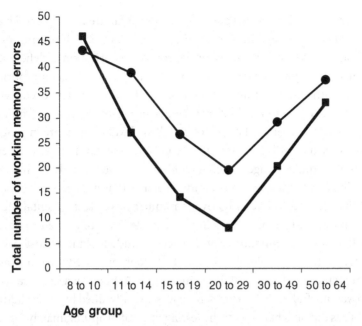

Fig. 4.1.   Total number of working memory errors as a function of age group for males (■) and females (●).

a rule that had been learned (representing failure at a simpler level of set-shifting ability). We have now examined patients very early in the course of the illness (mean illness duration of 95 days) and, despite obvious working memory difficulties, set-shifting ability is less impaired (Mahony *et al.*, 2001). Although there are no published longitudinal studies available using this task, these findings suggest that there is no or minimal impairment of set-shifting at first presentation, with a possible slow decline over continuing illness.

Working memory, a late emerging aspect of executive functions, is clearly impaired in patients with established illness (Pantelis *et al.*, 1997) and also at the first presentation of the disorder (Hutton *et al.*, 1998; Proffitt, 2001), with no progression over time (Proffitt, 2001). In addition, there are deficits in young people at ultra-high risk for psychosis prior to the onset of illness (Wood *et al.*, 2003), indicating that this ability has never been fully functional. Taken together with the relatively late development of spatial working memory in normal individuals (De Luca *et al.*, 2003), these findings suggest that functions which normally develop during the at-risk period for the development of psychosis manifest the most severe deficits.

An important aspect of the maturational changes in the expressed symptomatology of schizophrenia is the highly contested argument of whether impairments in cognitive functioning that present at the onset of psychosis represent a true regression in intellectual ability or, rather, a failure to progress developmentally. As stated at the beginning of this chapter, knowledge of the normal maturation of skills across the lifespan allows for improved categorization of deficits as a deterioration in functioning in contrast to a failure to make age-appropriate gains. Problems with extrapolating this information from study data occur when using age-corrected IQ values to look at changes in performance over childhood and early adolescence, a time when major cognitive developments are in progress. This method appears to disguise stability in performance over time, with equivalent raw scores at different ages placing children at opposite ends of the intelligence range. This view is supported by studies such as that of Jacobs et al. (2001), who found that despite decline in IQ over a number of years, the mental age scores of older children with spina bifida remained stable, reflecting a halt in development rather than a loss in function. Another recent study looking at post-psychotic IQ changes in patients with childhood-onset schizophrenia used raw scores as an index of dementia (Bedwell et al., 1999). Again, although there was a significant decline in post-psychotic full-scale IQ scores, the raw scores obtained by these children for all the subtests did not change over the testing interval of approximately 3 years. These findings provide strong support for the idea that the decline in IQ scores observed during adolescence for children with schizophrenia is the result of an inability to acquire new information and abilities (Bedwell et al., 1999) rather than reflecting cognitive deterioration. Such studies are important in addressing the ongoing debate about whether schizophrenia is a disorder of early or late neurodevelopment and/or involves neurodegenerative processes (Lieberman, 1999; Pantelis et al., 2003; Velakoulis et al., 2000).

Conclusions and future directions

The development of cognitive function is a lengthy process that is not complete until early adulthood, and during which different domains mature at different rates and times. An understanding of normal cognitive development is particularly important in order to appreciate the pattern of impairments in children and adolescents who suffer from illnesses of putative neurodevelopmental origin. In this chapter, we have discussed the gains in function made during adolescence, a time of major upheaval in behavioral and social domains. First, we reviewed the structural brain changes that occur during this time, after which we explored neuropsychological development, with a special focus on executive functions. The development of these skills is characterized by "spurts" beginning from as young as 12 months of age, with the majority of functions coming online around 8 years of age. However, evidence from our own and others' studies suggest that working memory in particular is slow to mature and may not reach maximal levels until early adulthood. We then discussed links between cognitive and cerebral development, with an emphasis on the impact of developmental lesions. Finally, we put forward a hypothesis explaining the neuropsychological deficits in schizophrenia as an interaction between the timing of illness onset and the timing of normal cognitive development. Specifically, we have suggested that cognitive functions that mature around the time when the illness first presents, such as working memory, are more impaired than those functions that mature earlier.

The study of cognitive development through adolescence is of great importance to our understanding of the neurobiology of disorders that first present at this time (Luna and Sweeney, 2001). However, in order to deepen our knowledge of the developmental period, it is now necessary to investigate how brain development is related to improvements in cognitive function. One way in which this is being done is through functional imaging (Casey *et al.*, 2000), which allows an exploration of the refinement of brain activation from childhood to adulthood. However, to date, these studies have been cross-sectional only, and longitudinal studies are now required to improve our understanding of the individual relationships between structural and functional brain development. In addition, our understanding of the distributed nature of the brain systems involved in higher-order cognition (Goldman-Rakic, 1988) means that our paradigms will need to explore the maturation of functional integration within these networks (Luna *et al.*, 2001).

Finally, we will need to explore new methods such as pharmacological MRI (Vaidya *et al.*, 1998) and carbon-13 spectroscopy (Shen *et al.*, 1999). Both techniques can potentially tell us about the development of neurotransmitter function in greater detail than has been possible up to now, allowing an understanding of adolescent development that will have enormous implications for the diagnosis and treatment of mental illness.

REFERENCES

Anderson, S. W., Bechara, A., Damasio, H., Tranel, D., Damasio, A. R. (1999). Impairment of social and moral behavior related to early damage in human prefrontal cortex. *Nat Neurosci* **2**: 1032–1037.

Anderson, S. W., Damasio, H., Tranel, D., Damasio, A. R. (2000). Long-term sequelae of prefrontal cortex damage acquired in early childhood. *Dev Neuropsychol* **18**: 281–296.

Anderson, V. (1988). Recovery of function in children: the myth of cerebral plasticity. In *Brain Impairment. Proceedings from the Thirteenth Annual Brain Impairment Conference*, ed. M. Matheson, H. Newman. Sydney: University of Sydney, pp. 223–247.

(1998). Assessing executive function in children: biological, psychological and developmental considerations. *Neuropsychol Rehab* **8**: 319–349.

Anderson, V., Jacobs, R. (2004). Frontal lobe damage in children: interruptions to normal development. In *Enfance and Neuropsychologie: Interface entre la Recherche et la Clinique*, ed. J.-P. Laurent. Quebec: Quebec University Press, in press.

Anderson, V., Lajoie, G., Bell, R. (1995). *Neuropsychological Assessment of the School-aged Child.* Department of Psychology, Melbourne: University of Melbourne.

Anderson, V. A., Anderson, P., Northam, E., Jacobs, R., Catroppa, C. (2001a). Development of executive functions through late childhood and adolescence in an Australian sample. *Dev Neuropsychol* 20: 385–406.

Anderson, V., Northam, E., Hendy, J., Wrennall, J. (2001b). *Developmental Neuropsychology.* Hove, UK: Psychology Press.

Ardila, A., Rosselli, M. (1994). Development of language, memory and visuospatial abilities in 5- to 12-year-old children using a neuropsychological battery. *Dev Neuropsychol* 10: 97–120.

Baddeley, A. (1998). Recent developments in working memory. *Curr Opin Neurol* 8: 234–238.

Barkley, R. A. (1996). Linkages between attention and executive functions. In *Attention, Memory and Executive Function*, ed. G. R. Lyon, A. Krasnegor. Baltimore, MD: Paul H. Brookes, pp. 307–326.

Bedwell, J. S., Keller, K., Smith, A. K., *et al.* (1999). Why does postpsychotic IQ decline in childhood-onset schizophrenia? *Am J Psychiatry* 156: 1996–1997.

Benes, F. M. (1989). Myelination of cortical–hippocampal relays during late adolescence. *Schizophr Bull* 15: 585–593.

Benes, F. M., Turtle, M., Khan, Y., Farol, P. (1994). Myelination of a key relay zone in the hippocampal formation occurs in the human brain during childhood, adolescence and adulthood. *Arch Gen Psychiatry* 51: 477–484.

Case, R. (1992). The role of the frontal lobes in the regulation of cognitive development. *Brain Cognit* 20: 51–73.

Casey, B. J., Giedd, J. N., Thomas, K. M. (2000). Structural and functional brain development and its relation to cognitive development. *Biol Psychiatry* 54: 241–257.

Chelune, G. J., Baer, R. (1986). Developmental norms of the Wisconsin Card Sorting Test. *J Clin Exp Neuropsychol* 8: 219–228.

Chugani, H., Phelps, M., Mazziotta, J. (1987). Positron emission tomography study of human brain functional development. *Ann Neurol* 22: 487–497.

De Luca, C. R., Wood, S. J., Anderson, V., *et al.* (2003). Normative data from the CANTAB. I: Development of executive function over the lifespan. *J Clin Exp Neuropsychol* 25: 242–254.

Dubas, J. (1991). Cognitive abilities and physical maturation. In *Encyclopedia of Adolescence*, Vol. 1, ed. R. Lerner *et al.* New York: Garland Publishing, pp. 133–138.

Elliott, R., Sahakian, B. J. (1995). The neuropsychology of schizophrenia: relations with clinical and neurobiological dimensions. *Psychol Med* 25: 581–594.

Eslinger, P. J., Damasio, A. R. (1985). Severe disturbance of higher cognition after bilateral frontal lobe ablation: Patient EVR. *Neurology* 35: 1731–1741.

Eslinger, P. J., Grattan, L. M., Damasio, H., Damasio, A. R. (1992). Developmental consequences of childhood frontal lobe damage. *Arch Neurol* 49: 764–769.

Eslinger, P., Biddle, K., Grattan, L. (1997). Cognitive and social development in children with prefrontal cortex lesions. In *Development of the Prefrontal Cortex: Evolution, Neurology, and Behavior*, ed. P. S. Goldman-Rakic. Baltimore, MD: Brookes, pp. 295–336.

Eslinger, P., Biddle, K., Pennington, B., Page, R. (1999). Cognitive and behavioral development up to 4 years after early right frontal lobe lesion. *Dev Neuropsychol* 15: 157–191.

Espy, K. (1997). The shape school: assessing executive function in preschool children. *Dev Neuropsychol* 13: 495–499.

Giedd, J. N., Blumenthal, J., Jeffries, N. O., *et al.* (1999). Brain development during childhood and adolescence: a longitudinal MRI study. *Nat Neurosci* 2: 861–863.

Golden, C. (1981). Luria Nebraska Children's Battery: theory and formulation. In *Neuropsychological Assessment of the School-aged Child*, ed. G. W. Hynd, J. E. Obzut. London: Grune and Stratton, pp. 277–302.

Goldman-Rakic, P. S. (1988). Topography of cognition: parallel distributed networks in primate association cortex. *Annu Rev Neurosci* 11: 137–156.

Happe, F., Frith, U. (1996). The neuropsychology of autism. *Brain* 119: 1377–1400.

Heilman, K., Valenstein, E., Watson, R. (1997). Disorders of attention. In *Contemporary Behavioral Neurology*, ed. M. Trimble, J. Cummings. London: Harcourt, pp. 127–138.

Hitch, G. J. (2002). Developmental changes in working memory: a multicomponent view. In *Lifespan Development of Human Memory*, ed. P. Graf, N. Ohta. Cambridge, MA: MIT Press, pp. 15–38.

Hitch, G. J., Towse, J., Hutton, U. (2001). What limits children's working memory span? Theoretical accounts and applications for scholastic development. *J Exp Psychol Gen* 130: 184–198.

Huttenlocher, P. (1984). Synapse elimination and plasticity in developing human cerebral cortex. *Am J Ment Defic* 88: 488–496.

Hutton, S. B., Puri, B. K., Duncan, L.-J., *et al.* (1998). Executive function in first-episode schizophrenia. *Psychol Med* 28: 463–473.

Jacobs, R., Northam, E., Anderson, V. (2001). Cognitive outcome in children with myelomeningocele and perinatal hydrocephalus. *J Dev Phys Disabil* 13: 389–405.

Klingberg, T., Vaidya, C. J., Gabrieli, J. D. E., Moseley, M. E., Hedehus, M. (1999). Myelination and organization of the frontal white matter in children: a diffusion tensor MRI study. *Neuroreport* 10: 2817–2821.

Klingberg, T., Forssberg, H., Westerberg, H. (2002). Increased brain activity in frontal and parietal cortex underlies the development of visuospatial working memory capacity during childhood. *J Cogn Neurosci* 14: 1–10.

Koski, L., Petrides, M. (2002). Distractibility after unilateral resections from the frontal and anterior cingulate cortex in humans. *Neuropsychologia* 40: 1059–1072.

Kwon, H., Reiss, A. L., Menon, V. (2002). Neural basis of protracted developmental changes in visuo-spatial working memory. *Proc Natl Acad Sci USA* 99: 13336–13341.

Leduc, M., Herron, J. E., Greenberg, D. R., Eslinger, P. J., Grattan, L. M. (1999). Impaired awareness of social and emotional competencies following orbital frontal lobe damage. *Brain Cogn* 40: 174–177.

Levin, H. S., Culhane, K. A., Hartmann, J., *et al.* (1991). Developmental changes in performance on tests of purported frontal lobe functioning. *Dev Neuropsychol* 7: 377–395.

Lieberman, J. A. (1999). Is schizophrenia a neurodegenerative disorder? A clinical and neurobiological perspective. *Biol Psychiatry* 46: 729–739.

Luciana, M., Nelson, C. A. (1998). The functional emergence of prefrontally guided working memory systems in four- to eight-year-old children. *Neuropsychologia* **36**: 273–293.

Luna, B., Sweeney, J. A. (2001). Studies of brain and cognitive maturation through childhood and adolescence: a strategy for testing neurodevelopmental hypotheses. *Schizophr Bull* **27**: 443–455.

Luna, B., Thulborn, K. R., Munoz, D. P., *et al.* (2001). Maturation of widely distributed brain function subserves cognitive development. *NeuroImage* **13**: 786–793.

Mahony, K., Pantelis, C., Proffitt, T., *et al.* (2001). Comparison of set-shifting ability in patients with first-episode psychosis and chronic schizophrenia. *Schizophr Res* **49**: 114–115.

Manly, T., Anderson, V., Nimmo-Smith, I., *et al.* (2001). The differential assessment of children's attention: The Test of Everyday Attention for Children (TEA-Ch). Normative sample and ADHD performance. *J Child Psychol Psychiatry* **42**: 1065–1087.

Marlowe, W. B. (1992). The impact of a right prefrontal lesion on the developing brain. *Brain Cogn* **20**: 205–213.

Mateer, C. A. (1990). Cognitive and behavioral sequalae of face and forehead injury in childhood. *J Clin Exp Neuropsychol* **12**: 95.

McKay, K., Halperin, J., Schwartz, S., Sharma, V. (1994). Developmental analysis of three aspects of information processing: sustained attention, selective attention and response organization. *Dev Neuropsychol* **10**: 121–132.

Meltzoff, A., Moore, M. (1977). Imitation of facial and manual gestures by human neonates. *Science* **198**: 74–78.

Murray, R. M., Lewis, S. (1987). Is schizophrenia a neurodevelopmental disorder? [Editorial] *Br Med J* **295**: 681–682.

Nichelli, F., Bulgheroni, S., Riva, D. (2001). Developmental patterns of verbal and visuospatial spans. *Neurol Sci* **22**: 377–384.

Owen, A. M., Roberts, A., Hodges, J., *et al.* (1993). Contrasting mechanisms of impaired attentional set-shifting in patients with frontal lobe damage or Parkinson's disease. *Brain* **116**: 1159–1175.

Pantelis, C., Barnes, T. R., Nelson, H. E., *et al.* (1997). Frontal-striatal cognitive deficits in patients with chronic schizophrenia. *Brain* **120**: 1823–1843.

Pantelis, C., Barber, F., Barnes, T. R., *et al.* (1999). Comparison of set-shifting ability in patients with chronic schizophrenia and frontal lobe damage. *Schizophr Res* **37**: 251–270.

Pantelis, C., Yücel, M., Wood, S. J., McGorry, P. D., Velakoulis, D. (2001). The timing and functional consequences of structural brain abnormalities in schizophrenia. *NeuroSci News* **4**: 36–46.

Pantelis, C., Wood, S. J., Maruff, P. (2002). Schizophrenia. In *Cognitive Deficits in Brain Disorders*, ed. A. M. Owen, J. Harrison. London: Martin Dunitz, pp. 217–248.

Pantelis, C., Yücel, M., Wood, S. J., McGorry, P. D., Velakoulis, D. (2003). Early and late neurodevelopmental disturbances in schizophrenia and their functional consequences. *Aust NZ J Psychiatry* **37**: 399–406.

Paus, T., Zijdenbos, A., Worsley, K., *et al.* (1999). Structural maturation of neural pathways in children and adolescents: in vivo study. *Science* **283**: 1908–1911.

Paus, T., Collins, D. L., Evans, A. C., *et al.* (2001). Maturation of white matter in the human brain: a review of magnetic resonance studies. *Brain Res Bull* **54**: 255–266.

Pentland, L., Todd, J. A., Anderson, V. (1998). The impact of head injury severity on planning ability in adolescence: a functional analysis. *Neuropsychol Rehab* **8**: 301–317.

Petersen, A. (1998). Adolescence. In *Behavioral Medicine and Women: A Comprehensive Handbook*, ed. E. Blechman, K. Brownell. New York: Guilford Press, pp. 45–50.

Piaget, J. (1965). *Moral Judgment of the Child.* New York: Free Press.

Price, B. H., Daffner, K. R., Stowe, R. M., Mesulam, M. M. (1990). The compartmental learning disabilities of early frontal lobe damage. *Brain* **113**: 1383–1393.

Proffitt, T. (2001). The stability of spatial working memory and problem solving deficits in first-episode psychosis and established psychotic illness. Ph.D. Thesis, University of Melbourne, Melbourne.

Rakic, P., Bourgeois, J.-P., Goldman-Rakic, P. S. (1994). Synaptic development of the cerebral cortex: implications for learning, memory and mental illness. In *Progress in Brain Research, The Self-organizing Brain: From Growth Cones to Functional Networks*, Vol. 102, ed. J. van Pelt, M. Corner, H. B. Uylings, F. Lopes de Silva. Amsterdam: Elsevier, pp. 227–243.

Rebok, G., Smith, C., Pascualvaca, D., *et al.* (1997). Developmental changes in attentional performance in urban children from eight to thirteen years. *Child Neuropsychol* **3**: 47–60.

Reiss, A. L., Abrams, M. T., Singer, H. S., Ross, J. L., Denckla, M. B. (1996). Brain development, gender and IQ in children: a volumetric imaging study. *Brain* **119**: 1763–1774.

Rezai, K., Andreasen, N. C., Alliger, R. J., *et al.* (1993). The neuropsychology of the prefrontal cortex. *Arch Neurol* **50**: 636–642.

Ridderinkhof, K., van der Molen, M. (1997). Mental resources, processing speed and inhibitory control: a developmental perspective. *Biol Psychol* **45**: 241–261.

Roberts, A., Robbins, T. W., Weiskrantz, L. (1998). Discussions and conclusions. In *The Prefrontal Cortex: Executive and Cognitive functions*, ed. A. Roberts, T. W. Robbins, L. Weiskrantz. Oxford: Oxford University Press, pp. 221–242.

Rubia, K., Overmeyer, S., Taylor, E., *et al.* (2000). Functional frontalisation with age: mapping neurodevelopmental trajectories with fMRI. *Neurosci Biobehav Rev* **24**: 13–19.

Shanab, M., Yasin, A. (1979). Intradimensional and extradimensional shifts by Jordanian students. *J Gen Psychol* **100**: 199–213.

Shen, J., Petersen, K. F., Behar, K. L., *et al.* (1999). Determination of the rate of the glutamate/glutamine cycle in the human brain by *in vivo* ^{13}C NMR. *Proc Natl Acad Sci USA* **96**: 8235–8340.

Sowell, E. R., Thompson, P. M., Holmes, C., Jernigan, T. L., Toga, A. (1999). In vivo evidence for post-adolescent brain maturation in frontal and striatal regions. *Nat Neurosci* **2**: 859–861.

Sowell, E. R., Thompson, P. M., Tessner, K. D., Toga, A. (2001a). Mapping continued brain growth and gray matter density reduction in dorsal frontal cortex: inverse relationships during postadolescent brain maturation. *J Neurosci* **21**: 8819–8829.

Sowell, E. R., Delis, D., Stiles, J., Jernigan, T. L. (2001b). Improved memory functioning and frontal lobe maturation between childhood and adolescence: a structural MRI study. *J Int Neuropsychol Soc* **7**: 312–322.

Sowell, E. R., Peterson, B. S., Thompson, P. M., *et al.* (2003). Mapping cortical change across the human life span. *Nat Neurosci* **6**: 309–315.

Spear, L. (2000). The adolescent brain and age-related behavioral manifestation. *Neurosci Biobehav Rev* **24**: 417–463.

Stuss, D. T. (1992). Biological and psychological development of executive functions. *Brain Cogn* **20**: 8–23.

Stuss, D. T., Benson, D. (1987). The frontal lobes and control of cognition and memory. In *The Frontal Lobes Revisited*, ed. E. Perecman. New York: Irbn Press, pp. 141–154.

Travis, F. (1998). Cortical and cognitive development in 4th, 8th and 12th grade students: the contribution of speed of processing and executive function to cognitive development. *Biol Psychol* **48**: 37–56.

Vaidya, C., Austin, G., Kirkorian, G., *et al.* (1998). Selective effects of methylphenidate in attention deficit hyperactivity disorder: a functional magnetic resonance study. *Proc Natl Acad Sci* **95**: 14494–14499.

Velakoulis, D., Wood, S. J., McGorry, P. D., Pantelis, C. (2000). Evidence for progression of brain structural abnormalities in schizophrenia: beyond the neurodevelopmental model. *Aust NZ J Psychiatry* **34**(Suppl.): S113–S126.

Walker, E., Savoie, T., Davis, D. (1994). Neuromotor precursors of schizophrenia. *Schizophr Bull* **20**: 441–451.

Weinberger, D. R. (1987). Implications of normal brain development for the pathogenesis of schizophrenia. *Arch Gen Psychiatry* **44**: 660–669.

Welsh, M. C., Pennington, B. F. (1988). Assessing frontal lobe functioning in children: views from developmental psychology. *Dev Psychol* **4**: 199–230.

Whitney, L., White, K. (1993). Dimensional shift and the transfer of attention. *Q J Exp Psychol* **46B**: 225–252.

Wood, S. J., Pantelis, C. (2001). Does a neurodevelopmental lesion involving the hippocampus explain memory dysfunction in schizophrenia? *Z Neuropsychol* **12**: 61–67.

Wood, S. J., Pantelis, C., Proffitt, T., *et al.* (2003). Spatial working memory ability is a marker of risk-for-psychosis. *Psychol Med* **33**: 1239–1247.

Yakovlev, P., Lecours, A. (1967). The myelogenetic cycles of regional maturation of the brain. In *Regional Development of the Brain in Early Life*, ed. A. Minkowski. Oxford: Blackwell, pp. 3–70.

5

Brain plasticity and long-term function after early cerebral insult: the example of very preterm birth

Matthew Allin, Chiara Nosarti, Larry Rifkin, and Robin M. Murray

Institute of Psychiatry, King's College, London, UK

Plastic: . . . easily influenced; impressionable . . . capable of being moulded or formed.

Collins Concise English Dictionary

Plasticity is an important phenomenon of vertebrate nervous systems throughout life and is an adaptation that allows an organism to adjust its behavior so as to deal with changes in its environment. In young animals, where both brain and behavior are rapidly changing as the animal grows, plasticity is particularly marked. In our own species, with our long period of postnatal development, plasticity allows for the experience-dependent tuning of neural networks that is required for the acquisition of complex behaviors such as our language and social interaction (Johnson, 2001). This chapter will be concerned with developmental plasticity rather than adult plasticity – indeed there is some evidence that these may have different underlying mechanisms (Linkenhoker and Knudsen, 2002). We will discuss the recovery, or sparing, of functions and the reorganization of brain structure that occurs as a consequence of early brain injury, using the example of preterm birth. This is of interest in the context of this book because of the neurodevelopmental theory of schizophrenia (Murray and Lewis, 1987; Weinberger, 1987) and of the link between obstetric complications and schizophrenia (Cannon *et al.*, 2002; Lewis and Murray, 1987; Lewis *et al.*, 1989).

A brief history of plasticity

The increased capacity of the immature brain to be 'moulded or formed' is part of everyday experience. For example, as most of us can attest, many schoolchildren and most adults find learning a second language very difficult. Those who

Neurodevelopment and Schizophrenia, ed. Matcheri S. Keshavan *et al.* Published by Cambridge University Press. © Cambridge University Press 2004.

grew up in a bilingual environment, by comparison, have no trouble speaking two languages fluently since they were exposed to both early in life, at a time when their brains were more plastic. This period of plasticity for language acquisition is relatively brief: infants respond to phonemes from widely disparate languages, but this ability begins to decline once they pass their first birthday, and they acquire a preference for the phonemes of their parents' language (Kolb, 1989). The "get them young" principle has also been applied to learning a musical instrument; for example, the intensive "Suzuki method" of teaching the violin starts in early childhood, the earlier the better (motto: "classical music from age zero").

This idea of a "critical period" for learning has caused some parents to play Mozart to their infants, both pre- and postnatally (Jones and Zigler, 2002). It will be interesting to see whether this leads to a cohort of gifted composers in the next two decades, since it is said that Mozart himself ". . . spent much time at the clavier, picking out thirds . . ." from the age of 3. Whether or not this curious experiment of fashion has any such effects, there is evidence to suggest that such early learning alters the brain in measurable ways. For example, Pantev et al. (1998) found that auditory cortex activation in response to the sound of a piano was greater in pianists who had started playing before they were 9 years old. Learning to play after this age did not have this effect. Early experience may also alter the structure of the brain, in a way that is gross enough to be visible on magnetic resonance imaging (MRI) scans later in life. For example Castro-Caldas et al. (1998) showed that the brains of those who learned to read and write in childhood are structurally different from those who did not (see also Frith, 1998).

The concept of "sensitive periods" in development dates back to Stockard's experiments in the 1920s in which he showed that embryos were better able to withstand hypoxia at some stages of development than at others. Wiesel and Hubel (1963) developed this concept in their classic experiments on the visual systems of cats. Kittens deprived of the use of one eye lost the pattern of ocular dominance columns in their visual cortex; adult cats do not reorganize their brains in this way. Similar results are found in many other experimental models (Linkenhoker and Knudsen, 2002). Different functions, and the areas of the brain that support them, mature at different rates and come "online" at different times; they may, therefore, have different "critical periods." For example, the acquisition of eye movement control in humans takes place during the first 6 months of life and may depend on the functional maturation of the parietal cortex (Johnson, 2001). At the other end of the scale, there is evidence for a late period for language acquisition, in adolescence, which may represent the fine tuning of frontal cortex and frontostriatal connections (Grimshaw et al., 1998; Sowell et al., 1999).

Plasticity after brain injury

The developmental plasticity of the young brain means that the effects of brain injuries in infancy and childhood are different to the effects of an equivalent injury in adulthood. One of the first scientific observations of this phenomenon was made by the nineteenth century surgeon, neurologist, and anthropologist Paul Broca (whose own brain has no further capacity for plasticity, residing as it does in a jar in the Musee de l'Homme in Paris). In 1863, Broca famously identified the area of left inferior frontal cortex that is necessary for the production of speech: if damaged by a stroke or other insult, the result would be expressive dysphasia. However, Broca also observed that if this area of the left hemisphere was damaged early in life, speech could be preserved. He suggested that in this case expressive language function could be taken over by the right hemisphere: the brain could remodel itself if the injury occurred sufficiently early in development. More recent research bears this out, suggesting that there is good functional recovery of language when brain damage is sustained to the left hemisphere in infancy. If the injury is sustained in middle childhood, however, adult-like aphasic symptoms occur (Hecaen, 1983).

It is now clear that the immature brain is capable of extensive reorganization, with preservation of function in the face of injury (see review by Payne and Lomber, 2001). This was elaborated in the 1930s by Margaret Kennard (1936) and became known as the Kennard principle, which states that the earlier in development the brain is damaged the less severe is the resulting behavioral disturbance (Kolb, 1989). This sparing of function could be the result of several processes: the recruitment of pre-existing alternative synaptic connections and axonal pathways, the development of new pathways so that the brain is 'rewired' (Elbert *et al.*, 2001; Kolk, 2000), or the learning of alternative cognitive strategies. There is some evidence for all three possibilities. Interestingly, the behavioral disturbances can also be mitigated somewhat in experimental animals by increasing the richness of the environment in which they are reared (Kolb, 1989; Kolb and Whishaw, 1989). The drive towards sparing functions is clearly a very strong one. Even children born with very little cerebral cortex as a result of hydranencephaly can demonstrate some behaviors and may be able to recognize faces even when primary visual (occipital) cortex is not present (Shewmon *et al.*, 1999).

However, there are some exceptions to the Kennard principle. For example, Goldman (1971) reported that frontal cortex lesions in infant monkeys had little effect on behavior initially but produced deleterious effects on behavior later in life, as the frontal cortex matured. Sams-Dodd *et al.* (1997) subjected newborn rats to lesions of the hippocampus. Again, these rats behaved apparently normally initially, but their behavior became grossly disturbed once they reached maturity. In humans, Anderson *et al.* (1999) studied two young adults who received focal non-progressive prefrontal damage before 16 months of age. These individuals showed no behavioral abnormalities up to the age of 3 years but had severely impaired social behavior despite normal basic cognitive abilities later on in life. Therefore, it seems that the very plasticity that enables the young brain to overcome injury so impressively, to reorganize its structure, and spare its essential functions may have an adverse effect on later development. The neurodevelopmental hypothesis of the etiology of schizophrenia postulates that a brain which is in some way abnormally "set up" as a result of an early insult may start to exhibit functional impairments later in life, particularly during the period of brain maturation and acquisition of adult cognitive capabilities in adolescence and young adulthood (Allin and Murray, 2002; Murray and Lewis, 1987; Weinberger, 1987). To examine these issues further, we have been studying a cohort of individuals who were subjected to risk of brain injuries around the time of birth as a result of being born preterm.

The example of very preterm birth

From the public health point of view, one of the most important challenges to early brain plasticity comes from preterm birth. Indeed, with the rapid advances in neonatal care, ever more and ever smaller babies are being rescued. They are at great risk of brain injury as a result of being born in an immature state, and their resilience is tested to the limit in the first few weeks of life. Unfortunately, relatively little is known about the long-term consequences of this. Do such individuals grow into adolescents and adults still showing the neuropsychological scars of their preterm birth?

The University College Hospital London study

We have been carrying out a longitudinal study of the consequences of preterm birth in collaboration with the University College Hospital London (UCHL) Department of Neonatal Paediatrics. This study combines detailed assessments of function from the first days of life, through childhood, and into adolescence, together with assessment of brain anatomy. In 1979–81, 172 infants born before 33 weeks of gestation (which we shall define as very preterm [VPT]) and admitted consecutively to the neonatal unit of UCHL within 5 days of birth survived and were discharged. Of this cohort, four died within 24 months; the remaining 168 were enrolled for long-term follow-up.

Follow-up

Prospective assessments of neurological and cognitive status of these children were carried out at 1, 4, and 8 years. At 14–15 years, 163 (97%) individuals were traced, including 16 who were living abroad. Of the 147 living in the UK, 118 (80%) agreed to attend for assessment. The cohort members who were unavailable for investigation did not differ from those studied in birth weight, gestational age at birth, sex ratio, mode of delivery, condition at birth, the need for mechanical ventilation, or neonatal cranial ultrasonographic findings. At 18 years, 102 of the VPT subjects were assessed again.

Patterns of perinatal brain injury

Being born before 33 weeks of gestation pitches a developmentally very immature infant into a hostile world. There they are prey to infections, which their immune systems are ill equipped to fight off. Their lungs are often immature, and they are unable to take in as much oxygen as they need. As a result, they frequently need supplementary oxygen, and even mechanical ventilation. It is difficult to provide them with sufficient nutrition. Their brains contain immature and delicate blood vessels, particularly in the remnants of their germinal matrix, and they do not autoregulate their cerebral blood flow effectively. Hypoxia, along with unprotected swings in systemic (and, therefore, cerebral) blood pressure, may cause these fragile blood vessels to break (Hoon, 1995; Rosenbloom and Sullivan, 1996).

Several patterns of brain lesions are thus associated with preterm birth. Hemorrhage may occur from immature vessels in the germinal matrix (germinal matrix hemorrhage [GMH]). This is the region adjacent to the ventricles that produces the new neurons that migrate out, along highways made of radial glia, to form the layers of the cerebral cortex. By 33 gestational weeks, the germinal matrix has largely involuted, but remnants of it are still present, particularly around the frontal horns of the lateral ventricles. GMH may also involve the ventricles (intraventricular hemorrhage [IVH]). These bleeds may also be associated with periventricular hemorrhagic infarction (PHI) of white matter in a localized and usually asymmetric distribution (Volpe, 1998). Diffuse white matter damage is also common and occurs adjacent to the ventricles (periventricular leukomalacia [PVL]) (Paneth et al., 1994). PVL is a necrotic lesion, causing the death of axons and their developing oligodendrocytes. It, therefore, also leads to incomplete and/or delayed myelination (Volpe, 1998) and is the lesion most likely to be associated with severe handicap – predominantly cerebral palsy. In addition to these lesions, vulnerable groups of neurons, which include those undergoing active mitosis or migration and those in an immature state of differentiation such as oligodendrocyte precursors, may be adversely, and diffusely, affected (Back et al., 2001, 2002; Johnston, 1998). The postmortem studies of Marin-Padilla (1996, 1997, 1999) have demonstrated that even localized lesions in the preterm brain can cause distant alterations of cell structure, dendritic arborization, and connectivity. So all these lesions may be expected to have both localized and diffuse effects on brain structure.

The UCHL VPT subjects were among the first infants to have neonatal ultrasound brain scanning performed, using relatively crude linear array apparatus. Even this imaging technique, with its relatively poor spatial resolution, showed a high prevalence of brain lesions: 43% had abnormal cranial ultrasound scans (Stewart *et al.*, 1983). A follow-up study by Roth *et al.* (1993) of 206 VPT infants reported the most frequently observed abnormality to be uncomplicated periventricular hemorrhage (PVH), which was present in 55 infants (27%). The next most common abnormality was ventricular dilatation, present in 21 infants (10%). In 13 of these infants, the dilatation had resolved on ultrasound by the time of discharge from the neonatal unit. Five infants developed hydrocephalus, and three of these required ventriculoperitoneal shunting. Thirteen (6%) had ultrasonographic evidence of cerebral atrophy. This was localized and associated with intraparenchymal PVH in seven infants but was more diffuse in six infants, in whom it was associated with PVH or cystic PVL. So, brain injuries are clearly common in VPT infants, but until recently it was not clear whether VPT individuals who survive the perinatal period continue to show both focal and diffuse abnormalities of brain structure later in life.

Can the sequelae of preterm birth still be seen in the brains of adolescents?

The relatively crude imaging resolution provided by ultrasound had demonstrated a significant amount of brain pathology at birth in the UCHL VPT cohort. However, some of these abnormalities had apparently resolved at the time of discharge, and the extent to which the brain damage suffered by these infants resulted in permanent change in brain structure was unclear. Therefore, at follow-up at 14–15 years, structural magnetic resonance imaging (MRI) of the brain was performed on all the participating VPT subjects. Stewart *et al.* (1999) reported on 72 VPT subjects and 21 full-term controls. The scans were "blindly" rated according to a structured format by two neuroradiologists. The scans were classified as normal (no detected abnormality), equivocal (negligible ventricular dilatation, or negligible thinning of the corpus callosum, or an isolated white matter hyperintensity), or abnormal (more than one parenchymal lesion plus definite ventricular dilatation, or definite thinning or atrophy of the corpus callosum plus reduced white matter or cortical volume plus multiple areas of white matter signal changes, or intraparenchymal cysts).

Only 24% of the scans of these VPT adolescents were rated as normal; 21% were equivocal and 56% abnormal. The equivalent percentages for the controls were 71% normal, 24% equivocal and 5% abnormal. In those preterm individuals with an MRI scan classified as abnormal, ventricular dilatation was observed in 80%, posterior trigonal dilatation in 73%, thinning of the corpus callosum (particularly involving the splenium) in 65%, abnormal white matter signal in 45%, and decreased white matter volume in 25%. Ventricular dilatation and thinning of the corpus callosum were correlated with each other and with other brain lesions and were considered to be markers of hypoxic–ischemic damage. The white matter signal abnormalities were thought to reflect scattered patchy gliosis secondary to ischemic damage (Hope *et al.*, 1988). In addition to these qualitative assessments of MRI scans, the volumes of the whole brain and of various brain regions and structures were determined using the Cavalieri stereological method, supported by the MEASURE software package (Johns Hopkins University, Baltimore, USA). The VPT subjects showed a 6.0% decrease in whole brain volume and a 11.8% decrease in total cortical gray matter volume. They also had a 42.0% increase in the size of the lateral ventricles. Those VPT adolescents who had experienced PVH in the neonatal period had a mean ventricular size twice as large as those who did not, indicating that these changes were the sequelae of the early damage. Additionally, those who had PVH and/or ventricular enlargement on neonatal ultrasound were especially likely to have decreased white matter volumes (Nosarti *et al.*, 2002). This is in agreement with Kuban *et al.* (1999), who found that both IVH and ventriculomegaly were powerful predictors of white matter damage in the first few weeks of life. Nosarti *et al.* (2002) also found a positive correlation between white matter volume and gestational age: the more immature the infant, the greater the damage to the white matter. This may be a reflection of the developmental vulnerability of white matter between 24 and 32 gestational weeks, when oligodendrocyte progenitors are immature and vulnerable to hypoxic injury (Back *et al.*, 2001, 2002; du Plessis and Volpe, 2002). Damage to these cell populations may disrupt the wave of white matter myelination, which normally rapidly increases after 29 weeks of gestation (Kinney *et al.*, 1988), leading to a reduction of white matter (and also possibly to an increase in ventricular volume).

In addition, the volumes of several brain structures were measured. VPT subjects had reduced volumes of left and right hippocampus, independent of overall brain volume reduction (Nosarti *et al.*, 2002). These findings are likely to be caused by hypoxic–ischemic damage (Kuchna, 1994; Mallard *et al.*, 1999). The volume of the cerebellum was also significantly smaller in VPT adolescents, again independent of total brain volume (Allin *et al.*, 2001). This may reflect damage to cerebellar granule cells at a sensitive period in their development, when they are actively dividing and migrating (Johnston, 1998; Sohma *et al.*, 1995). VPT individuals also had smaller corpora callosa, particularly in the posterior portion (the splenium) (Nosarti *et al.*, 2001a).

What are the consequences of persisting brain abnormality?

In the follow-up assessments of the UCHL VPT cohort, assessments were made of neurological, neuropsychological, and behavioral function. Some of these results are summarized below. In general, the VPT individuals showed good functional compensation in the face of abnormal brain structure, as might be predicted to be the result of a plastic response to early injury. However, there are some areas where function was compromised, sometimes in subtle ways, and there is evidence that VPT individuals are more likely to fail to match the educational performance of their term-born peers (Hadders-Algra *et al.*, 1988; Hall *et al.*, 1995; Msall *et al.*, 1998; Snider, 1998). They are more likely to be considered "clumsy" than their term-born classmates (Goyen *et al.*, 1998; Luoma *et al.*, 1998), a finding that has been termed "developmental coordination disorder" by some authors (Huh *et al.*, 1998).

Neurology

At 1 year of age, 10% of the UCHL cohort had minor neurological impairments not sufficient to cause disability, and 11% had major impairments with concomitant disability (Stewart *et al.*, 1989). The proportion of children in the cohort who showed major neurological impairments remained relatively constant at both 4 (15%) and 8 (12%) years, in agreement with other studies (Tin *et al.*, 1997). Ultrasound evidence of white matter damage, ventricular dilatation, or hydrocephalus were powerful predictors of major disability at 1, 4 and 8 years (Costello *et al.*, 1988; Roth *et al.*, 1993; Stewart *et al.*, 1983).

In contrast to the relative stability of major abnormalities, "minor" abnormalities increased in prevalence from 10% at age 1 to 23% at 8 years of age (Roth *et al.*, 1994). By the age of 14 years, 66% of the cohort had an abnormal or equivocal neurological examination (Stewart *et al.*, 1999). This may be because the range of motor skills that normal individuals can perform (and which can, therefore, be tested for) increases with age. An alternative explanation is that lesions of the brain acquired early in development may have a more significant deleterious effect when the affected neuronal systems reach developmental maturity, as discussed above (Goldman, 1971; Sams-Dodd *et al.*, 1997; see Ch. 4).

Neuropsychology

The mean full-scale intelligence quotient (IQ) of the VPT subjects was well within the normal range at 8 years, indicating that neural plasticity had succeeded in preserving function in spite of the abnormalities of brain structure reported above. However, evidence of more subtle deficits was present. Half of the VPT subjects showed neuropsychological evidence of poor interhemispheric interaction, and this was associated with poorer school performance (Stewart *et al.*, 1983). On initial investigation at 15 years, the VPT subjects were significantly impaired relative to controls on only two measures of cognitive function: cognitive flexibility and phonemic verbal fluency (Rushe *et al.*, 2001). Naming, spelling, IQ, visuomotor function, verbal memory, and visuospatial memory were not significantly impaired.

Behavior

Behavior was assessed at 15 years, using the Rutter behavioral scale (Rutter *et al.*, 1981) and the social adjustment scale of Cannon-Spoor and colleagues (1982). Behavioral abnormalities were significantly increased only in those preterm subjects with abnormal MRI scans. Social adjustment problems were increased in subjects with equivocal and abnormal MRI. Those with normal MRI scans showed similar social adjustment to controls. At 18 years, there was an increased prevalence of psychiatric illness in the VPT subjects compared with controls, but this difference did not reach statistical significance (Rooney *et al.*, 2001). In particular, there was a 2% rate of psychotic disorder in the VPT group, which exceeds the expected 0.2% population prevalence for this age. This result should be interpreted with caution in this relatively small study group but is of obvious interest in the context of the neurodevelopmental theory of schizophrenia.

The link between brain structure and brain function

In spite of the high prevalence of structural brain abnormality, the association between this and performance on specific cognitive and neurological tests is not straightforward. For example, Stewart *et al.* (1999) reported that the cognitive performance of the VPT subjects was unrelated to the presence of gross brain abnormality, except that reading age was lower in those preterm individuals with abnormal scans. The quantitative MRI results above were analyzed in relation to neurodevelopmental outcome at 14–15 years by Nosarti *et al.* (2002). They could not find a relationship between neurodevelopmental status and measures of brain structure, including whole brain volume, lateral ventricular volume, total gray and white matter volumes, and hippocampal volume. This may be because the presence of an early brain injury had altered brain structure such that functions had become aberrantly mapped in the brain (Moses and Stiles, 2002). As a result, the normal adult structure–function relationship may no longer hold.

There were some areas of brain structural abnormality, however, that proved to be more directly associated with functioning. Reduced cerebellar volume was significantly associated with deficits in executive and visuospatial function and language (Allin et al., 2001), findings that are broadly consistent with the "cerebellar cognitive–affective syndrome" described by Schmahmann and Sherman (1998). This suggests that cerebellar abnormalities may underlie some of the cognitive deficits found in VPT individuals. There was no association between cerebellar volume and motor neurological signs, however; perhaps suggesting that plasticity can allow motor functions to be spared, but at the expense of subtle abnormalities in cognitive performance.

VPT individuals have been reported to have poorer interhemispheric interaction (Roth et al., 1994), and it is possible that this is related to the reduced size of the corpus callosum, which is the major white matter tract connecting the two hemispheres. Nosarti et al. (2001a) found that verbal IQ, reading age, and verbal fluency scores were positively associated with reduced midsagittal area of the corpus callosum. Preliminary results of a functional MRI (fMRI) study conducted by our group showed that VPT boys with callosal thinning exhibited differential lateralization of phonological processing during a verbal fluency task compared with full-term controls (Rushe et al., 1999). Another fMRI study used visual and auditory tasks in a similar cohort of preterm boys in adolescence (Santhouse et al., 2002) and showed that the VPT subjects with damaged corpora callosa had significantly different activation patterns from the control group, and from a group of VPT adolescents without callosal damage. The findings suggest that the VPT brains are using alternative neural networks to circumvent the damaged corpus callosum. This could be a demonstration of "rerouting plasticity," as will be discussed below.

The left and right caudate nuclei were reduced in volume in VPT individuals, but this was not significant after controlling for total brain volume (Nosarti et al., 2001b). However, reduced bilateral caudate volumes were associated with higher scores on the "hyperactivity" index of the Rutter behavioral scale (Schachar et al., 1981). This characterizes the predominantly hyperactive/impulsive subtype of attention-deficit hyperactivity disorder (ADHD), defined by poor inhibitory regulation, limitations in perseverance, perseveration, restlessness, overactivity, and impaired self-awareness (Landau et al., 1999). This is consistent with evidence implicating the basal ganglia in the pathogenesis of ADHD (Semrud-Clikeman et al., 2000). This has been investigated further (Nosarti et al., 2002, 2004) in a group of 16-year-old VPT boys using a go–no-go fMRI paradigm. The findings again suggest that VPT individuals are activating different neural networks than controls and using alternative strategies when performing these cognitive tasks.

Possible mechanisms of brain reorganization and sparing of function

At the neuronal level

A brain that has been damaged in the perinatal period has lost neurons and synaptic connections in a focal and/or distributed pattern, and this represents a deficit in processing power that the brain seeks to mitigate. In response to injury, the brain produces growth factors that encourage adjacent neurons to sprout new neurites and so form new synaptic contacts. The developing brain has a greater potential for this kind of neuronal growth than the adult brain (Lindholm, 1994), and this may provide the substrate for the reconstitution of cortical circuits (Ide *et al.*, 1996). This mechanism has been demonstrated in a perinatal lesion model in rodents by Coltman *et al.* (1995), who observed collateral sprouting in the molecular layer of the hippocampal dentate gyrus as early as 6 days after a lesion. The developing brain has another advantage that may help it to repair itself: it already possesses more neurons and synapses than it needs. During normal development, the brain produces a large excess of both cells and synaptic connections (Chiron *et al.*, 1992). For example, the maximal density of synapses in human occipital cortex occurs at 4–12 months, and at this stage is around 150% of adult density (Johnson, 2001). Many of these "extra" connections are later removed: a process known as synaptic pruning (Black, 1998). These extra cells and synapses possess neurotrophin receptors, which may allow them to be rescued from pruning by the increased availability of growth factors released in response to injury (Lindholm, 1994). They could then be used to reconstitute damaged circuits. Indeed, there is histological evidence of alteration of cells, synapses and connections in preterm brains (Marin-Padilla, 1996, 1999). Synaptic pruning occurs at different ages in different parts of the brain. The frontal lobe is generally held to be the latest to mature; through synaptic pruning, the adult pattern is reached at approximately 18–20 years. In general, the earlier the injury to the brain occurs, the greater is the availability of alternative neural substrates to take over the role of any part that is damaged. However, there may be adverse consequences of this kind of reorganization. Aram and Eisele (1992) have suggested that one such consequence may be that complex cognitive functions which are acquired later in development suffer through a lack of synaptic sites.

At the level of neural networks

If a discrete perinatal lesion were to take out a particular cortical module, other areas of the brain may be able to take over the functions of the lost area. Studies on the visual system of the cat have demonstrated that this does occur in both adults and neonates, but functional preservation is more effective and complete in neonates (Spear, 1996). Much of modern neuroscience rests on the mapping of functions onto brain areas; this has been successful in many areas (a good example is Broca's area). This structure–function relationship, however, is altered in the case of early brain injury because functions may be remapped onto other undamaged areas of the brain (Moses and Stiles, 2002). Cioni *et al.* (2001) used fMRI to study two pairs of monozygotic twins, where one of each pair had suffered a focal hemispheric brain injury around the time of birth. They showed that the damaged area's duties had been taken over by undamaged areas in the same hemisphere adjacent to the injury site, and also by areas in the other (intact) hemisphere. Such remapping of functions can, therefore, occur locally and at more distant sites. The larger the lesion, the more likely it is that the contralateral hemisphere will take over (Payne and Lomber, 2001). This also depends on the maturational state of the system that is lesioned. For example, language can be acquired by the right hemisphere as late as 9 years if the left hemisphere is damaged (Vargha-Khadem *et al.*, 1997). Bates *et al.* (2001) compared language production in brain-injured children and adults. Adults with left-hemisphere lesions showed severe language impairment and those with right-hemisphere damage showed disinhibited and "empty" speech. Children with similar unilateral brain damage showed no language impairment whatever the side of the lesion (Rauschecker and Marler, 1987). However, this compensation may not be complete: the areas of the brain that have taken over functions may not have the right structural specialization to do the job as efficiently, and they may be diverted from other functions, which may suffer as a result. Some evidence that developmental compensation may not be complete comes from Weintraub and Mesulam (1983), who found that individuals born with right-sided brain lesions showed impairments later in life in spelling, arithmetic, prosody (the ability to vary speech to convey emotional meanings), and social interactions. This adds to the evidence that developmental plasticity may be a double-edged sword.

At the level of connectivity

If functions are remapped within the brain then, of necessity, the patterns of cortical wiring – the white matter – must be altered. Altered connectivity may thus be a secondary effect of particular neural networks being in a different location. However, it is also possible for changes in connectivity to be a primary adaptation to injury that may help to subserve effective performance. That is, rather than being remapped, functions may be rerouted (Kolk, 2000). The example of language is a good theoretical model of rerouting, as different pathways could be employed in order to achieve the same results (Neville *et al.*, 1993). For instance, sentence comprehension could be performed by using a syntactic (structurally based) or semantic (based on order and meaning of words) route, and reading aloud could be performed using lexical or non-lexical processes. Functional rerouting could be a consequence of two processes: *automatic* or *strategic* selection. In *automatic* selection, it is hypothesized that processing occurs in parallel along several routes and output competition exists between the routes. According to this model, if the route that normally secures output is impaired, another route takes its place. In *strategic* selection, the individual makes use of alternative information (e.g. from another sensory modality) (Finney *et al.*, 2001) in carrying out the function of the damaged area. Studies of reading aloud in dyslexic children (Hendrix and Kolk, 1996) and sentence production in agrammatic subjects (e.g., Kim and Thompson, 2000) have found evidence for strategic rerouting. The structural substrate underlying this rerouting is the white matter. Myelination of white matter begins around term and is not fully complete until well into adult life (Benes *et al.*, 1994; Girard *et al.*, 1991). This late maturation may allow for rerouting plasticity to occur.

The limits of brain plasticity

The results of the UCHL study indicate that brain injuries acquired around the time of birth in VPT babies cause abnormalities of brain structure that are still detectable in adolescence. Despite this, the level of functioning of those individuals who escape major physical disability is often not grossly impaired. In addition, it is not easy to predict patterns of functional deficit from abnormalities of brain structure in these individuals. This is most likely to be the result of developmental neural plasticity operating on any, or all, of the levels described above. This reorganization seems to have spared functions; however, there are hints that it may predispose to problems later in life. The animal studies mentioned above (Goldman, 1971; Sams-Dodd *et al.*, 1997) suggested that a brain lesion may remain relatively 'silent' until later in life, only causing functional compromise when the neural system involved reaches maturity. Some researchers have proposed similar mechanisms in humans (Anderson *et al.*, 1999; Rankin *et al.*, 1981; Weinberger, 1987). There is evidence that the prevalence of neuromotor and cognitive impairments increases with age in VPT individuals (Palfrey *et al.*, 1987; Roth *et al.*, 1994). It will be important to follow up this group into adulthood to determine whether they are at risk of late complications of their brain injuries, and if so, what could be done to mitigate the effects.

Conclusions

Plasticity is a fundamental property of vertebrate nervous systems. During development, a high degree of plasticity allows the nervous system to be moulded to best fit its environment, and this also enables the brain to compensate for injuries that would cause permanent loss of function in an adult. With increasing age, this capacity for plasticity begins to decline, with the eventual relative "crystallization" of brain and behavior, which allows the adult to display stable, adaptive behaviors. The enormous resilience of the young brain to injury is demonstrated by individuals born preterm, in whom functional impairments are relatively mild compared with the abnormalities of brain structure that they show. We have drawn attention to evidence that structural reorganization and remapping or rerouting of functions has occurred in the brains of these individuals. Given that important events of brain maturation and development continue into adulthood, there is the possibility that these structural changes may adversely affect function later in life. There is some evidence for this from animal models, and the severity of certain impairments in the preterm population seems to increase with age. It will be important to continue to follow up preterm individuals as they enter adulthood and to determine which factors are associated with poor outcome. There may be ways of using the residual plasticity of the child or even early adult brain to compensate for the late effects of early brain lesions.

REFERENCES

Allin, M., Murray, R. M. (2002). Schizophrenia: a neurodevelopmental or neurodegenerative disorder? *Curr Opin Psychiatry* **15**: 9–15.

Allin, M., Matsumoto, H., Santhouse, A. M., *et al.* (2001). Cognitive and motor function and the size of the cerebellum in adolescents born very preterm. *Brain* **124**: 60–66.

Anderson, S. W., Bechara, A., Damasio, H., Tranel, D., Damasio, A. R. (1999). Impairment of social and moral behavior related to early damage in human prefrontal cortex. *Nat Neurosci* **11**: 1032–1037.

Aram, D. M., Eisele, J. A. (1992). Plasticity and recovery of higher cognitive function following early brain damage. In *Handbook of Neuropsychology*, Vol. 6, ed. J. Boller, J. Grafman. Amsterdam: Elsevier, pp. 73–91.

Back, S. A., Luo, N. L., Borenstein, N. S., *et al.* (2001). Late oligodendrocyte precursors coincide with the developmental window of vulnerability for human perinatal white matter injury. *J Neurosci* **21**: 1302–1312.

Back, S. A., Han, B. H., Luo, N. L., *et al.* (2002). Selective vulnerability of late oligodendrocyte progenitors to hypoxia-ischaemia. *J Neurosci* **22**: 455–463.

Bates, E., Reilly, J., Wulfeck, B., *et al.* (2001). Differential effects of unilateral lesions on language production in children and adults. *Brain Lang* **79**: 223–265.

Benes, F. M., Turtle, M., Khan, Y., Farol, P. (1994). Myelination of a key relay zone in the hippocampal formation occurs in the human brain during childhood, adolescence, and adulthood. *Arch Gen Psychiatry* **51**: 477–484.

Black, J. E. (1998). How a child builds its brain: some lessons from animal studies of neural plasticity. *Prevent Med* **27**: 168–171.

Cannon, M., Jones, P. B., Murray, R. M. (2002). Obstetric complications and schizophrenia: historical and meta-analytical review. *Am J Psychiatry* **159**: 1080–1092.

Cannon-Spoor, H. E., Potkin, S. G., Wyatt, K. J. (1982). Measurement of premorbid adjustment in chronic schizophrenia. *Schizophr Bull* **8**: 470–484.

Castro-Caldas, A, Petersson, K. M., Reis, A., Stone-Elander, S., Ingvar, M. (1998). The illiterate brain: learning to read and write during childhood influences the structural organisation of the brain. *Brain* **121**: 1056–1063.

Chiron, C., Raynaud, C., Maziere, B., *et al.* (1992). Changes in regional cerebral blood flow during brain maturation in children and adolescents. *J Nucl Med* **33**: 696–703.

Cioni, G., Montanaro, D., Tosetti, M., Canapicchi, R., Ghelarduci, B. (2001). Reorganisation of the sensorimotor cortex after early focal brain lesion: a functional MRI study in monozygotic twins. *Neuroreport* **12**: 1335–1340.

Coltman, B. W., Earley, E. M., Shahar, A., Dudek, F. E., Ide, C. F. (1995). Factors influencing mossy fiber collateral sprouting in organotypic slice cultures of neonatal mouse hippocampus. *J Comp Neurol* **362**: 209–222.

Costello, A. M. de L., Hamilton, P. A., Baudin, J., *et al.* (1988). Prediction of neurodevelopmental impairment at four years from brain ultrasound appearance of very preterm infants. *Dev Med Child Neurol* **30**: 711–722.

du Plessis, A. J., Volpe, J. J. (2002). Perinatal brain injury in the preterm and term newborn. *Curr Opin Neurol* **15**: 151–157.

Elbert, T., Heim, S., Rockstroh, B. (2001). Neural plasticity and development. In *Handbook of Developmental Cognitive Neuroscience*, ed. C. A. Nelson, M. Luciana. Cambridge, MA: MIT Press, pp. 191–202.

Finney, E. M., Fine, I., Dobkins, K. R. (2001). Visual stimuli activate auditory cortex in the deaf. *Nat Neurosci* **4**: 1171–1173.

Frith, U. (1998). Literally changing the brain. *Brain* **121**: 1011–1012.

Girard, N., Raybaud, C., du Lac, P. (1991). MRI study of brain myelination. *J Neuroradiol* **18**: 291–307.

Goldman, P. S. (1971). Functional development of the prefrontal cortex in early life and the problem of plasticity. *Exp Neurol* **32**: 366–387.

Goyen, T-A., Lui, K., Woods, R. (1998). Visual–motor, visual–perceptual and fine motor outcomes in very-low-birth-weight children at 5 years. *Dev Med Child Neurol* **40**: 76–81.

Grimshaw, G. M., Adelstein, A., Bryden, M. P., MacKinnon, G. E. (1998). First-language acquisition in adolescence: evidence for a critical period for verbal language development. *Brain Lang* **63**: 237–255.

Hadders-Algra, M., Huisjes, H. J., Touwen, B. C. L. (1988). Perinatal risk factors and minor neurological dysfunction: significance for behaviour and school achievement at 9 years. *Dev Med Child Neurol* **30**: 482–491.

Hall, A., McLeod, A., Counsell, C., Thomson, L., Mutch, L. (1995). School attainment, cognitive ability and motor function in a total Scottish very-low-birthweight population at 8 years: a controlled study. *Dev Med Child Neurol* **37**: 1037–1050.

Hecaen, H. (1983). Acquired aphasia in childhood: revisited. *Neuropsychologia* **21**: 581–587.

Hendrix, A. W., Kolk, H. H. J. (1996). Strategic control in developmental dyslexia. *Cogn Neuropsych* **14**: 321–366.

Hoon, A. H. (1995). Neuroimaging in the high risk infant: relationship to outcome. *J Perinatol* **15**: 389–394.

Hope, P. L., Gould, S. J., Howard, S., *et al.* (1988). Precision of ultrasound diagnosis of pathologically verified lesions in the brain of very preterm infants. *Dev Med Child Neurol* **30**: 457–471.

Huh, J., Williams, H. G., Burke, J. R. (1998). Development of bilateral motor control in children with developmental coordination disorders. *Dev Med Child Neurol* **40**: 474–484.

Ide, C. F., Scripter, J. L., Coltman, B. W., *et al.* (1996). Cellular and molecular correlates to plasticity during recovery from injury in the developing mammalian brain. *Prog Brain Res* **108**: 365–377.

Johnson, M. H. (2001). Functional brain development in humans. *Nat Rev Neurosci* **2**: 475–483.

Johnston, M. V. (1998). Selective vulnerability in the neonatal brain. *Ann Neurol* **44**: 155–156.

Jones, S. M., Zigler, E. (2002). The Mozart effect: not learning from history. *J Appl Dev Psychol* **23**: 355–372.

Kennard, M. A. (1936). Age and other factors in motor recovery from precentral lesions in monkeys. *Am J Physiol* **115**: 138–146.

Kim, M., Thompson, C. K. (2000). Patterns of comprehension and production of nouns and verbs in agrammatism: implications for lexical organization. *Brain Lang* **74**: 1–25.

Kinney, H. C., Brody, B. A., Kloman, A. S., Gilles, F. H. (1988). Sequence of central nervous system myelination in human infancy. II. Patterns of myelination in autopsied infants. *J Neuropathol Exp Neurol* **47**: 217–234.

Kolb, B. (1989). Brain development, plasticity and behaviour. *Am Psychol* **44**: 1203–1212.

Kolb, B., Whishaw, I. Q. (1989). Plasticity in the neocortex: mechanisms underlying recovery from early brain damage. *Prog Neurobiol* **32**: 235–276.

Kolk, H. H. J. (2000). Multiple route plasticity. *Brain Lang* **71**: 129–131.

Kuban, K., Sanocka, U., Leviton, A., *et al.* (1999). White matter disorders of prematurity: association with intraventricular hemorrhage and ventriculomegaly. The Developmental Epidemiology Network. *J Pediatr* **134**: 539–546.

Kuchna, I. (1994). Quantitative studies of human newborns' hippocampal pyramidal cells after perinatal hypoxia. *Folia Neuropathol* **32**: 9–16.

Landau, Y. E., Gross-Tsur, V., Auerbach, J. G., van der Meere, J., Shalev, R. S. (1999). Attention-deficit hyperactivity disorder and developmental right-hemisphere syndrome: congruence and incongruence of cognitive and behavioral aspects of attention. *J Child Neurol* **14**: 299–303.

Lewis, S. W., Murray, R. M. (1987). Obstetric complications, neurodevelopmental deviance and risk of schizophrenia. *J Psychiatr Res* **21**: 413–422.

Lewis, S. W., Owen, M. J., Murray, R. M. (1989). Obstetric complications and schizophrenia: methodology and mechanisms. *Schizophrenia: Scientific Progress*, ed. S. Schutz, C. A. Tomminga. New York: Oxford University Press, pp. 56–68.

Lindholm, D. (1994). Role of neurotrophins in preventing glutamate induced neuronal cell death. *J Neurol* **242**: S16–S18.

Linkenhoker, B. A., Knudsen, E. I. (2002). Incremental training increases the plasticity of the auditory space map in adult barn owls. *Nature* **419**: 293–296.

Luoma, L., Herrgard, E., Martikainen, A. (1998). Neuropsychological analysis of the visuomotor problems in children born preterm at ≤ 32 weeks of gestation: a 5 year prospective follow-up. *Dev Med Child Neurol* **40**: 21–30.

Mallard, E. C., Rehn, A., Rees, S., Tolcos, M., Copolov, D. (1999). Ventriculomegaly and reduced hippocampal volume following intrauterine growth-restriction: implications for the aetiology of schizophrenia. *Schizophr Res* **40**: 11–21.

Marin-Padilla, M. (1996). Developmental neuropathology and impact of perinatal brain damage. I. Hemorrhagic lesions of neocortex. *J Neuropathol Exp Neurol* **55**: 758–773.

   (1997). Developmental neuropathology and impact of perinatal brain damage. II: white matter lesions of the neocortex. *J Neuropathol Exp Neurol* **56**: 219–235.

   (1999). Developmental neuropathology and impact of perinatal brain damage. III: gray matter lesions of the neocortex. *J Neuropathol Exp Neurol* **58**: 407–429.

Moses, P., Stiles, J. (2002). The lesion methodology: contrasting views from adult and child studies. *Dev Psychobiol* **40**: 266–277.

Msall, M. E., Buck, G. M., Schisterman, E. F., *et al.* (1998). Social and biomedical risks for 8 to 10 year educational outcomes of children born with extreme prematurity and without major disability. AACPDM Abstracts. *Dev Med Child Neurol Suppl* **H**: 27.

Murray, R. M., Lewis, S. W. (1987). Is schizophrenia a neurodevelopmental disorder? *Br Med J* **295**: 681–682.

Neville, H. J. (1993). Neurobiology of cognitive and language processing: Effects of early experience. In *Brain Development and Cognition: A Reader*, ed. M. H. Johnson. Oxford: Blackwell, pp. 424–448.

Nosarti, C., Rifkin, L., Rushe, T. M., *et al.* (2001a). Corpus callosum size in adolescents who were born very preterm. *Pediatr Res Special Suppl* **50**: 15A.

Nosarti, C., Allin, M., Al-Asady, M., *et al.* (2001b). Behavioural and cognitive consequences of caudate pathology in adolescents born very preterm. *Neuroimage*, **13**: 339.

Nosarti, C., Al-Asady, M. H. S., Frangou, S., *et al.* (2002). Adolescents who were born very preterm have decreased brain volumes. *Brain* **125**: 1616–1623.

Nosarti, C., Rubia, K., Frearson, S., Rifkin, L., Murray, R. M. (2004). Altered neuronal organisation of the brain of adolescents born very preterm during response inhibition. *Schizophr Res* **60**(Special Suppl.): 230.

Palfrey, J. S., Singer, J. D., Walker, D. A., Butler, J. A. (1987). Early identification of children's special needs: a study in five metropolitan communities. *J Pediatr* **111**: 651–659.

Paneth, N., Rudelli, R., Kazam, E., Monte, W. (1994). *Brain Damage in the Preterm Infant.* Cambridge: MacKeith Press/Cambridge University Press.

Pantev, C., Oostenveld, R., Engelien, A., *et al.* (1998). Increased auditory cortical representation in musicians. *Nature* **392**: 811–814.

Payne, B. R., Lomber, S. G. (2001). Timeline: reconstructing functional systems after lesions of cerebral cortex. *Nat Rev Neurosci* **2**: 911–919.

Rankin, J. M., Aram, D. M., Horwitz, S. J. (1981). Language ability in right and left hemiplegia children. *Brain Lang* **14**: 292–306.

Rauschecker, J. P., Marler, P. (1987). *Imprinting and Cortical Plasticity: Comparative Aspects of Sensitive Periods.* New York: Wiley.

Rooney, M., Allin, M., Rifkin, L., *et al.* (2001). Comparison of psychopathology in prematurely born adults from a 1979–1981 cohort, with full term born adults. *Schizophr Res* **49**: 41.

Rosenbloom, L., Sullivan, P. B. (1996). The nutritional and neurodevelopmental consequences of feeding difficulties in disabled children. In *Clinics in Developmental Medicine*, No. 104; *Feeding the Disabled Child*, ed. P. B. Sullivan, L. Rosenbloom. Cambridge, UK: MacKeith Press/Cambridge University Press, pp. 33–39.

Roth, S. C., Baudin, J., McCormick, D. C., *et al.* (1993). Relation between ultrasound appearance of the brain of very preterm infants and neurodevelopmental impairment at eight years. *Dev Med Child Neurol* **35**: 755–768.

Roth, S. C., Baudin, J., Pezzani-Goldsmith, M., *et al.* (1994). Relation between neurodevelopmental status of very preterm infants at one and eight years. *Dev Med Child Neurol* **36**: 1049–1062.

Rushe, T. M., Woodruff, P. W. R., Bullmore, E. B., *et al.* (1999). Lateralisation of language function in adults born very preterm. *Magn Reson Mater Phys, Biol Med* **8**(Suppl 1): 82.

Rushe, T. M., Rifkin, L., Stewart, A. L., *et al.* (2001). Neuropsychological outcome at adolescence of very preterm birth and its relation to brain structure. *Dev Med Child Neurol* **43**: 226–33.

Rutter, M., Tizard, J., Whitmore, K. (1981). *Education, Health and Behaviour.* Melbourne: Kreiger.

Sams-Dodd, F., Lipska, B. K., Weinberger, D. R. (1997). Neonatal lesions of the rat ventral hippocampus result in hyperlocomotion and deficits in social behaviour in adulthood. *Psychopharmacology* **132**: 303–310.

Santhouse, A. M., Ffytche, D. H., Howard, R. J., *et al.* (2002). The functional significance of perinatal corpus callosum damage: an fMRI study in young adults. *Brain* **125**: 1782–1792.

Schachar, R., Rutter, M., Smith, A. (1981). The characteristics of situationally and pervasively hyperactive children: implications for syndrome definition. *J Child Psychol Psychiatry* **22**: 375–392.

Schmahmann, J. D., Sherman, J. C. (1998). The cerebellar cognitive–affective syndrome. *Brain* **121**: 561–579.

Semrud-Clikeman, M., Steingard, R. J., Filipek, P., *et al.* (2000). Using MRI to examine brain–behavior relationships in males with attention deficit disorder with hyperactivity. *J Am Acad Child Adolesc Psychiatry* **39**: 477–484.

Shewmon, D. A., Holmes, G. L., Byrne, P. A. (1999). Consciousness in congenitally decorticate children: developmental vegetative state as a self-fulfilling prophecy. *Dev Med Child Neurol* **41**: 364–374.

Snider, L. M. (1998). Preschool performance skills of extremely low birth weight children. AACPDM Abstracts. *Dev Med Child Neurol Suppl* **H**: 27.

Sohma, O., Mito, T., Mizuguchi, M., Takashima, S. (1995). The prenatal age critical for the development of the pontosubicular necrosis. *Acta Neuropathol* **90**: 7–10.

Sowell, E. R., Thompson, P. M., Holmes, C. J., Jernigan, T. L., Toga, A. W. (1999). In vivo evidence for post-adolescent brain maturation in frontal and striatal regions. *Nat Neurosci* **2**: 859–861.

Spear, P. D. (1996). Neural plasticity after brain damage. *Prog Brain Res* **108**: 391–408.

Stewart, A. L., Thorburn, R. J., Hope, P. L., *et al.* (1983). Ultrasound appearance of the brain in very preterm infants and neurodevelopmental outcome at 18 months of age. *Arch Dis Child* **58**: 598–604.

Stewart, A. L., Costello, A. M., Hamilton, P. A., *et al.* (1989). Relationship between neurodevelopmental status of very preterm infants at 1 and 4 years. *Dev Med Child Neurol* **31**: 756–765.

Stewart, A. L., Rifkin, L., Amess, P. N., *et al.* (1999). Brain structure and neurocognitive and behavioural function in adolescents who were born very preterm. *Lancet* **353**: 1653–1657.

Tin, W., Wariyar, U., Hey, E. (1997). Changing prognosis for babies of less than 28 weeks' gestation in the north of England between 1983 and 1994. *Br Med J* **314**: 107–111.

Vargha-Khadem, F., Carr, L. J., Isaacs, E., *et al.* (1997). Onset of speech after left hemispherectomy in a nine-year-old boy. *Brain* **120**: 159–182.

Volpe, J. (1998). Neurologic outcome of prematurity. *Arch Neurol* **55**: 297–300.

Weinberger, D. R. (1987). Implications of normal brain development for the pathogenesis of schizophrenia. *Arch Gen Psychiatry* **44**: 660–669.

Weintraub, S., Mesulam, M. M. (1983). Developmental learning disabilities of the right hemisphere: emotional, interpersonal, and cognitive components. *Arch Neurol* **40**: 463–468.

Wiesel, T. N., Hubel, D. H. (1963). Single-cell responses in striate cortex of kittens deprived of vision in one eye. *J Neurophysiol* **26**: 1003–1017.

Part II

Etiological factors

6

Do degenerative changes operate across diagnostic boundaries? The case for glucocorticoid involvement in major psychiatric disorders

Carmine M. Pariante[1] and David Cotter[2]

[1] Institute of Psychiatry, King's College, London, UK
[2] Royal College of Surgeons, Dublin, Ireland

As it was initially proposed, the developmental theory of schizophrenia suggested that an early insult to the developing brain could result in cerebral changes that ultimately manifest as psychosis (Lewis and Murray, 1987; Weinberger, 1987). The success of this theory has been in its capacity to explain many of the known features of schizophrenia. Thus, the season of birth effect, the reported excess of obstetric complications, minor physical anomalies, dermatoglyphic abnormalities, and childhood developmental impairments may all be successfully and usefully explained by the influence of environmental and epigenetic factors on normal fetal brain development. Crucial supportive evidence for the theory was given by studies showing that classical degenerative brain changes were largely absent, by the presence of microscopic brain changes indicative of abnormal brain development, and by the absence of clear evidence for progressive ventricular dilatation among schizophrenia subjects.

However, these latter findings are no longer secure. For example, the absence of excess cortical gliosis is no longer accepted as indicating a lack of peri- or postnatal cerebral inflammation, and firm cytoarchitectural evidence of abnormal brain development has yet to be consistently presented (Harrison, 1999). Furthermore, some neuroimaging studies have shown evidence for progressive ventricular enlargement over time and others have shown that hippocampal volume reductions occur during the phase of a first psychotic episode (Lawrie et al., 2000; Pantellis et al., 2000). Reversibility of reductions in superior temporal gyrus volume has also been described during the first episode of psychosis (Keshavan et al., 1998), and progressive cortical reductions are observed in subjects with early-onset schizophrenia (Rappaport et al., 1999). Therefore, evidence is accumulating that supports the view that plastic changes in macroscopic cytoarchitecture may occur with illness.

Neurodevelopment and Schizophrenia, ed. Matcheri S. Keshavan *et al*. Published by Cambridge University Press. © Cambridge University Press 2004.

The microscopic basis of these cortical volume reductions are not known, but clues are provided by recent neuropathological studies that have shown reductions in cortical neuronal size, dendritic complexity, and synaptic proteins in schizophrenia (Harrison, 1999). Smaller neurons with fewer and less-elaborate branches would result in a diminution in the amount of neuropil, more compacted cells, and thus increased neuronal density. It is certainly feasible to suggest that these alterations underlie the regional cortical volume reductions observed in schizophrenia. The current challenge, however, is to understand the mechanism underlying these changes. The term atrophic is preferred over degenerative because evidence of cell death and of a gliotic response so characteristic of degenerative diseases is absent. However, regardless of what term is used, the findings necessitate a re-evaluation of the neurodevelopmental hypothesis of schizophrenia as it is currently understood.

Evidence for a common neuropathology in major depression, bipolar disorder, and schizophrenia

It is possible that the microscopic neuropathological changes described in schizophrenia may be vulnerability factors for schizophrenia. Alternatively, they could be an intrinsic component or a consequence of the illness. Neuropathological studies cannot tell which interpretation is correct. However, there are some important similarities in the neuropathology of schizophrenia, major depressive disorder (MDD) and bipolar disorder (BPD), which suggest that a common process of change is involved in each disorder.

Macroscopic neuroanatomical investigations of brain pathology in schizophrenia, BPD, and MDD show differences that are generally quantitative rather than qualitative. For example, ventricular dilatation and reduced hippocampal and frontal brain volumes are seen in schizophrenia, but they are also present to a lesser degree in MDD and BPD (McCarley et al., 1999). The single main departure from this pattern is that the volume of the amygdala may be specifically enlarged in BPD (Altshuler et al., 1998), possibly because of drug treatment. Microscopically, reductions in dendritic spine density (Rosoklija et al., 2000), neuronal size (Cotter et al., 2001; Rajkowska et al., 1999), and synaptic proteins (Eastwood and Harrison, 2001) have been described in mood disorders as well as in schizophrenia (Harrison, 1999). More recently, it has become apparent that glial cell loss may be a feature of MDD, BPD, and schizophrenia (Cotter et al, 2001; Rajkowska et al., 1999) depending, possibly, on the presence of coexisting affective symptoms and on which region of the brain is investigated.

This similar pattern of changes in cortical cellular architecture in schizophrenia and mood disorders suggests that a common pathophysiology may underlie aspects of these psychiatric diseases. What aspects of illness common to MDD, BPD, and schizophrenia could cause changes in keeping with the known cellular changes described above? Glucocorticoid-related neurotoxicity is one such candidate.

A role for glucocorticoids in the neuronal changes of mood disorders and schizophrenia?

There are several other lines of investigation that support the view that glucocorticoid-related neurotoxicity may be implicated in depression and schizophrenia. First, in vitro investigations have shown that high levels of glucocorticoid hormones result in reduced neuronal volume and dendritic arborization (Sapolsky, 2000), and these latter changes have been observed in both disorders. Second, elevated plasma glucocorticoid levels are associated with (largely reversible) hippocampal volume reductions in MDD, post-traumatic stress disorder (PTSD), Cushing's disease, and normal aging, and such reductions have been observed in the phase of a first psychotic episode (Lawrie *et al.*, 2000; Pantellis *et al.*, 2000). Third, the functional effect of glucocorticoids on reducing hippocampal glial cell activation and proliferation (Crossin *et al.*, 1997) mirrors the glial deficit observed in MDD, BPD, and possibly schizophrenia. Consequently, the glial deficit found in these disorders may also relate to glucocorticoid effects.

Hypothalamic–pituitary–adrenal axis abnormalities in major depression

There is substantial evidence that hyperactivity of the hypothalamic–pituitary–adrenal (HPA) axis is involved in the pathogenesis of mood disorder (Pariante, 2003; Pariante and Miller, 2001). A significant percentage of depressed patients have been shown to hypersecrete cortisol, the endogenous adrenal glucocorticoid in humans, as manifested by increased 24-hour urinary free cortisol and elevated plasma and cerebrospinal fluid (CSF) concentrations of cortisol (Dinan, 1996; Holsboer, 2000; McAllister-Williams *et al.*, 1998; McQuade and Young, 2000; Nemeroff, 1996). Adrenal hypertrophy and increased pituitary volume has also been described in these patients, and these findings have also been considered a marker of HPA axis activation (Axelson *et al.*, 1992; Nemeroff, 1996). Hyperactivity of the HPA axis in major depression is driven by the hypersecretion of corticotropin-releasing factor (CRF) in the hypothalamus (Holsboer, 2000; Nemeroff, 1996; Owens and Nemeroff, 1993). Most notable in this regard are the increased CSF concentrations of CRF consistently found in drug-free depressed patients, and the decreased number of CRF receptors in the frontal cortex of suicide victims (Banki *et al.*, 1987; Heuser *et al.*, 1998; Nemeroff, 1996; Nemeroff *et al.*, 1984; Owens and Nemeroff, 1993). Moreover, depressed patients exhibit increased CRF messenger RNA (mRNA) and protein in the paraventricular nucleus of the hypothalamus (postmortem samples)

(Purba *et al.*, 1995; Raadsheer *et al.*, 1995). Finally, a number of studies have provided evidence that CRF may play a role not only in the endocrinopathy of depression but also in the behavioral signs and symptoms of the disorder. Indeed, the behavioral effects of CRF after direct central nervous system administration are remarkably similar to the signs and symptoms of major depression (decreased libido, decreased appetite, psychomotor alterations, and disturbed sleep).

These increased levels of CRF in the hypothalamus are related, at least in part, to altered feedback inhibition by endogenous glucocorticoids (de Kloet *et al.*, 1998; Holsboer, 2000; McQuade and Young, 2000; Pariante and Miller, 2001; Pariante *et al.*, 2002). In fact, glucocorticoids interact with their receptors (the mineralocorticoid receptor [MR] and the glucocorticoid receptor [GR]) in HPA axis tissues, where they are responsible for feedback inhibition of the secretion of adrenocorticotropic hormone (ACTH) from the pituitary and CRF from the hypothalamus (de Kloet *et al.*, 1998; McEwen, 2000; Nemeroff, 1996; Young *et al.*, 1998). The MR has a high affinity for endogenous glucocorticoids and is believed to play a role in the regulation of circadian fluctuations of these hormones. In contrast to the MR, the GR has a lower affinity for endogenous glucocorticoids and is believed to be more important in the regulation of the response to stress, when endogenous levels of glucocorticoids are high (de Kloet *et al.*, 1998). Consistent with the fact that patients with major depression exhibit impaired HPA negative feedback in the context of elevated circulating levels of cortisol, when the negative feedback is largely mediated by the GR, many studies have demonstrated that GR-mediated feedback inhibition is impaired in major depression. Depressed patients have non-suppression of cortisol secretion following dexamethasone in the dexamethasone suppression test (DST), non-suppression of ACTH secretion following hydrocortisone (fast-feedback test), and lack of inhibition of ACTH responses to CRF following dexamethasone pretreatment (DEX/CRF test) (Heuser *et al.*, 1994, 1996; Holsboer, 2000; Nemeroff, 1996; Ribeiro *et al.*, 1993; Young *et al.*, 1991). The only study that specifically looked at MR-mediated negative feedback in depression found that this pathway is intact (or possibly oversensitive) in these patients (Young *et al.*, 2003). In further support of the suggestion that patients with major depression exhibit impaired GR-mediated HPA negative feedback, a number of studies have demonstrated that GR function is also reduced in other tissues of depressed patients, as shown by a decreased sensitivity to the effects of glucocorticoids on immune and metabolic functions (Pariante and Miller, 2001). While there is no consistent evidence of GR expression changes in blood mononuclear cells or fibroblasts from depressed patients (Pariante and Miller, 2001), three studies that have examined postmortem brains have found reduced corticosteroid receptor expression (Lopez *et al.*, 1998; Webster *et al.*, 2002; Xing *et al.*, 2004).

Hypothalamic–pituitary–adrenal axis abnormalities in schizophrenia

In contrast to depression, the evidence linking HPA hyperactivity and GR dysfunction with schizophrenia is less clear. Sachar et al. (1970) suggested that patients experiencing a first-episode psychosis were more likely to present with HPA abnormalities, because of the distress associated with its "dramatic and ego-dystonic" nature. Several studies have confirmed that patients who are in the acute phase of a psychotic disorder, with florid symptoms, newly hospitalized, or unmedicated, have an elevated HPA axis activity, as shown by raised cortisol levels (Sachar et al., 1970), non-suppression of cortisol secretion by dexamethasone in the DST and in the DEX/CRF test (Coryell and Tsuang, 1992; Herz et al., 1985; Lammers et al., 1995), elevated levels of CRF in the CSF (Banki et al., 1987), and abnormal volume of the pituitary gland (Pariante et al., 2004a). Moreover, cortisol levels are positively correlated with symptom severity in patients with psychosis or schizotypal personality disorder (Walder et al., 2000; Walker et al., 2001) and negatively correlated with performance on executive function and memory tasks (Walder et al., 2000). Prospective studies also showed that most non-suppressor patients convert into suppressors after a few weeks of antipsychotic treatment (Herz et al., 1985; Tandon et al., 1991). For example, Herz et al. (1985) described that 11 out of 15 newly hospitalized patients, who were acutely psychotic with "florid psychotic symptoms" following a relapse, were DST non-suppressor, and that four out of five of these non-suppressor patients converted to suppressor after a week of treatment. Finally, patients who are clinically stable and receiving treatment tend to have a normal HPA axis (Ismail et al., 1998; Tandon et al., 1991).

Interestingly, across studies, patients with schizophrenia seem to have "more" HPA axis activation than normal individuals, but "less" HPA axis activation than depressed patients. For example, Sharma et al. (1988) conducted a meta-analysis comparing the results at the DST in patients with schizophrenia with those in patients with major depression. They found that patients with schizophrenia had a 19% rate of non-suppression, which was higher than the 7% rate in normal controls but lower than the 51% rate in patients with major depression. Similarly, Banki et al. (1987) examined the CSF levels of CRF in controls, depressed patients, and patients with schizophrenia; while depressed patients had levels of CRF levels that were markedly elevated (double those of controls), patients with schizophrenia had CRF levels that were only slightly, but significantly, higher than control. Recently, Webster et al. (2002) and Xing et al. (2004) found decreased GR and MR mRNA in the frontal cortex and hippocampus not only of patients with non-psychotic depression but also in patients with BPD and schizophrenia. It is possible that HPA axis activation in depression is part of the pathogenesis of the disorder–the increased levels of CRF in the brain could be responsible for some of the depressive symptoms–while

HPA axis activation in schizophrenia is a temporary phenomenon and reflects a stress-related activation of the axis. However, even if this was not a primary patho-genetic event in schizophrenia, HPA axis activation could still have crucial clinical effects on brain function (Cotter and Pariante, 2002). Hence, there is a need to clar-ify whether there is HPA hyperactivity at any stage during the course of psychotic disorders, especially around the time of the onset.

Cortisol: hero or villain?

Despite this evidence supporting the view that the interactions between glucocorti-coid hormones and the brain may be abnormal in major depression and schizophre-nia, there remains one big unanswered question: does the fact that depressed patients have a hyperactive HPA axis actually mean that a lot of cortisol is flooding their brain, and that the depressive symptoms are a consequence of this putative "toxic" effect of cortisol? Or is the opposite true: that patients have a hyperactive HPA axis as a compensatory mechanism because their brain is resistant to the effects of circulating cortisol? The question is not trivial, especially in our quest for a more effective treatment. In the first scenario, our recommendation should be the low-ering of cortisol levels. In the second scenario, our recommendation should be the administering of more cortisol. The available data are still failing to give a defini-tive answer on this question, although certainly the evidence does not consistently support the hypothesis that an *excess* of cortisol can cause depressive symptoms and brain micro- and macroscopic changes. First, it is not at all clear whether the mechanism of neurotoxicity in vivo is mediated through elevated or lowered levels of cerebral glucocorticoids, for very low levels also have neurotoxic effects (Pariante, 2003; Sapolsky, 2000). Second, the reduction of GR levels in the brains of these patients, and the reduction of GR function in patients with depression and in subjects experiencing chronic stress (Avitsur *et al.*, 2001; Bauer *et al.*, 2000; Pariante and Miller, 2001) suggests that elevated plasma cortisol levels could rep-resent a compensatory strategy. Third, recent studies indicate that levels of cortisol in the brain of humans are regulated by efflux systems at the blood–brain barrier (de Kloet *et al.*, 1998; Pariante *et al.* 2001, 2003a,b), and that both GR and the cor-tisol efflux systems may be influenced by psychotropic drugs (Pariante and Miller 2001; Pariante *et al.*, 1997, 2001, 2003a,b, 2004b). This indicates that peripheral cor-tisol levels, as often assumed in studies, may not necessarily dictate cerebral levels. Finally, treatment with GR and MR agonists, including cortisol, has antidepressant effects in humans (Bouwer *et al.*, 2000), again suggesting that these patients may not necessarily experience "too much cortisol" in their brain (DeBattista *et al.*, 2000; Dinan *et al.*, 1997). In reality, whether patients with major depression (or schizophrenia) have elevated or lowered activation of the GR in the brain is yet to be fully elucidated.

Conclusions

Evidence is accumulating that there are brain changes occurring during and possibly after the period of the first acute psychosis: that is, changes that are not developmental in the traditional sense. Furthermore, these changes are not specific to schizophrenia, either in terms of macroscopic or microscopic brain structure, for they are also present, to a generally milder degree, in subjects with mood disorder, and they are in keeping with glucocorticoid-related brain changes. These brain changes may be epiphenomena secondary to stress-related changes in glucocorticoid hormones and not primary pathogenetic pathways. Nevertheless, they could have crucial clinical effects through diminishing neuronal and cortical function and so complicate recovery from the primary illness. These changes may possibly be reversed by therapies that protect from glucocorticoid-related neurotoxicity or which act to promote neuroprotective cell signaling pathways. What is clear, however, is that the developmental theory of schizophrenia as it was first presented (Lewis and Murray, 1987; Weinberger, 1987) is challenged, as it alone is insufficient to explain the neuroanatomy of the disorder. Consequently, it is now important to understand the illness in terms of both early and late events, which will involve both developmental and atrophic processes.

REFERENCES

Altshuler, L. L., Bartzokis, G., Grieder, T., Curran, J., Mintz, J. (1998). Amygdala enlargement in bipolar disorder and hippocampal reduction in schizophrenia: an MRI study demonstrating neuroanatomic specificity. *Arch Gen Psychiatry* **55**: 663–664.

Avitsur, R., Stark, J. L., Sheridan, J. F. (2001). Social stress induces glucocorticoid resistance in subordinate animals. *Horm Behav* **39**: 247–257.

Axelson, D. A., Doraiswamy, P. M., Boyko, O. B., *et al.* (1992). In vivo assessment of pituitary volume with magnetic resonance imaging and systematic stereology: relationship to dexamethasone suppression test results in patients. *Psychiatry Res* **44**: 63–70.

Banki, C. M., Bissette, G., Arato, M., O'Connor, L., Nemeroff, C. B. (1987). CSF corticotropin-releasing factor-like immunoreactivity in depression and schizophrenia. *Am J Psychiatry* **144**: 873–877.

Bauer, M. E., Vedhara, K., Perks, P., *et al.* (2000). Chronic stress in caregivers of dementia patients is associated with reduced lymphocyte sensitivity to glucocorticoids. *J Neuroimmunol* **103**: 84–92.

Bouwer, C., Claassen, J., Dinan, T. G., Nemeroff, C. B. (2000). Prednisone augmentation in treatment-resistant depression with fatigue and hypocortisolaemia: a case series. *Depress Anxiety* **12**: 44–50.

Coryell, W., Tsuang, D. (1992). Hypothalamic–pituitary–adrenal axis hyperactivity and psychosis: recovery during an 8-year follow-up. *Am J Psychiatry* **149**: 1033–1039.

Cotter, D., Pariante, C. M. (2002). Stress and the progression of the developmental hypothesis of schizophrenia. *Br J Psychiatry* **181**: 363–365.

Cotter, D., Mackay, D., Landau, S., Kerwin, R., and Everall, I. (2001). Glial cell loss and reduced neuronal size in the anterior cingulate cortex in major depressive disorder. *Arch Gen Psychiatry* **58**: 545–553.

Crossin, K. L., Tai, M. H., Krushel, L. A., Mauro, V. P., Edelman, G. M. (1997). Glucocorticoid receptor pathways are involved in the inhibition of astrocyte proliferation. *Proc Natl Acad Sci USA* **94**: 2687–2692.

de Kloet, E. R., Vreugdenhil, E., Oitzl, M. S., Joels, M. (1998). Brain corticosteroid receptor balance in health and disease. *Endocr Rev* **19**: 269–301.

DeBattista, C., Posener, J. A., Kalehzan, B. M., Schatzberg, A. F. (2000). Acute antidepressant effects of intravenous hydrocortisone and CRH in depressed patients: a double-blind, placebo-controlled study. *Am J Psychiatry* **157**: 1334–1337.

Dinan, T. G. (1996). Noradrenergic and serotonergic abnormalities in depression: stress-induced dysfunction? *J Clin Psychiatry* **57**(Suppl 4): 14–18.

Dinan, T. G., Lavelle, E., Cooney, J., *et al.* (1997). Dexamethasone augmentation in treatment-resistant depression. *Acta Psychiatr Scand* **95**: 58–61.

Eastwood, S. L., Harrison, P. J. (2001). Synaptic pathology in the anterior cingulate cortex in schizophrenia and mood disorders. A review and a western blot study of synaptophysin, GAP-43, and the complexins. *Brain Res Bull* **55**: 519–578.

Harrison, P. J. (1999). The neuropathology of schizophrenia: a critical review of the data and their interpretation. *Brain* **122**: 593–624.

Herz, M. I., Fava, G. A., Molnar, G., Edwards, L. (1985). The dexamethasone suppression test in newly hospitalized schizophrenic patients. *Am J Psychiatry* **142**: 127–129.

Heuser I. J., Yassouridis, A., Holsboer, F. (1994). The combined dexamethasone/CRH test: a refined laboratory test for psychiatric disorders. *J Psychiatr Res* **28**: 341–356.

Heuser, I. J., Schweiger, U., Gotthardt, U., *et al.* (1996). Pituitary–adrenal-system regulation and psychopathology during amitriptyline treatment in elderly depressed patients and normal comparison subjects. *Am J Psychiatry* **153**: 93–99.

Heuser, I. J., Bissette, G., Dettling, M., *et al.* (1998). Cerebrospinal fluid concentrations of corticotropin-releasing hormone, vasopressin, and somatostatin in depressed patients and healthy controls: response to amitriptyline treatment. *Depress Anxiety* **8**: 71–79.

Holsboer, F. (2000). The corticosteroid receptor hypothesis of depression. *Neuropsychopharmacology* **23**: 477–501.

Ismail, K., Murray, R. M., Wheeler, M. J., O'Keane, V. (1998). The dexamethasone suppression test in schizophrenia. *Psychol Med* **28**: 311–317.

Keshavan, M. S., Haas, G. L., Kahn, C. E., *et al.* (1998). Superior temporal gyrus and the course of early schizophrenia: progressive static or reversible? *J Psychiatr Res* **32**: 161–167.

Lammers, C. H., Garcia-Borreguero, D., Schmider, J., *et al.* (1995). Combined dexamethasone/corticotropin-releasing hormone test in patients with schizophrenia and in normal controls: II. *Biol Psychiatry* **38**: 803–807.

Lawrie, S. M., Whalley, H., Byrne, M., *et al.* (2000). Brain structure change and psychopathology in subjects at high risk of schizophrenia. *Schizophr Res* **41**: 11.

Lewis, S. W., Murray, R. M. (1987). Obstetric complications, neurodevelopmental deviance, and risk of schizophrenia. *J Psychiatr Res* **21**: 413–421.

Lopez, J. F., Chalmers, D. T., Little, K. Y., Watson, S. J. (1998). A. E. Bennett Research Award. Regulation of serotonin 1_A, glucocorticoid, and mineralocorticoid receptor in rat and human hippocampus: implications for the neurobiology of depression. *Biol Psychiatry* **43**: 547–573.

McAllister-Williams, R. H., Ferrier, I. N., Young, A. H. (1998). Mood and neuropsychological function in depression: the role of corticosteroids and serotonin. *Psychol Med* **28**: 573–584.

McCarley, R. W., Wible, C. G., Frumin, M., *et al.* (1999). MRI anatomy of schizophrenia. *Biol Psychiatry* **45**: 1099–1119.

McEwen, B. S. (2000). The neurobiology of stress: from serendipity to clinical relevance. *Brain Res* **886**: 172–189.

McQuade, R., Young, A. H. (2000). Future therapeutic targets in mood disorders: the glucocorticoid receptor. *Br J Psychiatry* **177**: 390–395.

Nemeroff, C. B. (1996). The corticotropin-releasing factor (CRF) hypothesis of depression: new findings and new directions. *Mol Psychiatry* **1**: 336–342.

Nemeroff, C. B., Widerlov, E., Bissette, G., *et al.* (1984). Elevated concentrations of CSF corticotropin-releasing factor-like immunoreactivity in depressed patients. *Science* **226**: 1342–1344.

Owens, M. J., Nemeroff, C. B. (1993). The role of corticotropin-releasing factor in the pathophysiology of affective and anxiety disorders: laboratory and clinical studies. *Ciba Found Symp* **172**: 296–308.

Pantellis, C., Velakoulis, D., Suckling, J., *et al.* (2000). Left medial temporal lobe volume reduction occurs during the transition from high risk to first episode psychosis. *Schizophr Res* **41**: 35.

Pariante, C. M. (2003). Depression, stress and the adrenal axis. *J Neuroendocrinol* **15**: 811–812.

Pariante, C. M., Miller, A. H. (2001). Glucocorticoid receptors in major depression: relevance to pathophysiology and treatment. *Biol Psychiatry* **49**: 391–404.

Pariante, C. M., Pearce, B. D., Pisell, T. L., Owens, M. J., Miller, A. H. (1997). Steroid-independent translocation of the glucocorticoid receptor by the antidepressant desipramine. *Mol Pharmacol* **52**: 571–581.

Pariante, C. M., Makoff, A., Lovestone, S., *et al.*, (2001). Antidepressants enhance glucocorticoid receptor function in vitro by modulating the membrane steroid transporters. *Br J Pharmacol* **134**: 1335–1343.

Pariante, C. M., Papadopoulos, A. S., Poon, L., *et al.* (2002). A novel prednisolone suppression test for the hypothalamic–pituitary–adrenal axis. *Biol Psychiatry* **51**: 922–930.

Pariante, C. M., Hye, A., Williamson, R., *et al.* (2003a). The antidepressant clomipramine regulates cortisol intracellular concentrations and glucocorticoid receptor expression in fibroblasts and rat primary neurones. *Neuropsychopharmacology* **28**: 1553–1561.

Pariante, C. M., Kim, R. B., Makoff, A., Kerwin, R. W. (2003b). The antidepressant fluoxetine enhances glucocorticoid receptor function in vitro by modulating membrane steroid transporters. *Br J Pharmacol* **139**: 1111–1118.

Pariante, C. M., Vassilopoulou, K., Velakoulis, D., *et al.* (2004a). Pituitary volume in psychosis. *Br J Psychiatry* **185**: 5–10.

Pariante, C. M., Thomas, S. A., Lovestone, S., Makoff, A., Kerwin, R. W. (2004b). Do antidepressants regulate how cortisol affects the brain? 2003 Curt Richter Award Paper. *Psychoneuroendocrinology* **29**: 423–447.

Purba, J. S., Raadsheer, F. C., Hofman, M. A., et al. (1995). Increased number of corticotropin-releasing hormone expressing neurons in the hypothalamic paraventricular nucleus of patients with multiple sclerosis. *Neuroendocrinology* **62**: 62–70.

Raadsheer, F. C., van Heerikhuize, J. J., Lucassen, P. J., et al. (1995). Corticotropin-releasing hormone mRNA levels in the paraventricular nucleus of patients with Alzheimer's disease and depression. *Am J Psychiatry* **152**: 1372–1376.

Rajkowska, G., Miguel-Hidalgo, J. J., Wei. J. (1999). Morphometric evidence for neuronal and glial prefrontal cell pathology in major depression. *Biol Psychiatry* **45**: 1085–1098.

Rappaport, J. L., Giedd, J. N., Blumenthal, J., et al. (1999). Progressive cortical change during adolescence in childhood-onset schizophrenia. A longitudinal magnetic resonance imaging study. *Arch Gen Psychiatry* **56**: 649–654.

Ribeiro, S. C., Tandon, R., Grunhaus, L., Greden, J. F. (1993). The DST as a predictor of outcome in depression: a meta-analysis. *Am J Psychiatry* **150**: 1618–1629.

Rosoklija, G., Toomayan, G., Ellis, S. P., et al. (2000). Structural abnormalities of subicular dendrites in subjects with schizophrenia and mood disorders. *Arch Gen Psychiatry* **57**: 349–356.

Sachar, E. J., Kanter, S. S., Buie, D., Engle, R., Mehlman, R. (1970). Psychoendocrinology of ego disintegration. *Am J Psychiatry* **126**: 1067–1078.

Sapolsky, R. (2000). The possibility of neurotoxicity in the hippocampus in major depression: a primer on neuron death. *Biol Psychiatry* **48**: 755–65.

Sharma, R. P., Pandey, G. N., Janicak, P. G., et al. (1988). The effect of diagnosis and age on the DST: a metaanalytic approach. *Biol Psychiatry* **24**: 555–568.

Tandon, R., Mazzara, C., DeQuardo, J., et al. (1991). Dexamethasone suppression test in schizophrenia: relationship to symptomatology, ventricular enlargement, and outcome. *Biol Psychiatry* **29**: 953–964.

Walder, D. J., Walker, E. F., Lewine, R. J. (2000). Cognitive functioning, cortisol release, and symptom severity in patients with schizophrenia. *Biol Psychiatry* **48**: 1121–1132.

Walker, E. F., Walder, D. J., Reynolds, F. (2001). Developmental changes in cortisol secretion in normal and at-risk youth. *Dev Psychopathol* **13**: 721–732.

Webster, M. J., Knable, M. B., O'Grady, J., Orthmann, J., Weickert, C. S. (2002). Regional specificity of brain glucocorticoid receptor mRNA alterations in subjects with schizophrenia and mood disorders. *Mol Psychiatry* **7**: 985–994, 924.

Weinberger, D. R. (1987). Implications of normal brain development for the pathogenesis of schizophrenia. *Arch Gen Psychiatry* **44**: 660–669.

Xing, G. Q., Russell, S., Webster, M. J., Post, R. M. (2004). Decreased expression of mineralo-corticoid receptor mRNA in the prefrontal cortex in schizophrenia and bipolar disorder. *Int J Neuropsychopharmacol* **7**: 143–153.

Young, E. A., Haskett, R. F., Murphy-Weinberg, V., Watson, S. J., Akil, H. (1991). Loss of gluco-corticoid fast feedback in depression. *Arch Gen Psychiatry* **48**: 693–699.

Young, E. A., Lopez, J. F., Murphy-Weinberg, V., Watson, S. J., Akil, H. (1998). The role of mineralocorticoid receptors in hypothalamic–pituitary–adrenal axis regulation in humans. *J Clin Endocrinol Metab* **83**: 3339–3345.

Young, E. A., Lopez, J. F., Murphy-Weinberg, V., Watson, S. J., Akil, H. (2003). Mineralocorticoid receptor function in major depression. *Arch Gen Psychiatry* **60**: 24–28.

7

Velo-cardio-facial syndrome (deletion 22q11.2): a homogeneous neurodevelopmental model for schizophrenia

Stephan Eliez[1] and Carl Feinstein[2]

[1] University of Geneva School of Medicine, Geneva, Switerland
[2] Stanford University School of Medicine, Stanford, USA

Since the pioneering reports by Barbara Fish in 1977 and of Daniel Weinberger in 1987, there has been increasing awareness that schizophrenia is most likely a neurodevelopmental disorder (Fish, 1977; Weinberger, 1987). According to this model of pathogenesis, there are underlying deviations already present in the early brain development of individuals who develop schizophrenia in adulthood. These neurodevelopmental abnormalities do not present as classical schizophrenia but as more subtle neurocognitive deficits. To test this theoretical model, several prospective longitudinal studies as well as other approaches that link earlier childhood clinical data to onset of schizophrenia in adulthood have been utilized in the search for early life indicators of vulnerability to this tragic disorder. Recent findings from these studies consistently indicate that children at high genetic risk for schizophrenia do, in fact, have significantly elevated rates of neurocognitive and behavioral problems (Cannon et al., 2002; Erlenmeyer-Kimling et al., 2000; Fish et al., 1992; Hans et al., 1999; Marcus et al., 1993). In addition, closely related research has demonstrated that, prior to the onset of schizophrenia in cohorts of adults, clear indicators of neurocognitive impairments were present earlier in life (Reichenberg et al., 2002). In a prospective longitudinal study of a population-based (non-high-risk) cohort, significant neuromotor, cognitive, and language impairments were present only among children who were later diagnosed with schizophreniform disorder or schizophrenia (Cannon et al., 2002). Most recently, subtle but similar neurocognitive impairments have been found in both non-schizophrenia children and adults with elevated familial risk for schizophrenia (Asarnow et al., 2002a,b). In summary, there is now a very impressive body of data supporting the neurodevelopmental hypothesis of schizophrenia.

Neurodevelopment and Schizophrenia, ed. Matcheri S. Keshavan *et al.* Published by Cambridge University Press. © Cambridge University Press 2004.

Just prior to the research findings summarized above, in 1992, Shprintzen and colleagues reported that children with velo-cardio-facial syndrome (VCFS), a genetic disability syndrome caused, in most cases, by a de novo 3 MB microdeletion at chromosome region 22q11.2, were at remarkably high risk for developing schizophrenia in adulthood. Of children with this medically complex chromosome 22 microdeletion syndrome, known mostly to pediatric specialists (and certainly obscure to most schizophrenia researchers), 30% developed schizophrenia or schizoaffective disorder by young adulthood. This finding has since been confirmed and extended by successive studies, which now indicate that approximately 2% of all individuals with adult-onset schizophrenia, and a possibly higher percentage of youngsters with childhood-onset schizophrenia, have VCFS, as confirmed by reliable laboratory-based genetic diagnostic methods.

There was initial reluctance among many mainstream researchers in schizophrenia to acknowledge this finding. Instead, it was argued that VCFS is a childhood developmental disability that, in adults, merely mimics the phenotype of "true" schizophrenia. Nevertheless, the accumulation of data confirming prior childhood neurodevelopmental impairments in adults with schizophrenia suggests that a more heuristic approach would be to view VCFS as a model type of disorder for studying the developmental pathogenesis of schizophrenia. Unlike the clusters of subtle neurocognitive deficits that are gradually emerging from other lines of research, VCFS has a known molecular genetic cause that can be biologically validated in earliest infancy. This makes possible detailed study of the interaction of known genetic factors with brain development from infancy through adulthood, as assayed by neuroimaging, neurophysiological, neuropsychological, and psychiatric diagnostic techniques. Through such studies, at least one biologically validated developmental pathway to the development of schizophrenia could be elucidated. This, in turn, would create opportunities to design early interventions for the prevention or amelioration of the schizophrenia before its most destructive symptoms appear. In this chapter, we summarize the available clinical, neuroimaging, and genetic information regarding VCFS, so that it may be available for clinical research in schizophrenia.

Medical aspects

VCFS was first described by Shprintzen *et al.* (1978) as a distinctive congenital pattern presenting in early childhood as hypernasal speech (associated either with cleft palate or submucosal cleft), cardiac defects, distinctive facial appearance, learning disabilities, and behavioral disturbances. Several other contemporaneous authors had also described children with conotruncal heart defects, palate malformations (and resulting hypernasal speech), numerous physical dysmorphisms, and both metabolic and hematological problems (Shprintzen, 1999). Consequently, a number of other names are still used for similar or overlapping medical syndromes, including DiGeorge syndrome, conotruncal anomaly face syndrome, and CATCH 22 (cardiac anomalies, abnormal facies, thymic hypoplasia, cleft palate, and hypocalcemia) (Bassett *et al.*, 1998; Driscoll *et al.*, 1993; Gong *et al.*, 1996; Scambler *et al.*, 1992). More recently, the term, 22q11.2 deletion syndrome has been used to describe this condition (Scambler *et al.*, 1992).

Well over 100 medical manifestations or physical anomalies are associated with VCFS, but there is great variability in the number, type, and severity of problems from individual to individual (Cohen *et al.*, 1999; Goldberg *et al.*, 1993; Golding-Kushner *et al.*, 1985; McDonald-McGinn *et al.*, 1999; Ryan *et al.*, 1997; Vantrappen *et al.*, 1999; a VCFS fact sheet published by R. Shprintzen can be downloaded at www.vcfsef.org). The most common clinical signs are clefting of the secondary palate, long facies, retrognathia, prominent nose, malar flattening, cardiac anomalies (ventriculoseptal defect, tetrology of Fallot, right-sided aortic arch), hypoparathyroidism, thymic hypoplasia, small stature, hypotonia, slender hands and digits, and learning disabilities or mental retardation. These medical anomalies are present at birth and often result in serious perinatal illness requiring surgery or other intensive intervention. However, mild cases, with no serious medical morbidity, may escape detection at infancy. Developmental delays in the preschool period may result in identification of VCFS at that time, but some children with VCFS and most adults whose condition was unrecognized in childhood are never identified, because of a low clinical index of suspicion.

Cognitive and behavioral phenotype in childhood developmental delays

Almost all toddler and preschool children with VCFS suffer from mild gross motor delays, severe expressive and receptive language delays, and characteristic disabling impairments in speech production (Gerdes *et al.*, 1999; Golding-Kushner *et al.*, 1985; McDonald-McGinn *et al.*, 1999; Scherer *et al.*, 1999; Swillen *et al.*, 1999). These delays are not accounted for by the frequently occurring palatal and related nasopharyngeal defects, and they are not associated with the presence or absence of severe cardiac defects (Gerdes *et al.*, 1999; Scherer *et al.*, 1999). Motor delays (particularly hypotonia) tend to be mild; however, early receptive and expressive language development is almost always severely delayed, with very little vocabulary development at 30 months of age (Gerdes *et al.*, 1999). Measures of overall intelligence in toddler and preschoolers with VCFS indicate a range of intelligence from near-average to mild/moderate retardation, with the overall mean trending towards the borderline to mildly retarded range by 30 months (Scherer *et al.*, 1999). Other relatively common findings in preschool VCFS children include microcephaly and feeding and swallowing problems.

School-age children and adolescents with VCFS suffer from decrements in overall cognitive ability, learning disabilities, and speech and language problems (Golding-Kushner *et al.*, 1985; McDonald-McGinn *et al.*, 1999; Moss *et al.*, 1999; Swillen *et al.*, 1999). Children ages 6 years and older with VCFS have intelligence quotients (IQ) that are lower than the population average. Approximately 40% perform in the mild to moderately mentally retarded range of intelligence (Goldberg *et al.*, 1993; Golding-Kushner *et al.*, 1985; Moss *et al.*, 1999; Ryan *et al.*, 1997; Swillen *et al.*, 1997). Learning disabilities are almost invariably present (Goldberg *et al.*, 1993; Moss *et al.*, 1999; Ryan *et al.*, 1997; Swillen *et al.*, 1997).

The cognitive profile of VCFS in this age range is complex, with an admixture of non-verbal learning disabilities and ongoing receptive and expressive language disorders (Golding-Kushner *et al.*, 1985; Moss *et al.*, 1999). By middle childhood, children with VCFS show considerable advances in aspects of their language development, particularly speech, vocabulary, reading, word recognition, and spelling. However, higher-order comprehension, abstract verbal understanding, and language formulation remained very deficient, characterized by "immature, concrete thought" (Golding-Kushner *et al.*, 1985). Speech almost invariably remains hypernasal. VCFS children have significantly lower mean performance IQ scores than verbal IQ scores (based on the Wechsler Intelligence Scale for Children version III), and it has been suggested that they might have a non-verbal learning disability (Moss *et al.*, 1999). However, scores on standardized measure of language functioning are often significantly lower than verbal IQ scores. Of children with VCFS, 50% meet full diagnostic criteria for specific language impairment. Therefore, it appears that VCFS children have distinctive impairments in higher-order language, abstract reasoning, visuaospatial reasoning, and arithmetic. Almost all require intensive, long-term special educational services.

Unfortunately, there are no prospective data available regarding the developmental trajectory of cognitive dysfunction from childhood to adulthood. Information about cognitive functioning in VCFS adults is very limited. A recent survey found that 94% had evidence of mental retardation or learning disability (Cohen *et al.*, 1999).

Childhood behavioral phenotype

Children with VCFS have a high rate of maladaptive behaviors and social traits. These include frequently occurring problems with overactive, impulsive, emotionally labile, and disorganized behaviors, and social problems such as shyness or disinhibition (Gerdes *et al.*, 1999; Golding-Kushner *et al.*, 1985; Swillen *et al.*, 1999). Papolos *et al.* (1996) reported that attention-deficit hyperactivity disorder is very common, and also described high rates of separation-anxiety disorder and obsessive–compulsive disorder. Dimensional behavior ratings utilizing the Child Behavioral Checklist noted abnormally high scores in the subscales for social problems, attention problems, thought problems, withdrawn behaviors, and anxiety/depression (Swillen *et al.*, 1997, 1999). Children with VCFS are at an increased risk for childhood-onset schizophrenia. Usiskin *et al.* (1999) recently reported that 6.4% of a cohort of youngsters with childhood-onset schizophrenia had VCFS.

However, it is also well known that rates of psychiatric disorder are elevated in children with borderline and mild mental retardation, developmental language disorders, and learning disabilities (Feinstein and Reiss, 1996; Feinstein and Weiner, 1997; Fraser and Nolan, 1994; Toppelberg and Shapiro, 2000). Consequently, it was not clear that the high rates of psychopathology in VCFS children were distinctively different from those of other children with similar degrees of developmental impairment. Feinstein *et al.* (2002) compared psychiatric findings in a group of VCFS children with a control group matched for reduced IQ and severe learning disabilities. They found very high rates of specific phobias, generalized anxiety disorder, major depressive disorder, oppositional defiant disorder, higher than expected rates of obsessive–compulsive disorder, and evidence of delusions and hallucinations in a few subjects. However, VCFS patients did not have significantly higher rates of any these disorders than the cognitively matched controls.

Despite the difficulties to date in finding specific cognitive or behavioral features in children with VCFS that are specific indicators of later-onset psychosis, it may be that a subset of symptoms within the total array are, indeed, specific markers. Further longitudinal study of children with VCFS into adulthood offers the best hope of identifying any specific markers present in childhood.

Psychiatric presentation in adulthood

Links between VCFS and adolescent- or adult-onset schizophrenia have been demonstrated through clinical research on both disorders. Shprintzen's group reported, one decade after their early papers on VCFS, that 20–30% of VCFS children 16 years or older had developed schizophrenia or schizoaffective disorder (Pulver *et al.*, 1994; Shprintzen *et al.*, 1992). Papolos *et al.* (1996) also noted a high rate of cyclothymia in adolescents with VCFS and reported that 64% met criteria for bipolar spectrum disorders. The issue of pathological mood lability in patients with VCFS remains a topic of interest, although it has been partially eclipsed for the moment by the more extensive documentation of increased risk for schizophrenia.

Karayiorgou *et al.* (1995) reported two patients with 22q11.2 deletions in a random sample of 100 schizophrenia patients. Gothelf *et al.* (1997) utilized a clinical ascertainment strategy to identify adult hospitalized schizophrenia patients with undiagnosed VCFS by selecting those patients with both heart and palate defects (or other significant congenital anomalies) and assaying for the VCFS chromosomal deletion. This approach identified three VCFS patients with schizophrenia from a pool of 20. Bassett and colleagues (Bassett and Chow, 1999; Bassett et al., 1998) have reported association between VCFS and schizophrenia, using a similar approach to that of Gothelf, identifying a group of 15 adult schizophrenia patients with at least two of five common physical or developmental phenotypic features of VCFS. Ten (67%) were found to have VCFS. The IQ scores of this group were within the borderline to mildly retarded range. In addition to delusions, hallucinations, social withdrawal, and adaptive impairment, most schizophrenia patients with VCFS had a cluster of associated behavioral features, including impulsivity, frequent aggressive or temper outbursts, mood lability, anxiety symptoms, and compulsive features.

Murphy et al. (1999) provided a decisive replication for previous findings of a high rate of schizophrenia in adults with VCFS employing a structured psychiatric research diagnostic algorithm for 50 VCFS patients: 30% were psychotic (24% schizophrenia, 2% schizoaffective, 2% psychosis [not otherwise specified], and 2% rapid cycling bipolar disorder) and 12% also had a lifetime history of major depressive disorder. The range of intelligence in the VCFS subjects was similar to other studies (mean IQ scores in the borderline retarded range). There was no statistical association between IQ, cardiac defects, or cleft palate problems and the presence or absence of psychosis. No association was found between psychosis and the allele for catechol-O-methyltransferase (COMT; see below).

Genetics

In 1992, Scambler et al. identified a microdeletion at chromosome 22q11.2 in a majority of patients presenting with VCFS, as well as the other similar named syndromes. Individuals with this deletion are hemizygous for all genes encompassed by the deletion site. The 22q11.2 deletion is estimated to occur in at least 1 per 2000 to 4500 live births (Tezenas Du Montcel et al., 1996). In most affected individuals, a de novo 3 Mb deletion at chromosome 22q11.2 is responsible for the syndrome; however, in 10–25%, VCFS is inherited from a parent with VCFS (Carlson et al., 1997a,b; Driscoll et al., 1993; Lindsay et al., 1995; Scambler et al., 1992; Shaikh et al., 2000). There is some evidence that patients with inherited VCFS may have more severe clinical manifestations (Ryan et al., 1997; Swillen et al., 1997). There also appears to be a preponderance of maternally transmitted inheritance, perhaps because of greater likelihood for having offspring in woman with VCFS (Murphy et al., 1999; Ryan et al., 1997).

In fact, several microdeletions of different sizes can occur (presumably involving different genes or different overlapping or non-overlapping regions in the deletion site) in VCFS, all sited within the larger and by far the most commonly occurring 3 Mb 22q11.2 deletion region (Shaikh *et al.*, 2000). The relationship between the size and genetic content of the deletion and the resulting phenotoype is not well understood. Moreover, not all patients presenting with features of VCFS have the 22q11.2 microdeletion. Clinic surveys have found the deletion in 76% of VCFS, 88% of those with DiGeorge syndrome, and 84% of those with conotruncal anomaly face syndrome (Driscoll *et al.*, 1993; Fokstuen *et al.*, 1998; Lindsay *et al.*, 1995). As diagnostic certainty will increase among clinicians, "non-deleted" individuals with VCFS might appear as exceptions. Nevertheless, the ability to test for the 22q11.2 microdeletion greatly facilitates identifying and classifying the somatic, cognitive, and psychiatric sequelae of hemizygosity for the chromosome 22q11.2 site.

At least 30 genes are encoded in the commonly deleted segment (Dunham *et al.*, 1999), a few of which are highly expressed in brain tissue and are likely to be essential for normal brain development (Funke *et al.*, 1997; Gottlieb *et al.*, 1997; Lachman *et al.*, 1996a; Roberts *et al.*, 1997; Yamagishi *et al.*, 1999). Certain specific genes within the 22q11.2 site have attracted intense interest because of their known relationship to central nervous system structure or functioning. These include the gene for the goosecoid-like protein (GSCL), the genes, *Es2*, *UFDIL*, the gene for proline dehydrogenase (PDH), *PIK4CA*, and the gene for COMT.

Both the *GSCL* and *ES2* genes play a role in mouse brain embryogenesis and thus could be related to structural brain abnormalities observed in VCFS (Funke *et al.*, 1997; Gottlieb *et al.*, 1997, 1998; Lindsay *et al.*, 1998; Saint-Jore *et al.*, 1998). Yamagishi *et al.* (1998) measured the expression of a newly identified gene, *UFDIL*, which has been localized to the commonly deleted region. Of 182 subjects with VCFS, all had that specific gene deleted. Findings from this study indicate that *UFDIL* plays a key role in the embryonic development of the heart, palate, frontonasal regions, and brain. Specific polymorphisms of *PIK4CA* (Saito *et al.*, 2003) and the gene for PDH (Jacquet *et al.*, 2002; Liu *et al.*, 2002a) have been found to be potentially more common among populations of individuals with schizophrenia or bipolar disorder. Therefore, polymorphisms of *PIK4CA* and the gene for PDH have been hypothesized to be also more frequent in individuals with VCFS and psychosis. So far, no reports have clearly established, within the VCFS population, a link between psychiatric symptoms and allelic variants.

More recently, three independent groups have targeted the T-box gene *Tbx1* for gene inactivation in mouse models (Jerome and Papaioannou, 2001; Lindsay *et al.*, 2001; Merscher *et al.*, 2001). *Tbx1* homozygosity was perinatally lethal and associated with several usual features of VCFS such as thymus and parathyroid gland aplasia, major ear malformations, cleft palate, and conotruncal heart defects

(McDermid and Morrow, 2002). Tbx1 is a member of the T-box-containing family of transcription factors and also may modulate brain expression of several genes expressed in gray and white matter brain tissue. More studies will be needed to elucidate the function in humans of the gene considered today as the strongest candidate for the malformative features associated with VCFS.

The *COMT* gene has attracted the greatest attention in psychiatry because of its key role in neurotransmitter function. Its expression produces the enzyme involved in the metabolism of catecholamines and catechol-containing drugs, including dopamine, epinephrine, and norepinephrine (Cooper *et al.*, 1996). The enzymic activity of COMT varies substantially in humans (Palmatier *et al.*, 1999; Weinshilboum, 1978) as a result of a single nucleotide polymorphism (known as the COMT158 polymorphism) in the gene. The two resulting different alleles, *COMT*^{M} and *COMT*^{V}, express two different versions of the COMT enzyme, with COMT^M having lower activity (three- to fourfold decreased) (Lachman *et al.*, 1996b). Individuals can have any of three combinations of the alleles, accounting for variability among humans in COMT enzyme activity. However, people with VCFS are hemizygous for the COMT allele and, therefore, are the only group where the possibility exists for possessing a single M allele (and, therefore, the only known human group having the lowest possible level of COMT enzyme activity) (Lachman *et al.*, 1996a).

There have been numerous studies concerning the potential association of low-enzymatic COMT polymorphism with psychiatric conditions, including bipolar disorder, schizophrenia, and attention-deficit hyperactivity disorder (Bilder *et al.*, 2002; Kirov *et al.*, 1998; Kunugi *et al.*, 1997; Lachman *et al.*, 1997, 1996b; Papolos *et al.*, 1998; Shifman *et al.*, 2002; Strous *et al.*, 1997; Weinberger *et al.*, 2001). VCFS has, at times, been referred to as a "human model" to assay the role of COMT polymorphisms in psychiatric disorders (Lachman *et al.*, 1996a; Papolos *et al.*, 1996; Shifman *et al.*, 2002). Unfortunately, findings from these studies are frequently contradictory and, therefore, the putative role of COMT in the pathogenesis of psychiatric disorders remains unclear.

Studies of the relationship between VCFS and schizophrenia have recently stimulated interest in further molecular genetic analysis of the 22q11.2 site, utilizing both family- and population-based schizophrenia samples. Most recently, Liu *et al.* (2002b,c), based on the VCFS data and on two independent schizophrenia genetic linkage reports of high-susceptibility loci for schizophrenia in the 22q11 region, reasoned that non-deletion variants of individual genes within the 22q11 region might be related to risk of schizophrenia (Chakravarti, 2002). They undertook a fine-grained molecular genetic search for schizophrenia susceptibility, utilizing linkage analysis of single nucleotide polymorphisms from a 1.5 MB "schizophrenia critical region" in the 22q11 region. Their findings indicated more than one haplotype within the segment, in which *PRODH2* and *DGCR6* are the only known genes, where the schizophrenia susceptibility variant(s) most likely resides.

Neuroimaging

Since the early 1990s, magnetic resonance imaging (MRI) methodologies have been utilized to investigate the effect of the 22q11.2 deletion on brain structure. Mitnick *et al.* (1994) reported brain abnormalities, most commonly small cerebellar vermises, among 9 of 11 children with VCFS. Reduced volume of the posterior fossa was found in four, and cysts adjacent to the anterior horns of the ventricles were found in three. Chow *et al.* (1999) studied 11 adults with VCFS and schizophrenia and found that 90% exhibited bilateral white matter hyperintensities, distributed mainly within the frontal lobes; 45% had either cavum septum pellucidum or cavum vergae, and 36% had cerebellar hypoplasia. More recently, several cases of cortical dysgenesis including uni/bilateral frontoparietal polymicrogyria have been reported in children with 22q11 deletion syndrome (Bingham *et al.*, 1998; Bird, 2001; Ghariani *et al.*, 2002; Kawame *et al.*, 2000; Worthington *et al.*, 2000), possibly resulting in hemiplegia and seizures in the most severely affected patient. The underlying pathogenic mechanism for the 22q11 deletion syndrome-associated cortical dysgenesis is still unclear. Abnormal neuronal migration is one proposed explanation, but vascular disruption has also been suggested as a potential mechanism (Bird, 2001).

There are only a limited number of publications presenting MRI quantitative data in VCFS (Chow *et al.*, 2002; Eliez *et al.*, 2000; Kates *et al.*, 2001; van Amelsvoort *et al.*, 2001). Eliez *et al.* (2000) first reported significant alterations in cerebral morphology among children and adolescents with VCFS; an 11% reduction in total brain volume was detected related to both gray and white matter reduction. Frontal lobe brain volume was relatively enlarged in subjects with VCFS. Most notable was a significant reduction of parietal lobe gray matter in the left hemisphere and alteration of cerebellar volumes and vermis (Eliez *et al.*, 2001a). The dissociation between the alteration of frontal and non-frontal regions in children with VCFS was confirmed by Kates *et al.* (2001) with white matter tissue affected to a greater extent than white matter. Interestingly, these authors also reported a reduction of white matter in the left temporal cortex.

Investigating differences between 10 adults with VCFS and 13 age- and IQ-matched controls (among which two met criteria for schizophrenia and four for mood disorder), van Amelsvoort *et al.* (2001) described reduction of gray matter in the cerebellum and left temporal lobe, and reduction of white matter in the superior medial regions of the frontal lobe and in the frontotemporal regions. Another study, comparing 14 adults with VCFS and schizophrenia with 14 normal gender- and

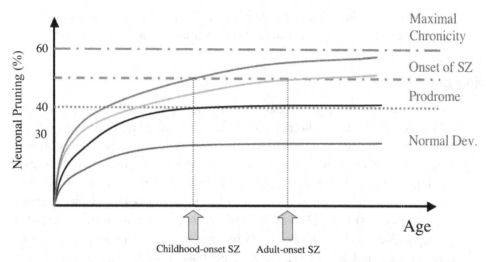

Fig. 7.1.   As suggested by several authors (McGlashan and Hoffman, 2000), the reduction of gray matter volumes in schizophrenia (SZ) is principally a result of abnormal dendritic arborization, giving rise to excessive pruning rather than decreased number of neurons. One might speculate that identical neurohistological characteristics are responsible for the gray matter volume decrease observed in individuals with the 22q11 deletion. To date, no detailed postmortem neuroanatomical and neurohistological studies have been published on human or animal models with velo-cardio-facial syndrome. These studies will be most valuable in order to understand the relation between genetic alteration and changes in white and gray matter tissue compartments.

age-matched controls (Chow *et al.*, 2002), reported an overall decrease of gray but not white matter. Lobar gray matter reduction was observed in the frontal and temporal lobes bilaterally and in the left parietal and occipital lobes. Ventricular cerebrospinal fluid was increased in individuals with VCFS and schizophrenia compared with controls. Most of the brain alterations described in VCFS are common to those reported in neuroimaging literature on schizophrenia (Shenton *et al.*, 2001).

A review of most of the available neuroimaging studies of children with VCFS would suggest that there is an early alteration of parietal lobe and cerebellum, and that the decrease of temporal lobe gray matter and hippocampus can be observed only in adults. However, in a study investigating volumetric changes with age in VCFS, Eliez *et al.* (2001b) found that accelerated decrease in volumes of gray matter in the temporal lobes and hippocampus already occurred during childhood and adolescence. The accelerated decrease of gray matter in temporal and mesiotemporal structures is likely to lead to significant volumetric differences by the time individuals with VCFS reach young adulthood. In another publication by the same group (Eliez *et al.*, 2001c), it has been suggested that individuals with a maternally derived 22q11.2 microdeletion have an accelerated decrease of gray matter, leading to significant reduction of total gray matter volumes and cognitive impairment (Glaser *et al.*, 2002). However, these results must be considered as preliminary since previous molecular studies did not show evidences for imprinting in the 22q11 region. Nevertheless, such findings emphasize the potential importance of epigenetic phenomenon like imprinting in the genetic factors contributing to brain development and function in schizophrenia.

Interestingly, in a recently reported longitudinal MRI study of individuals with early-onset schizophrenia, Thompson *et al.* (2001) showed that an alteration of cortical gray matter first developed in the parietal regions, then progressed towards frontal and temporal lobe, finally resulting in a severe overall gray matter reduction over a course of 4 years. In patients with adult-onset schizophrenia, gray matter volume reduction is already evident at the first clinical presentation of the disorder and appears to explain, at least partially, the morbid (Gold *et al.*, 1999; Gur *et al.*, 1999; Mohamed *et al.*, 1999; Thompson *et al.*, 2001) and premorbid cognitive features (Cannon *et al.*, 2002; Fuller *et al.*, 2002) associated with this condition. Further, differences in the size of the decrease in gray matter volume over time, modulated by parental origin of the deletion and other factors (yet to be identified), could explain the observed variability in the age of onset of schizophrenia in the VCFS population. Figure 7.1, concordant with a developmental model proposed by McGlashan and Hoffman (2000), illustrates the potential impact of gray matter decrease rate on age of onset of clinical symptoms, duration of prodromal phase before the expression of schizophrenia and the age at which the negative symptoms are predominant.

Conclusions

In summary, we have described the medical, genetic, cognitive, and behavioral phenotype of VCFS from infancy to adulthood, with particular emphasis on the variability of the phenotype and the strong association between the 22q11.2 chromosomal microdeletion and schizophrenia. VCFS represents a developmental model of a genetically homogeneous subtype of schizophrenia and a unique window to understand the interaction in children and adolescents between genes, brain, behavior, and cognition to lead to adult psychiatric disorders.

REFERENCES

Asarnow, R. F., Nuechterlein, K. H., Asamen, J., *et al.* (2002a). Neurocognitive functioning and schizophrenia spectrum disorders can be independent expressions of familial liability for schizophrenia in community control children: the UCLA family study. *Schizophr Res* **54**: 111–120.

Asarnow, R. F., Nuechterlein, K. H., Subotnik, K. L., *et al.* (2002b). Neurocognitive impairments in nonpsychotic parents of children with schizophrenia and attention-deficit/hyperactivity disorder: the University of California, Los Angeles Family Study. *Arch Gen Psychiatry* **59**: 1053–1060.

Bassett, A. S., Chow, E. W. (1999). 22q11 deletion syndrome: a genetic subtype of schizophrenia. *Biol Psychiatry* **46**: 882–891.

Bassett, A. S., Hodgkinson, K., Chow, E. W., *et al.* (1998). 22q11 deletion syndrome in adults with schizophrenia. *Am J Med Genet* **81**: 328–337.

Bilder, R., Volavka, J., Czobor, P., *et al.* (2002). Neurocognitive correlates of the COMT Val(158)Met polymorphism in chronic schizophrenia. *Biol Psychiatry* **52**: 701–707.

Bingham, P. M., Lynch, D., McDonald-McGinn, D., Zackai, E. (1998). Polymicrogyria in chromosome 22 delection syndrome. *Neurology* **51**: 1500–1502.

Bird, L. M. (2001). Cortical dysgenesis and 22q11 deletion. *Clin Dysmorphol* **10**: 77.

Cannon, M., Caspi, A., Moffitt, T. E., *et al.* (2002). Evidence for early-childhood, pan-developmental impairment specific to schizophreniform disorder: results from a longitudinal birth cohort. *Arch Gen Psychiatry* **59**: 449–456.

Carlson, C., Papolos, D., Pandita, R. K., *et al.* (1997a). Molecular analysis of velo-cardio-facial syndrome patients with psychiatric disorders. *Am J Hum Genet* **60**: 851–859.

Carlson, C., Sirotkin, H., Pandita, R., *et al.* (1997b). Molecular definition of 22q11 deletions in 151 velo-cardio-facial syndrome patients. *Am J Hum Genet* **61**: 620–629.

Chakravarti, A. (2002). A compelling genetic hypothesis for a complex disease, PRODHH2/DGCR6 variation leads to schizophrenia susceptibility. *Proc Natl Acad Sci USA* **99**: 4755–4756.

Chow, E., Zipursky, R. B., Mikulis, D., *et al.* (1999). MRI findings in adults with 22q11 deletion syndrome (22qDS) and schizophrenia. *Schizophr Res* **36**: 89.

Chow, E. W., Zipursky, R. B., Mikulis, D. J., Bassett, A. S. (2002). Structural brain abnormalities in patients with schizophrenia and 22q11 deletion syndrome. *Biol Psychiatry* **51**: 208–215.

Cohen, E., Chow, E., Weksberg, R., Bassett, A. S. (1999). Phenotype of adults with the 22q11 deletion syndrome. *Am J Med Genet* **86**: 359–365.

Cooper, J., Bloom, F., Roth, R. (1996): *The Biochemical Basis of Neuropharmacology*, 7th edn. New York: Oxford University Press.

Driscoll, D. A., Salvin, J., Sellinger, B., *et al.* (1993). Prevalence of 22q11 microdeletions in DiGeorge and velocardiofacial syndromes: implications for genetic counselling and prenatal diagnosis. *J Med Genet* **30**: 813–817.

Dunham, I., Shimizu, N., Roe, B. A., *et al.* (1999). The DNA sequence of human chromosome 22. *Nature* **402**: 489–495.

Eliez, S., Schmitt, J. E., White, C. D., Reiss, A. L. (2000). Children and adolescents with velocardiofacial syndrome: a volumetric MRI study. *Am J Psychiatry* **157**: 409–415.

Eliez, S., Schmitt, J. E., White, C. D., Wellis, V. G., Reiss, A. L. (2001a). A quantitative MRI study of posterior fossa development in velocardiofacial syndrome. *Biol Psychiatry* **49**: 540–546.

Eliez, S., Blasey, C. M., Schmitt, E. J., *et al.* (2001b). Velocardiofacial syndrome: are structural changes in the temporal and mesial temporal regions related to schizophrenia? *Am J Psychiatry* **158**: 447–453.

Eliez, S., Antonarakis, S. E., Morris, M. A., Dahoun, S. P., Reiss,, A. L. (2001c). Parental origin of the deletion 22q11.2 and brain development in velocardiofacial syndrome: a preliminary study. *Arch Gen Psychiatry* **58**: 64–68.

Erlenmeyer-Kimling, L., Rock, D., Roberts, S., *et al.* (2000). Attention, memory, and motor skills as childhood predictors of schizophrenia-related psychosis. *Am J Psychiatry* **157**: 1416–1422.

Feinstein, C., Reiss, A. L. (1996). Psychiatric disorders in mentally retarded children and adolescents. *Child Adolesc Psychiatr Clin N Am* **5**: 827–852.

Feinstein, C., Weiner, J. (1997). Developmental disorders of learning, motor skills, and communication. In *Textbook of Child and Adolescent Psychiatary*, ed. J. Weiner. Washington, DC: American Psychiatry Press, pp. 281–300.

Feinstein, C., Eliez, S., Blasey, C., Reiss, A. L. (2002). Psychiatric disorders and behavioral problems in children with velocardiofacial syndrome: usefulness as phenotypic indicators of schizophrenia risk. *Biol Psychiatry* **51**: 312–318.

Fish, B. (1977). Neurobiologic antecedents of schizophrenia in children. Evidence for an inherited, congenital neurointegrative defect. *Arch Gen Psychiatry* **34**: 1297–1313.

Fish, B., Marcus, J., Hans, S. L., Auerbach, J. G., Perdue, S. (1992). Infants at risk for schizophrenia: sequelae of a genetic neurointegrative defect. A review and replication analysis of pandysmaturation in the Jerusalem Infant Development Study. *Arch Gen Psychiatry* **49**: 221–235.

Fokstuen, S., Arbenz, U., Artan, S., *et al.* (1998). 22q11.2 deletions in a series of patients with non-selective congenital heart defects: incidence, type of defects and parental origin. *Clin Genet* **53**: 63–69.

Fraser, W., Nolan, M. (1994). Psychiatric disorders in mental retardation. In *Mental Health in Mental Retardation*, ed. N. Bouras. Cambridge: Cambridge University Press, pp. 79–92.

Fuller, R., Nopoulos, P., Arndt, S., *et al.* (2002). Longitudinal assessment of premorbid cognitive functioning in patients with schizophrenia through examination of standardized scholastic test performance. *Am J Psychiatry* **159**: 1183–1189.

Funke, B., Saint-Jore, B., Puech, A., *et al.* (1997). Characterization and mutation analysis of goosecoid-like (GSCL), a homeodomain-containing gene that maps to the critical region for VCFS/DGS on 22q11. *Genomics* **46**: 364–372.

Gerdes, M., Solot, C., Wang, P. P., *et al.* (1999). Cognitive and behavior profile of preschool children with chromosome 22q11.2 deletion. *Am J Med Genet* **85**: 127–133.

Ghariani, S., Dahan, K., Saint-Martin, C., *et al.* (2002). Polymicrogyria in chromosome 22q11 deletion syndrome. *Eur J Paediatr Neurol* **6**: 73–77.

Glaser, B., Mumme, D. L., Blasey, C., *et al.* (2002). Language skills in children with velocardiofacial syndrome (deletion 22q11.2). *J Pediatr* **140**: 753–758.

Gold, S., Arndt, S., Nopoulos, P., O'Leary, D. S., Andreasen, N. C. (1999). Longitudinal study of cognitive function in first-episode and recent-onset schizophrenia. *Am J Psychiatry* **156**: 1342–1348.

Goldberg, R., Motzkin, B., Marion, R., Scambler, P. J., Shprintzen, R. J. (1993). Velo-cardio-facial syndrome: a review of 120 patients. *Am J Med Genet* **45**: 313–319.

Golding-Kushner, K. J., Weller, G., Shprintzen, R. J. (1985). Velo-cardio-facial syndrome: language and psychological profiles. *J Craniofac Genet Dev Biol* **5**: 259–266.

Gong, W., Emanuel, B. B., Collins, J. E., *et al.* (1996). A transcription map of the DiGeorge and velocardiofacial syndrome minimal critical region. *Hum Mol Genet* 5: 789–800.

Gothelf, D., Frisch, A., Munitz, H., *et al.* (1997). Velocardiofacial manifestations and microdeletions in schizophrenic inpatients. *Am J Med Genet* 72: 455–461.

Gottlieb, S., Emanuel, B. S., Driscoll, D. A., *et al.* (1997). The DiGeorge syndrome minimal critical region contains a goosecoid-like (GSCL) homeobox gene that is expressed early in human development. *Am J Hum Genet* 60: 1194–1201.

Gottlieb, S., Hanes, S. D., Golden, J. A., Oakey, R. J., Budarf, M. L. (1998). Goosecoid-like, a gene deleted in DiGeorge and velocardiofacial syndromes, recognizes DNA with a bicoid-like specificity and is expressed in the developing mouse brain. *Hum Mol Genet* 7: 1497–1505.

Gur, R. E., Turetsky, B. I., Bilker, W. B., Gur, R. C. (1999). Reduced gray matter volume in schizophrenia. *Arch Gen Psychiatry* 56: 905–911.

Hans, S. L., Marcus, J., Nuechterlein, K. H., *et al.* (1999). Neurobehavioral deficits at adolescence in children at risk for schizophrenia: the Jersualem Infant Development Study. *Arch Gen Psychiatry* 56: 741–748.

Jacquet, H., Raux, G., Thibaut, F., *et al.* (2002). PRODH mutations and hyperprolinemia in a subset of schizophrenic patients. *Hum Mol Genet* 11: 2243–2249.

Jerome, L. A., Papaioannou, V. E. (2001). DiGeorge syndrome phenotype in mice mutant for the T-box gene, *Tbx1*. *Nat Genet* 27: 286–291.

Karayiorgou, M., Morris, M. A., Morrow, B., *et al.* (1995). Schizophrenia susceptibility associated with interstitial deletions of chromosome 22q11. *Proc Natl Acad Sci USA* 92: 7612–7616.

Kates, W. R., Burnette, C. P., Jabs, E. W., *et al.* (2001). Regional cortical white matter reductions in velocardiofacial syndrome: a volumetric MRI analysis. *Biol Psychiatry* 49: 677–684.

Kawame, H., Kurosawa, K., Akatsuka, A., Ochiai, Y., Mizuno, K. (2000). Polymicrogyria is an uncommon manifestation in 22q11.2 deletion syndrome. *Am J Med Genet* 94: 77–78.

Kirov, G., Murphy, K. C., Arranz, M., *et al.* (1998). Low activity allele of catechol-*O*-methyltransferase gene associated with rapid cylcing bipolar disorder. *Mol Psychiatry* 3: 342–345.

Kunugi, H., Vallada, H., Sham, P., *et al.* (1997). Catechol-*O*-methyltransferase polymorphisms and schizophrenia: a transmission disequilibrium study in multiply affected families. *Psychiatr Genet* 7: 97–101.

Lachman, H. M., Morrow, B., Shprintzen, R., *et al.* (1996a). Association of codon 108/158 catechol-*O*-methyltransferase gene polymorphism with the psychiatric manifestations of velo-cardio-facial syndrome. *Am J Med Genet* 67: 468–472.

Lachman, H. M., Papolos, D. F., Saito, T., *et al.* (1996b). Human catechol-*O*-methyltransferase pharmacogenetics: description of a functional polymorphism and its potential application to neuropsychiatric disorders. *Pharmacogenetics* 6: 243–250.

Lachman, H., Kelsoe, J., Moreno, L., Katz, S., Papolos, D. (1997). Lack of association of catechol-*O*-methyltransferase (COMT) functional polymorphism in bipolar affective disorder. *Psychiatr Genet* 7: 13–17.

Lindsay, E. A., Greenberg, F., Shaffer, L. G., *et al.* (1995). Submicroscopic deletions at 22q11.2: variability of the clinical picture and delineation of a commonly deleted region. *Am J Med Genet* 56: 191–197.

Lindsay, E. A., Harvey, E., Scambler, P., Baldini, A. (1998). *ES2*, a gene deleted in DiGeorge syndrome, encodes a nuclear protein and is expressed during early mouse development, where it shares an expression domain with a goosecoid-like gene. *Hum Mol Genet* **7**: 629–635.

Lindsay, E. A., Vitelli, F., Su, H., *et al.* (2001). *Tbx1* haploinsufficiency in the DiGeorge syndrome region causes aortic arch defects in mice. *Nature* **410**: 97–101.

Liu, H., Heath, S. C., Sobin, C., *et al.* (2002a). Genetic variation at the 22q11 *PRODH 2/DGCR6* locus presents an unusual pattern and increases susceptibility to schizophrenia. *Proc Natl Acad Sci USA* **99**: 3717–3722.

Liu, H., Abecasis, G. R., Heath, S. C., *et al.* (2002b). Genetic variation in the 22q11 locus and susceptibility to schizophrenia. *Proc Natl Acad Sci USA* **99**: 16859–16864.

Liu, H., Heath, S. C., Sobin, C., *et al.* (2002c). Genetic variation at the 22q11 *PRODH2/DGCR6* locus presents an unusual pattern and increases susceptibility to schizophrenia. *Proc Natl Acad Sci USA* **99**: 3717–3722.

Marcus, J., Hans, S. L., Auerbach, J. G., Auerbach, A. G. (1993). Children at risk for schizophrenia: the Jerusalem Infant Development Study II. Neurobehavioral deficits at school age. *Arch Gen Psychiatry* **50**: 797–809.

McDermid, H. E., Morrow, B. E. (2002). Genomic disorders on 22q11. *Am J Hum Genet* **70**: 1077–1088.

McDonald-McGinn, D. M., Kirschner, R., Goldmuntz, E., *et al.* (1999). The Philadelphia story: the 22q11.2 deletion. Report on 250 patients. *Genet Couns* **10**: 11–24.

McGlashan, T. H., Hoffman, R. E. (2000). Schizophrenia as a disorder of developmentally reduced synaptic connectivity. *Arch Gen Psychiatry* **57**: 637–648.

Merscher, S., Funke, B., Epstein, J. A., *et al.* (2001). *TBX1* is responsible for cardiovascular defects in velo-cardio-facial/DiGeorge syndrome. *Cell* **104**: 619–629.

Mitnick, R. J., Bello, J. A., Shprintzen, R. J. (1994). Brain anomalies in velo-cardio-facial syndrome. *Am J Med Genet* **54**: 100–106.

Mohamed, S., Paulsen, J. S., O'Leary, D., Arndt, S., Andreasen, N. (1999). Generalized cognitive deficits in schizophrenia: a study of first-episode patients. *Arch Gen Psychiatry* **56**: 749–754.

Moss, E. M., Batshaw, M. L., Solot, C. B., *et al.* (1999). Psychoeducational profile of the 22q11.2 microdeletion: a complex pattern. *J Pediatr* **134**: 193–198.

Murphy, K. C., Jones, L. A., Owen, M. J. (1999). High rates of schizophrenia in adults with velo-cardio-facial syndrome. *Arch Gen Psychiatry* **56**: 940–945.

Palmatier, M. A., Kang, A. M., Kidd, K. K. (1999). Global variation in the frequencies of functionally different catechol-*O*-methyltransferase alleles. *Biol Psychiatry* **46**: 557–567.

Papolos, D. F., Faedda, G. L., Veit, S., *et al.* (1996). Bipolar spectrum disorders in patients diagnosed with velo-cardio-facial syndrome: does a hemizygous deletion of chromosome 22q11 result in bipolar affective disorder? *Am J Psychiatry* **153**: 1541–1547.

Papolos, D. F., Veit, S., Faedda, G. L., Saito, T., Lachman, H. M. (1998). Ultra-ultra rapid cycling bipolar disorder is associated with the low activity catecholamine-*O*-methyltransferase allele. *Mol Psychiatry* **3**: 346–349.

Pulver, A. E., Nestadt, G., Goldberg, R., *et al.* (1994). Psychotic illness in patients diagnosed with velo-cardio-facial syndrome and their relatives. *J Nerv Ment Dis* **182**: 476–478.

Reichenberg, A., Weiser, M., Rabinowitz, J., *et al.* (2002). A population-based cohort study of premorbid intellectual, language, and behavioral functioning in patients with schizophrenia, schizoaffective disorder, and nonpsychotic bipolar disorder. *Am J Psychiatry* **159**: 2027–2035.

Roberts, C., Daw, S. C., Halford, S., Scambler, P. J. (1997). Cloning and developmental expression analysis of chick *Hira* (*Chira*), a candidate gene for DiGeorge syndrome. *Hum Mol Genet* **6**: 237–245.

Ryan, A. K., Goodship, J. A., Wilson, D. I., *et al.* (1997). Spectrum of clinical features associated with interstitial chromosome 22q11 deletions: a European collaborative study. *J Med Genet* **34**: 798–804.

Saint-Jore, B., Puech, A., Heyer, J., *et al.* (1998). Goosecoid-like (*Gscl*), a candidate gene for velocardiofacial syndrome, is not essential for normal mouse development. *Hum Mol Genet* **7**: 1841–1849.

Saito, T., Stopkova, P., Diaz, L., *et al.* (2003). Polymorphism screening of *PIK4CA*: possible candidate gene for chromosome 22q11-linked psychiatric disorders. *Am J Med Genet* **116**: 77–83.

Scambler, P. J., Kelly, D., Lindsay, E., *et al.* (1992). Velo-cardio-facial syndrome associated with chromosome 22 deletions encompassing the DiGeorge locus. *Lancet* **339**: 1138–1139.

Scherer, N. J., D'Antonio, L. L., Kalbfleisch, J. H. (1999). Early speech and language development in children with velocardiofacial syndrome. *Am J Med Genet* **88**: 714–723.

Shaikh, T. H., Kurahashi, H., Saitta, S. C., *et al.* (2000). Chromosome 22-specific low copy repeats and the 22q11.2 deletion syndrome: genomic organization and deletion endpoint analysis. *Hum Mol Genet* **9**: 489–501.

Shenton, M. E., Dickey, C. C., Frumin, M., McCarley, R. W. (2001). A review of MRI findings in schizophrenia. *Schizophr Res* **49**: 1–52.

Shifman, S., Bronstein, M., Sternfeld, M., *et al.* (2002). A highly significant association between a COMT haplotype and schizophrenia. *Am J Hum Genet* **71**: 1296–1302.

Shprintzen, R. J. (1999). Historic overview of VCFS. *Genet Couns* **10**: 1–2.

Shprintzen, R. J., Goldberg, R. B., Lewin, M. L., *et al.* (1978). A new syndrome involving cleft palate, cardiac anomalies, typical facies, and learning disabilities: velo-cardio-facial syndrome. *Cleft Palate J* **15**: 56–62.

Shprintzen, R. J., Goldberg, R., Golding-Kushner, K. J., Marion, R. W. (1992). Late-onset psychosis in the velo-cardio-facial syndrome. *Am J Med Genet* **42**: 141–142.

Strous, R., Bark, N., Parsia, S., Vovlavka, J., Lachman, H. (1997). Analysis of a functional catechol-O-methyltransferase gene polymorphism in schizophrenia: evidence for association with aggressive and antisocial behavior. *Psychiatr Res* **69**: 71–77.

Swillen, A., Devriendt, K., Legius, E., *et al.* (1997). Intelligence and psychosocial adjustment in velocardiofacial syndrome: a study of 37 children and adolescents with VCFS. *J Med Genet* **34**: 453–458.

(1999). The behavioural phenotype in velo-cardio-facial syndrome (VCFS): from infancy to adolescence. *Genet Couns* **10**: 79–88.

Tezenas Du Montcel, S., Mendizabai, H., *et al.* (1996). Prevalence of 22q11 microdeletion [letter]. *J Med Genet* **33**: 719.

Thompson, P. M., Vidal, C., Giedd, J. N., *et al.* (2001). Mapping adolescent brain change reveals dynamic wave of accelerated gray matter loss in very early-onset schizophrenia. *Proc Natl Acad Sci USA* **98**: 11650–11655.

Toppelberg, C., Shapiro, T. (2000). Language disorders: a 10-year research update review. *J Am Acad Child Adolesc Psychiatry* **39**: 143–152.

Usiskin, S. I., Nicolson, R., Krasnewich, D. M., *et al.* (1999). Velocardiofacial syndrome in childhood-onset schizophrenia. *J Am Acad Child Adolesc Psychiatry* **38**: 1536–1543.

van Amelsvoort, T., Daly, E., Robertson, D., *et al.* (2001). Structural brain abnormalities associated with deletion at chromosome 22q11: quantitative neuroimaging study of adults with velo-cardio-facial syndrome. *Br J Psychiatry* **178**: 412–419.

Vantrappen, G., Devriendt, K., Swillen, A., *et al.* (1999). Presenting symptoms and clinical features in 130 patients with the velo-cardio-facial syndrome. The Leuven experience. *Genet Couns* **10**: 3–9.

Weinberger, D. R. (1987). Implications of normal brain development for the pathogenesis of schizophrenia. *Arch Gen Psychiatry* **44**: 660–669.

Weinberger, D. R., Egan, M. F., Bertolino, A., *et al.* (2001). Prefrontal neurons and the genetics of schizophrenia. *Biol Psychiatry* **50**: 825–844.

Weinshilboum, R. M. (1978). Human biochemical genetics of plasma dopamine-beta-hydroxylase and erythrocyte catechol-*O*-methyltransferase. *Hum Genet Suppl* **1**: 101–112.

Worthington, S., Turner, A., Elber, J., Andrews, P. I. (2000). 22q11 deletion and polymicrogyria: cause or coincidence? *Clin Dysmorphol* **9**: 193–197.

Yamagishi, H., Garg, V., Matsuoka, R., Thomas, T., Srivastava, D. (1999). A molecular pathway revealing a genetic basis for human cardiac and craniofacial defects. *Science* **283**: 1158–1161.

8

Can structural magnetic resonance imaging provide an alternative phenotype for genetic studies of schizophrenia?

Colm McDonald and Robin M. Murray

Institute of Psychiatry, King's College, London, UK

There is overwhelming evidence from family, adoption, and twin studies that schizophrenia has a genetic component to its etiology. Estimates of the heritability of schizophrenia from modern twin studies are in the region of 80% (Cardno *et al.*, 1999), with the remaining variance attributed to non-shared environmental factors. Despite two decades of molecular genetics research, however, there has been slow progress towards identifying susceptibility genes for the illness, although there have been linkage findings replicated at some sites on the genome and potential suscep-tibility genes within these sites have recently been reported (Stefansson *et al.*, 2002; Straub *et al.*, 2002). The relative lack of success in identifying genes of major effect for the illness, combined with the pattern of inheritance of schizophrenia, has led many researchers to favor a multifactorial model for susceptibility, whereby liability is continuous within the population and multiple genes interact with environmental stressors to propel the individual over a threshold for illness expression (Gottesman, 1991). Unlike other multifactorial diseases, such as diabetes mellitus and coronary heart disease, genetic research into schizophrenia suffers from the added disad-vantages of having an uncertain phenotype with as yet no validating biological test, even at postmortem, and environmental risk factors that are unknown or of minor effect. There is growing interest, therefore, in utilizing other approaches in the search for susceptibility genes. Given a model of continuous liability within the population, the use of the qualitative phenotype (affected/unaffected) is often likely to be underpowered, but it may be possible to enhance the traditional categorical approach to phenotypic definition by identifying genetically valid traits that can be measured quantitatively. Candidates for such traits include symptom clusters or schizotypal traits as well as biological markers of neurobiological dysfunction or "endophenotypes."

Neurodevelopment and Schizophrenia, ed. Matcheri S. Keshavan *et al.* Published by Cambridge University Press. © Cambridge University Press 2004.

Endophenotypes are objectively measured neurobiological abnormalities that may represent more proximal effects of susceptibility genes than the clinical phenotype (Wickham and Murray, 1997). Such biological markers should fulfill a number of criteria to be useful in genetic studies (Gershon and Goldin, 1986; Leboyer *et al.*, 1998): (i) be heritable themselves, (ii) be associated with the illness in the general population, (iii) be state independent (i.e. be manifest whether or not the illness is active), (iv) cosegregate with the illness within families (i.e. among relatives who manifest the marker, the illness is more prevalent than among those relatives who do not), (v) be measurable in both affected and unaffected subjects, and (vi) be found more frequently among the biological relatives of patients than in healthy controls. Putative endophenotypes for schizophrenia include abnormalities of the auditory evoked response, such as the P300 and P50 waves (Frangou *et al.*, 1997a; Siegel *et al.*, 1984); oculomotor dysfunction, such as on smooth pursuit and anti-saccade tasks (Crawford *et al.*, 1998; Holzman *et al.*, 1988); neuropsychological deficits (Cannon *et al.*, 1994; Toulopoulou *et al.*, 2003); and abnormalities of brain structure. In this chapter, we review the value of structural brain deviations identified through magnetic resonance imaging (MRI) as potential endophenotypes in genetic studies of schizophrenia and the evidence to date that a number of specific brain deviations are linked to susceptibility genes for schizophrenia from studies of patients and their unaffected relatives.

The heritability of brain structure

One criticism of applying the endophenotypic approach to schizophrenia is that several of the putative markers have not yet themselves been demonstrated to be heritable. A powerful way of examining the extent to which a trait is heritable is to measure how commonly the trait is shared among monozygotic (MZ) twins, who have identical genotypes, compared with dizygotic (DZ) twins, who share on average 50% of their genes. One of the earliest studies of brain structure in normal twins was a computed tomographic (CT) study of subjects from the Maudsley Twin Series (Reveley *et al.*, 1982, 1984a). In this study, measurements of ventricular volume in normal MZ twins were much more highly correlated than those of DZ twins, indicating strong genetic control over ventricular size, with estimates of heritability for ventricular size using different methods all over 80%. There have been a number of similarly designed twin studies reported in recent years that use higher-resolution MRI and path analysis to model heritability. In contrast to the study by Reveley and colleagues, the heritability of lateral ventricular volume was reported to be low in two such studies (Baare *et al.*, 2001a; Wright *et al.*, 2002), with most variation in ventricular volume being a result of common environmental effects. However, Pfefferbaum *et al.* (2000) reported a high heritability of 79% for ventricular volume in 85 elderly twin pairs, and White *et al.* (2002) reported a correlation of 0.85 for ventricular volume among a sample of MZ pairs (although this did not significantly differ from the correlation in unrelated matched controls, 0.52, which was relatively high presumably because of the influence of age and gender over ventricular volume). Ventricular volume is known to be affected by environmental insults such as low birth weight (Nosarti *et al.*, 2002) and the true extent of genetic control over ventricular volume will require further studies.

Bartley and colleagues (1997) reported higher correlations among MZ than DZ twins for measures of cerebral volume, and subsequent statistical modeling demonstrated that this was most likely a result of additive genetic effects rather than shared environmental effects, with heritability estimated at 94%. This high degree of genetic control over brain volume has now been confirmed beyond doubt by several other MRI studies of twins (Baare *et al.*, 2001a; Carmelli *et al.*, 1998; Pennington *et al.*, 2000; Pfefferbaum *et al.*, 2000; Tramo *et al.*, 1998; White *et al.*, 2002). In one of the largest such studies to date, which included siblings of the twins in an attempt to dissect further the contribution of genetic as distinct from common environmental effects (since even DZ twins share the same prenatal environment), very high heritabilities were also found for global gray matter (82%) and white matter (88%) (Baare *et al.*, 2001a). In another large twin study, Pennington and colleagues (2000) demonstrated high genetic control over factors representing volumes of cortical and especially subcortical brain regions. In a sample of elderly male twins, there was evidence for high genetic control over lobar brain volumes, especially right frontotemporal regions, volume of white matter intensities, and the size of the corpus callosum (Carmelli *et al.*, 1998, 2002; Pfefferbaum *et al.*, 2000), but for lower genetic control over hippocampal volume compared with the other brain regions, the heritability of which was estimated at 40% (Sullivan *et al.*, 2001). As with ventricular volume, hippocampal volume is known to be susceptible to environmental insults such as early hypoxia (Rutherford *et al.*, 1995). A recent study of MZ twins found high correlations between twins for measures of gray matter, white matter, lobar volumes, cortical depth, cerebellum, thalamus, caudate, and putamen (White *et al.*, 2002). Other twin studies reported a high degree of genetic control over the size of the corpus callosum (Oppenheim *et al.*, 1989; Tramo *et al.*, 1998). By comparinson, there appears to be a poorer correlation between MZ twins for measures of cortical gyrification (Bartley *et al.*, 1997; Steinmetz *et al.*, 1994), gyral and sulcal curvature (White *et al.*, 2002), and asymmetry of the planum temporale (Steinmetz *et al.*, 1995), indicating less genetic control over these measures of brain structure.

Wright *et al.* (2002), in a reanalysis of the twins previously analyzed by Bartley *et al.* (1997) with whole brain voxel-based morphometry and more novel statistical analysis, found evidence for large genetic effects shared by several bilateral brain regions, especially paralimbic structures and the temporoparietal cortex. Also, using automated morphometry of the cortical surface, Thompson *et al.* (2001) reported a high degree of genetic control over large areas of gray matter encompassing the frontal lobes and the sensorimotor and linguistic neocortical regions. Consequently, there is considerable evidence for a high degree of genetic control over cerebral volume and many subregions within the adult human brain as assessed by volumetric measurement of MRI scans, which supports the value of exploring brain structure in vivo for potential endophenotypes of complex genetic illnesses like schizophrenia. Future twin studies will continue to dissect the genetic and environmental contributions towards other structures of interest to schizophrenia researchers.

Brain structure and schizophrenia

Despite heterogeneous patient samples and methodologies, neuroimaging studies consistently identify subtle volumetric deviations in a range of brain structures when schizophrenia patients are compared with controls. Enlargement of the lateral and third ventricles is the most prominent finding: a recent meta-analysis of 58 MRI studies reported a 26% enlargement of ventricular volume in schizophrenia subjects (Wright *et al.*, 2000). The illness is also characterized by a mild reduction (2%) in global cerebral volume and further volume reductions in a number of localized regions relative to cerebral volume. These regions include the hippocampus, amygdala, parahippocampal gyrus, superior temporal gyrus, prefrontal cortex, cingulate gyrus, thalamus, and insula (McCarley *et al.*, 1999; Wright *et al.*, 1999, 2000). In contrast to these volume reductions, increased volume of the basal ganglia is reported in schizophrenia. The basal ganglia are rich in dopaminergic input and the increased volume is usually attributed to the use of conventional antipsychotic medication, which potently blocks dopamine receptors, since it is not found in subjects who have had minimal antipsychotic treatment and the volume decreases on switching to an atypical antipsychotic (Chakos *et al.*, 1995). In general, the neuroimaging studies are supported by morphological findings from postmortem studies (Harrison, 1999).

Despite this evidence, the full nature and extent of structural abnormalities in schizophrenia has yet to be elucidated. Most studies to date have focused on a relatively small number of structures using a region-of-interest approach to morphometry, which is necessarily hypothesis driven and restricted to the particular regions the investigators choose to research; however, these studies ignore many brain regions not chosen for measurement and frequently amalgamate functionally distinct regions, for example within an entire lobe of the brain. More recently, some researchers have adopted alternative techniques involving whole brain analysis.

Goldstein *et al.* (1999), in a volumetric analysis of the entire neocortex divided into parcellation units, identified several regions of volume deficit, most prominently in the middle frontal gyrus, supramarginal gyrus, and paralimbic cortices, including the anterior cingulate, paracingulate gyri, and the insula. Other recent studies have used computational morphometry, a range of developing methodologies that involves automated whole brain analysis of MRI images at the voxel level. These studies have identified volumetric reduction in a range of distributed networks usually most prominent in fronto-temporolimbic areas and including the dorsolateral prefrontal cortex, frontomedial cortex, superior temporal gyrus, thalamus, cerebellum, insula, and limbic/paralimbic regions, as well as associated white matter tracts (Ananth *et al.*, 2002; Sigmundsson *et al.*, 2001; Suzuki *et al.*, 2002; Wilke *et al.*, 2001; Wright *et al.*, 1999).

State versus trait

Do the structural changes vary with the stage of the illness or its treatment? Some recent studies report greater deviation of structural changes as the illness advances, such as progressive ventricular and sulcal enlargement, and reduced volume of frontal and temporal regions, especially in the early stages of the illness or in those at the severe end of the spectrum (Gur *et al.*, 1998; Lieberman *et al.*, 2001). However, there are methodological difficulties associated with longitudinal quantitative neuroimaging studies, including different resolution of imaging techniques, small sample sizes, and inadequate matching of controls and subjects; further longitudinal studies are required to elucidate fully whether brain deviations worsen over the course of the illness (Weinberger and McClure, 2002).

Whether or not certain brain changes become more extensive over time, it is apparent that they are not solely dependent on the presence of symptomatic episodes to become manifest. Indeed various lines of evidence indicate that several of the structural deviations result from impairment of normal neurodevelopment.

First, many brain abnormalities are detectable in patients at or near the onset of psychosis, including enlargement of the lateral and third ventricles and reduced volume of cortical gray matter, the thalamus, the left hippocampus/amygdala, and the left posterior superior temporal gyrus (DeLisi *et al.*, 1991; Fannon *et al.*, 2000; Hirayasu *et al.*, 1998).

Second, some of the morphological abnormalities identified in adult schizophrenia patients suggest pathophysiological processes affecting the early developing brain. These include uncommon developmental brain lesions such as aqueduct stenosis, arachnoid and septal cysts, and agenesis of the corpus callosum, which occur with excess frequency in schizophrenia (Lewis, 1990). Normal structural cerebral asymmetries such as those of the planum temporale and fronto-occipital petalias also develop during fetal life, and some studies have reported loss or reversal of such asymmetries in schizophrenia (Bilder *et al.*, 1994; Falkai *et al.*, 1995). Similarly, gyrification of the prefrontal cortex achieves stability soon after birth and right frontal cortical hypergyrification has been reported in schizophrenia (Vogeley *et al.*, 2001).

Third, a series of correlations have been reported between early environmental risk factors for schizophrenia and structural deviations in the adult brain. These include early reports (Murray *et al.*, 1985) of an association between increased ventricle-to-brain ratio on CT scans and exposure to obstetric complications, although other studies did not find a relationship between obstetric complications and lateral ventricular enlargement (McGrath and Murray, 1995). Other structural abnormalities, such as reduced hippocampal volume, have also been linked to obstetric complications (McNeil *et al.*, 2000; Stefanis *et al.*, 1999).

Fourth, some of the brain abnormalities have also been reported in the unaffected relatives of patients, which would indicate that such abnormalities are not restricted to the pathological process of psychosis but are a manifestation of familial risk factors, the most likely candidates being genes influencing neurodevelopment (see below). Therefore, several of the brain deviations linked to schizophrenia are probably related to aberrant neurodevelopment. Since at least some of the susceptibility genes for schizophrenia are likely to influence neurodevelopmental processes (Jones and Murray, 1991), such brain deviations could present suitable alternative phenotypes to utilize in the search for such genes.

Brain abnormalities in unaffected relatives

First-degree relatives of schizophrenia subjects share 50% of their genes with their affected relative on average; therefore, neurobiological traits of the illness that are linked to susceptibility genes should be found more commonly among such relatives. Three types of study design have examined the extent of structural brain abnormalities in unaffected first-degree relatives. (i) Family studies assess unaffected adult relatives, usually siblings and parents who tend to have lived beyond the usual age of onset. (ii) High-risk studies assess offspring or adolescents with first-degree relatives with schizophrenia; usually assessment is before the age of onset of schizophrenia and hence 10–15% of these subjects would be expected to develop the illness over time. (iii) Twin studies usually include groups of discordant MZ twins and are thus designed to identify non-genetic traits of the illness, but abnormalities in unaffected co-twins compared with normal twins could represent manifestations of genetic risk, especially if also found more commonly in MZ than DZ unaffected co-twins.

Ventricles

Unaffected first-degree relatives of schizophrenia patients were first included in CT studies as a comparison group for patients in order to reduce the considerable genetic variation of ventricular size that exists in the population. These studies generally demonstrated greater ventricular enlargement in patients than in their unaffected relatives (DeLisi *et al.*, 1986; Reveley *et al.*, 1982; Silverman *et al.*, 1998; Weinberger *et al.*, 1981; Zorrilla *et al.*, 1997). Most did not include an independent control group and thus were not able to determine whether unaffected relatives themselves displayed greater ventricular enlargement than controls. Of those sibling CT studies that did include an independent control group, Weinberger *et al.* (1981) reported significantly increased ventricle-to-brain ratio in unaffected siblings compared with controls, whereas no significant differences were found in studies by DeLisi *et al.* (1986) and Silverman *et al.* (1998) (the latter study also failing to detect a significant difference in this ratio between the schizophrenia subjects and controls). Reveley *et al.* (1982) reported a non-significant trend for the unaffected twins from a small group of MZ pairs discordant for schizophrenia to have larger ventricle-to-brain ratio than healthy twins. In a Danish cohort study of 97 adult offspring of mothers with schizophrenia (who had actually largely lived through the risk period for schizophrenia, with a mean age of 42 years) and 60 controls (Cannon *et al.*, 1993), the offspring had ventricular enlargement that increased in accordance with likely genetic risk: from having no parent with schizophrenia, to one parent affected, to both parents affected with a schizophrenia spectrum disorder.

This finding that ventricular enlargement is most prominent in those unaffected relatives more likely to carry susceptibility genes for schizophrenia is supported by the Maudsley Family Study, which used high-resolution MRI and volumetric assessments of ventricular size (McDonald *et al.* 2002; Sharma *et al.*, 1998). McDonald *et al.* (2002) analysed MRI measurements that were performed on 66 subjects with schizophrenia, 96 of their unaffected first-degree relatives, and 68 controls. A gradient of likely genetic risk was provided by these families since the patients were divided into those from multiply affected families and those with no family history of psychosis. The relatives of patients from multiply affected families included a group of parents who were considered especially likely to be unaffected gene carriers ("presumed obligate carriers"), since they appeared to transmit the liability for schizophrenia to their affected children by virtue of also having a sibling and/or parent affected. The patients had significantly enlarged lateral ventricles, and so did the presumed obligate carriers, whereas those relatives from singly affected families had similar ventricular volume to the controls. Other MRI studies do not report significant lateral ventricular enlargement in relatives of schizophrenia patients (Cannon *et al.*, 1998; Lawrie *et al.*, 1999; Seidman *et al.*, 1999; Staal *et al.*, 2000), although mild ventricular enlargement that falls short of significance is often noted. Since these studies did not focus on relatives from multiply affected families, the lack of significant results is unsurprising. The finding that ventricular volume enlargement is present only in those relatives most likely to carry susceptibility genes is consistent with data from another MRI study on offspring, which reported no overall significant difference in ventricular volume between relatives and controls, but increasing ventricular enlargement in unaffected relatives with a stronger family history of schizophrenia (Lawrie et al., 1999). There is also evidence from twin studies that non-genetic factors such as obstetric complications contribute to larger lateral ventricles in schizophrenia (Baare et al., 2001b; McNeil et al., 2000; Reveley et al., 1984b; Suddath et al., 1990). Recent family studies point to an interaction between genetic risk for schizophrenia and hypoxic birth events upon ventricular volume, since subjects most likely to be gene carriers demonstrate the greatest ventricular enlargement in association with obstetric complications (Cannon et al., 1993, 2002a; McDonald et al., 2002).

Third ventricular volume tends to correlate with lateral ventricular volume, and several studies on relatives have found that third ventricular volume is increased in size (Keshavan et al., 1997; Lawrie et al., 2001; Seidman et al., 1999; Staal et al., 2000). As with lateral ventricular volume, there is evidence that third ventricular volume increases with likelihood of carrying susceptibility genes in unaffected relatives (Lawrie et al., 1999; McDonald et al., 2002).

Global cerebral and tissue volumes

Baare et al. (2001b) studied a number of morphometric measures in 15 MZ and 14 DZ twin pairs discordant for schizophrenia and 29 matched control twin pairs; they report that both patients with schizophrenia from discordant MZ twin pairs and their co-twins display decrements in intracranial volume compared with normal twins, which are not shared by DZ discordant twin pairs. The authors interpreted their findings as indicating that reduced early brain growth is linked to schizophrenia susceptibility genes. Whole brain volume was reduced in both patients and unaffected co-twins from MZ and DZ twins pairs compared with control twins, suggesting either a genetic or a shared environmental effect on brain size. Keshavan et al. (2002) reported a trend for reduced brain volume in high-risk offspring. However, several other studies did not find unaffected relatives to have reduced cerebral volume compared with controls (Lawrie et al., 2001; McDonald et al., 2002; Noga et al., 1996; Seidman et al., 2002; Staal et al., 2000).

In the Danish cohort study, Cannon et al. (1993) also found that the offspring had enlargement of sulcal cerebrospinal fluid (CSF) spaces (implying reduced volume of the cerebral cortex), which increased in accordance with their likely genetic risk (i.e. in a stepwise fashion from controls to those with one parent affected, to those having both parents affected with a schizophrenia spectrum disorder). In contrast to ventricular volume, there was no evidence for an interaction between genetic risk and birth complications upon CSF spaces in this study. In a later MRI study of 75 probands with schizophrenia, 60 of their siblings and 56 controls from a Finnish cohort, Cannon *et al.* (1998) found that siblings had a similar decrement in global gray matter and increase in CSF as probands, especially in frontotemporal regions, whereas only patients, and not their siblings, had reduced white matter volume. In a proportion of this cohort, fetal hypoxia was associated with reduced volume of gray matter and increased sulcal spaces in siblings and probands, especially in the temporal region (Cannon *et al.*, 2002a), indicating a gene–environment interaction similar to that reported for ventricular volume. Other studies did not detect reduced global gray matter or white matter volumes in unaffected relatives (Cannon *et al.*, 2002a; Seidman *et al.*, 1999; Sharma *et al.*, 1998; Staal *et al.*, 2000).

Subcortical structures

Studies of unaffected siblings and offspring have found the thalamus to be reduced in volume compared with controls (Lawrie *et al.*, 2001; Seidman *et al.*, 1999; Staal *et al.*, 1998), consistent with the increased volume of the third ventricle identified in the same studies. There was little evidence for abnormalities of the caudate or lentiform nuclei from these studies (Lawrie *et al.*, 2001; Seidman *et al.*, 1999; Staal *et al.*, 2000).

Temporal lobe

No evidence has been reported in unaffected relatives for abnormality of the total temporal lobe volume (Lawrie *et al.*, 2001; McDonald *et al.*, 2002; Schreiber *et al.*, 1999) nor for the superior temporal gyrus (Frangou *et al.*, 1997b). However, several groups have reported that the amygdala-hippocampal formation or the hippocampus is reduced in volume in unaffected relatives or offspring (Baare *et al.*, 2001b; O'Driscoll *et al.*, 2001; Schreiber *et al.*, 1999; Steel *et al.*, 2002; van Erp *et al.*, 2002), especially on the left (Lawrie *et al.*, 2001, Keshavan *et al.*, 2002; Seidman *et al.*, 2002). There have also been negative studies (Staal *et al.*, 2000) and one study reporting an enlarged hippocampus in those relatives likely to be transmitting genetic risk (Harris *et al.*, 2002). Schulze *et al.* (2003) also failed to detect reduced volume of the hippocampus in unaffected relatives who took part in the Maudsley Family Study but found that a history of obstetric complications was associated with reduced volume of the left hippocampus. Evidence for a gene – environment interaction for birth complications upon hippocampal volume, similar to that found for ventricular volume in the same sample, was provided by van Erp *et al.* (2002), who found that fetal hypoxia was associated with reduced volume of the hippocampus in probands only and not in their siblings or controls.

Frontal lobe

No evidence has been reported for abnormality of the prefrontal lobe comparing groups of unaffected siblings or offspring of schizophrenia subjects with controls (Keshavan *et al.*, 2002; Lawrie *et al.*, 2001; Schreiber *et al.*, 1999; Staal *et al.*, 2000). However Baare *et al.* (2001b) reported that both patients with schizophrenia from discordant MZ twin pairs and their co-twins display decrements in frontal lobe volume compared with normal twins whereas DZ discordant twin pairs do not, strongly suggestive of a genetic etiology. Furthermore, although no group differences were found, Lawrie *et al.* (2001) reported that the prefrontal lobe volume reduces as likelihood of carrying susceptibility genes increases among high risk adolescents. Cannon *et al.* (2002b), in a computational morphometry study of three-dimensional cortical maps from the MRI scans of 10 MZ and 10 DZ twin pairs discordant for schizophrenia and 20 matched control twin pairs from a Finnish cohort, reported evidence for reduced volume predominantly of the anterior and superior prefrontal cortex in accordance with likely genetic risk among unaffected twins.

Other structures

Sharma *et al.* (1999) reported that unaffected relatives from multiply affected families had loss of normal fronto-occipital brain asymmetries compared with controls, to a lesser degree than that found in affected probands, although a subsequent study from the same Maudsley group, using a similar design, failed to replicate this finding (Chapple *et al.*, 2004). There is no evidence for abnormal volume of the cerebellum in unaffected relatives compared with controls (McDonald *et al.*, 2002; Seidman *et al.*, 1999; Staal *et al.*, 2000) nor for midsagittal area reduction of the corpus callosum (Chua *et al.*, 2000; Narr *et al.*, 2002). In the Finnish twin study, significant vertical displacement of the corpus callosum (which was associated with lateral ventricular enlargement) was found in the unaffected co-twins as well as in the co-twins affected with schizophrenia in MZ twins but was not found in unaffected DZ twins, suggesting that this structural deviation also represents a genetic marker for schizophrenia (Narr *et al.*, 2002).

The true nature of the morphological phenotype of schizophrenia is likely to involve more widespread networks than those chosen for analysis by the region-of-interest studies performed to date on unaffected relatives, and future studies using whole brain analysis are likely to be helpful in more comprehensively investigating these. In a recent paper, Faraone *et al.* (2003) studied volumetric measurements of the whole brain divided into parcellation units in relatives of patients with schizophrenia and in controls. They identified three factors loaded by several parcellation units throughout the neocortical ribbon as well as in subcortical and limbic regions that could be used to describe an MRI phenotype which succeeded in discriminating relatives from controls and was most deviant in relatives from more densely affected families.

The varying morphometric deviations reported in unaffected relatives most likely reflect the effect of differing study designs, samples, and methodologies, as well as the limited statistical power associated with many of the studies: since deviations in relatives tend to be even more subtle than those found in probands, larger numbers of subjects are required to demonstrate a statistically significant result in studies of relatives than when comparing only probands with controls. Despite these disagreements, work to date in this field does demonstrate that unaffected relatives frequently display abnormalities of brain structure compared with controls that are similar in nature to, but less severe than, those associated with schizophrenia. The greatest evidence to date is for increased ventricular volume; reduced gray matter volume, especially in frontotemporal regions; reduced volume of the thalamus; and reduced volume of the amygdala–hippocampal complex. These "familial" abnormalities identified in probands and unaffected relatives are presumably genetic in etiology but could also represent the impact of shared environmental factors. Further evidence for the likely genetic origin of such traits can be inferred if they are found most commonly in those relatives who are more likely to be gene carriers. Studies that have examined likely genetic loading of unaffected relatives, based on number of affected relatives or genetic relatedness to the proband, have generally found the structural abnormalities in unaffected relatives to be more prominent in those with a higher genetic loading (Cannon et al., 1993, 2002b; Faraone et al., 2003; Lawrie et al., 1999, 2001; McDonald et al., 2002; Seidman et al., 2002). This finding of increased impairment in relatives in accordance with their genetic loading is in keeping with the predictions of the multifactorial model for transmission of the illness. Given the impact that the known environmental risk factor of obstetric complications may have on ventricular and hippocampal volume, which may act interactively with susceptibility genes, future studies should collect such information where feasible.

Molecular genetics

Few published studies to date have attempted to link measures of brain morphology in schizophrenia with specific genetic factors. Shihabuddin et al. (1996) found that those family members with a marker allele on chromosome 5p14.1–13.1, which had previously been linked to schizophrenia-related disorders in a single pedigree, had larger ventricle-to-brain ratios and greater fronto-parietal sulcal atrophy than those who lacked the marker allele. Other studies have examined relationships between different allele frequencies of polymorphisms in genes likely to have a role in neurodevelopment and MRI morphometric measures. In a small sample of patients with psychosis, Kunugi et al. (1999) reported that hippocampal volume was reduced in patients with schizophrenia who were carriers, compared with non-carriers, of the *A3* allele of a dinucleotide repeat polymorphism in the neurotrophin 3 gene. Wassink and colleagues (1999, 2000) examined the relationship between brain morphometry and alleles of polymorphisms in the genes for brain-derived neurotrophic factor and tumor necrosis factor receptor II in patients with schizophrenia, their parents, and controls. The polymorphisms were not related to the clinical schizophrenia phenotype, but subjects with at least one copy of "allele 1" of the brain-derived neurotrophic factor polymorphism had larger parietal lobes than those who did not (Wassink *et al.*, 1999). Subjects with schizophrenia who were homozygous for "allele 1" of the tumor neurosis factor receptor II polymorphism had larger ventricles and smaller frontal lobes than subjects with at least one copy of "allele 2" (Wassink *et al.*, 2000). Meisenzahl *et al.* (2001) examined the association of MRI measurements from a sample of male patients with schizophrenia and controls with a polymorphism in the promoter region of the gene for interleukin-1β. The polymorphism had no influence on brain morphology in controls, but schizophrenia patients who were "allele 2" carriers of the polymorphism had gray matter volume deficits in frontotemporal regions and generalized white matter deficits compared with non-carriers. In a similar sample, Rujescu *et al.* (2002) examined a common biallelic polymorphism, Met129Val, in the gene coding the prion protein (PRNP). Allele frequencies did not differ between patients and controls, but homozygosity for methionine was significantly associated with decreased white matter volume and enlarged CSF volume in the subjects, independent of diagnosis.

The results of these molecular genetic studies must be considered very tentative in the absence of replication. However, they demonstrate the value of using brain morphometry as an alternative phenotype in genetic studies of schizophrenia and suggest that a richer understanding of the actions of potential susceptibility genes could be achieved through such a design.

Conclusions

The study of the relationship between genetics and neuroimaging represents an emerging field of research in complex neuropsychiatric disorders. Further studies using more advanced methodology are likely to help to clarify the brain structural manifestations of schizophrenia susceptibility genes. Research to date indicates that there is a high degree of genetic control over brain morphometry, that schizophrenia is associated with several subtle deviations of brain morphology, which are frequently neurodevelopmental in origin, and that unaffected relatives also demonstrate some of these deviations. The brain morphological phenotype of schizophrenia is likely to be increasingly used as a valuable alternative to the clinical phenotype in molecular genetic studies and should help to simplify the genetic and biological complexity of the illness, and thus facilitate the search for susceptibility genes.

REFERENCES

Ananth, H., Popescu, I., Critchley, H. D., *et al.* (2002). Cortical and subcortical gray matter abnormalities in schizophrenia determined through structural magnetic resonance imaging with optimized volumetric voxel-based morphometry. *Am J Psychiatry* **159**: 1497–1505.

Baare, W. F., Hulshoff Pol, H. E., Boomsma, D. I., *et al.* (2001a). Quantitative genetic modeling of variation in human brain morphology. *Cereb Cortex* **11**: 816–824.

Baare, W. F., van Oel, C. J., Hulshoff Pol, H. E., *et al.* (2001b). Volumes of brain structures in twins discordant for schizophrenia. *Arch Gen Psychiatry* **58**: 33–40.

Bartley, A. J., Jones, D. W., Weinberger, D. R. (1997). Genetic variability of human brain size and cortical gyral patterns. *Brain* **120**: 257–269.

Bilder, R. M., Wu, H., Bogerts, B., *et al.* (1994). Absence of regional hemispheric volume asymmetries in first-episode schizophrenia. *Am J Psychiatry* **151**: 1437–1447.

Cannon, T. D., Mednick, S. A., Parnas, J., *et al.* (1993). Developmental brain abnormalities in the offspring of schizophrenic mothers. I. Contributions of genetic and perinatal factors. *Arch Gen Psychiatry* **50**: 551–564.

Cannon, T. D., Zorrilla, L. E., Shtasel, D., *et al.* (1994). Neuropsychological functioning in siblings discordant for schizophrenia and healthy volunteers. *Arch Gen Psychiatry* **51**: 651–661.

Cannon, T. D., van Erp, T. G. M., Huttunen, M., *et al.* (1998). Regional gray matter, white matter, and cerebrospinal fluid distributions in schizophrenic patients, their siblings, and controls. *Arch Gen Psychiatry* **55**: 1084–1091.

Cannon, T. D., van Erp, T. G., Rosso, I. M., *et al.* (2002a). Fetal hypoxia and structural brain abnormalities in schizophrenic patients, their siblings, and controls. *Arch Gen Psychiatry* **59**: 35–41.

Cannon, T. D., Thompson, P. M., van Erp, T. G., *et al.* (2002b). Cortex mapping reveals regionally specific patterns of genetic and disease-specific gray-matter deficits in twins discordant for schizophrenia. *Proc Natl Acad Sci USA* **99**: 3228–3233.

Cardno, A. G., Marshall, E. J., Coid, B., *et al.* (1999). Heritability estimates for psychotic disorders: the Maudsley twin psychosis series. *Arch Gen Psychiatry* **56**: 162–168.

Carmelli, D., DeCarli, C., Swan, G. E., *et al.* (1998). Evidence for genetic variance in white matter hyperintensity volume in normal elderly male twins. *Stroke* **29**: 1177–1181.

Carmelli, D., Swan, G. E., DeCarli, C., *et al.* (2002). Quantitative genetic modeling of regional brain volumes and cognitive performance in older male twins. *Biol Psychol* **61**: 139–155.

Chakos, M. H., Lieberman, J. A., Alvir, J., *et al.* (1995). Caudate nuclei volumes in schizophrenic patients treated with typical antipsychotics or clozapine. *Lancet* **345**: 456–457.

Chapple, B., Grech A., Sham, P., *et al.* (2004). Normal cerebral asymmetry in familial and non-familial schizophrenic probands and their unaffected relatives. *Schizophr Res* **67**: 33–40.

Chua, S. E., Sharma, T., Takei, N., *et al.* (2000). A magnetic resonance imaging study of corpus callosum size in familial schizophrenic subjects, their relatives, and normal controls. *Schizophr Res* **41**: 397–403.

Crawford, T. J., Sharma, T., Puri, B. K., *et al.* (1998). Saccadic eye movements in families multiply affected with schizophrenia: the Maudsley Family Study. *Am J Psychiatry* **155**: 1703–1710.

DeLisi, L. E., Goldin, L. R., Hamovit, J. R., *et al.* (1986). A family study of the association of increased ventricular size with schizophrenia. *Arch Gen Psychiatry* **43**: 148–153.

DeLisi, L. E., Hoff, A. L., Schwartz, J. E., *et al.* (1991). Brain morphology in first-episode schizophrenic-like psychotic patients: a quantitative magnetic resonance imaging study. *Biol Psychiatry* **29**: 159–175.

Falkai, P., Bogerts, B., Schneider, T., *et al.* (1995). Disturbed planum temporale asymmetry in schizophrenia. A quantitative post-mortem study. *Schizophr Res* **14**: 161–176.

Fannon, D., Chitnis, X., Doku, V., *et al.* (2000). Features of structural brain abnormality detected in first-episode psychosis. *Am J Psychiatry* **157**: 1829–1834.

Faraone, S. V., Seidman, L. J., Kremen, W. S., *et al.* (2003). Structural brain abnormalities among relatives of patients with schizophrenia: implications for linkage studies. *Schizophr Res* **60**: 125–140.

Frangou, S., Sharma, T., Alarcon, G., *et al.* (1997a). The Maudsley Family Study, II: endogenous event-related potentials in familial schizophrenia. *Schizophr Res* **23**: 45–53.

Frangou, S., Sharma, T., Sigmudsson, T., *et al.* (1997b). The Maudsley Family Study IV. Normal planum temporale asymmetry in familial schizophrenia – A volumetric MRI study. *Br J Psychiatry* **170**: 328–333.

Gershon, E. S. Goldin, L. R. (1986). Clinical methods in psychiatric genetics. I. Robustness of genetic marker investigative strategies. *Acta Psychiatr Scand* **74**: 113–118.

Goldstein, J. M., Goodman, J. M., Seidman, L. J., *et al.* (1999). Cortical abnormalities in schizophrenia identified by structural magnetic resonance imaging. *Arch Gen Psychiatry* **56**: 537–547.

Gottesman, I. I. (1991). *Schizophrenia Genesis: The Origins of Madness.* New York: H Freeman.

Gur, R. E., Cowell, P., Turetsky, B. I., *et al.* (1998). A follow-up magnetic resonance imaging study of schizophrenia. Relationship of neuroanatomical changes to clinical and neurobehavioral measures. *Arch Gen Psychiatry* **55**: 145–152.

Harris, J. G., Young, D. A., Rojas, D. C., *et al.* (2002). Increased hippocampal volume in schizophrenics' parents with ancestral history of schizophrenia. *Schizophr Res* **55**: 11–17.

Harrison, P. J. (1999). The neuropathology of schizophrenia: a critical review of the data and their interpretation. *Brain* **122**: 593–624.

Hirayasu, Y., Shenton, M. E., Salisbury, D. F., *et al.* (1998). Lower left temporal lobe MRI volumes in patients with first-episode schizophrenia compared with psychotic patients with first-episode affective disorder and normal subjects. *Am J Psychiatry* **155**: 1384–1391.

Holzman, P. S., Kringlen, E., Matthysse, S., *et al.* (1988). A single dominant gene can account for eye tracking dysfunctions and schizophrenia in offspring of discordant twins. *Arch Gen Psychiatry* **45**: 641–647.

Jones, P., Murray, R. M. (1991). The genetics of schizophrenia is the genetics of neurodevelopment. *Br J Psychiatry* **158**: 615–623.

Keshavan, M. S., Montrose, D. M., Pierri, J. N., *et al.* (1997). Magnetic resonance imaging and spectroscopy in offspring at risk for schizophrenia: Preliminary studies. *Prog Neuropsychopharmacol Biol Psychiatry* **21**: 1285–1295.

Keshavan, M. S., Dick, E., Mankowski, I., *et al.* (2002). Decreased left amygdala and hippocampal volumes in young offspring at risk for schizophrenia. *Schizophr Res*, **58**: 173–183.

Kunugi, H., Hattori, M., Nanko, S., *et al.* (1999). Dinucleotide repeat polymorphism in the neurotrophin-3 gene and hippocampal volume in psychoses. *Schizophr Res* **37**: 271–273.

Lawrie, S. M., Whalley, H., Kestelman, J. N., *et al.* (1999). Magnetic resonance imaging of brain in people at high risk of developing schizophrenia. *Lancet* **353**: 30–33.

Lawrie, S. M., Whalley, H. C., Abukmeil, S. S., *et al.* (2001). Brain structure, genetic liability, and psychotic symptoms in subjects at high risk of developing schizophrenia. *Biol Psychiatry* **49**: 811–823.

Leboyer, M., Bellivier, F., Nosten-Bertrand, M., *et al.* (1998). Psychiatric genetics: search for phenotypes. *Trends Neurosci* **21**: 102–105.

Lewis, S. W. (1990). Computerised tomography in schizophrenia 15 years on. *Br J Psychiatry* **9**(Suppl.): 16–24.

Lieberman, J., Chakos, M., Wu, H., *et al.* (2001). Longitudinal study of brain morphology in first episode schizophrenia. *Biol Psychiatry* **49**: 487–499.

McCarley, R. W., Wible, C. G., Frumin, M., *et al.* (1999). MRI anatomy of schizophrenia. *Biol Psychiatry* **45**: 1099–1119.

McDonald, C., Grech, A., Toulopoulou, T., *et al.* (2002). Brain volumes in familial and non-familial schizophrenic probands and their unaffected relatives. *Am J Med Genet* **114**: 616–625.

McGrath, J., Murray, R. (1995). Risk factors for schizophrenia: from conception to birth. In *Schizophrenia*, ed. S. Hirsch, D. R., Weinberger. Oxford: Blackwell Scientific, pp. 187–205.

McNeil, T. F., Cantor-Graae, E., Weinberger, D. R. (2000). Relationship of obstetric complications and differences in size of brain structures in monozygotic twin pairs discordant for schizophrenia. *Am J Psychiatry* **157**: 203–212.

Meisenzahl, E. M., Rujescu, D., Kirner, A., *et al.* (2001). Association of an interleukin-1beta genetic polymorphism with altered brain structure in patients with schizophrenia. *Am J Psychiatry* **158**: 1316–1319.

Murray, R. M., Lewis, S. W., Reveley, A. M. (1985). Towards an aetiological classification of schizophrenia. *Lancet* **i**: 1023–1026.

Narr, K. L., Cannon, T. D., Woods, R. P., *et al.* (2002). Genetic contributions to altered callosal morphology in schizophrenia. *J Neurosci* **22**: 3720–3729.

Noga, J. T., Bartley, A. J., Jones, D. W., *et al.* (1996). Cortical gyral anatomy and gross brain dimensions in monozygotic twins discordant for schizophrenia. *Schizophr Res* **22**: 27–40.

Nosarti, C., Al-Asady, M. H., Frangou, S., *et al.* (2002). Adolescents who were born very preterm have decreased brain volumes. *Brain* **125**: 1616–1623.

O'Driscoll, G. A., Florencio, P. S., Gagnon, D., *et al.* (2001). Amygdala-hippocampal volume and verbal memory in first-degree relatives of schizophrenic patients. *Psychiatry Res* **107**: 75–85.

Oppenheim, J. S., Skerry, J. E., Tramo, M. J., *et al.* (1989). Magnetic resonance imaging morphology of the corpus callosum in monozygotic twins. *Ann Neurol* **26**: 100–104.

Pennington, B. F., Filipek, P. A., Lefly, D., *et al.* (2000). A twin MRI study of size variations in human brain. *J Cogn Neurosci* **12**: 223–232.

Pfefferbaum, A., Sullivan, E. V., Swan, G. E., *et al.* (2000). Brain structure in men remains highly heritable in the seventh and eighth decades of life. *Neurobiol Aging* **21**: 63–74.

Reveley, A. M., Reveley, M. A., Clifford, C. A., *et al.* (1982). Cerebral ventricular size in twins discordant for schizophrenia. *Lancet* **i**: 540–541.

Reveley, A. M., Reveley, M. A., Chitkara, B., *et al.* (1984a). The genetic basis of cerebral ventricular volume. *Psychiatr Res* **13**: 261–266.

Reveley, A. M., Reveley, M. A., Murray, R. M. (1984b). Cerebral ventricular enlargement in non-genetic schizophrenia: a controlled twin study. *Br J Psychiatry* **144**: 89–93.

Rujescu, D., Meisenzahl, E. M., Giegling, I., *et al.* (2002). Methionine homozygosity at codon 129 in the prion protein is associated with white matter reduction and enlargement of CSF compartments in healthy volunteers and schizophrenic patients. *Neuroimage* **15**: 200–206.

Rutherford, M. C., Pennock, J. M., Schwieso, J. E., *et al.* (1995). Hypoxic ischaemic encephalopathy: early magnetic resonance findings and their evolution. *Neuropediatrics* **26**: 183–191.

Schreiber, H., Baur-Seack, K., Kornhuber, H. H., *et al.* (1999). Brain morphology in adolescents at genetic risk for schizophrenia assessed by qualitative and quantitative magnetic resonance imaging. *Schizophr Res* **40**: 81–84.

Schulze, K., McDonald, C., Frangou, S., *et al.* (2003). Hippocampal volume in familial and nonfamilial schizophrenic probands and their unaffected relatives. *Biol Psychiatry* **53**: 562–570.

Seidman, L. J., Faraone, S. V., Goldstein, J. M., *et al.* (1999). Thalamic and amygdala–hippocampal volume reductions in first-degree relatives of patients with schizophrenia: an MRI-based morphometric analysis. *Biol Psychiatry* **46**: 941–954.

Seidman, L. J., Faraone, S. V., Goldstein, J. M., *et al.* (2002). Left hippocampal volume as a vulnerability indicator for schizophrenia: a magnetic resonance imaging morphometric study of nonpsychotic first- degree relatives. *Arch Gen Psychiatry* **59**: 839–849.

Sharma, T., Lancaster, E., Lee, D., *et al.* (1998). Brain changes in schizophrenia – volumetric MRI study of families multiply affected with schizophrenia: The Maudsley Family Study 5. *Br J Psychiatry* **173**: 132–138.

Sharma, T., Lancaster, E., Sigmundsson, T., *et al.* (1999). Lack of normal pattern of cerebral asymmetry in familial schizophrenic patients and their relatives: the Maudsley Family Study. *Schizophr Res* **40**: 111–120.

Shihabuddin, L., Silverman, J. M., Buchsbaum, M. S., *et al.* (1996). Ventricular enlargement associated with linkage marker for schizophrenia-related disorders in one pedigree. *Mol Psychiatry* **1**: 215–222.

Siegel, C., Waldo, M., Mizner, G., *et al.* (1984). Deficits in sensory gating in schizophrenic patients and their relatives. Evidence obtained with auditory evoked responses. *Arch Gen Psychiatry* **41**: 607–612.

Sigmundsson, T., Suckling, J., Maier, M., *et al.* (2001). Structural abnormalities in frontal, temporal, and limbic regions and interconnecting white matter tracts in schizophrenic patients with prominent negative symptoms. *Am J Psychiatry* **158**: 234–243.

Silverman, J. M., Smith, C. J., Guo, S. L., *et al.* (1998). Lateral ventricular enlargement in schizophrenic probands and their siblings with schizophrenia-related disorders. *Biol Psychiatry* **43**: 97–106.

Staal, W. G., Hulshoff, H. E., Schnack, H., *et al.* (1998). Partial volume decrease of the thalamus in relatives of patients with schizophrenia. *Am J Psychiatry* **155**: 1784–1786.

Staal, W. G., Pol, H. E. H., Schnack, H. G., *et al.* (2000). Structural brain abnormalities in patients with schizophrenia and their healthy siblings. *Am J Psychiatry* **157**: 416–421.

Steel, R. M., Whalley, H. C., Miller, P., *et al.* (2002). Structural MRI of the brain in presumed carriers of genes for schizophrenia, their affected and unaffected siblings. *J Neurol Neurosurg Psychiatry* **72**: 455–458.

Stefanis, N., Frangou, S., Yakeley, J., *et al.* (1999). Hippocampal volume reduction in schizophrenia: effects of genetic risk and pregnancy and birth complications. *Biol Psychiatry* **46**: 697–702.

Stefansson, H., Sigurdsson, E., Steinthorsdottir, V., *et al.* (2002). Neuregulin 1 and susceptibility to schizophrenia. *Am J Hum Genet* **71**: 877–892.

Steinmetz, H., Herzog, A., Huang, Y., *et al.* (1994). Discordant brain-surface anatomy in monozygotic twins. *N Engl J Med* **331**: 951–952.

Steinmetz, H., Herzog, A., Schlaug, G., *et al.* (1995). Brain asymmetry in monozygotic twins. *Cereb Cortex* **5**: 296–300.

Straub, R. E., Jiang, Y., MacLean, C. J., *et al.* (2002). Genetic variation in the 6p22.3 gene *DTNBP1*, the human ortholog of the mouse dysbindin gene, is associated with schizophrenia. *Am J Hum Genet* **71**: 337–348.

Suddath, R. L., Christison, G. W., Torrey, E. F., *et al.* (1990). Anatomical abnormalities in the brains of monozygotic twins discordant for schizophrenia. *N Engl J Med* **322**: 789–794.

Sullivan, E. V., Pfefferbaum, A., Swan, G. E., *et al.* (2001). Heritability of hippocampal size in elderly twin men: equivalent influence from genes and environment. *Hippocampus* **11**: 754–762.

Suzuki, M., Nohara, S., Hagino, H., *et al.* (2002). Regional changes in brain gray and white matter in patients with schizophrenia demonstrated with voxel-based analysis of MRI. *Schizophr Res* **55**: 41–54.

Thompson, P. M., Cannon, T. D., Narr, K. L., *et al.* (2001). Genetic influences on brain structure. *Nat Neurosci* **4**: 1253–1258.

Toulopoulou, T., Morris, R. G., Rabe-Hesketh, S., *et al.* (2003). Selectivity of verbal memory deficit in schizophrenic patients and their relatives. *Am J Med Genet* **116**: 1–7.

Tramo, M. J., Loftus, W. C., Stukel, T. A., *et al.* (1998). Brain size, head size, and intelligence quotient in monozygotic twins. *Neurology* **50**: 1246–1252.

van Erp, T. G., Saleh, P. A., Rosso, I. M., *et al.* (2002). Contributions of genetic risk and fetal hypoxia to hippocampal volume in patients with schizophrenia or schizoaffective disorder, their unaffected siblings, and healthy unrelated volunteers. *Am J Psychiatry* **159**: 1514–1520.

Vogeley, K., Tepest, R., Pfeiffer, U., *et al.* (2001). Right frontal hypergyria differentiation in affected and unaffected siblings from families multiply affected with schizophrenia: a morphometric MRI study. *Am J Psychiatry* **158**: 494–496.

Wassink, T. H., Nelson, J. J., Crowe, R. R., *et al.* (1999). Heritability of BDNF alleles and their effect on brain morphology in schizophrenia. *Am J Med Genet* **88**: 724–728.

Wassink, T. H., Crowe, R. R., Andreasen, N. C. (2000). Tumor necrosis factor receptor-II: heritability and effect on brain morphology in schizophrenia. *Mol Psychiatry* **5**: 678–682.

Weinberger, D. R., McClure, R. K. (2002). Neurotoxicity, neuroplasticity, and magnetic resonance imaging morphometry: what is happening in the schizophrenic brain? *Arch Gen Psychiatry* **59**: 553–558.

Weinberger, D. R., DeLisi, L. E., Neophytides, A. N., *et al.* (1981). Familial aspects of CT scan abnormalities in chronic schizophrenic patients. *Psychiatry Res* **4**: 65–71.

White, T., Andreasen, N. C., Nopoulos, P. (2002). Brain volumes and surface morphology in monozygotic twins. *Cereb Cortex* **12**: 486–493.

Wickham, H. Murray, R. M. (1997). Can biological markers identify endophenotypes predisposing to schizophrenia? *Int Rev Psychiatry* **9**: 355–364.

Wilke, M., Kaufmann, C., Grabner, A., *et al.* (2001). Gray matter-changes and correlates of disease severity in schizophrenia: a statistical parametric mapping study. *Neuroimage* **13**: 814–824.

Wright, I. C., Ellison, Z. R., Sharma, T., *et al.* (1999). Mapping of grey matter changes in schizophrenia. *Schizophr Res* **35**: 1–14.

Wright, I. C., Rabe-Hesketh, S., Woodruff, P. W. R., *et al.* (2000). Meta-analysis of regional brain volumes in schizophrenia. *Am J Psychiatry* **157**: 16–25.

Wright, I. C., Sham, P., Murray, R. M., *et al.* (2002). Genetic contributions to regional variability in human brain structure: methods and preliminary results. *Neuroimage* **17**: 256–271.

Zorrilla, L. T., Cannon, T. D., Kronenberg, S., *et al.* (1997). Structural brain abnormalities in schizophrenia: a family study. *Biol Psychiatry* **42**: 1080–1086.

9

Nutritional factors and schizophrenia

Sahebarao P. Mahadik

Medical College of Georgia and VA Medical Center, Augusta, USA

Proper nutrition, in biological terms, is the dietary intake of essential nutrients, including amino acids, lipids, minerals, vitamins, and an adequate energy supply for every cell type in the body. Such nutrition enables each cell to make the unique proteins, lipids, and nucleic acids to carry out its function from conception to death as dictated by the genetic program. Additionally, properly nourished cells can adapt (i.e. change their cellular machinery through changes in gene expression) in response to environmental factors such as heat, cold, infections, toxins, hypoxia, etc. Poor nutrition can be considered as undernutrition, a significant reduction in caloric intake in general rather than of one or more essential nutrients, or malnutrition, a lack of essential nutrients with no accompanying lack in caloric intake, is a state in which a cell lacks or has a reduced intake of one or more essential nutrients. This state can impair the ability of the cell to adapt to altered environmental situations and can lead to the disruption of normal physiological function, which is a disease state (e.g. cardiovascular, hepatic, diabetic, or brain disorders/diseases) depending on the cell type.

The role of nutrition in the development and maintenance of a healthy body and mind has been considered throughout the ages. The ancient Indian scripture *Bhagavad Gita* (*c.* 600 BC) (Ch. 6, verse 17, and Ch. 17 verses 6, 8, 9 and 10) stated that proper nutrition builds the "noble character," which can further improve the nutrition, from existing knowledge and experimentation and becomes a nutritional standard for better civilization. There is a prevailing general belief that the body and mind have synergistic influences on the choice of food eaten and thus on nutrition. The role of nutritional factors in schizophrenia has been considered for a long time. One hypothesis states that schizophrenia may be a developmental systemic metabolic disorder involving membrane phospholipids (Horrobin, 1996, 1998; Horrobin *et al.*, 1994; Rotrosen and Wolkin, 1987). However, schizophrenia has been primarily characterized as a brain disorder giving rise

Neurodevelopment and Schizophrenia, ed. Matcheri S. Keshavan *et al.* Published by Cambridge University Press. © Cambridge University Press 2004.

to serious behavioral disturbances, which cause the patient major suffering and disability.

At this stage, the role of nutrition in the etiology of schizophrenia is circumstantial and speculative; however, nutrition may play a critical role in its variable course and outcome. Large nutritional differences, resulting from the quality and quantity of food available, exist between cultures and socioeconomic classes (Mahadik et al., 1999a). Cultures evolve by selection of food that supports the healthy body and mind. An editorial by Murphy (1984) suggested that diseases such as general paresis, peptic ulcer, and schizophrenia could be caused as well as cured by civilization. Civilization, which is conceived through a process rather than established as a state, combines single human individuals into one great unity (Freud, 1961). Torrey (1980) has suggested a close correlation between the prevalence of schizophrenia and the degree to which a civilization has advanced; he favored a viral theory of the etiology of schizophrenia, since specific types of virus can be propagated, modified, and transmitted from generation to generation. Others have blamed the diet of a civilization for the diseases it suffers. The pathogenic factors that cause these diseases may be incidental, rather than an essential aspect of civilization. The nutrition, lifestyle, and viruses are unique and essential aspects of each culture and socioeconomic class. However, since the incidence of schizophrenia is similar in all cultures, while the course and outcome vary widely (see below), nutritional factors may influence the underlying pathophysiology of the disease to varying degrees.

Multinational studies coordinated by the World Health Organization (WHO) have found that the incidence, prevalence, and manifestation of schizophrenia are similar across different countries and cultures, but the course and outcome of the disease vary widely from mild in developing countries to chronic in developed countries (Jablensky et al., 1991; Sartorius et al., 1986; WHO, 1973). These findings have led to the notion of a "universality" of schizophrenia prevalence but variability in outcome. Several studies also have shown that the outcome of schizophrenia is related to the socioeconomic class of the patient within a culture (Eaton, 1985; Nandi et al., 1980). Several variables, such as social stigma, family support, type of treatment, and family history, examined in the WHO studies could not satisfactorily account for the cross-national/cross-cultural variability in outcome (Craig et al., 1997; Edgerton and Cohen, 1994; Karno and Jenkins, 1993). Recently, the influence of culture and socioeconomic classes on various facets (i.e. epidemiology, etiology, phenomenology, course, and outcome) of schizophrenia has been discussed extensively (Kulhara and Chakrabarti, 2001). In addition to these factors, viral infections, famines, and season of birth, which have all been found to be associated with schizophrenia and its course and outcome, can significantly affect the availability and metabolism of essential nutrients during the early stages of human development (Horrobin *et al.*, 1994; Mahadik *et al.*, 1999a). Therefore, this chapter will focus primarily on the role of essential nutritional factors such as amino acids, lipids, vitamins, and minerals on the course and outcome of schizophrenia.

Nutrition in brain and behavioral development and maintenance

Both under- and malnutrition have been found to impair the brain and behavioral development, as well as affect the health of the body and mind in the adult (Chafetz, 1990; Coleman and Gillberg, 1996; Dhopeshwarkar, 1983; Edelson, 1988). Generally, undernutrition refers to a significant reduction in caloric intake and not to a reduction in essential nutrients. Although severe prenatal undernutrition has been found to affect the brain growth and maturation of the fetus, often resulting in cognitive and psychomotor retardation, undernutrition per se may not be related to schizophrenia, since schizophrenia patients who have adequate caloric intake, both in developed countries and in the upper socioeconomic classes of underdeveloped countries, can suffer from a more unfavorable course and outcome. However, it is likely that undernutrition during infections or famine may also result in malnutrition at critical stages of fetal brain development. This may explain the higher incidence of schizophrenia reported in a population in the decades following a viral epidemic (Mednick *et al.*, 1988) or famine (Hoek *et al.*, 1998; Hulshoff *et al.*, 2000). Malnutrition refers to the lack of essential nutrients, such as essential amino acids, lipids, vitamins, and trace elements and may be more relevant to schizophrenia than undernutrition. It is suggested that schizophrenia may be associated with the reduced availability or lack of some essential nutrients during a critical stage of brain development, and a continued lack of these essential nutrients after birth and through adolescence may contribute to an unfavorable course and outcome of the disease.

Nutritional factors and schizophrenia

As indicated above, establishing the direct role of specific nutritional factors in the etiology of schizophrenia and identifying strategies to prevent the disease can be very difficult tasks at present. However, knowledge of the specific nutritional factors that can improve the course and outcome of the disease may be critical. Based on the nutritional data of the Food and Drug Administration (FDA), there should be relatively less malnutrition in the USA (in those citizens receiving the recommended daily allowance of essential amino acids, vitamins, and minerals) (e.g. selenium, zinc, copper, manganese). However, the dietary intake of omega-3 essential fatty acids (EFAs) and antioxidant vitamins (e.g. vitamins C and E) has steadily declined since the 1950s, primarily because of a decline in food resources containing these nutrients and the intake of these foods (Simopoulos, 1991).

Furthermore, studies indicate that the need for these nutrients has increased because of significant changes in lifestyle during this period. Therefore, dietary availability of essential amino acids and most vitamins and minerals may not be relevant to schizophrenia. Nevertheless, a low prenatal vitamin D hypothesis for schizophrenia has been proposed (McGrath, 1999). However, since this hypothesis is primarily based on the higher prevalence of schizophrenia among individuals born in winter months or at higher latitudes, this may still be related to some other dietary factors (e.g. EFAs and antioxidants) that are reduced under these circumstances (Mahadik *et al.*, 1999a). Furthermore malnutrition is probably not related to defective utilization (absorption, transport, and incorporation into biologically active molecules) of amino acids, vitamins, and minerals, since such defects are often fatal. This brings us to the primary issue of dietary availability of essential lipids, specifically essential polyunsaturated fatty acids (EPUFAs) and antioxidants. The former are needed to synthesize membrane phospholipids, particularly neural membrane phospholipids, which are highly enriched in EPUFAs (Horrocks *et al.*, 1982). Antioxidants are needed to protect these EPUFAs from alteration by free radicals (Mahadik and Gowda, 1996; Mahadik *et al.*, 2001).

Since the 1950s, schizophrenia has been treated with a wide range of antipsychotic drugs, and these are going to be the drugs of choice for the treatment of schizophrenia for a long time. However, Khan *et al.* (2001) recently analyzed the full FDA database on clinical trials of antipsychotic drugs and reported that the average reduction in symptoms was 17.3% when a conventional antipsychotic drug was administered, and 16.6% when a newer antipsychotic drug was administered. This, and the earlier finding by Hegarty *et al.* (1994) that long-term favorable outcomes in terms of employment and reintegration into the community do not significantly differ from 100 years ago, suggests that current therapeutic strategies have limitations in correcting the neuropathophysiology of schizophrenia and in improving the psychopathology associated with the disease. In addition, antipsychotic treatments, in general, are associated with numerous morbidities, including weight gain, insulin resistance, cardiovascular problems, and abnormal lipid metabolism, which result in a diminished quality of life and even in increased mortality (McIntyre *et al.*, 2001). Increasing evidence suggests that dietary supplementation with selective essential nutritional factors, such as, essential fatty acids and antioxidants, may significantly improve the course and outcome of schizophrenia (Fenton *et al.*, 2000; Horrobin, 1998; Mahadik and Evans, 1997; Mahadik and Gowda, 1996; Mahadik and Scheffer, 1996; Mahadik *et al.*, 2001; Reddy and Yao, 1996).

Essential polyunsaturated fatty acids and schizophrenia

Burr and Burr (1929) established the dietary essentiality of the EPUFAs. There are two types, omega-6 and omega-3, so named for the position of the carbon-6 and carbon-3 chemical double bonds on each molecule, respectively. Algae and plants exclusively make these EPUFAs. All animals actually consume the precursors of EPUFAs (linolenic acid [LA; C18:2n6] and α linolenic acid [ALA; C18:3n3] or their predominant functional analogs (arachidonic acid [AA] and docosahexaenoic acid [DHA], respectively). AA and DHA make 50% of the fatty acids that are attached to brain phospholipids, which comprise almost 60% of brain mass (Suzuki, 1981).

Altered fatty acid metabolism in schizophrenia

Extensive work on membrane phospholipids and their EPUFAs in schizophrenia has established that AA and DHA metabolism is altered beginning in the very early stages of schizophrenia (Horrobin, 1998; Horrobin et al., 1994; Keshavan et al., 1993; Mahadik et al., 1994, 1996a,b; Rotrosen and Wolkin, 1987; Yao, 1999; Yao et al., 1994). Christinsen and Christinsen (1988) were the first to identify the relationship between the outcomes of schizophrenia patients and variation in the intake of dietary fat. They observed that 98% of the variation in the course of schizophrenia could be explained by variations in fat intake. The course of schizophrenia was better in developing countries with a low-fat diet in which the major dietary source of fat was from vegetables and seafood (low saturated fatty acid and high EPUFA contents) compared with the course of the disease in developed countries, with high-fat diets in which the major source of the fat consumed was from land animals and birds (high saturated fatty acids and low EPUFA contents). Glen et al. (1994) reported reduced levels of AA and DHA in patients with predominantly negative symptoms. Recently, a few studies have found that the levels of AA and DHA in the membranes of red blood cells correlated with the severity (based on symptomatic scores) of schizophrenia (Arvindakshan et al., 2003a; Khan et al., 2002); such changes parallel changes in brain membranes under a variety of pathophysiological conditions. In addition, improving the levels of AA and DHA in red blood cell membranes by supplementation or by increased dietary intake has been found to correlate with improved clinical outcomes in patients with schizophrenia (Arvindakshan, 2003; Arvindakshan et al., 2003a; Peet and Horrobin, 2002; Peet et al., 1995, 2001). These studies strongly indicate that AA and DHA may have a critical role in the pathophysiology and symptomatology of schizophrenia. However, the Western diet is very rich in AA. Therefore, only DHA, and its precursors ALA and eicosapentaenoic acid (EPA) may be critical for schizophrenia.

Precursors of brain phospholipids and neurodevelopment in schizophrenia

Both AA and DHA are critical for brain and behavioral development (Innis, 1991; Simopoulos, 1991; Wainwright, 1992), which has consistently been found to be abnormal in patients with schizophrenia (Bloom, 1993; Keshavan and Murray, 1997; Murray, 1994; Raedler et al., 1998; Weinberger, 1996). Dietary depletion of AA and DHA during pregnancy in animals, and the resulting lack of availability to the fetus, has been shown to cause reduced body weight, head size, brain weight, and cognitive deficits (Crawford, 1992; Neuringer et al., 1986; Wainwright, 1992; Yamomoto et al., 1987). Similar changes, including cognitive deficits, are also found in patients with schizophrenia (Chua and McKenna, 1995; Lawrie and Abukmeil, 1998; Tollefson, 1996). Specifically, these studies indicate differential reductions in volumes of certain brain regions (probably secondary to reduced number of neurons and their processes), disorganized neuronal networks, and increased ventricular size; all of which are believed to predate the onset of illness. In addition, an increased "pruning" (excessive removal of nerve endings and processes during pubertal maturation) has been proposed (Feinberg, 1990; Keshavan et al., 1994), which is supported by postmortem studies (Glantz and Lewis, 2000; Selemon et al., 1995). AA and DHA are selectively enriched in the neuropils and synapses of the cortex, hippocampus, and basal ganglia (Carlson et al., 1986; O'Brien and Sampson, 1965). Schizophrenia has been associated with significant morphological abnormalities in these brain regions (Heckers, 1997).

Membrane signal transduction

AA and DHA are critical constituents of neuronal membrane phospholipids (Horrocks et al., 1982; Thompson, 1992). Using nuclear magnetic resonance spectroscopy, altered brain membrane phospholipid metabolism has been reported in both first-episode psychotic patients and chronic medicated schizophrenia patients (Fukuzako et al., 1996; Pettegrew et al., 1991; Stanley et al., 1995). These phospholipids are critical for maintaining membrane fluidity appropriate for functioning of membrane receptors. Specific phospholipids are hydrolyzed by receptor-mediated processes, generating intermediates that act as second messengers (e.g. diacylglycerol, inositol polyphosphates, AA, prostaglandins, and cytokines) (Axelrod, 1990; Berridge, 1981; Horrobin et al., 1994; Rana and Hokin, 1990). Particularly, dopamine receptor activation of the AA cascade seems to be a basis for D_1/D_2 receptor synergism (Piomelli et al., 1991). Several investigators have also reported altered phosphoinositol turnover after thrombin receptor activation of platelets in schizophrenia (Essali et al., 1990; Kaiya et al., 1989; Yao et al., 1992). Altered membrane receptor-mediated signal transduction of several neurotransmitters and growth factors has been considered in schizophrenia (Hudson et al., 1993). This is probably a result of alterations in second messenger-derived membrane phospholipids, since the effects of several transmitters (e.g. dopamine, serotonin, acetylcholine, norepinephrine, glutamate, and gamma-aminobutyric acid) (Axelrod, 1990) and growth factors (Virdee *et al.*, 1994) are mediated by these mechanisms.

Other physiological roles of phospholipid precursors relevant to schizophrenia

In addition to the possible role of AA and DHA in the structure and function of neural membranes in schizophrenia, these fatty acids, combined with antioxidants, play critical roles in several important cellular processes and medical morbidities. DHA has been shown to prevent apoptosis under a variety of pathophysiological conditions (Akbar and Kim, 2002; Brand *et al.*, 2000). This may be important since increased apoptosis has been proposed in schizophrenia (Margolis *et al.*, 1994). DHA is effectively converted into EPA, a precursor for prostaglandins that plays an important role as an anti-inflammatory factor; abnormal prostaglandin metabolism has been reported in schizophrenia (Horrobin *et al.*, 1994). DHA has also been found to regulate a large number of genes for transcription factors, genes involved in sterol, including cholesterol metabolism, and neuroprotective genes such as trophic factors and anti-apoptotic factors (Ntambi and Bene, 2001). The role of DHA in apoptosis and inflammatory processes, combined with its beneficial effects in controlling weight gain, diabetes, hypertension, autoimmune disorders, certain cancers, and preventing neurodegeneration (Simopoulos, 1991), makes it a very important nutritional factor in schizophrenia, which is associated with many of these morbidities.

Factors affecting membrane polyunsaturated fatty acid metabolism in schizophrenia

Intake of polyunsaturated fatty acids

Both prenatal and postnatal membrane EPUFA status is critical in the etiology of schizophrenia. Many factors influence the dietary intake of EPUFAs by an individual: the season in which a person is conceived and born (which significantly affects the availability of food rich in EPUFAs), family size, birth order, whether the person was breast-fed as an infant, culture, socioeconomic status, and domicile (urban or rural) (Mahadik *et al.*, 1999a). Breast-feeding (mother's milk is very rich in DHA, which was not present in bottle formula until recently) has been thought to be associated with lower incidence and better outcome of schizophrenia (McCreadie, 1997). Similarly, the levels of EPUFA in membranes are influenced by a patient's dietary availability and intake of EPUFAs and antioxidants, lifestyle, medications, family support, and illness (Mahadik and Evans, 1997; Mahadik *et al.*, 1999a). This is particularly important since the quality and quantity of a patient's diet depends on the family or care providers. Lifestyle, which includes habits such as alcohol consumption, smoking, and drug use, and level of physical activity influences the metabolism of EPUFAs (Mahadik *et al.*, 2001). However, since the 1970s with increased migration of population and very significant changes in food production and delivery, some of the influences of season, culture, and family-related factors are being attenuated.

Oxidative breakdown of polyunsaturated fatty acids

Peroxidative breakdown of EPUFA by free radicals, also called reactive oxygen species (e.g. $O_2^{\bullet-}$, $^{\bullet}OH$, OH^-, $^{\bullet}NO$ and $ONOO^-$), may be a very important factor in the pathophysiology of schizophrenia (Mahadik and Mukherjee, 1996; Reddy and Yao, 1996). EPUFAs are selectively susceptible to peroxidation. Increased oxidative stress and lipid peroxidation is associated with schizophrenia (Mahadik *et al.*, 1999b). Furthermore, typical antipsychotic drugs have pro-oxidant effects and atypical drugs have antioxidant effects (Parikh *et al.*, 2002). Membrane AA and DHA levels in patients treated with atypical antipsychotic drugs such as clozapine have been found be higher than levels in patients taking haloperidol (Horrobin, 1999; Khan *et al.*, 2002). In addition, some newer antipsychotic drugs have been found to increase the patient's caloric intake significantly, which can increase the oxidative stress and peroxidative EPUFA breakdown. This drug effect is unhealthy and pro-oxidant, particularly when combined with a lifestyle involving little or no exercise, high levels of smoking and drinking alcohol, and a high-fat diet (Brown *et al.*, 1999; Scottish Schizophrenia Research Group, 2000). In animals, caloric restriction has been shown to reduce the oxidative cellular damage associated with a regular high-caloric diet (Sohal *et al.*, 1994) and also to improve learning and memory (Forster *et al.*, 1996). However, peroxidative breakdown of EPUFA can be effectively prevented by dietary supplementation of antioxidants such as β-carotene, quinones, flavones, lycopenes, and vitamins E and C, which contain antioxidants to prevent oxidative damage to the membrane lipid (hydrophobic) and cytosolic (hydrophilic) constituents of the EPUFA (Mahadik and Gowda, 1996). Several studies have reported that supplementation with vitamin E primarily improves the tardive dyskinesia symptomatology (Adler *et al.*, 1999; Mahadik and Gowda, 1996; Mahadik and Scheffer, 1996 Reddy and Yao, 1996). Only one study found that supplementation with vitamin E reduced the lipid peroxides, increased the membrane EPUFAs, and improved the clinical outcome of schizophrenia (Peet *et al.*, 1993). Recent studies have found that reduced levels of EPUFAs and increased levels of peroxides correlated with the severity of schizophrenia (Arvindakshan *et al.*, 2003a; Khan *et al.*, 2002). The antioxidants primarily prevent the peroxidation of EPUFAs. Therefore, dietary supplementation with a combination of antioxidants (e.g. vitamin E and C) and EPUFAs, particularly EPA and DHA, has been suggested to improve the outcome of schizophrenia (Mahadik *et al.*, 2001). One study that used such supplementation has reported very significantly improved and sustained outcomes in a racially homogenous group of schizophrenia patients (Arvindakshan *et al.*, 2003b).

Strategies to address nutritional deficits in schizophrenia

At present the primary concerns for nutritional factors in schizophrenia relate to intake of EPUFAs, particularly the omega-3 EFAs, and antioxidants, such as vitamins E and C. It may be important to examine the therapeutic value of these supplements as an adjunctive to pharmacotherapy. However, all the EPUFA supplementation studies so far have been carried out with patients with chronic schizophrenia, who have been treated with a variety of antipsychotic drugs. These studies have indicated several critical issues that must be considered in designing and carrying out further research.

Factors influencing supplementation
Age and duration of illness

The age of the patient may be an important issue, since age has been associated with the body's antioxidant defense. Furthermore, the number of years of illness and treatment, particularly with typical antipsychotic drugs, may lead to a state of membrane pathology that may be difficult to correct. Fenton *et al.* (2000), who did not find any therapeutic effect from administering EPUFAs, have suggested supplementation in younger patients in their early stages of illness.

Adjunctive medication

Typical antipsychotic drugs such as haloperidol have pro-oxidant properties (Jeding *et al.*, 1995). These medications can also affect EPUFA metabolism (Horrobin *et al.*, 1994). The newer atypical antipsychotic drugs have antioxidant effects, particularly clozapine, which has been found to improve membrane EPUFA levels (Arvindakshan *et al.*, 2003a; Horrobin, 1999; Khan *et al.*, 2002). Recently, we have found that haloperidol reduced the antioxidant enzymes and increased the lipid peroxides in the rat brain; however, none of the atypical drugs such as clozapine, olanzapine, and risperidone did this (Parikh *et al.*, 2002).

Type of essential polyunsaturated fatty acid

Earlier studies have reported the efficacy of administering omega-6 fatty acids (Vaddadi *et al.*, 1989). Recently, Peet and Horrobin (2002) reported that the omega-3 fatty acid EPA alone might be adequate to correct the membrane EPUFA deficits and improve psychopathology in schizophrenia. However, the use of a mixture of EPA and DHA may still be preferred, since a large percentage of EPA is converted to prostaglandin and may not be adequate as a substrate for DHA, which is a predominant omega-3 fatty acid in neuronal membranes.

Dose and the quality of omega-3 fatty acid

Dose is significantly influenced by the patient's lifestyle and dietary status. Furthermore, since the omega-3 EPUFA preparations are unstable, the quality must be carefully monitored. If not balanced with dietary antioxidants, high doses of EPUFAs may increase the levels of peroxides, which are known to be toxic to several plasma membrane functions including neurotransmitter signal transduction (Rafalowska *et al.*, 1989).

Duration of treatment

Earlier studies have suggested that supplementation for at least 4 months is required to restore the level of EPUFA in red blood cells and brain membranes to a steady state (Mahadik and Evans, 1997). However, one study indicated that supplementation with EPA had therapeutic effects within a few weeks, indicating a possible indirect role for EPA and/or its metabolites (Peet and Horrobin, 2002).

Placebo control

Since psychiatric disorders show a significant placebo effect on symptom reduction, well-designed, placebo-controlled, dose-ranging replication studies would be critical to establish the therapeutic benefits of omega-3 EPUFAs (Peet and Horrobin, 2002).

Preferred supplementation components

Based on the concept that the ongoing oxidative breakdown of cell membrane EPUFAs must be stopped and their levels maintained to restore and preserve neural membrane function in schizophrenia, the use of a combination of antioxidants to prevent peroxidative damage and EPUFAs to restore membrane phospholipids may be necessary for optimal treatment of schizophrenia. Unfortunately, studies reported so far involve the administration of either an antioxidant, which has been exclusively vitamin E alone (Adler *et al.*, 1999; Mahadik and Mukherjee, 1996; Reddy and Yao, 1996), or of EPUFAs accompanied by only trace amounts of antioxidants (Fenton *et al.*, 2000; Mahadik and Evans, 1997). Only one study has reported using a dietary supplementation with EPA (180 mg) and DHA (120 mg) plus vitamins E (400 iu) and C (500 mg) (Arvindakshan *et al.*, 2003b). There was a highly significant reduction in symptomatology in patients with chronic schizophrenia after taking the supplement twice a day for 4 months. It is also important to note that all the patients in the study were racially homogeneous, and they had previously had a very similar dietary intake of EPUFAs (based on diet questionnaire) and lifestyle.

When and what should be treated with antioxidants and essential polyunsaturated fatty acids?

The above discussion indicates that oxidative cell injury and altered EPUFA metabolism could conceivably predate the illness, contribute to the onset of psychopathologies, and continue and even worsen during the course of schizophrenia. Supplementation with antioxidants and EPUFAs may, therefore, play a critical role in altering the onset and improving the course and outcome of schizophrenia. Since typical antipsychotic drugs are still the drugs of choice for the effective control of psychosis, the most serious symptom of schizophrenia, adjunctive treatment with antioxidants and EPUFAs may prove important in the early course of schizophrenia, in its outcome, and in the reduction of serious comorbidities. EPUFAs have also been found to be lower in children with attention-deficit hyperactivity disorder (Arnold et al., 1994; Stevens and Burgess, 1999), a disorder that may be a premorbid indicator of a person's risk for developing schizophrenia (Keshavan et al., 2003a). Interestingly, a recent study has suggested that children at genetic risk for schizophrenia had evidence for decreased membrane phospholipid metabolism in the prefrontal cortex, as examined by phosphorus-31 magnetic resonance spectroscopy (Keshavan et al., 2003b). These alterations were more marked in children and adolescents with attention-deficit hyperactivity disorder and other neurodevelopmental disorders. These observations suggest the possible benefit of very early supplementation with antioxidants and EPUFAs early in schizophrenia and in individuals at risk for this illness.

Conclusions

Since proper nutrition regulates the normal development of body and mind, and maintains their health throughout a person's life, it can play a critical role in influencing the pathophysiology, and thereby the psychopathology, of schizophrenia. However, based on global epidemiological data, nutrition can primarily be considered as a means of improving the course and outcome of the disease. Proper nutrition is a complex issue, particularly for schizophrenia patients, whose dietary intake can be affected by lifestyle, illness, medications, support services, and other yet unknown metabolic genetic defects. Reports on diet in developed countries such as the USA indicate that there is malnutrition (lack or reduced intake) with respect to dietary intake of omega-3 EPUFAs and antioxidants. This and the increased oxidative stress and reduced levels of membrane phospholipid omega-3 EFAs from very early stages of schizophrenia illness suggest that early nutritional supplementation of omega-3 EFAs and antioxidants could significantly improve the clinical course and outcome of patients; such supplementation may also potentially diminish the likelihood of other medical morbidities such as weight gain, hypertension, diabetes, immune disorders, and some cancers associated with schizophrenia.

REFERENCES

Adler, L. A., Rotrosen, J., Edson, R., *et al.* (1999). Vitamin E treatment for tardive dyskinesia. *Arch J Psychiatry* **56**: 836–841.

Akbar, M., Kim, H. Y. (2002). Protective effects of docosahexaenoic acid in staurosporine-induced apoptosis: involvement of phosphatidylinositol-3 kinase pathway. *J Neurochem* **82**: 655–665.

Arnold, L. E., Kleykamp, D., Votolato, N., Gibson, R. A., Horrocks, L. (1994). Potential link between dietary intake of fatty acids and behavior: pilot exploration of serum lipids in attention-deficit hyperactivity disorder. *J Child Adoles Psychopharmacol* **4**: 171–182.

Arvindakshan, M. (2003). The role of membrane essential fatty acids in schizophrenia outcome. Ph.D. Thesis, Pune University India.

Arvindakshan, M., Sitasawad, S., Debsikdar, V., *et al.* (2003a). Membrane essential polyunsaturated fatty acids (EPUFA) and schizophrenia outcome: EPUFA and lipid peroxide levels in never-medicated and medicated schizophrenics. *Biol Psychiatry* **53**: 56–64.

Arvindakshan, M., Ghate, M., Ranjekar, P. K., Evans, D. R., Mahadik, S. P. (2003b). Supplementation with a combination of omega-3 fatty acids and antioxidants (vitamins E and C) improves the outcome of schizophrenia. *Schizophr Res* **62**: 195–204.

Axelrod, J. (1990). Receptor-mediated activation of phospholipase A_2 and arachidonic acid release in signal transduction. *Biochem Soc Trans* **18**: 503–507.

Berridge, M. J. (1981). Phosphatidylinositol hydrolysis: a multifunctional transducting mechanism. *Mol Cell Endocrinol* **24**: 115–140.

Bloom, F. (1993). Advancing neurodevelopmental origin for schizophrenia. *Arch Gen Psychiatry* **50**: 224–227.

Brand, A., Gil, S., Yavin, E. (2000). N-Methyl bases of ethanolamine prevent apoptotic cell death induced by oxidative stress in cells of oligodendroglia origin. *J Neurochem* **74**: 1596–1604.

Brown, S., Birtwistle, J., Roe, L., Thompson, C. (1999). The unhealthy lifestyle of people with schizophrenia. *Psychol Med* **29**: 697–701.

Burr, G. O., Burr, M. M. (1929). A new deficiency disease produced by the rigid exclusion of fat from the diet. *J Biol Chem* **82**: 345–367.

Carlson, S. E., Rhodes, P. G., Ferguson, M. G. (1986). Docosahexaenoic acid status of preterm infants at birth and following feeding with human milk or formula 1–3. *Am J Clin Nutr* **44**: 798–804.

Chafetz, M. D. (1990). *Nutrition and Neurotransmitters: The Nutrient Bases of Behavior.* Englewood Cliffs, NJ: Prentice Hall.

Christinsen, O., Christinsen, E. (1988). Fat consumption and schizophrenia. *Acta Psychiatr Scand* **78**: 587–591.

Chua, S. E., McKenna, P. J. (1995). Schizophrenia: a brain disease? A critical review of structural and cerebral abnormalities in the disorder. *Br J Psychiatry* **166**: 563–582.

Coleman, M., Gillberg, C. (1996). *The Schizophrenias. A Biological Approach to the Schizophrenia Spectrum Disorders.* New York: Springer.

Craig, T. J., Siegel, C., Hopper, K., Lin, S., Sartorius, N. (1997). Outcome in schizophrenia and related disorders compared between developing and developed countries. *Br J Psychiatry* **170**: 229–233.

Crawford, M. A. (1992). Essential fatty acids and neurodevelopmental disorder. In *Neurobiology of Essential Fatty Acids*, ed. N. G. Bazan. New York: Plenum Press, pp. 307–314.

Dhopeshwarkar, G. A. (1983). *Nutrition and Brain Development.* New York: Plenum Press.

Eaton, W. W. (1985). Epidemiology of schizophrenia. *Epidemiol Cal Rev* **7**: 105–126.

Edelson, E. (1988). *Nutrition and the Brain.* New York: Chelsea House.

Edgerton, R. B., Cohen, A. (1994). Culture and schizophrenia: the DOSMD challenge. *Br J Psychiatry* **164**: 222–231.

Essali, M. A., Das, R., de Belleroche, J., Hirsch, S. R. (1990). The platelets polyphosphoinositide system in schizophrenia: the effects of neuroleptic treatment. *Biol Psychiatry* **28**: 478–487.

Feinberg, I. (1990). Cortical pruning and the development of schizophrenia. *Schizophr Bull* **16**: 567–568.

Fenton, W. S., Hibbeln, J., Knable, M. (2000). Essential fatty acids, lipid membrane abnormalities, and the diagnosis and treatment of schizophrenia. *Biol Psychiatry* **47**: 8–21.

Forster, M. J., Dubey, A., Dawson, K. M., *et al.* (1996). Age-related losses of cognitive and motor skills in mice are associated with oxidative protein damage in the brain. *Proc Natl Acad Sci, USA* **93**: 4765–4769.

Freud, S. (1961). Civilization and its discontents. In *The Standard Edition of the Complete Psychological Work of Sigmund Freud*, Vol. 21, ed. J. Strachey. New York: Norton, pp. 59–145.

Fukuzako, H. Fukuzako, T., Takeuchi, K., *et al.* (1996). Phosphorus magnetic resonance spectroscopy in schizophrenia: correlation between membrane PL metabolism in the temporal lobe and positive symptoms. *Progr Neuropsychopharmacol Biol Psychiatry* **20**: 629–640.

Glantz, L. A., Lewis, D. A. (2000). Decreased dendritic spine density on prefrontal cortical pyramidal neurons in schizophrenia. *Arch Gen Psychiatry* **57**: 65–73.

Glen, A. I. M., Glen, E. M. T., Horrobin, D. F., *et al.* (1994). A red cell membrane abnormality in a subgroup of schizophrenic patients: evidence for two diseases. *Schizophr Res* **12**: 53–61.

Heckers, S. (1997). Neuropathology of schizophrenia: cortex, thalamus, basal ganglia, and neurotransmitter-specific projection system. *Schizophr Bull* **23**: 403–421.

Hegarty, J. D., Baldessarini, R. J., Tohen, M., Waternaux, C., Oepen, G. (1994). One hundred years of schizophrenia: a meta-analysis of the outcome literature. *Am J Psychiatry* **151**: 1409–1416.

Hoek, H. W., Brown, A. S., Susser, E. (1998). The Dutch famine and schizophrenia spectrum disorders. *Soc Psychiatry Psychiatr Epidemiol* **33**: 373–379.

Horrobin, D. F. (1996). Schizophrenia as a membrane lipid disorder which is expressed throughout the body. *Prostaglandins, Leukot Essent Fatty Acids* **55**: 3–8.

(1998). The membrane phospholipid hypothesis as a biochemical basis for the neurodevelopmental concept of schizophrenia. *Schizophr Res* **30**: 193–208

(1999). The effects of antipsychotic drugs on membrane phospholipids: a possible novel mechanism of action of clozapine. In *Phospholipid Spectrum Disorders in Psychiatric*, ed. M. Peet, A. L. Glen, D. Horrobin. Carnforth, UK: Marius Press, pp. 113–117.

Horrobin, D. F., Glen, A. I. M., Vaddadi, K. S. (1994). The membrane hypothesis of schizophrenia. *Schizophr Res* 13: 195–208.

Horrocks, L. A., Ansell, G. B., Porcellati, G. (ed.) (1982). *Phospholipids in the Nervous System*, Vol. 1, *Metabolism*. New York: Raven Press.

Hudson, C. J., Young, L. T., Li, P. P., Warsh, J. J. (1993). CNS signal transduction in the pathophysiology and pharmacology of affective disorders and schizophrenia. *Synapse* 13: 278–293.

Hulshoff Pol, H. E., Hoek, H. W., Susser, E., *et al.* (2000). Prenatal exposure to famine and brain morphology in schizophrenia. *Am J Psychiatry* 157: 1170–1172.

Innis, S. M. (1991). Essential fatty acids in growth and development. *Progr Lipid Res* 30: 39–103.

Jablensky, A., Sartorius, N., Ernberg, G., *et al.* (1991). Schizophrenia: manifestations, incidence and course in different cultures. *Psychol Med Monogr Suppl* 20: 1–97.

Jeding, I., Evans, P. J., Akanmu, D., *et al.* (1995). Characterization of the potential antioxidant and pro-oxidant actions of some neuroleptic drugs. *Biochem Pharmacol* 49: 359–365.

Kaiya, H., Nishida, A., Imai, A., Nakashima, S., Nozawa, Y. (1989). Accumulation of diacylglycerol in platelet phosphoinositides turnover in schizophrenia: a biological marker of good prognosis? *Biol Psychiatry* 26: 669–676.

Karno, M., Jenkins, J. H. (1993). Cross-cultural issues in the course and treatment of schizophrenia. *Psych Clin North Am* 16: 339–350.

Keshavan, M. S., Murray, R. M. (1997). *Neurodevelopment and Adult Psychopathology*. Cambridge, UK: Cambridge University Press.

Keshavan, M. S., Mallinger, A. G., Pettegrew, J. W., Dippold, C. (1993). Erythrocyte membrane phospholipids in psychotic patients. *Psychiatr Res* 49: 9–95.

Keshavan, M. S., Anderson, S., Pettegrew, J. W. (1994). Is schizophrenia due to excessive synaptic pruning in the prefrontal cortex? The Feinberg hypothesis revisited. *J Psychiatr Res* 28: 239–265.

Keshavan, M. S., Sujata, A., Mehra, M., Montrose, D. M., Sweeney, J. A. (2003a). Psychosis proneness and ADHD in young relatives of schizophrenia patients. *Schizophr Res* 59: 85–92.

Keshavan, M. S., Stanley, J. A., Montrose, D. M., Minshew, N. J., Pettegrew, J. W. (2003b). Prefrontal membrane phospholipid metabolism of child and adolescent offspring at risk for schizophrenia or schizoaffective disorder: an in vivo ^{31}P MRS study. *Mol Psychiatry* 8: 316–323.

Khan, A., Khan, S. R., Leventhal, R. M., Brown, W. A. (2001). Symptom reduction and suicide risk among patients treated with placebo in antipsychotic clinical trials: an analysis of the Food and Drug Administration database. *Am J Psychiatry* 158: 1449–1454.

Khan, M. M., Evans, D. R., Gunna, V., *et al.* (2002). Reduced erythrocyte membrane essential fatty acids increased lipid peroxides in schizophrenia at the never-medicated first-episode of psychosis and after years of treatment with antipsychotics. *Schizophr Res* 58: 1–10.

Kulhara, P., Chakrabarti, S. (2001). Culture and schizophrenia and other psychotic disorders. *Psychiatr Clin North Am* **24**: 449–464.

Lawrie, S. M., Abukmeil, S. S. (1998). Brain abnormality in schizophrenia: a systematic and quantitative review of volumetric magnetic resonance imaging studies. *Br J Psychiatry* **172**: 119–120.

Mahadik, S. P., Evans, D. (1997). Essential fatty acids in the treatment of schizophrenia. *Drugs Today* **33**: 5–17.

Mahadik, S. P., Gowda, S. (1996). Antioxidants in the treatment of schizophrenia. *Drugs Today* **32**: 1–13.

Mahadik, S. P., Mukherjee, S. (1996). Free radical pathology and the antioxidant defense in schizophrenia. *Schizophr Res* **19**: 1–18.

Mahadik, S. P., Scheffer, R. E. (1996). Oxidative injury and potential use of antioxidants in schizophrenia. *Prostaglandins, Leukot Essent Fatty Acids* **55**: 45–54.

Mahadik, S. P., Mukherjee, S., Correnti, E., *et al.* (1994). Distribution of plasma membrane phospholipids and cholesterol in skin fibroblasts from drug-naive patients at the onset of psychosis. *Schizophr Res* **13**: 239–247.

Mahadik, S. P., Mukherjee, S., Horrobin, D., *et al.* (1996a). Plasma membrane phospholipid fatty acid composition of cultured skin fibroblasts from schizophrenic patients: comparison with bipolar and normal controls. *Psychiatr Res* **63**: 133–142.

Mahadik, S. P., Shendarkar, N. S., Scheffer, R., Mukherjee, S., Correnti, E. E. (1996b). Utilization of precursor essential fatty acids in culture by skin fibroblasts from schizophrenic patients and normal controls. *Prostaglandins, Leukot Essent Fatty Acids* **55**: 65–70.

Mahadik, S. P., Mulchandani, M., Hegde, M. V., Ranjekar, P. K. (1999a). Cultural and socioeconomic differences in dietary intake of essential fatty acids and antioxidants-effects on the outcome. In *Phospholipid Spectrum Disorders in Psychiatric*, ed. D., Horrobin, A. L. Glen, M. Peet. Carnforth, UK: Marius Press, pp. 167–179.

Mahadik, S. P., Sitasawad, V., Mulchandani, M. (1999b). Membrane peroxidation and the neuropathology of schizophrenia. In *Phospholipid Spectrum Disorders in Psychiatric*, ed. D. Horrobin, A. L. Glen, M. Peet. Carnforth, UK: Marius Press, pp. 99–111.

Mahadik, S. P., Evans, D., Lal, H. (2001). Oxidative stress and the role of antioxidant and ω-3 essential fatty acid supplementation in schizophrenia. *Prog Neuropsychopharmacol Biol Psychiatry* **25**: 463–493.

Margolis, R. L., Chung, D.-M., Post, R. M. (1994). Programmed cell death: Implications for neuropsychiatric disorders. *Biol Psychiatry* **35**: 946–956.

McCreadie, R. G. (1997). The Nithsdale Schizophrenia Surveys 16: breast-feeding and schizophrenia: preliminary results and hypothesis. *Br J Psychiatry* **170**: 334–337.

McGrath, J. (1999). Hypothesis: is low vitamin D a risk-modifying factor for schizophrenia? *Schizophr Res* **40**: 173–177.

McIntyre, R. S., McCann, S. M., Kennedy, S. H. (2001). Antipsychotic metabolic effects: weight gain, diabetes mellitus and lipid abnormalities. *Can J Psychiatr* **46**: 272–281.

Mednick, S. A., Machon, R. A., Huttunen, M. O., Bonett, D. (1988). Adult schizophrenia following prenatal exposure to an influenza epidemic. *Arch Gen Psychiatry* **45**: 189–192.

Murphy, H. B. M. (1984). Editorial: diseases of civilization? *Psychol Med* **14**: 487–490.

Murray, R. M. (1994). Neurodevelopmental schizophrenia: the rediscovery of dementia precox. *Br J Psychiatry* **165**(Suppl. 25): 6–12.

Nandi, D. N., Mukherjee, S. P., Boral, G. C., *et al.* (1980). Socioeconomic status and mental morbidity in certain tribes and castes in India: a cross-cultural study. *Br J Psychiatry* **136**: 73–85.

Neuringer, M. Connor, W. E., Lin, D. S., Barstad, L., Luck, S. (1986). Biochemical and functional effect of prenatal and postnatal omega-3 fatty acid deficiency on retina and brain in rhesus monkeys. *Proc Natl Acad Sci* USA **83**: 4021–4025.

Ntambi, J. M., Bene, H. (2001). Polyunsaturated fatty acid regulation of gene expression. *J Mol Neurosci* **16**: 273–278.

O'Brien, J. S., Sampson, E. L. (1965). Lipid composition of the normal human brain: gray matter, white matter, and myelin. *J Lipid Res* **6**: 537–544.

Parikh, V. Khan, M. M., Mahadik, S. P. (2002). Differential effects of antipsychotics on expression of antioxidant enzymes and membrane lipid peroxidation in rat brain. *J Psychiatr Res* **37**: 43–51.

Peet, M., Laugharne, J., Rangarajan, N., Renolds, G. P. (1993). Tardive dyskinesia, lipid peroxidation, and sustained amelioration with vitamin E treatment. *Int Clin Psychopharmacol* **8**: 151–153.

Peet, M., Laugharne, J., Mellor, J. E., Ramchand, C. N. (1995). Essential fatty acid deficiency in erythrocyte membranes from chronic schizophrenic patients, and the clinical effects of dietary supplementation. *Prostaglandins, Leukotr Essent Fatty Acids* **55**: 119–122.

Peet, M., Brind, J., Ramchand, C. N., Shah, S., Vankar, G. K. (2001). Two double-blind placebo-controlled pilot studies of eicosapentaenoic acid in the treatment of schizophrenia. *Schizophr Res* **49**: 243–251.

Peet, M., Horrobin, D. F., in association with the E-E Multicenter Study Group (2002). A dose-ranging exploratory study of the effects of ethyl-eicosapentaenoate in patients with persistent schizophrenic symptoms. *J Psychiatric Res* **36**: 7–18.

Pettegrew, J. W., Keshavan, M. S., Minshew, N. J. (1991). Alterations in brain high-energy phosphate and membrane phospholipid metabolism in first-episode, drug-naive schizophrenics. A pilot study of the dorsal prefrontal cortex using in vivo phosphorus 31 nuclear magnetic resonance spectroscopy. *Arch Gen Psychiatry* **48**: 563–568.

Piomelli, D., Pilon, C., Giros, B., *et al.* (1991). Dopamine activation of the arachidonic acid cascade as a basis for D_1/D_2 receptor synergism. *Nature* **353**: 164–167.

Raedler, T. J., Knable, M. B., Weinberger, D. R. (1998). Schizophrenia as a developmental disorder of the cerebral cortex. *Curr Opin Neurobiol* **8**: 157–161.

Rafalowska, U., Liu, G.-J., Floyd, R. A. (1989). Peroxidation induced changes in synaptosomal transport of dopamine and gamma-aminobutyric acid. *Free Rad Biol Med* **6**: 485–492.

Rana, R. S., Hokin, L. E. (1990). Role of phosphoinositols in transmembrane signaling. *Physiol Rev* **70**: 115–164.

Reddy, R., Yao, J. (1996). Free radical pathology in schizophrenia: a review. *Prostaglandins, Leukot Essent Fatty Acids* **55**: 33–43.

Rotrosen, J., Wolkin, A. (1987). Phospholipid and prostaglandin hypotheses of schizophrenia. In *Psychopharmacology: The Third Generation of Progress*, ed. H. Y. Meltzer. New York. Raven Press, pp. 759–764.

Sartorius, N., Jablensky, A., Korten, A., *et al.* (1986). Early manifestations and first-contact incidence of schizophrenia in different cultures. *Psychol Med* 16: 909–928.

Scottish Schizophrenia Research Group (2000). Smoking habits and plasma lipid peroxides and vitamin E in never medicated first-episode schizophrenic patients with schizophrenia. *Br J Psychiatry* 176: 290–293.

Selemon, L. D., Rajkowska, G., Goldman-Rakic, P. S. (1995). Abnormally high neuronal density in the schizophrenic cortex. *Arch Gen Psychiatry* 52: 805–818.

Simopoulos, A. P. (1991). Omega-3 fatty acids in health and disease, and in growth and development. *Am J Clin Nutr* 54: 438–463.

Sohal, R. S., Ku, H.-H., Agarwal, S., Forster, M. J., Lal, H. (1994). Oxidative damage, mitochondrial oxidant generation and antioxidant defenses during aging, and in response to food restriction in the mouse. *Mech Aging Dev* 74: 121–133.

Stanley, J. A., Williamson, P. C., Drost, D. J., *et al.* (1995). An in vivo study of the prefrontal cortex of schizophrenic patients at different age of illness via phosphorous magnetic resonance spectroscopy. *Arch Gen Psychiatry* 52: 399–406.

Stevens, L. J., Burgess, J. R. (1999). Essential fatty acids in children with attention-deficit/hyperactivity disorder. In *Phospholipid Spectrum Psychiatric Disorders*, ed. D. Horrobin, A. L. Glen, M. Peet. Carnforth, UK: Marius Press, pp. 263–269.

Suzuki, K. (1981). Chemistry and metabolism of brain lipids. In *Basic Neurochemistry*, 3rd edn, ed. D. J. Seigel, R. W. Albers, B. W. Agranoff, *et al.* Boston, MA: Little Brown, pp. 355–370.

Tollefson, G. D. (1996). Cognitive function in schizophrenic patients. *J Clin Psychiatry* 57(Suppl. 11): 31–39.

Thompson, G. A. (1992). *The Regulation of Membrane Lipid Metabolism*, 2nd edn. Boca Raton, FL: CRC Press.

Torrey, E. F. (1980). *Schizophrenia and Civilization*. New York: Jason Aronson.

Vaddadi, K. S., Courtney, P., Gilleard, C. S., Manku, M. S., Horrobin, D. F. (1989). A double-blind trial of essential fatty acid supplementation in patients with tardive dyskinesia. *Psychiatr Res* 27: 313–323.

Virdee, K., Brown, B. L., Dobson, P. R.-M. (1994). Stimulation of arachidonic acid release from Swiss 3T3 cells by recombinant basic fibroblast growth factor: independence from phosphoinositide turnover. *Biochim Biophys Acta* 16: 193–205.

Wainwright, P. E. (1992). Do essential fatty acids play a role in brain and behavioral development? *Neurosci Biobehav Rev* 16: 193–205.

Weinberger, D. R. (1996). On the plausibility of "the neurodevelopmental hypothesis" of schizophrenia. *Neuropsychopharmacology* 14: 1S–11S.

WHO (World Health Organization) (1973). *The International Pilot Study of Schizophrenia*, Vol. 1. Geneva: World Health Organization.

Yamamoto, N., Saitoh, M., Moriuchi, A., Nomura, M., Okuyama, H. (1987). Effect of dietary γ-linolenate/linoleate balance on brain lipid compositions and learning ability of rats. *J Lipid Res* 28: 144–151.

Yao, J. K. (1999). Red blood cell and platelet fatty acid metabolism in schizophrenia. In *Phospho-lipid Spectrum in Psychiatric Disorders*, ed. D. Horrobin, A. L. Glen, M. Peet. Carnforth, UK: Marius Press, pp. 57–71.

Yao, J. K., Yasaei, P., van Kammen, D. P. (1992). Increased turnover of platelet phosphatidylinositol in schizophrenia. *Prostaglandins, Leukotr Essent Fatty Acids* **46**: 39–46.

Yao, J. K., van Kammen, D. P., Welker, J. A. (1994). Red cell membrane dynamics in schizophrenia: II fatty acid composition. *Schizophr Res* **13**: 217–226.

10

Schizophrenia, neurodevelopment, and epigenetics

Arturas Petronis

Centre for Addiction and Mental Health, Toronto, Canada

The neurodevelopmental theory of schizophrenia is based on the hypothesis that early brain insults affect brain development and eventually cause dysfunction of the mature brain, predisposing to schizophrenia. The basis for these ideas formed early in the twentieth century when clinical psychiatrists insightfully speculated that schizophrenia could be resulting from cerebral maldevelopment (Kraepelin, 1919). Over the last several decades, a myriad of clinical, epidemiological, morphological, and molecular studies have investigated brain development to find evidence concerning possible neurodevelopmental changes in schizophrenia (reviewed in Lewis and Levitt, 2002; Woods, 1998). Although the results of such studies are not necessarily fully consistent, there is converging evidence that at least a subgroup of schizophrenia patients exhibit subtle developmental abnormalities that presumably occur during embryogenesis. Changes have been detected in brain asymmetry, neuronal cell migration and clustering, density of neurons in various brain regions, and their cytoarchitectural organization and synapse formation. Schizophrenia-associated morphological differences of the brain have also been documented at the macroscopic level, including larger lateral brain ventricules and changes of the volume of cortex and subcortical structures. Consistently with the brain morphological aberrations, prospective and retrospective behavioral studies of schizophrenia patients showed that, long before they became affected, such individuals exhibited a higher incidence of minor neuromotor abnormalities, delayed attainment of developmental milestones, and various other subtle behavioral and intellectual abnormalities. Beyond the brain, schizophrenia patients are also reported to have a higher prevalence of minor physical anomalies, such as low-set ears, furrowed tongue, high-arched palate, curved fingers, and greater distance between the eyes, among numerous others. Since both the skin and the brain originate from the ectoderm, the minor physical anomalies can be considered as external signs of damage to

Neurodevelopment and Schizophrenia, ed. Matcheri S. Keshavan *et al.* Published by Cambridge University Press. © Cambridge University Press 2004.

the ectoderm during embryogenesis, which serves as indirect support for aberrant neurodevelopment.

What could be the cause(s) of the above brain development and schizophrenia-related aberrations? A large group of putative etiological factors has been suggested, investigated, and categorized into environmental and genetic groups. The first group includes various obstetric complications such birth traumas, maternal viral infection during pregnancy, pre-eclampsia, and deficiencies in nutrition. The second group puts the emphasis on DNA sequence variation in the genes that may play a role in neurodevelopment. So far, none of the above factors has been proven to be in a cause–effect relationship with schizophrenia. In this chapter, the idea that developmental changes in schizophrenia can be caused and/or mediated by epigenetic factors is suggested. It is argued that shifting the emphasis from the traditional "gene–environment" dichotomy to epigenetics may provide a cohesive theoretical framework for the myriad of fragmented phenomenological and molecular findings in schizophrenia and lead to a series of new molecular strategies, designs, and approaches.

The basics of epigenetics

By definition, epigenetics refers to regulation of gene expressions that are controlled by heritable but potentially reversible changes in DNA methylation and/or chromatin structure (Henikoff and Matzke, 1997) (Fig. 10.1). In most organisms, cytosines can be of two functional states: unmodified cytosines (C) and cytosines that are methylated at the 5-position of the pyrimidine ring (^{met}C). DNA methylation is an enzymatic reaction performed by several types of DNA methyltransferase, namely DNMT1, DNMT3A, and DNMT3B (reviewed in Bestor, 2000). DNMT1 is ubiquitously expressed and its primary role is maintaining the DNA methylation pattern in the somatic cells by methylating hemimediated CpG sites after DNA replications. DNMT3A and DNMT3B are required to initiate de nova methylation and establish new DNA methylation patterns (Bestor, 2000). The evidence for DNA demethylase has been controversial so far. It is interesting to note that, although the overwhelming majority of organisms from single-cell prokaryotes to complex multicellular mammals have cytosine methylation, among the rare exceptions that do not exhibit DNA methylation there are three major model organisms: *Drosophila*, yeast, and *Caenorhabditis elegans*. A large number of genes exhibit an inverse correlation between the degree of methylation and gene expression, which supports an increasing body of experimental evidence suggesting that epigenetic modification is intimately involved in the regulation of expression of genes (Holliday, 1996; Jackson-Grusby *et al.*, 2001; Razin and Shemer, 1999; Siegfried *et al.*, 1999; Singal

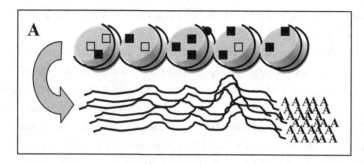

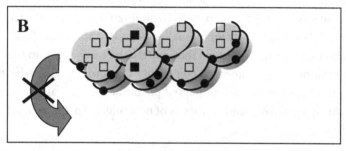

Fig. 10.1.   DNA and histone modifications in regulation of gene expression. DNA is wrapped around histone complexes (gray cylinders) to form nucleosomes. Depending on DNA and histone modifications (small circles and squares) chromatin can be transcriptionally competent (A) or not (B). PolyA sequences represent mRNA molecules.

and Ginder, 1999; Stancheva and Meehan, 2000; Yeivin and Razin, 1993) although this is not universal (Walsh and Bestor, 1999).

One of the mechanisms of epigenetic regulation of genes is related to methylation of the binding sites for transcription factors, serving to change the affinity of these factors for the regulatory sequences of these specific genes (Riggs *et al.*, 1998). In addition to the "critical site" effects of ^{met}C, the overall ratio of ^{met}Cs over unmethylated cytosines in a gene-regulatory region also contributes to gene activity. This type of regulation seems to be linked to another mechanism of epigenetic regulation, namely various types of histone modification. Histones are key components of nucleosomes represented by four highly conservative proteins: H2A, H2B, H3, and H4. The role of mediators between DNA modification and chromatin modification is performed by a group of ^{met}C-binding proteins such as MECP2, MBD1, and MBD2, among others (reviewed in Li, 2002). The ^{met}C-binding proteins recruit different chromatin remodeling proteins and transcription complexes to the loci of methylated DNA. For example, MECP2 binds to methylated DNA and attracts histone deacetylases that hypoacetylate histones. Transcriptionally competent chromatin is normally enriched with acetylated histones, while transcriptionally silent chromatin is deacetylated (reviewed in Robertson and Wolffe, 2000). The interaction of DNA methylation and histone acetylation demonstrates that the two types of epigenetic regulation act in concert. In addition to acetylation, nucleosomal histones can be modified by methylation, phosphorylation, ubiquitylation, and possibly other, yet undiscovered, ways. It is important to note that histone modification targets are numerous residues of lysine, arginine, and serine. For example, Lys9, Lys14, Lys18, and Lys23 of H3 and Lys5, Lys8, Lys12, and Lys16 of H4, together with lysines on H2A and H2B, can be acetylated; whereas Lys4, Lys9, Lys27, Arg2, Arg17, and Arg26 of H3 and Lys20 and Arg3 of H4 can be methylated (Li, 2002). It is evident that a large number of combinations of various types of histone modification are possible even over a short stretch of chromatin. Furthermore, the same DNA sequence may be in a wide variety of functional states. This provided the basis for the concept of the "histone code" (Jenuwein and Allis, 2001).

In addition to their putative role in regulation of autosomal biallelically expressed genes, epigenetic mechanisms of transcriptional repression are of primary importance for X chromosome inactivation and genomic imprinting, as well as in the transcriptional inactivation of endogenous retroviruses and other "parasitic" sequences (reviewed in Wolffe and Matzke, 1999). Furthermore, epigenetic factors play a role in DNA mutagenesis and repair as well as in DNA recombination and possibly replication.

Epigenetic patterns are transmitted similarly to DNA sequences, from maternal chromatids to daughter chromatids during mitotic divisions, and transmission of the epigenetic status is called the *epigenetic inheritance system* (Maynard Smith, 1990). Unlike DNA sequences, which exhibit nearly complete interclonal fidelity, epigenetic status usually exhibits only partial stability; over time, this can result in substantial changes across identical sequences. DNA and chromatin modifications do react to the extracellular environment. Stochastic factors in the cell also contribute to epigenetic differences in the cells of the same line. After mitotic division, the daughter chromosomes do not necessarily carry identical epigenetic patterns in comparison with the parental chromosomes, and, although belonging to the same group of cells (myocytes, lymphocytes, and epithelial cells), these cells exhibit small quantitative differences in terms of their phenotypes and functions. Over time, substantial epigenetic differences may be accumulated across the cells of the same cell line or the same tissue (Riggs *et al.*, 1998). This represents a fundamental difference between epigenetic systems and DNA sequence-based hereditary factors. The partial stability of epigenetic modification is called *epigenetic metastability*. Epigenetic metastability also applies to the germline. Although it has been generally accepted that the parental epigenetic profile is replaced by a new one during the maturation of gametes, there is increasing evidence demonstrating that some epigenetic signals escape erasure and can be transmitted from one generation to another (Rakyan *et al.*, 2002).

Relevance of epigenetics to schizophrenia

Two key aspects of epigenetic modification of the genome make epigenetics very relevant to schizophrenia (as well as numerous other complex non-Mendelian diseases) (Petronis [2001] and references therein for this section). First, epigenetic modifications of DNA and chromatin "orchestrate" the activity of the genome, including regulation of gene expression. While a DNA sequence provides the information of what specific protein has to be synthesized, it is absolutely necessary that each gene is regulated accordingly to the type and the needs of a specific cell. While relatively small deviations in the expression pattern account for normal individual variations, more significant ones can be as detrimental to a cell as the mutant DNA sequences that encode dysfunctional proteins.

Epigenetic metastability is the second aspect that makes epigenetics relevant to various non-Mendelian irregularities of schizophrenia. Epigenetic regulation of genes undergoes significant reorganization during development and aging as well as under the influence of extracellular factors (e.g. hormonal status of an organism) or environmental factors (reviewed in Jablonka and Lamb, 1995). Epigenetic regulation represents the dynamic feature of a gene and genome, whereas most of the DNA sequences (especially the coding ones) do not change during the life of an individual.

Age-dependent epigenetic changes may shed a new light on the relatively late age of onset in schizophrenia as well as the periods of critical age of susceptibility (early twenties and late sixties in both sexes, plus late forties in women). It is evident that the ages of the increased incidence coincide with major hormonal rearrangements in the organism. Epigenetic status of a gene is one of the targets of hormone action. Changes in endocrine status may lead to significant epigenetic rearrangements. Various hormones, including sex hormones, have a significant impact on gene expression, and this is achieved by changing chromatin conformation and/or local patterns of gene methylation. A disease process may be provoked by hormone-mediated epigenetic changes in the critical genes. In the absence of solid evidence for the involvement of the X chromosome, the same mechanism may contribute to the clinical differences of schizophrenia in males and females (reviewed in Seeman, 1997; see Ch. 18). In this respect, changes in the hormonal milieu during maturation and involution can substantially affect the regulation of genes, which at least to some extent is achieved via their epigenetic modifications.

Parent-of-origin effects present with differential risk to the offspring of being affected with a disease depending on which of the two parents is affected with that specific disease. In molecular genetic studies, parental effects present with cosegregation of the disease with either maternal or paternal alleles and/or with differences in the lod scores (measure of genetic linkage) in the families with maternal versus paternal transmission of the disease (reviewed in Petronis, 2000). Parental origin effect is one of the classical epigenetic mechanisms of differential regulation of gene activity, called genomic imprinting.

Epigenetic metastability may shed a new light on the non-Mendelian mode of transmission of schizophrenia as well as on the presence of both sporadic and familial cases of the disease (in the absence of phenotypic differences between the two groups). As a rule, the clinical phenotypes in sporadic schizophrenia are indistinguishable from familial ones. Meiotically stable epimutations can segregate like quasi-Mendelian factors and may represent familial disease, while the epimutations that are erased during gametogenesis may be the cause of sporadic cases. In summary, the epigenetic theory puts the emphasis on epigenetic changes (or absence of such changes) in specific genomic loci during meiosis, while the traditional DNA sequence-oriented paradigm infers that different genes are operating in familial and sporadic cases (major genes and minor genes, respectively).

The most straightforward example of the value of the epigenetic theory is the new interpretation of discordance of monozygotic twins, one of the key mysteries in complex traits. The rate of monozygotic twin discordance in schizophrenia in a combined twin sample is about 50% (Cardno and Gottesman, 2000). Although two co-twins contain the same DNA sequence in the overwhelming majority of somatic cells, substantial epigenetic differences may be accumulated over numerous cell divisions during development and aging in such co-twins. The epigenetic non-identity may result in differential epigenetic regulation of disease-relevant genes, which would result in only one twin reaching the "threshold" of clinical symptoms (Petronis *et al.*, 2003).

In addition, the putative epigenetic misregulation-based disease mechanisms are consistent with numerous epidemiological, clinical, and molecular findings (Chen *et al.*, 2002; Petronis *et al.*, 2002; Tremolizzo *et al.*, 2002). Of particular interest to the topic of this book is the contribution of epigenetic factors in embryogenesis and development with regard to premorbid changes in the brains of schizophrenia patients. The next section is dedicated to the overview of the role of epigenetic factors in development.

Epigenetics and development

There are numerous links between development and epigenetics. Etymologically, the term *epigenetics* originates from *epigenesis*, a theory of development, which proposed that the embryo at its early stage of development is not differentiated and embryogenesis proceeds by increasing levels of complexity (Holliday, 1994). Epigenesis contrasted with preformation, a theory which assumed that complexity already existed in the very early embryo.

The idea of a putative relationship between gene activity and development was entertained by numerous biologists during the twentieth century. For example, T. H. Morgan hypothesized that "genes . . . are changing in some way as development proceeds in response to that part of the protoplasm in which they lie, and that these changes have reciprocal influence on the protoplasm" (Morgan, 1934). In the 1950s, C. H. Waddington coined the term "epigenetics," which referred to the developmental processes that "connect" the genotype to phenotype, or the processes by which genotype gives a rise to phenotype (reviewed in Slack, 2002). These ideas originated long before the advent of molecular biology and represented predominantly a theoretical, although inspiring, framework that influenced various other fields of scientific activity including psychiatric research (Gottesman and Shields, 1982; Woolf, 1997). Waddington is best known for the concept of "epigenetic landscape." The uneven surface of the landscape with "hills" and "valleys" represents a simplified version of multidimensional and intricate non-linear interactions of various molecules within the cell during the embryonic development (Fig. 10.2A). The rolling ball symbolizes a phenotype of a differentiating cell, which at each developmental step acquires new features. The end result of this process is a huge variety of highly specialized cells (Fig. 10.2B).

The idea of the primary role of epigenetic factors in development was raised again in two seminal papers published in 1975 (Holliday and Pugh, 1975; Riggs, 1975). At that time, the presence of epigenetic DNA modification (methylation) was already known and there was experimental evidence suggesting that epigenetic modification may have an impact on the regulation of gene activity. The two papers represented the first systematic attempt to synthesize the available evidence regarding linkage of epigenetic regulation to both differentiation of cells and maintenance of the differentiated cell states. There are two key questions. First, how do the pluripotent undifferentiated embryonic cells become highly specialized. Second, how is the specific phenotype of a specialized cell maintained over numerous mitotic divisions. For example, ectoderm cells differentiate into two very different phenotypes, neurons and keratocytes, and the latter would never convert into the former, and vice versa. What keeps the cell "locked" in a particular regulated state? Understanding the molecular principles of the developmental programs remains one of the main challenges for developmental biologists. Although there are no final answers, epigenetics seems to be one of the best candidates for a molecular mechanism that would be consistent with a wide variety of developmental events in a cell.

Maintenance of the epigenetic profile is consistent with the phenotypic stability of somatic cells. In mammals, methylation occurs predominantly at the symmetrical dinucleotide CpG positions, which after DNA replication become hemimethylated. This hemimethylated DNA is the favored substrate for DNMT1, which efficiently

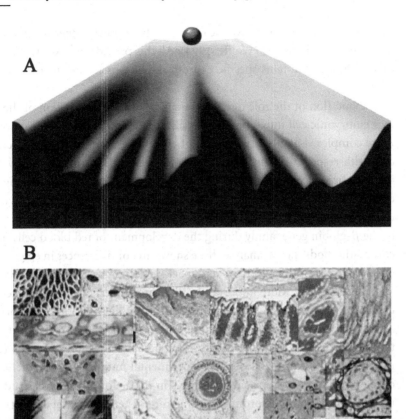

Fig. 10.2.   Epigenetics and cell differentiation. (A) Waddington's epigenetic landscape represents the imaginary path of an undifferentiated pluripotent embryonic cell during development. (B) The end result of cell differentiation is a wide variety of highly specialized cells that look different and perform different functions, although they contain the same DNA sequences. For a colour version of this figure, see www.cambridge.org/9780521126595.

recognizes unmethylated CpGs in the newly synthesized strands that are complementary to the methylated CpG and proceeds to methylate them (Bestor, 2000). In tissue culture, fidelity of maintenance methylation in mammalian cells was 97–99.9% and de novo methylation activity was 3–5% per mitosis (Riggs *et al.*, 1998). Fidelity of maintenance methylation in different types of cell in vivo is unknown but it is very possible that it is sufficient to assure clonal continuity of myocytes, hepatocytes, and the many other kinds of specialized cell. The ways by which various types of epigenetic modification of histones can be inherited in mitotic cells have also been discussed (Wolffe, 1994). All this provides an excellent mechanism that faithfully maintains specific expression patterns in various types of somatic cell.

The question of the role of epigenetic factors in differentiation of the pluripotent embryonic cell into a highly specialized one in the developing embryo is far more complex. Longitudinal studies of epigenetic changes in specific embryonic cells with respect to their increasing differentiation are still technically challenging and there have been only a few studies investigating the relationship between epigenetic changes in the specific genes and changes in such gene activity during cell differentiation. The best known case is the epigenetic changes in regulation of the β-globin gene family during the development of red blood cells. DNA and chromatin modification analyses have shown major differences in epigenetic regulation of transcriptionally active and inactive globin genes (Litt *et al.*, 2001; Singal and Ginder, 1999). More importantly, there are suggestions that such cell-specific epigenetic changes in the chromatin structure of the β-globin locus precede the activation of individual genes; therefore, transcriptional competence (the potential for expression) is detected before the actual transcription occurs (reviewed in Wolffe and Barton, 2000). Such experimental findings are consistent with the developmental role of epigenetic changes in the genome. However, studies of the methylation state of the promoter of the mouse gene for skeletal α-actin showed no correlation between methylation and expression patterns during development and differentiation (Warnecke and Clark, 1999). It is important to note that only a relatively small genomic region of the gene was investigated; consequently, given our very superficial understanding the critical regions of epigenetic regulation, rejection of the role of epigenetic factors is premature.

Indirect evidence implicating the role of epigenetic modifications in development derives from the surprising complexity of epigenetic changes during gametogenesis and embryogenesis (Fig. 10.3). The spermatozoon and oocyte genomes exhibit major differences in their methylation patterns. In mice studies, mRNA for Dnmt1 is present at high levels in post-mitotic germ cells but undergoes alternative splicing of sex-specific 5′ exons, which controls the production and localization of enzyme during specific stages of gametogenesis (Mertineit *et al.*, 1998). An oocyte-specific 5′ exon is associated with the production of very large amounts of active Dnmt1 protein, which is truncated at the N-terminus and sequestered in the cytoplasm during the later stages of oocyte growth, while a spermatocyte-specific 5′ exon interferes with translation and prevents production of mouse Dnmt1 during the prolonged crossing-over stage of male meiosis (Mertineit *et al.*, 1998). During embryonic development, the genome is subjected to major changes in epigenetic regulation (reviewed in Reik *et al.*, 2001). There are developmental periods of reprogramming

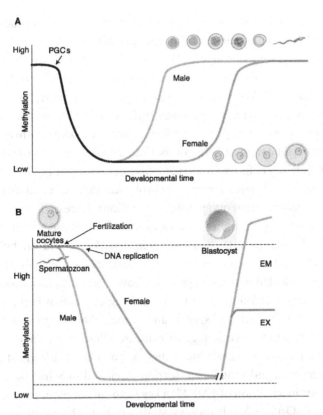

Fig. 10.3.   (A) Methylation reprogramming in the germline. Primordial germ cells (PGCs) in the mouse become demethylated early in development. Remethylation begins in pro-spermatogonia in male germ cells and after birth in growing oocytes. Some stages of germ cell development are shown. (B) Methylation reprogramming in preimplantation embryos. The paternal genome is demethylated by an active mechanism immediately after fertilization. The maternal genome is demethylated by a passive mechanism that depends on DNA replication. Both are remethylated around the time of implantation to different extents in embryonic (EM) and extraembryonic (EX) lineages. Methylated imprinted genes and some repeat sequences (upper dashed line) do not become demethylated. Unmethylated imprinted genes (lower dashed line) do not become methylated. (Reproduced with permission from Reik, W., Dean, W., and Walter, J. (2001). Epigenetic reprogramming in mammalian development. *Science*, **293**: 1089–1093. Copyright 2001 American Association for the Advancement of Science.)

of methylation patterns in vivo, when a substantial part of the genome is demethylated and after some time remethylated in a cell- or tissue-specific pattern. Reprogramming of DNA methylation in early embryos occurs both by active and passive mechanisms (Reik *et al.*, 2001).

It is highly unlikely that such a sophisticated machinery of epigenetic changes would be operating for no reason or that such a reason would not be related to development. Consistent with this idea, genome-wide alterations in methylation induced by knockouts of the genes encoding the epigenetic regulators often result in embryo death or developmental defects. For example, inactivation of Dnmt1 in the *Dnmt1-/-* knockouts resulted in a significant reduction of total ^{met}C in the genome after several rounds of DNA replication and developmental arrest at an early stage of embryogenesis (reviewed in Li, 2002). Interestingly, it has been shown that Dnmt3a, and Dnmt3b are also required for the stable inheritance of DNA-methylation parent in mouse embryonic stem cells. By comparison, *Mbd2-/-* knockouts were viable and fertile but showing defective maternal behavior (reviewed in Li, 2002). Animals lacking MeCP2 exhibited complex neurological defects, including tremor, ataxia, hindlimb clasping, stereotypic forelimb motions, increased anxiety-related behavior, and seizures. In humans, mutations of *MECP2* cause a neurodevelopmental disorder known as Rett syndrome (van den Veyver and Zoghbi, 2001). *MECP2* is located on the X chromosome, with male carriers of mutant *MECP2* being lethal. Girls affected with Rett syndrome have normal development for the first 18 months, which is followed by a period of regression that is characterized by loss of purposeful hand use and speech, and by mental handicap. In addition to Rett syndrome, two other classical epigenetic diseases, Prader–Willi and Angelman syndromes, exhibit numerous brain anomalies such as abnormal cortical development, microencephaly, and ventricular dilation (reviewed in Schumacher, 2001). Finally, epigenetic inactivation of *FMR1* is a key factor in etiopathogenesis of fragile X syndrome (El-Osta, 2002). Pathology, studies from the brains of patients and from *Fmr1* knockout mice show abnormal dendritic spines and altered synaptic plasticity (El-Osta *et al.*, 2001).

Further supportive evidence for the role of epigenetic changes in development derives from nuclear cloning experiments in mammals. Although a somatic cell nucleus from adult tissue can initiate embryonic development after being transplanted into an enucleated oocyte, cloning is extremely inefficient. Most cloned embryos die shortly after implantation and the few that survive to birth frequently have developmental abnormalities (Rideout *et al.*, 2001). Studies of DNA methylation have shown that genome-wide demethylation before implantation is less efficient in cloned embryos, and that de novo methylation occurs at an earlier stage in cloned embryos than in normal embryos (Reik *et al.*, 2001). The abnormal reprogramming of DNA methylation could result in the failed reactivation of the genes that are essential for embryonic development.

Further evidence relating epigenetics and embryogenesis derives from the action of some teratogenic agents, changing epigenetic regulation. An example could be sodium valproate, a medication commonly used for treatment of epilepsy that also exhibits teratogenic effects. It has been recently shown that valproic acid inhibits histone deacetylase, causing hyperacetylation of histones in cultured cells, which results in activation of transcription from diverse exogenous and endogenous promoters (Gottlicher *et al.*, 2001; Phiel *et al.*, 2001). Non-teratogenic analogs of valproic acid do not affect histone deacetylase and do not activate transcription. Based on these observations, it can be proposed that inhibition of histone deacetylase is the cause of valproic acid-induced developmental defects.

All the above considerations provide the basis for further elaboration and experimental analysis of the ideas suggested by Morgan and Waddington (Morgan, 1934; Slack, 2002). Morgan's "dynamic genes" can now be seen as "hard core" coding DNA sequences packed in their malleable epigenetic environment, which regulates the activity of such sequences. Waddington suggested that the epigenetic landscape is formed by the action of various genes and on the "underside" of the landscape, such genes can be visualized as pegs stuck in the ground, each with a longer or shorter rope attached to the peaks and troughs, respectively (see Fig. 3C in Slack, 2002). Since it is now known that DNA sequences do not change during development and that such sequences are identical nearly in all somatic cells of an individual, it is more likely that the peaks and troughs are formed by the epigenetic modifications of such genes (Fig. 10.4).

In conclusion, although direct proof of the role of epigenetics in development is yet to come, epigenetic regulation may serve as a convenient candidate for the mechanistic explanation of cell differentiation and development.

The synthesis: epigenetics, development, and schizophrenia

The putative role of epigenetic factors in development adds an important aspect to the epigenetic theory of schizophrenia. Since embryogenesis is related to major epigenetic rearrangements and the genesis of highly specialized cells includes thousands and thousands of small epigenetic steps, it is very likely that deviation from the "ideal" epigenetic scenario is quite common. Because of its complexity, the brain is likely to be the most susceptible organ and even mild epigenetic malfunction might lead to a wide variety of small morphological and functional changes in the developing brain. Epigenetic aberrations (epimutations) may originate from any of the three sources acting individually or in combination. First, because of epigenetic metastability, epimutations can be inherited through the germline. Second, epigenetic misregulation can be caused by environmental factors, such as exposure of an embryo or fetus to various toxic agents, some medications, malnutrition, or a mother's infections during pregnancy. Third, epigenetic aberrations may be generated by stochastic events in the embryonic cells. In the last case, there is neither inherited predisposition nor exposure to the hazardous factors but the developmental program goes awry for various non-deterministic events of the molecular world. An example of a stochastic event is where hemimethylated DNA

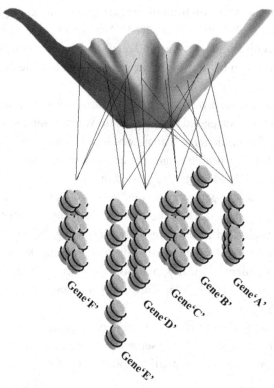

Fig. 10.4.   Waddington's epigenetic landscape: a view from "behind." The peaks and troughs are formed by the epigenetic status of various genes (A, B, C, etc.) in the cell, and this determines cellular phenotype and functions.

remained asymmetrically methylated because there was no DNMT1 in the close vicinity at that specific time; this effect would be amplified during the subsequent mitotic divisions. Prenatal epigenetic misregulation would cause subtle aberrations in neuronal cell migration, density of neurons, and their cytoarchitectural organization but would not lead to major dysfunction of brain activity. Since the age of onset in most psychoses is delayed for a relatively long time, it is possible that inherited and/or acquired epimutations are "tolerated" by the brain cells during the childhood and adulthood of an individual at risk. It takes several decades of age-dependent epigenetic changes (which are also a part of the postnatal developmental program) until the epigenetic misregulation of a critical gene(s) reaches a sufficient level that the compensatory mechanisms of a cell are not able to deal with the problem, resulting in the manifestation of psychotic symptoms. External factors such as stress, other diseases, and urban life may or may not play a role in adding to the "critical mass" of epigenetic misregulation. It is more likely, however, that the endogenous environment of an individual (i.e. changes in the gonadal and adrenal hormone homeostasis during puberty) is the key factor that changes from a predisposing epimutation to a disease-causing one. Environmental factors may contribute to the progression of pre-epimutation, but it is more likely that developmental changes and stochastic events play a more important role (Petronis, 2001). Consistent with the latter, some first episodes of schizophrenia come without any herald of the disease and in the absence of hazardous environmental factors. Severity of epigenetic misregulation may fluctuate over time, which in clinical terms will be treated as disease remissions and relapses. The age-dependent epigenetic changes may reach epigenetic reversion to a near normal state, which is seen as a decline of psychotic symptoms and partial recovery from the disease (Petronis, 2001).

There is one key issue that the epigenetic theory treats differently to the neurodevelopmental approach. From the epigenetic point of view, age- and hormone-dependent neurochemical changes rather than structural changes in the brain are the main disease mechanism. Brain morphological aberrations are more likely to be just the reporters of mild deviation in the developmental program rather than factors causing or predisposing to schizophrenia. There is strong reason to believe that those early and minor developmental aberrations can be fully compensated by the developing brain, which exhibits surprising plasticity and compensatory potential (Kolb, 1995; Woods, 1998). The shift from the brain structural peculiarities to the functional ones is consistent with the rare but very informative cases of monozygotic twins discordant for schizophrenia, where brain anomalies are more severe in the unaffected twin (Torrey et al., 1999, Fig. 6.4 on p. 114). The subtle localized non-progressive prenatal brain developmental aberrations are just like superficial scars, which do not do any harm but only remind of an old minor injury. The problem of latency of the neurodevelopmental changes – one of the main unclear issues in the neurodevelopmental theory – can now be reformulated into the latency of epigenetic misregulation of some critical genes.

The heuristic value of the epigenetic model of schizophrenia lies in the possibility of integrating a variety of unrelated data into a new theoretical framework that provides the basis for new experimental approaches in the study of this disease. As it was attempted to show above, epigenetics is likely to be intimately related to development and, therefore, represents an important aspect in the interpretation of the neurodevelopmental findings in schizophrenia. In one of her seminal papers on "dynamic genome," Barbara McClintock (1951) wrote: "If the ordered processes of development are deranged, then genes which usually become active at very specific times may instead be activated spasmodically or in random fashion during development." Fifty years later we raise a reverse question: can abnormally expressed genes derange development? The answer to this question should provide new insights into the mystery of schizophrenia.

Acknowledgements

I thank Dr. A. Wong and Mr. Z. A. Kaminsky (CAMH, Toronto, Canada) for their valuable comments and advice. This work was supported by grants from the Ontario Mental Health Foundation, the National Alliance for Research on Schizophrenia and Depression, and the Stanley Foundation.

REFERENCES

Bestor, T. H. (2000). The DNA methyltransferases of mammals. *Hum Mol Genet* **9**: 2395–2402.

Cardno, A. G., Gottesman, I. I. (2000). Twin studies of schizophrenia: from bow-and-arrow concordances to Star Wars Mx and functional genomics. *Am J Med Genet* **97**: 12–17.

Chen, Y., Sharma, R. P., Costa, R. H., Costa, E., Grayson, D. R. (2002). On the epigenetic regulation of the human reelin promoter. *Nucl Acids Res* **30**: 2930–2939.

El-Osta, A. (2002). FMR1 silencing and the signals to chromatin: a unified model of transcriptional regulation. *Biochem Biophys Res Commun* **295**: 575–581.

El-Osta, A., Baker, E. K., Wolffe, A. P. (2001). Profiling methyl-CpG specific determinants on transcriptionally silent chromatin. *Mol Biol Rep* **28**: 209–215.

Gottesman, I., Shields, J. (1982). *Schizophrenia: The Epigenetic Puzzle*. Cambridge, UK: Cambridge University Press.

Gottlicher, M., Minucci, S., Zhu, P., *et al.* (2001). Valproic acid defines a novel class of HDAC inhibitors inducing differentiation of transformed cells. *EMBO J* **20**: 6969–6978.

Henikoff, S., Matzke, M. A. (1997). Exploring and explaining epigenetic effects. *Trends Genet* **13**: 293–295.

Holliday, R. (1994). Epigenetics: an overview. *Dev Genet* **15**: 453–457.

(1996). DNA methylation in eukaryotes: 20 years on. In *Epigenetic Mechanisms of Gene Regulation*, ed. V. Russo, R. Martienssen, A. Riggs. Cold Spring Harbor, NY: Cold Spring Harbor Laboratory Press, pp. 5–27.

Holliday, R., Pugh, J. E. (1975). DNA modification mechanisms and gene activity during development. *Science* **187**: 226–232.

Jablonka, E., Lamb, M. (1995). *Epigenetic Inheritance and Evolution*. Oxford: Oxford University Press.

Jackson-Grusby, L., Beard, C., Possemato, R., *et al.* (2001). Loss of genomic methylation causes p53-dependent apoptosis and epigenetic deregulation. *Nat Genet* **27**: 31–39.

Jenuwein, T., Allis, C. D. (2001). Translating the histone code. *Science* **293**: 1074–1080.

Kolb, B. (1995). *Brain Plasticity and Behavior*. Mahwah, NJ: Lawrence Erlbaum Associates.

Kraepelin, E. (1919). *Dementia Praecox and Paraphrenia*. Edinburgh: Livingstone.

Lewis, D. A., Levitt, P. (2002). Schizophrenia as a disorder of neurodevelopment. *Annu Rev Neurosci* **25**: 409–432.

Li, E. (2002). Chromatin modification and epigenetic reprogramming in mammalian development. *Nat Rev Genet* **3**: 662–673.

Litt, M. D., Simpson, M., Gaszner, M., Allis, C. D., Felsenfeld, G. (2001). Correlation between histone lysine methylation and developmental changes at the chicken beta-globin locus. *Science* **293**: 2453–2455.

Maynard Smith, J. (1990). Models of a dual inheritance system. *J Theor Biol* **143**: 41–53.

McClintock, B. (1951). Chromosome organization and genic expression. *Genes and Mutations. Cold Spring Harb Symp Quant Biol* **XVI**: 13–47.

Mertineit, C., Yoder, J. A., Taketo, T., *et al.* (1998). Sex-specific exons control DNA methyltransferase in mammalian germ cells. *Development* **125**: 889–897.

Morgan, T. H. (1934). *Embryology and Genetics.* New York: Columbia University Press.

Petronis, A. (2000). The genes for major psychosis: aberrant sequence or regulation? *Neuropsychopharmacology* **23**: 1–12.

   (2001). Human morbid genetics revisited: relevance of epigenetics. *Trends Genet* **17**: 142–146.

Petronis, A., Paterson, A. D., Kennedy, J. L. (1999). Schizophrenia: an epigenetic puzzle? *Schizophr Bull* **25**: 639–655.

Petronis, A., Popendikyte, V., Kan, P. X., Sasaki, T. (2002). Major psychosis and chromosome 22: genetics meets epigenetics. *CNS Spectrums* **7**: 209–214.

Petronis, A., Gottesman, I. I., Kan, P. X., *et al.* (2003). Monozygotic twins exhibit numerous epigenetic differences: clues to twin discordance? *Schizophr Bull* **29**: 169–178.

Phiel, C. J., Zhang, F., Huang, E. Y., *et al.* (2001). Histone deacetylase is a direct target of valproic acid, a potent anticonvulsant, mood stabilizer, and teratogen. *J Biol Chem* **276**: 36734–36741.

Rakyan, V. K., Blewitt, M. E., Druker, R., Preis, J. I., Whitelaw, E. (2002). Metastable epialleles in mammals. *Trends Genet* **18**: 348–351.

Razin, A., Shemer, R. (1999). Epigenetic control of gene expression. *Results Probl Cell Differ* **25**: 189–204.

Reik, W., Dean, W., Walter, J. (2001). Epigenetic reprogramming in mammalian development. *Science* **293**: 1089–1093.

Rideout, III, W. M., Eggan, K., Jaenisch, R. (2001). Nuclear cloning and epigenetic reprogramming of the genome. *Science* **293**: 1093–1098.

Riggs, A., Xiong, Z., Wang, L., LeBon, J. M. (1998). Methylation dynamics, epigenetic fidelity and X chromosome structure. In *Epigenetics*, Vol. *Novartis Foundation Symposium 214: Epigenetics*, ed. A. Wolffe. Chichester, UK: Wiley, pp. 214–227.

Riggs, A. D. (1975). X inactivation, differentiation, and DNA methylation. *Cytogenet Cell Genet* **14**: 9–25.

Robertson, K. D., Wolffe, A. P. (2000). DNA methylation in health and disease. *Nat Rev Genet* **1**: 11–19.

Schumacher, A. (2001). Mechanisms and brain specific consequences of genomic imprinting in Prader–Willi and Angelman syndromes. *Gene Funct Dis* **1**: 7–25.

Seeman, M. V. (1997). Psychopathology in women and men: focus on female hormones. *Am J Psychiatry* **154**: 1641–1647.

Siegfried, Z., Eden, S., Mendelsohn, M., *et al.* (1999). DNA methylation represses transcription in vivo. *Nat Genet* **22**: 203–206.

Singal, R., Ginder, G. D. (1999). DNA methylation. *Blood* **93**: 4059–4070.

Slack, J. M. (2002). Conrad Hal Waddington: the last Renaissance biologist? *Nat Rev Genet* **3**: 889–895.

Stancheva, I., Meehan, R. R. (2000). Transient depletion of xDnmt1 leads to premature gene activation in *Xenopus* embryos. *Genes Dev* **14**: 313–327.

Torrey, E. F., Bowler, A. E., Taylor, E. H., Gottesman, I. I. (1999). *Schizophrenia and Manic Depressive Disorder. The Biological Roots of Mental Illness as Revealed by the Landmark Study of Identical Twins.* New York: Basic Books.

Tremolizzo, L., Carboni, G., Ruzicka, W. B., *et al.* (2002). An epigenetic mouse model for molecular and behavioral neuropathologies related to schizophrenia vulnerability. *Proc Natl Acad Sci USA* **99**: 17095–17100.

van den Veyver, I. B., Zoghbi, H. Y. (2001). Mutations in the gene encoding methyl-CpG-binding protein 2 cause Rett syndrome. *Brain Dev* **23**(Suppl. 1): S147–S151.

Walsh, C. P., Bestor, T. H. (1999). Cytosine methylation and mammalian development. *Genes Dev* **13**: 26–34.

Warnecke, P. M., Clark, S. J. (1999). DNA methylation profile of the mouse skeletal alpha-actin promoter during development and differentiation. *Mol Cell Biol* **19**: 164–172.

Wolffe, A. P. (1994). Inheritance of chromatin states. *Dev Genet* **15**: 463–470.

Wolffe, A. P., Barton, M. C. (2000). Developmental regulation of chromatin function and gene expression. In *Chromatin Structure and Regulation*, ed. S. C. R. Elgin, J. L. Workman. Oxford: Oxford University Press, pp. 182–202.

Wolffe, A. P., Matzke, M. A. (1999). Epigenetics: regulation through repression. *Science* **286**: 481–486.

Woods, B. T. (1998). Is schizophrenia a progressive neurodevelopmental disorder? Toward a unitary pathogenetic mechanism. *Am J Psychiatry* **155**: 1661–1670.

Woolf, C. M. (1997). Does the genotype for schizophrenia often remain unexpressed because of canalization and stochastic events during development? *Psychol Med* **27**: 659–668.

Yeivin, A., Razin, A. (1993). Gene methylation patterns and expression. In *DNA Methylation: Molecular Biology and Biological Significance*, ed. J. Jost, H. Saluz. Basel: Birkhauser Verlag, pp. 523–568.

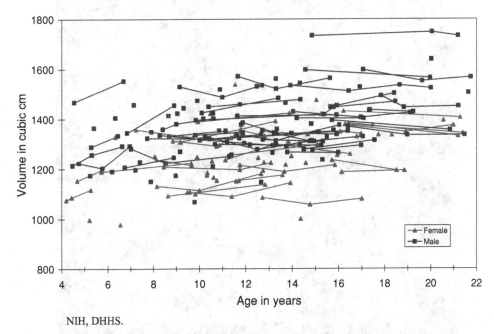

NIH, DHHS.

Fig. 2.1.   Total cerebral volume for 145 children and adolescents (ages 4–22) based on 243 brain magnetic resonance imaging scans. (Jay N. Giedd, Child Psychiatry Branch, NIMH, NIH, DHHS.)

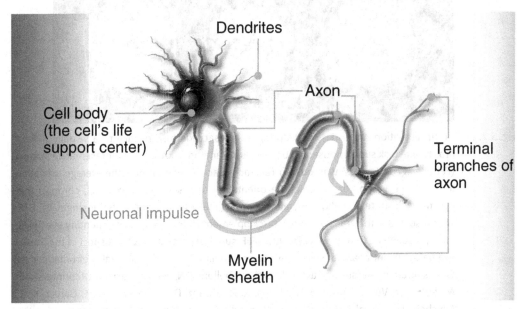

Fig. 2.2.   The neuron. (Donald Bliss, NIH Medical Arts and Photography Branch for Jay N. Giedd, Child Psychiatry Branch, NIMH, NIH, DHHS.)

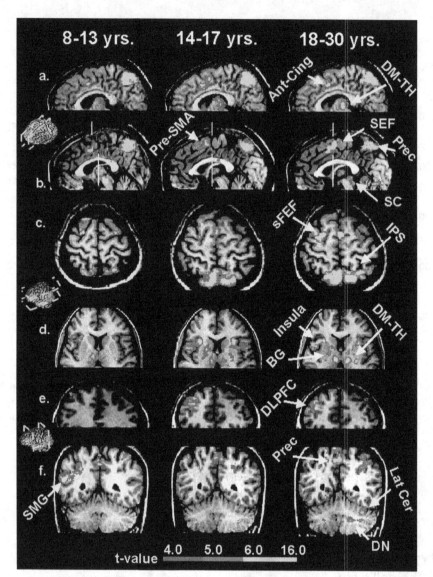

Fig. 3.2.   Group activation maps (t ≥ 4.0) during an antisaccade task relative to a visually guided prosaccade task superimposed on the structural anatomic image of a representative subject (Female aged 26 years) warped into Talairach space. Columns show the average activation for each age group. Rows depict the orientation (a,b, sagittal; d, axial; e,f, coronal) that optimally illustrate activation in brain regions of interest. Ant-Cing, anterior cingulate; DM-TH, dorsomedial thalamus; Pre-SMA, presupplementary area; SEF, supplementary eye fields; Prec, precuneus; SC, superior colliculus; sFEF, superior precentral sulcus aspect of the frontal eye field; IPS, intraparietal sulcus; BG, basal ganglia; DLPFC, dorsolateral prefrontal cortex; SMG, supramarginal sulcus; Lat Cer, lateral cerebellum; DN, dentate nucleus. (Reprinted from *NeuroImage*, Vol. 13, Luna, B., Thulborn, K. R., Munoz, D. P., Merriam, E. P., Garver, K. E., Minshew, N. J., *et al.*, "Maturation of widely distributed brain function subserves cognitive development" 786–793, Copyright 2001, with permission from Elsevier.)

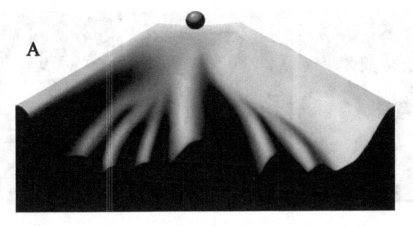

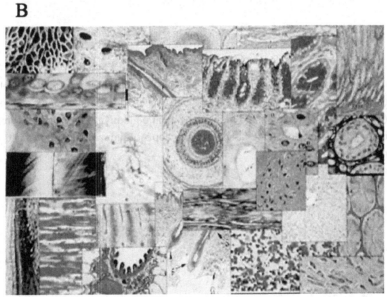

Fig. 10.2.   Epigenetics and cell differentiation. (A) Waddington's epigenetic landscape represents the imaginary path of an undifferentiated pluripotent embryonic cell during development. (B) The end result of cell differentiation is a wide variety of highly specialized cells that look different and perform different functions, although they contain the same DNA sequences.

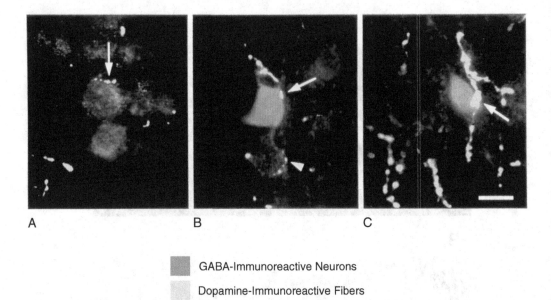

GABA-Immunoreactive Neurons

Dopamine-Immunoreactive Fibers

Fig. 16.4.   A series of confocal photomicrographs showing colocalization of gamma-aminobutyric acid (GABA) neurons (green) and dopamine fibers (yellow) in rat medial prefrontal cortex before (A) and after (B) weaning and in the early adult period (C). There is an apparent increase in the number of dopamine fibers and they appear to form increased contacts with GABA neurons.

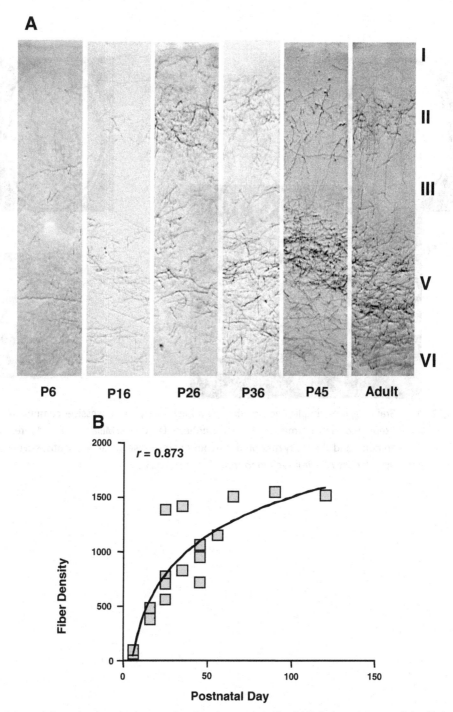

Fig. 16.5. Amygdala projections to the anterior cingulate cortex after birth in rats. (A) Amygdalar fibers visualized with anterograde tracing show a marked increase in layers II and V during the postnatal period. (B) The increase in fiber density shows a highly significant curvilinear rise between birth (postnatal day 0) and adulthood (postnatal day 120) in layer II.

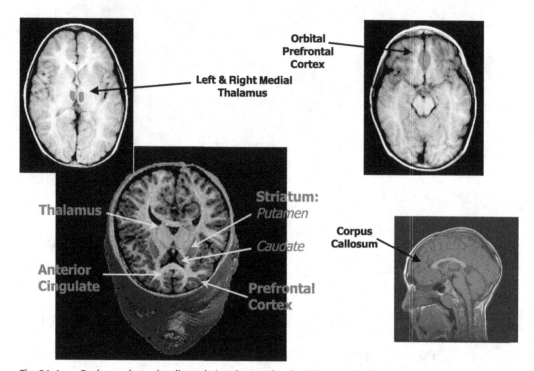

Fig. 21.4.   Brain regions implicated in the pathophysiology of obsessive–compulsive disorder. (Reprinted with permission from Rosenberg, D. R., MacMillan, S. N., Moore, G. J. Brain anatomy and chemistry may predict treatment response in paediatric obsessive–compulsive disorder. *Int J Neuropsychopharmacol* **4**: 179, 2001.)

11

Early environmental risk factors for schizophrenia

Mary Cannon[1,2], Kimberlie Dean[1], and Peter B. Jones[3]

[1] Institute of Psychiatry, King's College, London, UK
[2] Royal College of Surgeons in Ireland, Dublin, Ireland
[3] University of Cambridge, UK

The existence of early environmental risk factors for schizophrenia is central to the notion of schizophrenia as a neurodevelopmental disorder (Marenco and Weinberger, 2000; McDonald *et al.*, 2000) and these risk factors represent some of the most challenging and interesting targets of schizophrenia epidemiology. This chapter discusses prenatal and perinatal risk factors for schizophrenia. Childhood developmental impairment and later environmental and psychosocial risk factors are dealt with in Chs. 22 and 13, respectively.

Prenatal risk factors for schizophrenia

Time and place of birth

The risk of developing schizophrenia has consistently been found to be increased (1.5 to 2-fold) among those born in cities compared with those born in rural areas (Lewis *et al.*, 1992; Marcelis *et al.*, 1998; Mortensen *et al.*, 1999; Takei *et al.*, 1995; Torrey and Bowler, 1990). Studies that have teased apart the effects of urban birth and urban living (Marcelis *et al.*, 1999) have found that the greatest risk was for those born in urban areas, with no additional effect of later urban residence, indicating that the urban risk factor or factors associated with an increase in risk of schizophrenia appear to act in early life rather than around the time of illness onset. Linear trends for risk of schizophrenia with increasing population density of area of birth have been noted (Marcelis *et al.*, 1998; Mortensen *et al.*, 1999). There is also consistent evidence for a small (5–8%) winter–spring excess of births for both schizophrenia and mania/bipolar disorder (Cotter *et al.*, 1996; McGrath and Welham, 1999; Mortensen *et al.*, 1999; Torrey *et al.*, 1997). The cause or causes of the "season of birth" effect and the "urban birth" effects are not as yet clear. Both are proxy variables that could encompass a large

Neurodevelopment and Schizophrenia, ed. Matcheri S. Keshavan *et al*. Published by Cambridge University Press. © Cambridge University Press 2004.

number of possible risk factors, including prenatal and childhood infections, the prevalence of which tends to increase with increasing population density and in winter.

Prenatal influenza

The early evidence regarding the role of prenatal infections has come from ecological, or population-association studies. In 1988, Mednick and colleagues demonstrated that the offspring of women who were in the second trimester of pregnancy during the 1957–8 influenza A_2 pandemic in Helsinki were about twice as likely to be hospitalized with a diagnosis of schizophrenia as those not exposed during pregnancy or exposed earlier or later in pregnancy. There have been many attempts to replicate this finding for the 1957 epidemic using an ecological design (Erlenmeyer-Kimling et al., 1994; Izumoto et al., 1999; Kendell and Adams, 1991; Kendell and Kemp, 1989; Kunugi et al., 1995; McGrath et al., 1994; Mednick et al., 1990; O'Callaghan et al., 1991; Torrey et al., 1992). The effect sizes demonstrated in these studies are small: somewhere between 1.5 and 2.0 (Cannon and Jones, 1996), and not all ecological studies replicated the association (Kendell and Kemp, 1989; Selten and Slaets, 1994; Selten et al., 1999; Susser et al., 1994; Torrey et al., 1988; Westergaard et al., 1999). However, the balance of evidence does suggest that prenatal exposure to the 1957 epidemic was associated with a raised incidence of schizophrenia, particularly if the exposure occurred in the second trimester of pregnancy (reviewed by McGrath et al., 1995a; Wright et al., 1999). Studies of longer-term trends in the association between the timing of influenza epidemics and the birth dates of people with schizophrenia have yielded generally positive results in most (Adams et al., 1993; Barr et al., 1990; Sham et al., 1992; Takei et al., 1994) but not all (Morgan et al., 1997; Selten and Slaets, 1994; Torrey et al., 1988) cases. In most studies where the sexes are examined separately, the positive association was found mainly or exclusively in females (Adams et al., 1993; Izumoto et al., 1999; Kendell and Kemp, 1989; McGrath et al., 1994; Mednick et al., 1990; O'Callaghan et al., 1991; Takei et al., 1994), but no satisfactory explanation has yet been offered for this.

The ecologic design has undoubted limitations, including the so-called "ecological fallacy" (we cannot be certain that the individuals in the population who were exposed to influenza in utero are the same individuals who are diagnosed with schizophrenia as adults) and the possibility of unknown confounding with other factors, such as maternal fever or medication.

However, the application of cohort and case–control methodology has not shed much light on the problem. Two case–control studies replicated the association between second-trimester exposure to influenza and later schizophrenia but relied on maternal recall for information about the exposure (Stöber et al., 1992;

Wright *et al.*, 1995). Two cohort studies have failed to support the influenza–schizophrenia association (Cannon *et al.*, 1996; Crow and Done, 1992) but had low power to examine this effect (Adams and Kendell, 1996).

Prenatal rubella and other prenatal infections

Interest in prenatal infection as a risk factor for schizophrenia is not restricted to influenza. Influenza lends itself to study because of the frequent occurrence of well-defined epidemics. Brown *et al.* (2000a) showed that second-trimester exposure to a wide variety of respiratory infections (including influenza, pneumonia, tuberculosis and acute bronchitis among others) was associated with significant (twofold) increased risk of schizophrenia spectrum disorders. These results indicate that several infections, both bacterial and viral, may increase the risk of schizophrenia through some common pathogenic mechanism.

Brown and colleagues (2000b) investigated a cohort of individuals who were serologically documented to have sustained in utero exposure to rubella and found that the rubella-exposed subjects, most of whom were exposed in the first trimester, had a substantially higher risk (relative risk, 5.2) of developing non-affective psychoses than those who were not exposed, independent of hearing status. The cohort methodology with proof of individual exposure status is robust and the effect size for the association between prenatal rubella and schizophrenia is much larger than that reported for prenatal influenza. These findings suggest that non-affective psychosis may be a remote neuropsychiatric consequence of prenatal rubella. An ecological study from Finland by Suvisaari and colleagues (1999) found an association between second-trimester exposure to poliovirus infection and later schizophrenia. Jones and colleagues (1999) have followed a large group of individuals whose mothers were identified during pregnancy as suffering from identified viral infections (Fine *et al.*, 1985) and have found evidence relating neurotropic virus exposure with a range of adverse central nervous system (CNS) outcomes, including mental retardation, epilepsy, and psychosis.

The availability of stored prenatal serum from birth cohorts in the USA who are now in the period of risk for schizophrenia has opened up a new research avenue for investigating prenatal infection as a risk factor for psychiatric illness (Susser *et al.*, 2000). Using stored prenatal serum samples from the Providence cohort of the National Collaborative Perinatal Project, Buka *et al.* (2001) found a strong association between maternal antibodies to herpes simplex virus type 2 gG2 glycoprotein and later psychosis (odds ratio, 5.8; 95% confidence interval, 1.7–19.3), and have subsequently replicated this finding in another sample from the same cohort (Buka *et al.*, 2003). Analysis of prenatal serum from a birth cohort in Oakland, California (Prenatal Determinants of Schizophrenia Study) has produced the first serological evidence of an association between prenatal influenza infection in the first half of pregnancy and an increased (threefold) risk of adult schizophrenia (Brown *et al.*, 2003).

Neonatal and early childhood infection

The time window during which early exposure to infection may exert an effect appears to extend into childhood. The North Finland 1966 Birth Cohort contains all live births (12 058 in total), to women in northern Finland (Oulu and Lapland provinces) during 1966 (Rantakallio, 1969). Rantakallio and colleagues (1997) identified through record linkage all cohort members who had been hospitalized during childhood for a CNS infection (mainly encephalitis and meningitis). They then identified those members of the cohort who had been hospitalized for psychiatric illness. Of 145 in the group with serologically diagnosed childhood CNS infections who had survived to age 16 years, four (2.8%) developed schizophrenia, compared with 0.7% of the unexposed majority. This fourfold relative risk may even underestimate the true risk because of the restriction to severe exposure. An estimate of the population attributable fraction (the amount by which the population burden of schizophrenia would be reduced if the effect of the exposure, if causal, were removed) is around 4%. As with any causal inference, one must consider the possibility of reverse causality. The CNS may already have been abnormal in the individuals who developed infection and schizophrenia, and these abnormalities may have made them liable to CNS infection. Unknown genetic or epigenetic factors may be necessary components of the causal pathway.

Prenatal malnutrition

A series of ecological studies of exposure to prenatal famine (Susser and Lin, 1992, 1994; Susser *et al.*, 1996) have demonstrated dose–response relationships between maternal nutritional deprivation during the Nazi blockade of the Netherlands in the winter of 1944–5 and risk of later schizophrenia in the offspring. The initial finding to emerge from these studies was that birth cohorts exposed to the famine in early but not late gestation had a twofold increase in risk for schizophrenia (Susser and Lin, 1992; Susser *et al.*, 1996). A subsequent study using military conscription data demonstrated that prenatal famine during early gestation was associated with a twofold elevation in risk for schizoid or schizotypal personality disorders (Hoek *et al.*, 1996). The authors postulated that severe nutritional deprivation is the etiological mechanism involved (Butler *et al.*, 1999; Hoek *et al.*, 1999). This possibility has received indirect support from a finding that a short interval between siblings is associated with an increased risk of schizophrenia (Westergaard *et al.*, 1999). There is biological plausibility for this putative cause; congenital CNS defects in this population were related to famine exposure in a similar fashion (Susser *et al.*,

1985). Interaction with maternal genetic effects or exposure to maternal stress may also be components of any causal association (Koenig *et al.*, 2002).

Rhesus incompatibility

Rhesus (Rh) incompatibility, characterized by an Rh-negative mother pregnant with an Rh-positive fetus, has been associated with an elevated risk for schizophrenia. Hollister *et al.* (1996) used data on males from the Danish Perinatal Cohort Study and found an elevated risk for schizophrenia among offspring of Rh-incompatible pregnancies compared with Rh-compatible pregnancies. Rhesus incompatibility can give rise to hemolytic disease of the newborn, which results, among other things, in childhood neuromotor abnormalities and behavioral disorders such as emotional instability. It is possible that schizophrenia is yet another possible consequence of rhesus hemolytic disease (Hollister and Brown, 1999). Rhesus hemolytic disease occurs most commonly in mothers who have already delivered a Rh-positive child, thus triggering the production of the antibody against the Rh(D) antigen. As hypothesized, the risk for schizophrenia among males in the Danish Perinatal Cohort Study was increased over threefold in second and later-born offspring from Rh-incompatible pregnancies, but there was no increased risk for first-born offspring (Hollister *et al.*, 1996).

Minor physical anomalies

The term minor physical anomalies (MPAs) is used to refer to a group of subtle but observable defects of the head, face, hands, and feet. The concept encompasses both qualitative and quantitative abnormalities, such as facial asymmetries, the presence of clefts, misshapen appendages, and a variety of abnormal skull measurements. These MPAs are known to arise from abnormalities occurring in ectodermal development before the third trimester of pregnancy. The precise cause of such abnormal development is not yet known but is likely to involve the interacting effects of both genes and the prenatal environment. Examination of MPAs is ideally suited to gaining insight into the prenatal period because, once produced in utero, they persist largely unchanged throughout life. MPAs can act as a marker of neurodevelopmental disorder since the brain is also ectodermally derived.

There is now a strong body of evidence demonstrating that the prevalence of MPAs is elevated in sufferers of schizophrenia compared with controls (Gualtieri *et al.*, 1982; Ismail *et al.*, 1998, 2000; Lane *et al.*, 1997; McGrath *et al.*, 1995b, 2002). These findings lend weight to the neurodevelopmental model of schizophrenia. Patients with schizophrenia demonstrate an excess of multiple dysmorphic features of the craniofacial and skull base regions (Lane *et al.*, 1997; McGrath *et al.*, 2002), including high palate, abnormal palatal ridges, abnormal supraorbital ridges, presence of bifid tongue, presence of epicanthus, narrow mouth, widened anterior ear helix, ear protrusion, abnormal eye fissure inclination, abnormal binocular diameter, wide skull base, and hypoplastic ear lobe size. A novel method for studying craniofacial dymorphology is the use of three-dimensional laser surface scanning and geometric morphometric analysis (Hennessy *et al.*, 2002), and its application to psychosis is in progress. Elevated rates of MPAs have also been reported in other psychoses (McGrath *et al.*, 2002) and disorders such as schizotypal personality disorder (Weinstein *et al.*, 1999); MPAs appear to be relatively independent of obstetric complications in their association with later development of schizophrenia (McNeil and Cantor-Graae, 1999, 2000). MPAs are increased in those at genetic risk for schizophrenia in some (Lawrie *et al.*, 2001; Schiffman *et al.*, 2002) but not all (Griffiths *et al.*, 1998) studies that have examined this issue. The association between MPAs and schizophrenia does not appear to be confounded by ethnicity (Dean *et al.*, 2003).

Prenatal exposure to stress

Maternal experience of extremely stressful events, such as death of spouse (Huttunen and Niskanen, 1978), war (van Os and Selten, 1998), tornado (Kinney *et al.*, 1999), or nuclear explosion (Imamura *et al.*, 1999) appears to increase the risk of schizophrenia in offspring who are in midgestation at the time (for review see Kinney, 2001). More subtle forms of prenatal stress may also have an effect. In the 1966 North Finland Birth Cohort, both maternal depression in late pregnancy (Jones *et al.*, 1998) and "un-wantedness" of a pregnancy by the mother (Myhrman *et al.*, 1996) were independently associated with a modest increase in the risk of schizophrenia in the offspring. Many potential confounders, such as maternal age, physical conditions, and socioeconomic status, were taken into account, but a diluted genetic effect cannot be excluded.

There is a considerable animal literature concerning the effects of prenatal stress on brain development and behavior of the offspring (reviewed by Koenig *et al.*, 2002; Suomi, 1997). Animals exposed to prenatal stress produce elevated levels of cortisol in response to stressful situations, indicative of enhanced hypothalamic–pituitary–adrenal axis reactivity. These effects are robust and persistent, indicating that this axis can be "programmed" during fetal life. Prenatal stress is associated with smaller head circumference, neonatal neurological impairment (Lou *et al.*, 1994), and behavior problems in childhood (O'Connor *et al.*, 2002). Stress during birth also appears to have an effect (Taylor *et al.*, 2000). Prenatal stress in human subjects is also associated with neonatal neurological impairment (Lou *et al.*, 1994), increased response of the infant to stress (Taylor *et al.*, 2000), and behavior problems in childhood (O'Connor *et al.*, 2002), which further support the heuristic value of a prenatal stress model for schizophrenia. Prenatal stress is associated with low birth weight and preterm birth (Lou *et al.*, 1994), which have been reported as risk factors for schizophrenia. This effect is possibly mediated by uterine artery vasoconstriction and reduced placental blood flow (Teixeira *et al.*, 1999). Prenatal stress may be particularly pathogenic in those already at genetic risk of schizophrenia (Mednick and Schulsinger, 1968; Mednick *et al.*, 1971).

Perinatal risk factors: obstetric complications

There is a large literature on the possible role of obstetric complications in schizophrenia (reviewed by Cannon, 1997; McNeil, 1988, 1995; McNeil *et al.*, 2000). Before 1997, most of the studies showing an association were of case–control design using maternal recall for assessment of the exposure. They also had small sample sizes and were prone to various forms of bias. Geddes and Lawrie (1995) carried out a meta-analysis of the results published from 16 case–control studies and two cohort studies and reached three main conclusions: (i) a pooled odds ratio of 2.0 (95% confidence interval 1.6–2.4) suggested that obstetric complications did have a small effect on increasing risk for schizophrenia; (ii) there was evidence for selection and publication bias; (iii) there was significant heterogeneity between the results from the case–control studies and the two birth cohort studies.

Because of methodological problems associated with the classic case–control design, particularly when measuring such early exposures, cohort and population-based study designs have now been exploited to investigate the relationship between obstetric complications and later schizophrenia. Results of these population-based studies are given in Table 11.1. They all have the following characteristics: large and psychiatrically well-defined samples of schizophrenia patients were drawn from population-based registers; standardized, prospectively collected obstetric information was obtained from birth records or registers; controls were from the general population with obstetric complication information from the same source and context; demographic confounding factors were controlled through either matching or statistical adjustment. It can be seen from Table 11.1 that these methodological advances have not confirmed the earlier findings. Moreover, although the designs of these studies are broadly similar, their results are quite diverse and no consensus has yet been reached. The methodological reasons for this include lack of definition of exposures, confounding by period and cohort effects, and insufficient statistical power (for further detail see Zornberg *et al.* (2000a) and Cannon *et al.* (2002a)). The issue of interactive effects is especially problematic. Pregnancy, birth, and neonatal complications do not act independently of each other. Pregnancy factors that have been associated with schizophrenia, such as rhesus incompatibility and prenatal stress (see above), can increase the risk for hypoxic–ischemic damage during delivery. Current studies have negligible statistical power to detect such interactive effects. Some studies try to overcome these problems by examining only

Table 11.1. Summary of results of population-based studies of obstetric complications and schizophrenia

Study	Country	Design (cohort or case–control)	Findings
Done *et al.* (1991)	UK	Cohort: NCDS	No overall association between risk factors for perinatal death and later schizophrenia. Low maternal weight and medications given to baby were associated with narrowly defined schizophrenia
Buka *et al.* (1993)	US	Cohort: NCPP (Providence center)	Non-significant increased risk of psychosis in those exposed to chronic fetal hypoxia (OR, 2.6)
Sacker *et al.* (1995)	UK	Cohort: NCDS	Re-analysis of Done *et al.* (1991). The following variables were associated with increased risk of narrowly defined schizophrenia: low maternal weight; maternal psychological problems; smoking in pregnancy; poor antenatal attendance; rhesus negative; parity > 2; previous births < 2500 g; bleeding in pregnancy; untrained person delivering; baby's weight < 2500 g; other drugs given to baby
Jones *et al.* (1998)	Finland	Cohort: 1966 North Finland Birth Cohort	Low birth weight (OR, 2.4; CI, 1–5.6): combination of low birth weight and prematurity (OR, 3.5; CI, 1.3–9.6) and perinatal brain damage (OR, 6.9; CI, 2.9–16.3) were associated with schizophrenia
Hultman *et al.* (1999)	Sweden	Case–control	Schizophrenia was associated with multiparity (OR, 2.0); bleeding during pregnancy (OR, 3.5); winter birth (OR, 1.4); SGA (males only OR, 3.2); parity > 4 (males only OR, 3.6)
Dalman *et al.* (1999)	Sweden	Cohort	Increased risk of pre-eclampsia (OR, 2.5); vacuum extraction (OR, 1.7); malformations (OR, 2.4); parity of 1 (OR, 1.3); bleeding during pregnancy (OR, 2.0); threatened premature delivery (OR, 2.3); gestational age < 32 weeks (OR, 2.7); prolonged delivery (OR, 1.6); uterine inertia (OR, 2.4; ponderal index < 20 (OR, 3.4); respiratory illness (OR, 1.5); birth weight < 2500 g (males only OR, 2.2); birth weight < 1500 g (females only OR, 6.0); SGA (males only OR, 1.9). Preeclampsia remained significant after adjusting for all other complications
Kendell *et al.* (2000)	Scotland	Case–control	No association found between any OC and schizophrenia
Kendell *et al.* (2000)	Scotland	Case–control	Emergency Cesarian section (OR, 3.7; CI, 1.02–13.1) and labor > 12 hours were associated with subsequent schizophrenia

Table 11.1. (*cont.*)

Study	Country	Design (cohort or case–control)	Findings
Byrne *et al.* (2000)	Ireland	Case–control	No overall differences in complication rates. Cesarian section and narrow maternal pelvis commoner among cases. Males with early-onset schizophrenia had greater frequency and severity of OCs than controls.
Cannon *et al.* (2000)	US	Cohort: NCPP (Philadephia center)	Hypoxia-related complications > 3 increased the risk of schizophrenia (OR, 3.84) and particularly early-onset schizophrenia (OR, 7.3)
Rosso *et al.* (2000)	Finland	Case–control	Risk of early-onset schizophrenia increased (OR, 2.16; CI, 1.3–3.5) per hypoxia-related OC
Zornberg *et al.* (2000b)	US	Cohort: NCPP (Providence centre)	Re-analysis of Buka *et al.* (1993). Composite variable entitled "hypoxic–ischaemia-related fetal/neonatal complications" associated with schizophrenia (OR, 4.56; CI, 2.42–8.6)
Dalman *et al.* (2001)	Sweden	Case–control	Signs of asphyxia at birth were associated with increased risk for schizophrenia (OR, 4.4; CI, 1.9–10.3) after adjusting for other complications and confounders

NCPP, National Collaborative Perinatal Project: NCDS, National Child and Development Study; OR, odds ratio; CI, confidence interval; SGA, small for gestational age; OC, obstetric complication.

one exposure based on a prior hypothesis, and these have showed significant effects for the putative risk increasing mechanism of hypoxic–ischemic damage (Buka *et al.*, 1993; Cannon *et al.*, 2000; Rosso *et al.*, 2000; Zornberg *et al.*, 2000b).

The standardized fashion of reporting results and the methodological similarities of the population-based studies listed in Table 11.1 lend themselves to a meta-analytic approach. Meta-analysis provides a method for integrating quantitative data from multiple studies by using a weighted average of the results in which larger studies have more influence than smaller studies. It improves the estimates of effect size, increases the statistical power, and helps to make sense out of studies with conflicting conclusions (Egger *et al.*, 1997; Fleiss, 1993).

Cannon *et al.* (2002a) carried out a meta-analytic synthesis of the prospective "population-based" studies that had published data on individual obstetric complications and found that three groups of complications were significantly associated with schizophrenia: (i) complications of pregnancy (bleeding, diabetes, rhesus incompatibility, pre-eclampsia); (ii) complications of delivery (uterine atony, asphyxia, emergency cesarean section); and (iii) abnormal fetal growth and development (low birth weight, congenital malformations, reduced head circumference).

Pooled estimates of effect sizes were generally small (odds ratios 2). Interactive effects and independence of obstetric risk factors could not be examined using this design. An individual patient-data meta-analysis on these population-based studies, such as that carried out by Geddes *et al.* (1999) on case–control studies, may help to elucidate such issues.

The period of risk during which hypoxic brain damage may lead to later schizophrenia appears to extend beyond birth. In the North Finland 1966 cohort, a group of CNS insults that had hypoxia as a common mechanism was identified and termed perinatal brain damage (Rantakallio *et al.*, 1987). Of 125 survivors of such perinatal brain damage, six (4.8%) developed schizophrenia in adult life: a sevenfold relative risk (Jones *et al.*, 1998). The estimate of the proportion of schizophrenia in the general population that may be attributable to this mechanism was 5–8% in this study.

Neonatal risk factors: early rearing environment

Human brain development does not stop after birth; the brain continues to develop substantially during the first 2 years of life, during which time it is particularly susceptible to adverse environmental effects, not only those of a physical nature but also from interpersonal affective experiences (Schore, 2001; Siegel, 2001). The central role of the early rearing environment in influencing later emotional and psychological outcomes has long been recognized (Bowlby *et al.*, 1944; Kendler *et al.*, 1992; Murray *et al.*, 1996; Nemeroff, 1999; Rutter, 2002) and is also relevant to schizophrenia (Schiffman *et al.*, 2001). Unwantedness of the pregnancy (Myhrman *et al.*, 1996), antenatal depression (Jones *et al.*, 1998), atypical mother–infant interaction (Cannon *et al.*, 2002b), poor mothering (Jones *et al.*, 1994), and early parental loss (Agid *et al.*, 1999) have been variously associated with increased risk of schizophrenia. Conversely, a good adoptive family environment appears to act as a protective factor among adoptees at genetic risk for the disorder (Tienari, 1991; Wahlberg *et al.*, 1997).

Conclusions

It seems that many pre- and perinatal risk factors are somehow involved in increasing the risk for schizophrenia in later life. The best evidence to date is for prenatal (probably second-trimester) exposure to influenza and other respiratory infections, prenatal rubella, hypoxia-related obstetric complications and low birth weight or intrauterine growth retardation. Evidence is less secure for prenatal stress or prenatal malnutrition, principally because of the difficulties in obtaining suitable samples in which to examine these exposures.

Table 11.2. Estimate of approximate effect sizes for pre- and perinatal risk factors for schizophrenia

Pre- or perinatal risk factor	Approximate effect size (RR or OR)
Place or time of birth	
Winter birth	1.15
Urban birth	1.5–2.4
Infection	
Prenatal influenza	2.0
Prenatal respiratory infection (2°)	2.1
Prenatal rubella	5.2
Prenatal poliovirus (2°)	1.05
Neonatal and childhood CNS infection	4.0
Malnutrition	
Prenatal famine (1°)	2.0
Prenatal stress	
Bereavement of spouse	6.2
Flood (2°)	1.8
War (2°)	
"Unwantedness"	2.4
Maternal depression (3°)	1.8
Obstetric complications	
General	2.0
Rhesus incompatibility	2.8
Hypoxia-related	2.1–4.4
Perinatal brain damage	7.0
Low birth weight (< 2500 g)	1.6
Pre-eclampsia	2.5

RR, relative risk; OR, odds ratio; 1°, 2°, 3°, first, second, and third trimester, respectively.

The effect sizes for these prenatal and perinatal risk factors are small, with odds ratios or relative risks of approximately 2 (Table 11.2). Similarly, genetic studies since the early 1990s have suggest that multiple genes with small effect sizes are involved in causation of schizophrenia. These and other findings indicate that we are likely to be dealing with interactive effects of prenatal and genetic factors (Jones and Murray, 1991; Tsuang, 2000). Recent findings confirm earlier reports that increasing paternal age is associated with an increased risk of schizophrenia (Hare and Moran, 1979; Malaspina *et al.*, 2001). The most parsimonious interpretation attributes the effect to mutations in the male sperm line prior to conception. These mutations, in turn, are to a large extent environmentally determined, by both the cumulative life experience (age) and specific environmental exposures (e.g. toxins) of the biological father.

Techniques for investigating genetic and environmental risk factors are beginning to converge, with case–control and cohort designs being used for genetic association studies. Molecular genetic studies are including measures of environment and cohort studies are collecting both DNA samples and information on early and later environmental risk factors (Caspi *et al.*, 2002, 2003). Over the next few years, we should see the first reports of studies examining precisely measured genetic and early environmental causes of schizophrenia in the same populations.

Acknowledgements

This work was made possible by the support of the Wellcome Trust (MC), NARSAD (MC) and the Theodore and Vada Stanley Foundation (PBJ).

REFERENCES

Adams, W., Kendell, R. E. (1996). Influenza and schizophrenia (letter). *Br J Psychiatry* **169**: 791–792.

Adams, W., Kendell, R. E., Hare, E. H. (1993). Epidemiological evidence that maternal influenza contributes to the aetiology of schizophrenia: an analysis of Scottish, English and Danish data. *Br J Psychiatry* **163**: 522–534.

Agid, O., Shapira, B., Zislin, J., *et al.* (1999). Environment and vulnerability to major psychiatric illness: a case control study of early parental loss in major depression, bipolar disorder and schizophrenia. *Mol Psychiatry* **4**: 163–172.

Barr, C. E., Mednick, S. A., Munk-Jorgensen, P. (1990). Exposure to influenza epidemics during gestation and adult schizophrenia: a 40 year study. *Arch Gen Psychiatry* **47**: 869–874.

Bowlby, J. (1944). Forty four juvenile thieves: their characters and home life. *Int J Psychoanalysis* **25**: 19–52, 107–127.

Brown, A. S., Cohen, P., Greenwald, S., Susser, E. (2000a). Nonaffective psychosis after prenatal exposure to rubella. *Am J Psychiatry* **157**: 438–443.

Brown, A. S., Schaefer, C. A., Wyatt, R. J., *et al.* (2000b). Maternal exposure to respiratory infections and adult schizophrenia spectrum disorders: a prospective birth cohort study. *Schizophr Bull* **26**: 287–296.

Brown, A. S., Begg, M., Gravenstein, S., *et al.* (2003). Serologic evidence for prenatal influenza in the etiology of schizophrenia. *Schizophr Res* **60**: 34.

Buka, S. L., Tsuang, M. T., Lipsitt, L. P. (1993). Pregnancy/delivery complications and psychiatric diagnosis. A prospective study. *Arch Gen Psychiatry* **50**: 151–156.

Buka, S. L., Tsuang, M. T., Torrey, E. F., *et al.* (2001). Maternal infections and subsequent psychosis among offspring. *Arch Gen Psychiatry* **58**: 1032–1037.

Buka, S. L., Tsuang, M. T., Goldstein, J. M., *et al.* (2003). Maternal exposure to herpes simplex virus type 2 and psychosis among adult offspring: replication and reanalysis. *Schizophr Res* **60**: 35.

Butler, P. D., Printz, D., Klugewicz, D., Brown, A. S., Susser, E. S. (1999). Plausibility of early nutritional deficiency as a risk factor for schizophrenia. In *Prenatal Exposures in Schizophrenia*, ed. E. S. Susser, A. S. Brown, J. M. Gorman. Washington, DC: American Psychiatric Press, pp. 163–193.

Byrne, M., Browne, R., Mulryan, N., *et al.* (2000). Labour and delivery complications and schizophrenia. Case–control study using contemporaneous labour ward records. *Br J Psychiatry* **176**: 531–536.

Cannon, M., Jones, P. (1996). Schizophrenia: neuroepidemiology of schizophrenia. *J Neurol Neurosurg Psychiatry* **61**: 604–613.

Cannon, M., Cotter, D., Sham, P. C., *et al.* (1996). Schizophrenia in an Irish sample following prenatal exposure to the 1957 influenza epidemic: a case-controlled, prospective follow-up study. *Schizophr Res* **11**: 95.

Cannon, M., Jones, P. B., Murray R. M. (2002a). Obstetric complications and schizophrenia. Historical and meta-analytic review. *Am J Psychiatry* **159**: 1080–1092.

Cannon, M., Caspi, A., Moffott, T. E., *et al.* (2002b). Evidence for early-childhood, pan-developmental impairment specific to schizophreniform disorder. Results from a longitudinal birth cohort. *Arch Gen Psychiatry* **59**: 449–456.

Cannon, T. D. (1997). On the nature and mechanisms of obstetric influences in schizophrenia: a review and synthesis. *Int Rev Psychiatry* **9**: 387–397.

Cannon, T. D., Rosso, I. M., Hollister, J. M., *et al.* (2000). A prospective cohort study of genetic and perinatal influences in the etiology of schizophrenia. *Schizophr Bull* **26**: 351–366.

Caspi, A., McClay, J., Moffitt, T. E., *et al.* (2002). Role of genotype in the cycle of violence in maltreated children. *Science* **297**: 851–854.

Caspi A., Sugden, K., Moffitt, T. E., *et al.* (2003). Influence of life stress on depression: moderation by a polymorphism in the 5-HTT gene. *Science* **301**: 386–389.

Cotter, D., Larkin, C., Waddington, J. L., O'Callaghan, E. (1996). Season of birth in schizophrenia: clue or cul-de-sac. In *The Neurodevelopmental Basis of Schizophrenia*, ed. J. L. Waddington, P. B. Buckley. Austin, TX: Landes, pp. 17–33.

Crow, T. J., Done, J. (1992). Prenatal exposure to influenza does not cause schizophrenia. *Br J Psychiatry* **161**: 390–393.

Dalman, C., Allebeck, P., Culberg, J., Grunewald, C., Köster, M. (1999). Obstetric complications and the risk of schizophrenia: a longitudinal study of a national birth cohort. *Arch Gen Psychiatry* **56**: 234–240.

Dalman, C., Thomas, H. V., David, A. S., *et al.* (2001). Signs of asphyxia at birth increase the risk of schizophrenia. A population-based case–control study. *Br J Psychiatry* **179**: 403–408.

Dean, K., Fearon, P., Dazzan, P., *et al.* (2003). Increased minor physical anomalies in all ethnic groups in the AESOP first-onset study. *Schizophr Res* **60**.

Done, J., Johnstone, E. C., Frith, C. D., *et al.* (1991). Complications of pregnancy and delivery in relation to psychosis in adult life: data from the British Perinatal Mortality Survey. *Br Med J* **302**: 1576–1580.

Egger, M., Davey Smith, G., Phillips, A. N. (1997). Meta-analysis: principles and procedures. *Br Med J* **315**: 1533–1537.

Erlenmeyer-Kimling, L., Folnegovic, Z., Hrabic-Zerjavic. V., Borcic, B., Folnegovic-Smalc, V. (1994). Schizophrenia and prenatal exposure to the 1957 influenza epidemic in Croatis. *Am J Psychiatry* **151**: 1496–1498.

Fine, P. E. M., Adelstein, A. M., Snowman, J., Clarkson, J. A., Evans, S. M. (1985). Long term effects of exposure to viral infections in utero. *Br Med J* **290**: 509–511.

Fleiss, J. L. (1993). The statistical basis of meta-analysis. *Stat Meth Med Res* **2**: 121–145.

Geddes, J. R., Lawrie, S. M. (1995). Obstetric events in schizophrenia: a meta-analysis. *Br J Psychiatry* **167**: 786–793.

Geddes, J. R., Verdoux, H., Takei, N., *et al.* (1999). Schizophrenia and complications of pregnancy and labor: an individual-patient data meta-analysis. *Schizophr Bull* **25**: 413–423.

Griffiths, T. D., Sigmundsson, T., Takei, N., *et al.* (1998). Minor physical anomalies in familial and sporadic schizophrenia: the Maudsley family study. *J Neurol Neurosurg Psychiatry* **64**: 56–60.

Gualtieri, C. T., Adams, A., Shen, C. D., Loiselle, D. (1982). Minor physical anomalies in alcoholic and schizophrenic adults and hyperactive and autistic children. *Am J Psychiatry* **139**: 640–643.

Hare, E. H., Moran, P. A. (1979). Raised parental age in psychiatric patients: evidence for the constitutional hypothesis, *Br J Psychiatry* **134**: 169–177.

Hennessy, R. J., Kinsella, A., Waddington, J. L. (2002). 3D laser surface scanning and geometric morphometric analysis of craniofacial shape as an index of cerebro-craniofacial morphogenesis: initial application to sexual dimorphism. *Biol Psychiatry* **51**: 507–514.

Hoek, H. W., Susser, E., Buck, K. A., *et al.* (1996). Schizoid personality disorder after prenatal exposure to famine. *Am J Psychiatry* **153**: 1637–1639.

Hoek, H. W., Brown, A. S., Susser, E. S. (1999). The Dutch famine studies: prenatal nutritional deficiency and schizophrenia. In *Prenatal Exposures in Schizophrenia*, ed. E. S. Susser, A. S. Brown, J. M. Gorman. Washington, DC: American Psychiatric Press, pp. 135–161.

Hollister, J. M., Brown, A. S. (1999). Rhesus incompatibility and schizophrenia. In *Prenatal Exposures in Schizophrenia*, ed. E. S. Susser, A. S. Brown, J. M. Gorman. Washington, DC: American Psychiatric Press, pp. 197–214.

Hollister, J. M., Laing, P., Mednick, S. A. (1996). Rhesus incompatibility as a risk factor for schizophrenia in male adults. *Arch Gen Psychiatry* **53**: 19–24.

Hultman, C. M., Sparen, P., Takei, N., Murray, R. M., Cnattingius, S. (1999). Prenatal and perinatal risk factors for schizophrenia, affective psychosis and reactive psychosis of early onset: case–control study. *Br Med J* **318**: 421–426.

Huttunen, M., Niskanen, P. (1978). Prenatal loss of father and psychiatric disorders. *Arch Gen Psychiatry* **35**: 427–431.

Imamura, Y., Nakane, Y., Ohta, Y., Kondo, H. (1999). Lifetime prevalence of schizophrenia among individuals exposed to atomic bomb radiation in Nagasaki. *Acta Psychiatr Scand* **100**: 344–349.

Ismail, B., Cantor-Graae, E., McNeil, T. F. (1998). Minor physical anomalies in schizophrenic patients and their siblings. *Am J Psychiatry* **155**: 1695–1702.

    (2000). Minor physical anomalies in schizophrenia: cognitive, neurological and other clinical correlates. *J Psychiatr Res* **34**: 45–56.

Izumoto, Y., Inoue, S., Yasuda, N. (1999). Schizophrenia and the influenza epidemics of 1957 in Japan. *Biol Psychiatry*, **46**: 119–124.

Jones, P., Murray, R. (1991). The genetics of schizophrenia is the genetics of neurodevelopment, *Br J Psychiatry* **158**: 615–623.

Jones, P., Rodgers, B., Murray, R., Marmot, M. (1994). Childhood developmental risk factors for schizophrenia in the British 1946 birth cohort. *Lancet* **344**: 1398–1402.

Jones, P. B., Rantakallio, P., Hartikainen, A. L., *et al.* (1998). Schizophrenia as a long-term outcome of pregnancy, delivery and perinatal complications: a 28-year follow-up of the 1966 North Finland general population birth cohort. *Am J Psychiatry* **155**: 355–364.

Jones, P. B., Pang, D., Piriach, S., Fine, P. E. M. (1999). Prenatal viral infection and subsequent mental illness: a long-term cohort study of 6152 subjects. *Schizophr Res* **36**: 45.

Kendell, R. E., Adams, W. (1991). Unexplained fluctuations in the risk for schizophrenia by month and year of birth. *Br J Psychiatry* **158**: 758–763.

Kendell, R. E., Kemp, J. W. (1989). Maternal influenza in the aetiology of schizophrenia. *Arch Gen Psychiatry* **46**: 878–882.

Kendell, R. E., McInneny, K., Jusczak, E., Bain, M. (2000). Obstetric complications and schizophrenia: two case–control studies based on structured obstetric records. *Br J Psychiatry* **174**: 516–522.

Kendler, K. S., Neale, M. C., Kessler, R. C., Heath, A. C., Eaves, L. J. (1992). Childhood parental loss and adult psychopathology in women. A twin study perspective. *Arch Gen Psychiatry* **49**: 109–116.

Kinney, D. K. (2001). Prenatal stress and risk for schizophrenia. *Int J Mental Health* **29**: 62–71.

Kinney, D. K., Hyman, W., Greetham, C., Tramer, S. (1999). Increased relative risk for schizophrenia and prenatal exposure to a severe tornado. *Schizophr Res* **36**: 45–46.

Koenig, J. I., Kirkpatrick, B., Lee, P. (2002). Glucocorticoid hormones and early brain development in schizophrenia. *Neuropsychopharmacology* **27**: 309–318.

Kunugi, H., Nanko, S., Takei, N., *et al.* (1995). Schizophrenia following in utero exposure to the 1957 influenza epidemics in Japan. *Am J Psychiatry* **152**: 450–452.

Lane, A., Kinsella, A., Murphy, P., *et al.* (1997). The anthropometric assessment of dysmorphic features in schizophrenia as an index of its developmental origins. *Psychol Med* **27**: 1155–1164.

Lawrie, S. M., Byrne, M. Miller, P. *et al.* (2001). Neurodevelopmental indices and the development of psychotic symptoms in subjects at high risk of schizophrenia. *Br J Psychiatry* **178**: 524–530.

Lewis, G., David, A., Andreasson, S., Allebeck, P. (1992). Schizophrenia and city life. *Lancet* **340**: 137–140.

Lou, H., Hansen, D., Nordentoft, M., *et al.* (1994). Prenatal stressors of human life affect fetal brain development. *Dev Med Child Neurol* **36**: 826–832.

Malaspina, D., Harlap, S., Fennig, S., *et al.* (2001). Advancing paternal age and the risk of schizophrenia. *Arch Gen Psychiatry* **58**: 313–412.

Marcelis, M., Takei, N., van Os, J. (1999). Urbanization and risk for schizophrenia: does the effect operate before or around the time of illness onset? *Psychol Med* **29**: 1197–1203.

Marcelis, M., Navarro-Mateu, F., Murray, R., Selten, J. P., van Os, J. (1998). Urbanization and psychosis: a study of 1942–1978 birth cohorts in the Netherlands. *Psychol Med* **28**: 871–879.

Marenco, S., Weinberger, D. R. (2000). The neurodevelopmental hypothesis of schizophrenia: following a trail of evidence from cradle to grave. *Dev Psychopathol* **12**: 501–527.

McDonald, C., Fearon, P., Murray, R. M. (2000). Neurodevelopmental hypothesis of schizophrenia 12 years on: data and doubts. In *Childhood Onset of Adult Psychopathology*, ed. J. L. Rapaport. Washington, DC: American Psychiatric Press, pp. 193–222.

McGrath, J. J., Welham, J. L. (1999). Season of birth and schizophrenia: a systematic review and meta-analysis of data from the Southern Hemisphere. *Schizophr Res* **35**: 237–242.

McGrath, J. J., Pemberton, M. R., Welham, J. L., Murray, R. M. (1994). Schizophrenia and the influenza epidemics of 1954, 1957 and 1959: a southern hemisphere study. *Schizophr Res* **14**: 1–8.

McGrath, J. J., Castle, D., Murray, R. M. (1995a). How can we judge whether or not prenatal exposure to influenza causes schizophrenia. In *Neural Development and Schizophrenia. Theory and Research*, ed. S. A. Mednick, J. M., Hollister. New York: Plenum Press, pp. 203–214.

McGrath, J. J., van Os, J., Hoyos, C., *et al.* (1995b). Minor physical anomalies in psychoses: associations with clinical and putative aetiological variables. *Schizophr Res* **18**: 9–20.

McGrath, J., El-Saadi, O., Grim, V., *et al.* (2002). Minor physical anomalies and quantitative measures of the head and face in patients with psychosis. *Arch Gen Psychiatry* **59**: 458–464.

McNeil, T. F. (1988). Obstetric factors and perinatal injuries. In *Handbook of Schizophrenia*, Vol. 3: *Nosology, Epidemiology and Genetics*, ed. M. T. Tsuang, J. C. Simpson. North Holland: Elsevier Science, pp. 319–311.

(1995). Perinatal risk factors and schizophrenia: selective review and methodological concerns. *Epidemiol Rev* **17**: 107–112.

McNeil, T. F., Cantor-Graae, E. (1999). Does preexisting abnormality cause labor–delivery complications in fetuses who will develop schizophrenia? *Schizophr Bull* **25**: 425–435.

(2000). Minor physical anomalies and obstetric complications in schizophrenia. *Aust NZ J Psychiatry* **34**(Suppl.): S65–S73.

McNeil, T., Cantor-Graae, E., Ishmail, B. (2000). Obstetric complications and congenital malformations in schizophrenia. *Brain Res Rev* **31**: 166–178.

Mednick, S. A., Schulsinger F. (1968). Some premorbid characteristics related to breakdown in children with schizophrenic mothers. *J Psychiat Res* **6**(Suppl. 1): 267–291.

Mednick, S. A., Mura, E., Schulsinger, F., Mednick, B. (1971). Perinatal conditions and infant development in children with schizophrenic parents. *Soc Biol* **18**: S103–S113.

Mednick, S. A., Machon, R. A., Huttunen, M. O., Bonett, D. (1988). Adult schizophrenia following prenatal exposure to an influenza epidemic. *Arch Gen Psychiatry* **45**: 189–192.

Mednick, S. A., Machon, R. A., Huttunen, M. O. (1990). An update on the Helsinki influenza project. Letter to Editor. *Arch Gen Psychiatry* **47**: 292.

Morgan, V., Castle, D., Page, A., *et al.* (1997). Influenza epidemics and incidence of schizophrenia, affective disorders and mental retardation in Western Australia: no evidence of a major effect. *Schizophr Res* **26**: 25–39.

Mortensen, P. B., Pedersen, C. B., Westergaard, T., *et al.* (1999). Effects of family history and place and season of birth on the risk of schizophrenia. *N Engl J Med* **340**: 603–608.

Murray, L., Fiori-Crowley, A., Hooper, R., Cooper P. J. (1996). The impact of post natal depression and associated adversity on early mother–infant interactions and later infant outcome. *Child Dev* **67**: 2512–2526.

Myhrman, A., Rantakallio, P., Isohanni, M., Jones, P. B., Partanen, U. (1996). Unwantedness of a pregnancy and schizophrenia in the child. *Br J Psychiatry* **169**: 637–640.

Nemeroff, C. (1999). The pre-eminent role of early untoward experience on vulnerability to major psychiatric disorders: the nature–nurture controversy revisited and soon to be resolved. *Mol Psychiatry* **4**: 106–108.

O'Callaghan, E., Sham, P., Takei, N., Glover, G., Murray, R. M. (1991). Schizophrenia after prenatal exposure to 1957 A2 influenza epidemic. *Lancet* **337**: 1248–1250.

O'Connor, T., Heron, J., Golding, J., Beveridge, M., Glover, V. (2002). Maternal antenatal anxiety and children's behavioural/emotional problems at 4 years. *Br J Psychiatry* **180**: 502–508.

Rantakallio, P. (1969). Groups at risk in low birth weight infants and perinatal mortality. *Acta Paediatr Scand Suppl* **193**: 1–71.

Rantakallio, P., von Wendt, L., Koivu, M. (1987). Prognosis of perinatal brain damage: a prospective study of a one year birth cohort of 12 000 children. *Early Hum Dev* **15**: 75–84.

Rantakallio, P., Jones, P., Moring, J., von Wendt, L. (1997). Association between central nervous system infections during childhood and adult onset schizophrenia and other psychoses: a 28-year follow-up. *Int J Epidemiol* **26**: 837–843.

Rosso, I. M., Cannon, T. D., Huttunen, T., *et al.* (2000). Obstetric risk factors for early-onset schizophrenia in a Finnish birth cohort. *Am J Psychiatry* **157**: 801–807.

Rutter, M. (2002). The interplay of nature, nurture and development. *Arch Gen Psychiatry* **59**: 996–1001.

Sacker, A., Done, D. J., Crow, T. J., Golding, J. (1995). Antecedents of schizophrenia and affective illness: obstetric complications. *Br J Psychiatry* **166**: 734–741.

Schiffman, J., Abrahamson, A., Cannon, T., *et al.* (2001). Early rearing factors in schizophrenia. *Int J Mental Health* **30**: 3–16.

Schiffman, J., Ekstrom, M., LaBrie, J., *et al.* (2002). Minor physical anomalies and schizophrenia spectrum disorders: a prospective investigation. *Am J Psychiatry* **159**: 238–243.

Schore, A. N. (2001). Effects of early relational trauma on right brain development, affect regulation, and infant mental health. *Infant Ment Health J* **22**, 201–269.

Selten, J. P. C. J., Slaets, J. P. J. (1994). Evidence against maternal infection as a risk factor for schizophrenia. *Br J Psychiatry* **164**: 674–676.

Selten, J. P., van der Graaf, Y., van Duursen, R., Gispen-de Wied, C. C., Kahn, R. S. (1999). Psychotic illness after prenatal exposure to the 1953 Dutch Flood Disaster. *Schizophr Res* **35**: 243–245.

Sham, P. C., O'Callaghan, E., Takei, N., *et al.* (1992). Schizophrenia following pre-natal exposure to influenza epidemics between 1939 and 1960. *Br J Psychiatry* **160**: 461–466.

Siegel, D. J. (2001). Toward an interpersonal neurobiology of the developing mind: attachment relationships, "mindsight", and neural integration. *Infant Ment Health J* **22**: 67–94.

Stöber, G., Franzek, E., Beckmann, J. (1992). The role of maternal infectious diseases during pregnancy in the aetiology of schizophrenia in offspring. *Eur Psychiatry* **7**: 147–152.

Suomi, S. J. (1997). Long-term effects of different early rearing experiences on social, emotional, and physiological development in nonhuman primates. In M. S. Keshavan and R. M. Murray (Eds.) *Neurodevelopment and Adult Psychopathology*, Ch. 8, ed. M. S. Keshavan, R. M. Murray. Cambridge: Cambridge University Press, pp. 104–116.

Susser, E., Lin, S. P. (1992). Schizophrenia after prenatal exposure to the Dutch Hunger Winter of 1944–1945. *Arch Gen Psychiatry* **49**: 983–988.

(1994). Schizophrenia after prenatal exposure to the Dutch hunger winter of 1944–1945. *Arch Gen Psychiatry* **51**: 333–334.

Susser, E. S., Lin, S. P., Brown, A. S., Lumey, L. H., Erlenmeyer-Kimling, L. (1994). No relation between risk of schizophrenia and prenatal exposure to influenza in Holland. *Am J Psychiatry* **151**: 922–924.

Susser, E. S., Neugebauer, R., Hoek, H. W., *et al.* (1996). Schizophrenia after prenatal famine. *Arch Gen Psychiatry* **53**: 25–31.

Susser, E. S., Schaefer, C., Brown, A., Begg, M., Wyatt, R. J. (2000). The design of the Prenatal Determinants of Schizophrenia Study (PDS). *Schizophr Bull* **26**: 257–273.

Susser, M., Hauser, W. A., Keity, J. L., Paneth, N., Stein, Z. (1985). Quantitative estimates of prenatal and perinatal risk factors for perinatal mortality, cerebral palsy, mental retardation and epilepsy. In *Prenatal and Perinatal Factors Associated with Brain Disorder*, ed. J. Freeman. Washington, DC: Institute of Health, pp. 359–432.

Suvisaari, J., Haukka, J., Tanskanen, A., Hovi, T., Lönnqvist, J. (1999). Association between prenatal exposure to poliovirus infection and adult schizophrenia. *Am J Psychiatry* **156**: 1100–1102.

Takei, N., Sham, P., O'Callaghan, E., *et al.* (1994). Prenatal exposure to influenza and the development of schizophrenia: is the effect confined to females? *Am J Psychiatry* **151**: 117–119.

Takei, N., Sham, P., O'Callaghan, E., Glover, G., Murray, R. M. (1995). Schizophrenia: increased risk associated with winter and city birth: a case–control study in 12 regions within England and Wales. *J Epidemiol Community Health* **49**: 106–107.

Taylor, A., Fisk, N., Glover, V. (2000). Mode of delivery and later stress response. *Lancet* **355**: 120.

Teixeira, J. M. A., Fisk, N. M., Glover, V. (1999). Association between maternal anxiety in pregnancy and increased uterine artery resistance index: cohort based study. *Br Med J* **318**: 153–157.

Tienari, P. (1991). Interaction between genetic vulnerability and family environment: the Finnish adoptive family study of schizophrenia. *Acta Psychiatr Scand* **84**: 460–465.

Torrey, E. F., Bowler, A. (1990). Geographical distribution of insanity in America: evidence for an urban factor. *Schizophr Bull* **16**: 591–604.

Torrey, E. F., Rawlings, R., Waldman, I. N. (1988). Schizophrenic births and viral diseases in two states. *Schizophr Res* **1**: 73–77.

Torrey, E. F., Bowler, A. E., Rawlings, R. (1992). Schizophrenia and the 1957 influenza epidemic. *Schizophr Res* **6**: 100–107.

Torrey, E. F., Miller, J., Rawlings. R., Yolken, R. H. (1997). Seasonality of birth in schizophrenia and bipolar disorder: a review. *Schizophr Res* **28**: 1–38.

Tsuang, M. (2000). Schizophrenia: genes and environment. *Biological Psychiatry* **47**: 210–220.

van Os, J., Selten, J.-P. (1998). Prenatal exposure to maternal stress and later schizophrenia: the May 1940 invasion of the Netherlands. *Br J Psychiatry* **172**: 324–326.

Wahlberg, K.-E., Wynne, L. C., Oja, H., *et al.* (1997). Gene–environment interaction in vulnerability to schizophrenia: findings from the Finnish Adoptive Family Study of Schizophrenia. *Am J Psychiatry* **154**: 355–362.

Weinstein, D. D., Diforio, D., Schiffman, J., Wlaker, E., Bonsall, R. (1999). Minor physical anomalies, dermatoglyphic asymmetries and cortisol levels in adolescents with schizotypal personality disorder. *Am J Psychiatry* **156**: 617–623.

Westergaard, T., Mortensen, P. B., Pedersen, C. B., Wohlfahrt, J., Melbye, M. (1999). Exposure to prenatal and childhood infections and the risk of schizophrenia. *Arch Gen Psychiatry* **56**: 993–998.

Wright, P., Rifkin, L., Takei, N., Murray, R. (1995). Maternal influenza, obstetric complications and schizophrenia. *Am J Psychiatry* **152**: 1714–1720.

Wright, P., Takei, N., Murray, R. M., Sham, P. C. (1999). Seasonality, prenatal influenza exposure and schizophrenia. In *Prenatal Exposures in Schizophrenia*, ed. E. S. Susser, A. S. Brown, J. M. Gorman. Washington, DC: American Psychiatric Press, pp. 89–112.

Zornberg, G., Buka, S. L., Tsuang, M. T. (2000a). The problem of obstetrical complications and schizophrenia. *Schizophr Bull* **26**: 249–256.

(2000b). Hypoxic-ischaemia-related fetal/neonatal complications and risk of schizophrenia and other nonaffective psychoses: a 19 year longitudinal study. *Am J Psychiatry* **157**: 196–202.

12

Transcriptomes in schizophrenia: assessing altered gene expression with microarrays

David A. Lewis[1], Karoly Mirnics[1], and Pat Levitt[2]

[1] University of Pittsburgh, Pittsburgh, USA
[2] Vanderbilt University, Nashville, USA

The diversity of implicated etiological factors and the heterogeneity of clinical features in schizophrenia have been associated, not surprisingly, with a wide variety of findings regarding the nature of the brain abnormalities that underlie the pathophysiology of this illness (Lewis and Lieberman, 2000). Because all of these abnormalities are either caused by, or reflected in, changes at the molecular level, the molecular neuropathology of schizophrenia is certain to provide keys to improved treatment in the near term and disease prevention in the more distant future. Characterizing the molecular neuropathology of schizophrenia requires, at least in part, knowledge of the full complement of genes showing altered expression in the brains of affected individuals. The advent of new technology has made it possible to determine transcriptomes: the collection of all mRNA transcripts expressed in a given brain region or cell type. As the product of genomic DNA, the transcriptome is a central determinant of the phenotype of a given brain region or cell type (Brown and Bottenstein, 1999; Duggan et al., 1999). Therefore, determining the schizophrenia-related transcriptomes is likely to provide critical insight into the pathogenetic and pathophysiological processes of this illness. In this chapter, we review the current status of the technology to assess transcriptomes, its associated strengths and limitations, and initial findings resulting from the use of this approaches to study schizophrenia.

Assessing transcriptomes with microarrays

Although a variety of approaches are available to assess transcriptomes, this review will focus on the use of DNA microarrays: high-density arrangements of single- or double-stranded DNA sequences (termed "probes") that are immobilized at specific locations on a solid surface or membrane (DeRisi et al., 1996; Lockhart

Neurodevelopment and Schizophrenia, ed. Matcheri S. Keshavan et al. Published by Cambridge University Press. © Cambridge University Press 2004.

et al., 1996; Schena *et al.*, 1995). Microarray technology is based on the well-established principle of complementary hybridization between nucleic acids; each microarray probe is capable of recognizing the complementary sequence through base pairing (Southern *et al.*, 1999). The "target" (e.g. mRNA extracted from a tissue sample) is hybridized to the immobilized DNA sequence probes on the array surface, an approach made possible by the miniaturization process and development of high-throughput printing robots. After a series of high-stringency washes, only the highly complementary probe–target complexes remain tightly bound. The amount of the retained label is then quantified over each probe spot, with the amount of retained label or the signal intensity providing a direct reflection of the abundance of that mRNA species in the sample (Cheung *et al.*, 1999).

Thus, microarrays permit an extensive and relatively rapid screening of the expression levels of thousands of mRNA transcripts. Indeed, it is now possible to analyze the expression profile in cells from a schizophrenia patient using microarrays that represent a majority of the human genome. Although this approach is not informative regarding the potential contribution of translational or post-translational processing events to the disease state, proteins in the postmortem brain are likely to be less intact than mRNA, and their large-scale analysis is much more complex. Furthermore, microarrays analyze transcripts that are intrinsic to the harvested brain region, whereas protein profiles reflect intrinsic and extrinsic sources, making it more difficult to discern the anatomical source of the observed disease-related changes.

Two types of microarray platform have been used in studies of schizophrenia. Complementary DNA (cDNA) microarrays are composed of relatively long cDNA probes (typically ranging from approximately 100 to 2000 base pairs) that are usually DNA clones amplified by the polymerase chain reaction (PCR) or expressed sequence tags (ESTs) derived from the 3′ end of RNA targets. Thousands of these probes are each deposited or synthesized in very small, unique locations on a solid support (e.g. glass or membrane structure) (Duggan *et al.*, 1999; Schena and Davis, 1999). The sample analysis can be performed using a single label or a dual fluorescent method. In a dual-color analysis, two different fluorescent tags (e.g. cyanin 3 and 5 [Cy3 and Cy5, respectively]) are used to label, through a reverse transcription procedure (Schena *et al.*, 1996; DeRisi *et al.*, 1997), the mRNA species present in each of the two tissue samples to be compared (e.g. a subject with schizophrenia and a matched normal control). The samples containing the labeled targets are combined and hybridized together onto the same microarray. Using two independent scans that are selective for each of two incorporated fluorescent tags' emission wavelengths, a high-resolution fluorescent intensity measurement is obtained from each spot on the microarray. This signal is quantified, standardized, and compared between the two images, and the intensity differences are interpreted as relative differences in transcript abundance between the two samples (e.g. schizophrenia and control).

The other general type of platform, synthetic oligonucleotide probe arrays, consists of high-density, two-dimensional arrays of synthetic oligonucleotides. The GeneChip®, manufactured under the proprietary technology of Affymetrix, is currently the most widely utilized (Lockhart and Barlow, 2001). These glass-supported arrays are constructed by spatially arranging light-directed combinatorial chemical synthesis of thousands of different oligonucleotides (Lipshutz *et al.*, 1999; Lockhart *et al.*, 1996). This photochemical, solid-phase technology facilitates a high spatial resolution and precision of probe placement, which thus permits very high-density throughput for gene expression analyses. For example, the human U133 GeneChip® contains probe spots as small as $324\ \mu m^2$ on a single $1.28\ cm \times 1.28\ cm$ array, such that up to 80% of the human genome is represented across two arrays. The expression of each gene is interrogated with multiple probes, and the presence of the transcript of interest is detected using a sophisticated mathematical modeling process. Then, after a routine standardization procedure, expression differences across different arrays (i.e. each array interrogates one sample) are detected using a statistical algorithm.

Experimental design in microarray studies

The study of gene expression in human brain tissue, the area of interest in schizophrenia, requires the use of postmortem human brain specimens. Thus, such studies require an understanding of both the advantages and the limitations intrinsic to the use of postmortem material. First, the successful application of microarray technology to the study of schizophrenia depends upon the use of well-characterized tissue specimens, in which potential confounds are identified and addressed in the experimental design (Lewis, 2002). Three general issues are important to consider.

First, the relevant demographic and diagnostic information needs to be obtained in a standardized fashion for both cases and comparison subjects. Ideally, this information is acquired from both the review of available medical records and through structured interviews conducted with surviving relatives and other informants (Glantz and Lewis, 1997). The latter typically provides data that are not available from the medical records, as well as an additional way to verify the information in these records through collateral sources. In addition to demographic variables, these investigations yield the clinical characterization of the illness (e.g. diagnostic signs and symptoms, age of onset, duration of illness, family history of illness), the treatment of the illness (e.g. medications at the time of death, history of treatment with other medications, length and number of hospitalizations), and factors that may be comorbid with the primary diagnosis of interest (e.g. history of alcohol or other substance abuse, nicotine exposure). This information is essential for the selection of appropriate comparison subjects, including both normal controls and subjects with other disorders who share some features (e.g. medication history) with the schizophrenia subjects under investigation. In addition, the detailed clinical information suggests the types of parallel study that may need to be conducted in animal model systems, where factors such as medication exposure can be assessed in a controlled fashion. For example, we have used macaque monkeys treated chronically with antipsychotic drugs in a manner that directly mimics their use in humans as one way of assessing the potential contribution of these therapeutic agents to our microarray findings in subjects with schizophrenia (Mirnics et al., 2000).

Second, in order to avoid the introduction of potential confounds secondary to geographic factors, differences in the handling of tissue specimens, or other variables, all tissue specimens ideally are obtained from the same source. A standardized approach to blocking the brain facilitates examination and sampling for neuropathological studies and permits a uniform dissection of the region(s) of interest at the time that a microarray study is initiated. Photographic documentation of the tissue blocks provides a means to confirm and record that the same macroscopic landmarks are present in the tissue blocks from all subjects. These procedures also facilitate the design of cutting and sampling procedures to best approximate the acquisition of systematic and uniform random samples of the region of interest. In addition, the preparation of slide-mounted sections from the tissue blocks that are used for the isolation of RNA provides Nissl-stained material that can be used to verify that the tissue block contains the characteristic cytoarchitecture of the brain region targeted for study. Other sections are used to confirm array findings for individual transcripts by in situ hybridization.

Third, it is important to assess variables that may affect the expression or integrity of mRNA. These variables include agonal state events, the cause and manner of death, and the postmortem interval (PMI), the period between the time of death and the freezing of the tissue specimens. Although most mRNA species exhibit minimal to modest degradation following PMIs of more than 24 hours (comparable to freshly frozen animal brain tissue), premortem events can have a substantial negative impact. In particular, antemortem hypoxia and/or acidosis, conditions frequently found in individuals who die in hospital following medical complications or sustained periods of illness, appear to be associated with the loss of at least some mRNA species. Available studies suggest that postmortem brain pH provides an easily measured and reliable assessment of the severity of these factors (Harrison et al., 1995). Because the factors monitored by brain pH or PMI may not have linear effects on mRNA integrity, we prefer to match individual pairs of subjects as closely as possible on these variables, in addition to including pre- and postmortem conditions as covariates in statistical analyses.

Microarray data analysis and interpretation

Biological sensitivity differs from the nominal microarray sensitivity of microarrays. That is, at a sensitivity of 1 in 250 000 copies of mRNA, both cDNA and oligonucleotide microarrays can theoretically detect even the lowest abundance mRNA species in a uniform cell population. However, the complexity introduced by the many different cell types present in a given region of the brain can result in a dilution effect such that the relative abundance of mRNAs expressed in only a subset of cells falls below microarray detection limits. Consequently, the biological sensitivity may be substantially lower than the nominal microarray sensitivity, and some relatively rare transcripts (e.g. neurotransmitter receptors), which are readily identified by other molecular techniques, such as *in situ* hybridization, will not be detected by microarrays. Furthermore, cross-hybridization between RNA species can obscure differences in expression levels for the transcript of interest.

Initially, microarray experiments used "fold change" (i.e. the ratio of the expression level for a given gene in a subject with schizophrenia relative to that of the matched control subject) as a descriptor of the magnitude of the measurement difference across samples. Unfortunately, the reliability of "fold changes" depends on many parameters, such as probe length and properties, absolute abundance of a molecule, data standardization, modeling, type of tissue specimen, and array platform. In addition, "fold changes" may be relatively insensitive to marked disease processes. For example, the loss of 20% of the neurons in a region may produce only a 0.2-fold change in the transcripts that are expressed in all neurons. Consequently, other statistical approaches are being developed and used (see below) to uncover expression changes of modest magnitude that, nonetheless, may have great importance for the disease process under study.

Microarray studies of brain regions do not reveal the cellular source or cause of any changes in gene expression. For example, a given decrease in the level of a transcript could be the result of a consistent downregulation of expression across all cells or the complete absence of expression in a subset of cells. Furthermore, parallel expression changes in different transcripts may occur in the same cell type or may be present in different, but functionally related, cell classes. Obviously, obtaining this type of information is critical for the biological interpretation of the findings, and it demonstrates the need for microarray data to be supplemented with anatomically based molecular approaches.

Although changes in protein levels may occur without expression changes in the underlying transcripts, changes in gene expression usually result in protein level changes, albeit not necessarily of the same magnitude. However, the sources of proteins and transcripts may be different in a given brain region. That is, mRNA signal originates predominantly from cell bodies in the harvested tissue, whereas proteins are also found in the axon terminals that project to a given region.

Consequently, apparent discrepancies in transcript versus the protein change in tissue homogenates may reflect differences in the anatomical source of the change, rather than the absence of a change in protein level in association with a change in transcript expression.

Gene expression changes associated with schizophrenia

In postmortem brain specimens from subjects with schizophrenia, a difference in the expression level of one or a cluster of genes may have several different meanings. First, given the apparent polygenic nature of schizophrenia, some transcript differences may result from DNA sequence variants that confer disease susceptibility through changes in expression level of the encoded mRNA. Second, some changes may represent secondary effects that either contribute to the pathophysiology of the illness or represent a compensatory response. Finally, some expression changes may result from the treatment of schizophrenia or be associated with factors that frequently accompany schizophrenia (e.g. depression, substance abuse or nicotine exposure). Therefore, in this section, we review existing transcriptome findings from studies of schizophrenia and consider their potential significance from these perspectives.

The first microarray study of schizophrenia used a cDNA platform containing about 8000 genes and ESTs to examine area 9 of the dorsolateral prefrontal cortex (Mirnics *et al.*, 2000). The initial evaluation of these data involved the a-priori categorization of the represented transcripts into approximately 250 gene groups. This approach was used in order to exploit the power of microarray data to reveal the presence of disease-related transcriptome changes among functionally related genes, relationships that are not apparent from examining lists of "most-changed" genes or conducting classical hierarchical analyses. In our own studies, we used a supervised approach, assuming that a single gene expression deficit in a functional pathway would be associated with altered expression of the other genes belonging to the same pathway. Although 95% of detectable transcripts showed normal levels of expression in schizophrenia, this analysis revealed a prominent deficit in the expression of members of a group of genes (termed the *PSYN* group) whose protein products contribute to the mechanisms involved in the presynaptic release of neurotransmitters. These findings appear to be related to the disease process of schizophrenia and are not a consequence of its treatment, since (i) comparable findings were observed in individuals with schizophrenia who were on or off antipsychotic medications at the time of death, and (ii) no deficits in the expression of *PSYN* genes were found in monkeys exposed chronically to haloperidol in a manner, and with serum levels, that mimiced clinical use. In addition to a highly significant effect at the level of the gene group, the expression deficits of individual genes within the *PSYN* group appeared to be subject specific. That is, although all subjects with schizophrenia showed decreased expression of multiple *PSYN* genes, the specific combination of affected transcripts varied from subject to subject. This phenotypic diversity may reflect a continuum of molecular phenotypes in schizophrenia, perhaps similar to the variability in the clinical manifestations of the illness across subjects. In addition to this general molecular diversity seen across subjects, consistent expression deficits in several genes, such as those for *N*-ethylmaleimide-sensitive factor (NSF), synapsin 2, and vesicular ATPase, were found in almost all subjects with schizophrenia. NSF and its attachment proteins are critical to provide energy for synaptic vesicle fusion; synapsin II regulates vesicle availability for exocytosis; and vesicular ATPase is responsible for synaptic vesicle homeostasis. These expression deficits were confirmed by *in situ* hybridization, indicating that they did not represent artifacts of the microarray data analysis or interpretation procedures.

Associated with these alterations in *PSYN* genes, robust decreases were also found in two groups comprising much smaller numbers of genes represented on the arrays. These two gene groups encode proteins that are specifically related to neurotransmission for gamma-aminobutyric acid (GABA) and glutamate, which together account for over 95% of cortical synapses. In the glutamate transmission gene group, glutamate receptor 2 (AMPA2) showed the largest expression decrease, and the 67 kDa isoform of glutamic acid decarboxylase (GAD_{67}) was the most robustly and consistently affected gene related to GABA neurotransmission (Mirnics *et al.*, 2000). These single gene findings replicated previous reports using more conventional methods (Akbarian *et al.*, 1995; Eastwood *et al.*, 1995; Volk *et al.*, 2000). The etiology of these changes remains unknown, yet it is possible that these group-wise changes reflect changes secondary to the broader alterations in presynaptic function. For example, a reduction in synaptic activity may lead to the findings of reduced prefrontal brain-derived neurotrophic factor (BDNF) signaling in schizophrenia (Hashimoto *et al.*, 2002; Weickert *et al.*, 2003). This, in turn, may account for the marked and selective reduction in GAD_{67} mRNA expression observed in the subpopulation of prefrontal GABA neurons (Hashimoto *et al.*, 2003) that express TrkB, the receptor for BDNF.

Because of the high metabolic demands placed on neurons by the processes involved in synaptic communication, and given the in vivo evidence for alterations in prefrontal cortical metabolism in schizophrenia (Berman *et al.*, 1986; Buchsbaum *et al.*, 1992), we used the well-accepted listing of metabolic groups from the *Kyoto Encyclopedia of Genes and Genomes* (KEGG) to identify 70 different clusters of genes whose protein products are involved in metabolic functions (Middleton *et al.*, 2002). Remarkably, only five of these metabolic gene groups displayed significant alteration in expression in the prefrontal cortex of subjects with schizophrenia.

These included the mitochondrial malate shuttle system, transcarboxylic acid cycle, ornithine/polyamine, aspartate/alanine, and ubiquitin metabolism groups. Verification of these microarray data by *in situ* hybridization confirmed reduced mRNA levels for soluble malate dehydrogenase (MAD1), mitochondrial glutamate–oxaloacetate transaminase type 2, ornithine decarboxylase antizyme inhibitor, and ornithine aminotransferase. Interestingly, assessment of expression levels of individual genes in these pathways for changes in haloperidol-exposed monkeys revealed an unexpected increase in the expression of MAD1, raising the intriguing possibility that the antipsychotic treatment may counteract the MAD1 expression decrease observed in schizophrenia. The MAD1 expression increase was most prominent in the deep cortical layers, including layer 5, which contains the highest density of dopamine D_2 receptors (Lidow *et al.*, 1989). Together, these findings suggest that altered prefrontal metabolism may be an important component of the disease process in schizophrenia, contributing to or reflecting alterations in presynaptic function in the same brain region, and that the reversal of at least some of these abnormalities may be involved in the therapeutic effects of antipsychotic medications.

The same microarray data set also revealed multiple changes in genes that play a role in chemical neurotransmission from the postsynaptic side. In addition to changes in a subset of glutamate and GABA receptors, we found a marked and highly consistent reduction in the transcript for a regulator of G-protein signaling protein (RGS4) (Mirnics *et al.*, 2001a). RGS proteins are GTPase-activating proteins that facilitate hydrolysis of GTP bound to G_α-protein and thus limit the duration and timing of signaling through G-protein-coupled receptors (De Vries *et al.*, 2000). Hence, downregulation of RGS4 may compensate for decreased synaptic efficacy in the prefrontal cortex by increasing the duration of signaling following activation of G-protein-coupled receptors. However, a similar magnitude of RGS4 transcript reduction was also present in motor and visual cortices of the same subjects with schizophrenia, regions that differ substantially from the prefrontal cortex in structure, connectivity, and function. In addition, these changes in RGS4 expression were not observed in the prefrontal cortex of subjects with major depression or in monkeys exposed chronically to haloperidol. Consequently, these findings suggest that decreased RGS4 expression in schizophrenia is not restricted to the prefrontal cortex, and that this decrease may be specific to the disease process and not a consequence of potentially confounding factors such as comorbid depression or antipsychotic medications. Together, these observations support the hypothesis that RGS4 represents a schizophrenia susceptibility gene. Interestingly, RGS4 is present at chromosomal locus 1q21–22, which has been linked to schizophrenia in some cohorts (Brzustowicz *et al.*, 2000). Consistent with this hypothesis, evidence of association between allelic variations in the 5′ region of RGS4 and schizophrenia was found in three family samples, although the pattern of transmission differed across them (Chowdari et al., 2002). Although replication studies are required to confirm this finding, these studies do exemplify how expression information from microarray studies, in concert with positional and functional data, can be used to identify schizophrenia susceptibility genes.

The concomitant reduction in expression of presynaptic, energy metabolism, and postsynaptic genes in the same subjects strongly suggests that these findings are interrelated components of the disease process of schizophrenia, although the direction of causality among them is unclear at present. It is possible that a primary deficit in the PSYN group, leading to decreased or inefficient synaptic activity, could lead to secondary downregulation of energy metabolism and altered signaling at the postsynaptic membrane. Indeed, we have proposed a testable model (Mirnics et al., 2001b) which argues that a primary reduction in synaptic efficacy could account for both the developmental trajectory of schizophrenia and the findings of decreased markers of cortical synaptic number (Glantz and Lewis, 1997, 2000). Specifically, we suggested that impaired synaptic function in certain cortical circuits would initially be compensated, at least to a certain degree, by the normal exuberant production of synapses, but that these connections would be rendered more vulnerable to additional alterations as a result of later developmental events. For example, the adolescence-related pruning of cortical excitatory synapses (Huttenlocher, 1979; Rakic et al., 1986) would not only reduce the total complement of cortical synapses but might also do so to a greater degree than normal because of the diminished function of the affected circuits (Mirnics et al., 2001b). In this regard, the evidence of cognitive abnormalities during childhood of individuals who later become ill with schizophrenia may be considered to reflect both the disease process and a risk factor for later developmental disturbances required for the clinical manifestations of the illness (Lewis and Levitt, 2002). Once pruning is completed, normally during the second decade of life (although the temporal trajectory could itself be altered in schizophrenia), the manifestations of the illness would be expected to be relatively stable; however, the effects of normal aging might be more severe, perhaps accounting for the non-Alzheimer's dementia seen in elderly individuals with schizophrenia (Arnold et al., 1998). Consistent with this hypothesis, altering neuronal excitability during synaptogenesis has a profound effect on the numbers of synapses that form, but this effect is not seen if excitability is altered after synaptogenesis (Burrone et al., 2002).

As in all studies of schizophrenia, replication of findings in additional subjects and by other investigators is essential. Other investigators, using different cohorts of subjects, observed some of our microarray findings. For example, Sklar and co-workers (Sklar, 2001) reported that NSF was decreased in the prefrontal cortex of schizophrenia subjects; an analysis of single cells from subjects with schizophrenia showed decreased expression levels of several synaptic markers (Hemby *et al.*, 2002); and altered expression of genes involved in ubiquitinization was reported by Vawter and colleagues (2001, 2002). Such replication studies are challenging for microarray techniques for a variety of reasons including a lack of standardized methods and modes of analysis and differences in sensitivity of different platforms. Indeed, the rapid advances in microarray technology suggest that in the short-term we are more likely to see improvement in, rather than replication of, results (Branca, 2003). One of the biggest challenges to replication of findings from gene investigators at present is the fact that different sets of gene are represented on different microarrays. For example, using a microarray containing 1127 brain-related genes to probe prefrontal area 9 from subjects with schizophrenia, Vawter *et al.* (2002) found reduced expression of several of the *PSYN* (e.g. NSF, vesicular ATPase, synaptogyrin), GABA (e.g. GAD_{67}), and glutamate (e.g. AMPA2) genes identified in our initial study. However, perhaps because the specific genes constituting these groups in this study were different and smaller in number than those used in our study, significant effects at the level of gene groups were not observed.

The impact that the genes represented on the arrays can have on the outcome of a study may also be reflected in a study using a different platform, the Affymetrix GeneChip. Investigators from the Mt Sinai group reported deficient expression of six genes whose protein products are thought to play important roles in myelination (Hakak *et al.*, 2001). Consistent with these observations, we found reduced expression of proteolipid protein 1 (PLP1) across the majority of subjects with schizophrenia (Pongrac *et al.*, 2002). This PLP1 expression deficit did not appear to be related to antipsychotic medication since it was not found in haloperidol-treated monkeys. PLP1 appears to have a dual function, participating in both glial cell development and the assembly of myelin (Schneider *et al.*, 1992). These deficits in myelin-related genes also raise the interesting question of the possible factors that may account for such an alteration in the transcriptome. Although such deficits are frequently discussed as evidence of alterations in transcription, they may be caused by more fundamental problems. For example, the Mt Sinai group has also observed a decreased number of glial cells in layer 3 and the underlying white matter in area 9 of subjects with schizophrenia (Hof *et al.*, 2003), suggesting that the reduction in myelin-related transcripts may be the consequence of a process that leads to decreased numbers of oligodendrocytes.

Another major study, using a custom-made candidate gene array comprising 300 genes, found upregulated expression of members of the apo L lipoprotein family (apo L1, apo L2 and apo L4, which play a central role in cholesterol transport) in several independent cohorts of subjects with schizophrenia (Mimmack *et al.*, 2002). Although the function of apo L proteins in the brain is unknown, the findings are of particular interest given that the genes for apo L proteins are located on chromosome 22q12, a susceptibility locus for schizophrenia (Waterworth *et al.*, 2002).

Conclusions and future directions

The application of transcriptome-based methods to studies of the molecular neuropathology of schizophrenia are clearly in their infancy, and like newborns they offer great promise for the future. However, careful rearing is essential to fulfill this promise. Ongoing improvements in the number of genes represented on arrays, in the sensitivity for detecting rare transcripts within samples and subtle differences between samples, and for the statistical management of data mining and interpretation are certain to advance the field. In addition, single cells of defined phenotypes from the diseased brain can now also be analyzed for complex gene expression patterns in a high-throughput fashion. Using laser-capture dissection or sharp electrode harvest of identified single cells, members of a subclass of cells can be pooled and analyzed using high-throughput genomic techniques (Hemby *et al.*, 2002; Kamme *et al.*, 2003; Luo *et al.*, 1999). The characterization of gene expression patterns in neuronal populations defined by a shared axonal projection target and/or electrophysiological properties will advance our understanding of specific neuronal phenotypes by placing them in the context of circuits and neural networks, and thus inform how transcriptome alterations may contribute to the disturbances in brain functions that are manifest as schizophrenia.

Acknowledgements

The interactions between our laboratories that are reflected in this chapter were supported by NIMH Conte Center Grant MH45156 and by MH43784.

REFERENCES

Akbarian, S., Kim, J. J., Potkin, S. G., *et al.* (1995). Gene expression for glutamic acid decarboxylase is reduced without loss of neurons in prefrontal cortex of schizophrenics. *Arch Gen Psychiatry* **52**: 258–266.

Arnold, S. E., Trojanowski, J. Q., Gur, R. E., *et al.* (1998). Absence of neurodegeneration and neural injury in the cerebral cortex in a sample of elderly patients with schizophrenia. *Arch Gen Psychiatry* **55**: 225–232.

Berman, K. F., Zec, R. F., Weinberger, D. R. (1986). Physiological dysfunction of dorsolateral prefrontal cortex in schizophrenia. II. Role of neuroleptic treatment, attention and mental effort. *Arch Gen Psychiatry* **43**: 126–135.

Branca, M. (2003). Genetics and medicine: putting gene arrays to the test. *Science* **300**: 238.

Brown, P. O., Bottenstein, D. (1999). Exploring the new world of the genome with DNA microarrays. *Nat Genet* **21S**: 33–37.

Brzustowicz, L. M., Hodgkinson, K. A., Chow, E. W. C., Honer, W. G., Bassett, A. S. (2000). Location of a major susceptibility locus for familial schizophrenia on chromosome 1q21–q22. *Science* **288**: 678–682.

Buchsbaum, M. S., Haier, R. J., Potkin, S. G., *et al.* (1992). Frontrostriatal disorder of cerebral metabolism in never-medicated schizophrenics. *Arch Gen Psychiatry* **49**: 935–942.

Burrone, J., O'Byren, M., Murthy, V. N. (2002). Multiple forms of synaptic plasticity triggered by selective suppression of activity in individual neurons. *Nature* **420**: 414–418.

Cheung, V. G., Morley, M., Aguilar, F., *et al.* (1999). Making and reading microarrays. *Nat Genet* **21S**: 20–32.

Chowdari, K. V., Mirnics, K., Semwal, P., *et al.* (2002). Association and linkage analyses of *RGS4* polymorphisms in schizophrenia. *Hum Mol Genet* **11**: 1373–1380.

DeRisi, J., Iyer, V. R., Brown, P. O. (1997). Exploring the metabolic and genetic control of gene expression on a genomic scale. *Science* **278**: 680–686.

DeRisi, J., Penland, L., Brown, P. O., *et al.* (1996). Use of a cDNA microarray to analyse gene expression patterns in human cancer. *Nat Genet* **14**: 457–460.

De Vries, L., Zheng, B., Fischer, T., Elenko, E., Farquhar, M. G. (2000). The regulator of G protein signaling family. *Annu Rev Pharmacol Toxicol* **40**: 235–271.

Duggan, D. J., Bittner, M., Chen, Y., Meltzer, P., Trent, J. M. (1999). Expression profiling using cDNA microarrays. *Nat Genet* **21S**: 10–14.

Eastwood, S. L., McDonald, B., Burnet, P. W. J., *et al.* (1995). Decreased expression of mRNAs encoding non-NMDA glutamate receptors GluR1 and GluR2 in medial temporal lobe neurons in schizophrenia. *Mol Brain Res* **29**: 211–223.

Glantz, L. A., Lewis, D. A. (1997). Reduction of synaptophysin immunoreactivity in the prefrontal cortex of subjects with schizophrenia: regional and diagnostic specificity. *Arch Gen Psychiatry* **54**: 943–952.

   (2000). Decreased dendritic spine density on prefrontal cortical pyramidal neurons in schizophrenia. *Arch Gen Psychiatry* **57**: 65–73.

Hakak, Y., Walker, J. R., Li, C., *et al.* (2001). Genome-wide expression analysis reveals dysregulation of myelination-related genes in chronic schizophrenia. *Proc Natl Acad Sci USA* **98**: 4746–4751.

Harrison, P. J., Heath, P. R., Eastwood, S. L., *et al.* (1995). The relative importance of premortem acidosis and postmortem interval for human brain gene expression studies: selective mRNA vulnerability and comparison with their encoded proteins. *Neurosci Lett* **200**: 151–154.

Hashimoto, T., Volk, D. W., Buchheit, S. E., Lewis, D. A. (2002). Expression of BDNF and trkB mRNAs in prefrontal cortex of subjects with schizophrenia. *Soc Neurosci Abstr* **28**: 703.7.

Hashimoto, T., Volk, D. W., Eggan, S. M., *et al.* (2003). Gene expression deficits in a subclass of GABA neurons in the prefrontal cortex of subjects with schizophrenia. *J Neurosci* **23**: 6315–6326.

Hemby, S. E., Ginsberg, S. D., Brunk, B., *et al.* (2002). Gene expression profile for schizophrenia: discrete neuron transcription patterns in the entorhinal cortex. *Arch Gen Psychiatry* **59**: 631–640.

Hof, P. R., Haroutunian, V., Friedrich, Jr., V. L., *et al.* (2003). Loss and altered spatial distribution of oligodendrocytes in the superior frontal gyrus in schizophrenia. *Biol Psychiatry* **53**: 1075–1085.

Huttenlocher, P. R. (1979). Synaptic density in human frontal cortex: developmental changes and effects of aging. *Brain Res* **163**: 195–205.

Kamme, F., Salunga, R., Yu, J., *et al.* (2003). Single-cell microarray analysis in hippocampus CA1: demonstration and validation of cellular heterogeneity. *J Neurosci* **23**: 3607–3615.

Lewis, D. A. (2002). The human brain revisited: opportunities and challenges in postmortem studies of psychiatric disorders. *Neuropsychopharmacology* **26**: 143–154.

Lewis, D. A., Levitt, P. (2002). Schizophrenia as a disorder of neurodevelopment. *Annu Rev Neurosci* **25**: 409–432.

Lewis, D. A., Lieberman, J. A. (2000). Catching up on schizophrenia: natural history and neurobiology. *Neuron* **28**: 325–334.

Lidow, M. S., Goldman-Rakic, P. S., Rakic, P., Innis, R. B. (1989). Dopamine D(2) receptors in the cerebral cortex: distribution and pharmacological characterization with [(3)H]raclopride. *Proc Natl Acad Sci USA* **86**: 6412–6416.

Lipshutz, R. J., Fodor, S. P. A., Gingeras, T. R., Lockhart, D. J. (1999). High density synthetic oligonucleotide arrays. *Nat Genet* **21S**: 20–24.

Lockhart, D. J., Barlow, C. (2001). DNA arrays and gene expression analysis in the brain. In *Methods in Genomic Neuroscience*, ed. H. R. Chin, S. Moldin. New York: CRC Press, pp. 143–170.

Lockhart, D. J., Dong, H., Byrne, M. C., *et al.* (1996). Expression monitoring by hybridization to high-density oligonucleotide arrays. *Nat Biotechnol* **14**: 1675–1680.

Luo, L., Salunga, R. C., Guo, H., *et al.* (1999). Gene expression profiles of laser-captured adjacent neuronal subtypes. *Nat Med* **5**: 117–122.

Middleton, F. A., Mirnics, K., Pierri, J. N., Lewis, D. A., Levitt, P. (2002). Gene expression profiling reveals alterations of specific metabolic pathways in schizophrenia. *J Neurosci* **22**: 2718–2729.

Mimmack, M. L., Ryan, M., Baba, H., *et al.* (2002). Gene expression analysis in schizophrenia: reproducible up-regulation of several members of the apolipoprotein L family located in a high-susceptibility locus for schizophrenia on chromosome 22. *Proc Natl Acad Sci USA* **99**: 4680–4685.

Mirnics, K., Middleton, F. A., Marquez, A., Lewis, D. A., Levitt, P. (2000). Molecular characterization of schizophrenia viewed by microarray analysis of gene expression in prefrontal cortex. *Neuron* **28**: 53–67.

Mirnics, K., Middleton, F. A., Stanwood, G. D., Lewis, D. A., Levitt, P. (2001a). Disease-specific changes in regulator of G-protein signaling 4 (RGS4) expression in schizophrenia. *Mol Psychiatry* **6**: 293–301.

Mirnics, K., Middleton, F. A., Lewis, D. A., Levitt, P. (2001b). Analysis of complex brain disorders with gene expression microarrays: schizophrenia as a disease of the synapse. *Trends Neurosci* **24**: 479–486.

Pongrac, J., Middleton, F. A., Lewis, D. A., Levitt, P., Mirnics, K. (2002). Gene expression profiling with DNA microarrays: advancing our understanding of psychiatric disorders. *Neurochem Res* **27**: 1049–1063.

Rakic, P., Bourgeois, J. P., Eckenhoff, M. F., Zecevic, N., Goldman-Rakic, P. S. (1986). Concurrent overproduction of synapses in diverse regions of the primate cerebral cortex. *Science* **232**: 232–235.

Schena, M., Davis, R. W. (1999). Microgenes, genomes and chips. In *DNA Microarrays: A Practical Approach*, ed. M. Schena. Oxford: Oxford University Press, pp. 1–16.

Schena, M., Shalon, D., Davis, R. W., Brown, P. O. (1995). Quantitative monitoring of gene expression patterns with a complementary DNA microarray. *Science* **270**: 467–470.

Schena, M., Shalon, D., Heller, R., *et al.* (1996). Parallel human genome analysis: microarray-based expression monitoring of 1000 genes. *Proc Natl Acad Sci USA* **93**: 10614–10619.

Schneider, A., Montague, P., Griffiths, I., *et al.* (1992). Uncoupling of hypomyelination and glial cell death by a mutation in the proteolipid protein gene. *Nature* **358**: 758–761.

Sklar, P. (2001). Microarray analysis of the Stanley brain collection. Abstract. In *7th Symposium on the Neurobiology and Neuroimmunology of Schizophrenia and Bipolar Disorder*. Washington, DC: *Stanley Foundation.*

Southern, E., Mir, K., Shchepinov, M. (1999). Molecular interactions on microarrays. *Nat Genet* **21**: 5–9.

Vawter, M. P., Barrett, T., Cheadle, C., *et al.* (2001). Application of cDNA microarrays to examine gene expression differences in schizophrenia. *Res Bull* **55**: 641–650.

Vawter, M. P., Crook, J. M., Hyde, T. M., *et al.* (2002). Microarray analysis of gene expression in the prefrontal cortex in schizophrenia: a preliminary study. *Schizophr Res* **58**: 11–20.

Volk, D. W., Austin, M. C., Pierri, J. N., Sampson, A. R., Lewis, D. A. (2000). Decreased GAD_{67} mRNA expression in a subset of prefrontal cortical GABA neurons in subjects with schizophrenia. *Arch Gen Psychiatry* **57**: 237–245.

Waterworth, D. M., Bassett, A. S., Brzustowicz, L. M. (2002). Recent advances in the genetics of schizophrenia. *Cell Mol Life Sci* **59**: 331–348.

Weickert, C. S., Hyde, T. M., Lipska, B. K., *et al.* (2003). Reduced brain-derived neurotrophic factor in prefrontal cortex of patients with schizophrenia. *Mol Psychiatry* **8**: 592–610.

13

Is there a role for social factors in a comprehensive developmental model for schizophrenia?

Jane Boydell[1], Jim van Os[2], and Robin M. Murray[1]

[1] Institute of Psychiatry King's College London, UK
[2] Maastricht University, Maastricht, the Netherlands

In the 1950s and 1960s, there was much extravagant discussion of the role of social factors in the etiology of schizophrenia. However, there was little scientific basis to this speculation, and it was swept away by the demonstration that people with schizophrenia showed abnormalities of brain structure on computed tomographic scans (Johnstone *et al.*, 1976). A decade later, the neurodevelopmental model of schizophrenia was proposed, and it subsequently became the dominant etiological and pathogenetic model (Murray and Fearon, 1999; Murray *et al.*, 1992). As a result of these two developments, researchers have come to regard schizophrenia as a brain disease, and social factors have been largely ignored as putative etiological agents.

It is increasingly clear, however, that the neurodevelopmental model, an essentially neurological concept, does not explain all the available data about schizophrenia. One consequence has been a revival during the 1990s, particularly in Europe, of research into the role of social factors as causal agents in schizophrenia. It is opportune, therefore, to draw together this disparate research and to examine critically whether any of it stands up to scientific scrutiny. We will review both those social factors that are postulated to operate early in life and those which may act more proximal to the onset of the disorder (see Table 13.1 for an overview). First we will briefly consider how animal research has informed on psychiatric conditions.

Animal models of isolation rearing and social stress

Brain development is to an important degree dependent on experience (Wiesel and Hubel, 1974); conversely, altered brain development can influence the way individuals interact with their environment (Fishbein, 2000). Some of the strongest

Neurodevelopment and Schizophrenia, ed. Matcheri S. Keshavan *et al.* Published by Cambridge University Press. © Cambridge University Press 2004.

Table 13.1. Selected social risk factors for schizophrenia

Risk factor	Measure of effect	Effect size (95% CI)	Outcome	Type of study	Author
Unwanted child	OR	2.4 (1.2–4.8)	DSM III-R schizophrenia	Birth cohort	Myhrman et al. (1996)
Poor mothering	OR	2.65 (1.2–5.6)	Schizophreniform disorders DSM IV	Birth cohort	Cannon et al. (2002)
Early parental loss	OR	3.8*	DSM III-R schizophrenia	Case–control	Agid et al. (1999)
Childhood abuse	OR	7.3 (1.1–49)	Positive psychotic symptoms reaching clinical significance	Population cohort	Janssen et al. (2003)
City birth	RR	2.4 (2.13–2.7)	ICD 8 schizophrenia	Population cohort	Mortensen et al. (1999)
City upbringing	RR	2.75 (2.31–3.28)	ICD 8 schizophrenia	Population cohort	Pedersen and Mortensen (2001)
Ethnic minority status	IRR	4.4 (2.49–7.75)	RDC Schizophrenia	Ecological	Boydell et al. (2001)
Racial harassment (verbal abuse)	OR	2.86 (1.69–4.83)	Psychosis diagnosed by semistructured interview	Cross-sectional	Karlsen and Nazroo (2002)

CI, confidence interval; OR, odds ratio; RR, relative risk; IRR, incidence rate ratio; DSM III-R, *Diagnostic and Statistical Manual III–Revised*; ICD, *International Statistical Classification of Diseases, Injuries, and Causes of Death*.
* $p = 0.001$.

evidence for the role of social factors in brain development has come from animal experiments. For example, there is ample evidence that rats reared in isolation for a period after birth have structural and physiological differences in their hippocampi compared with rats reared in groups (Whitaker-Azmitia et al., 2000). Isolation reared rats also show behavioral changes, anxiety, learning deficits, and sensory changes. Furthermore, Matthews et al. (2001) found increased levels of dopamine in the dorsal and ventral striatum in adult rats who were separated from their mothers early in life. There is also evidence that rats reared in isolation, but not other rats, respond to antipsychotic drugs in such a way as to normalize their behavior (Heidbreder et al., 2001).

Therefore, by analogy, these data suggest that the social factors in the environment of the developing child may similarly affect physical brain development. These factors are now being revisited by psychiatric researchers searching for the brain–environment interactions that shape vulnerability to conditions such as psychosis. For example, experiences embedded in social relationships may alter the prefrontal brain systems that mediate emotional self-regulation (Lyons *et al.*, 2002); similarly, the early social environment appears to program aspects of neurobiological development that, in turn, affect behavioral, emotional, cognitive, and physiological development (Sanchez *et al.*, 2001). The early social environment has been shown to induce synaptic changes that may be indicative, and perhaps the cause, of alterations of behavioral and cognitive capacities (Ovtscharoff and Braun, 2001).

Although much of this work comes from animal research, there is evidence that the early social environment can mediate the establishment of neural networks that regulate a child's response to stress and capacity for self-control (DiPietro, 2000). Furthermore, studies of exposure to institutional deprivation have shown dramatic effects on a range of child behavioral outcomes, with clear dose–response relationships between adverse outcomes and length of exposure (Beckett *et al.*, 2002). As Eisenberg (1995) states "The human brain is constructed socially."

Family factors

Mother–child relationship

The British 1946 cohort study followed up all children (5362) born in 1 week in the UK. By age 43, there were 30 cases of schizophrenia. The quality of the mother-child relationship at 4 years of age, as rated by health visitors, was one of the most powerful risk factors for later schizophrenia; a poor relationship (less skilled and less understanding of the child) carried a sixfold increase in risk of schizophrenia (Jones *et al.*, 1994). Similarly, the Dunedin study (Cannon *et al.*, 2002), which followed up about 1000 children from birth to age 26 with comprehensive medical and psychiatric assessments, found that the mothers of children who developed schizophreniform disorders were rated as having poorer attitudes and behavior towards their children at age 3 (odds ratio [OR], 2.65; 95% confidence interval [CI], 1.2–5.6).

The British 1946 and the Dunedin studies are particularly interesting as they are population-based and not high-risk studies. However, we do not know the direction of the relationship. Is the increased risk an effect of poor mothering or is it that the preschizophrenic child could not form a normal relationship with the mother?

Unwantedness

Several studies have claimed that being an unwanted child is associated with emotional and social deprivation (Kubicka *et al.*, 1995; Myhrman, 1992). Myhrman *et al.* (1996), therefore, investigated whether unwantedness of pregnancy was a risk factor for schizophrenia in the child as defined in the Diagnostic and Statistical

Manual III (DSM III-R; American Psychiatric Association, 1987). Their sample was the Northern Finland 1966 Birth Cohort, which comprised 11 017 individuals who were followed up until they were 28. Their mothers had been asked by a midwife (when 6 or 7 months pregnant) whether the pregnancy was wanted, mistimed but wanted, or unwanted. The risk of schizophrenia among the unwanted group was considerably raised even after adjusting for sociodemographic, pregnancy (including depression), and perinatal variables (OR, 2.4; 95% CI, 1.2–4.8). Unfortunately, genetic risk was not considered in the study and, as with much social research, there may have been residual confounding.

Family communication deviance

In the 1950s, several research groups (Bateson *et al.*, 1956; Lidz, 1958; Wynne *et al.*, 1958) claimed that communication deviance in parents of people with schizophrenia had a causal role in the development of the disorder. However, Hirsch and Leff (1975), who comprehensively reviewed this work, were not convinced by the methodology used in much of it. Furthermore, most authorities have considered that, if such abnormalities do exist, they reflect an expression of genetic loading rather than independent causal factors. One recent study, however, has suggested that family communication deviance may be of etiological importance. Wahlberg *et al.* (1997, 2000) found a significant interaction between high genetic risk for schizophrenia and communication deviance in their adoptive parents. The high risk but not the control adoptees showed greater evidence of thought disorder if their adoptive parents showed communication deviance. This provocative claim awaits replication, and the reader could be forgiven for being skeptical given the previous history of research on this topic.

Dysfunctional family environment

In the Finnish Adoptive Family Study, the risk of developing schizophrenia spectrum disorders was higher in those adopted-away offspring of schizophrenia parents who were exposed to a dysfunctional adoptive family-rearing environment (Tienari, 1991). The most recent report from this study suggests that the adopted-away offspring may have lower risk than children who remain with their schizophrenia parents (Tienari *et al.*, 2000). Similarly, the Danish–American adoption studies suggested that the high-risk adopted-away offspring had a lower chance of later developing schizophrenia than those who remained with their biological parents (Rosenthal *et al.*, 1971).

Communal upbringing

In the Israeli High Risk Study, Mirsky *et al.* (1985) carried out a follow-up study of 46 children with high genetic risk, half of whom were brought up communally on a kibbutz (where their parents lived) and half in family homes, and compared them with controls. Children with known genetic risk for schizophrenia were significantly more likely to develop a psychotic disorder and, interestingly, also an affective disorder if they were brought up on a kibbutz, rather than a family home. The control kibbutz children did not have a higher risk (although the numbers were small), suggesting genetic vulnerability to the social environment in the high-risk children. Similar findings emerged from the Copenhagen High Risk Project, which followed up 207 high-risk children and compared them with controls (Mednick *et al.*, 1987). The high-risk children who had been separated from their parents were either brought up in public care institutions or foster placements with families. The latter group had a better outcome (especially for males) but of course the placement was not random. Nevertheless, these two high-risk studies are among the few studies into social factors during childhood that are less likely to have been confounded by the inherited characteristics of the child.

Early parental loss

Another aspect of childhood that has been examined is parental loss through death or separation. Agid *et al.* (1999), in a case–control study, found that permanent parental loss before the age of 8 years was significantly associated with later schizophrenia (OR, 4.3), particular for loss of the mother (OR, 6). The association was stronger for parental death than separation, making confounding less likely as an explanation for the findings. The DSM III-R diagnoses were based on structured interviews, making misdiagnosis less likely. Similarly, Mallett *et al.* (2002) found that separation from both parents in childhood distinguished UK African–Caribbean subjects with schizophrenia from African–Caribbean controls (OR, 5; 95% CI, 1.09 22.82).

Expressed emotion

It is well known that social overstimulation (Wing, 1978) and high expressed emotion within families (Vaughn and Leff, 1976, 1982) are associated with relapse in schizophrenia. Some assume that these factors are also implicated in the first episode (Wing, 1978). As far as we are aware, there is no evidence to support or refute this.

Childhood abuse

Several investigators have claimed an association between trauma and psychosis (Read *et al.*, 2001). First, studies of patients with psychosis have demonstrated that they recall a high incidence of trauma in their lifetimes (Ross *et al.*, 1994), and those who experience positive symptoms of schizophrenia are especially likely to give a history of childhood trauma (Ellason and Ross, 1997; Ross *et al.*, 1994). Conversely, patients who give a history of abuse are particularly likely to experience positive symptoms (Heins *et al.*, 1990; Sansonnet-Hayden *et al.*, 1987). In a recent study, childhood abuse was a significant predictor of hallucinations, even in the absence of adult abuse (Read *et al.*, 2003).

Second, in patients with other diagnoses, such as bipolar disorder (Hammersley *et al.*, 2003; Read and Argyle, 1999) or post-traumatic shock disorder (Butler *et al.*, 1996), a history of child abuse has also been found to "cooccur" with a high frequency of auditory hallucinations and delusions. Dissociative identity disorder, which is assumed to be a disturbance resulting from severe childhood abuse (Putnam *et al.*, 1986), may present with Schneiderian first rank symptoms, particularly in the form of auditory hallucinations (Ross *et al.*, 1989). It has even been suggested that, of all diagnostic categories, psychosis displays the strongest associations with child abuse (Bryer *et al.*, 1987; Swett *et al.*, 1990).

The experience of abuse may create a biological (Read *et al.*, 2001) or psychological (Garety *et al.*, 2001) vulnerability for the development of psychotic symptoms, including subclinical psychotic experiences such as low-grade delusional ideation and isolated auditory hallucinations (Johns and van Os, 2001). In the general population, childhood sexual abuse is related to schizotypy, including perceptual aberrations (Startup, 1999), which are 10 times more common in adults who were maltreated as children (Berenbaum, 1999). In both clinical and non-clinical populations, the diagnostic group with the highest rate of childhood abuse consistently reported the most Schneiderian symptoms (Ross and Joshi, 1992). In a population-based cross-sectional study, Bebbington (2003) found increased odds of psychosis (diagnosed by semistructured interview) in those reporting childhood sexual abuse and other forms of trauma. Therefore, several studies have now found evidence for an association between abuse and psychotic experiences in non-clinical samples (Ross and Joshi, 1992; Startup, 1999).

The difficulty with almost all of the above studies is that they are cross-sectional in nature and rely on psychotic people giving an accurate picture of their childhood. However, there have been attempts to go beyond such bias-prone studies. For example, in a recent 3 year longitudinal study of a general population sample of 4045 subjects aged 18–64 years with no previous lifetime presence of psychotic or psychosis-like symptoms, baseline reported childhood abuse predicted development of clinically relevant positive psychotic symptoms associated with need for care (OR, 11.5; 95% CI, 2.6–51.6). This association remained after adjustment for demographic variables, a range of other reported risk factors, and presence of any lifetime psychiatric diagnosis at baseline (OR, 7.3; 95% CI, 1.1–49.0) (Janssen *et al.*, 2004).

The urban effect

City birth

Many studies have found an increased incidence of schizophrenia in cities (e.g. Farris and Dunham, 1939). For decades it was suggested that this could be because people at higher risk or in the early stages of schizophrenia moved into the city (social drift). Now several studies have shown a significant effect for urban birth and/or urban upbringing (Allardyce *et al.*, 2001; Lewis *et al.*, 1992; Marcelis *et al.*, 1998, 1999). One of the most impressive was carried out by Mortensen *et al.* (1999), who investigated the effect of place on risk of admission with schizophrenia, as defined by the *International Statistical Classification of Diseases, Injuries and Causes of Death* (ICD) 8 (World Health Organization, 1967), in a large Danish population-based cohort of 1.75 million. The relative risk associated with birth in Copenhagen compared with birth in rural areas was 2.40 (95% CI, 2.13–2.7), and there was a clear dose–response relationship for urbanicity in that the larger the town of birth, the greater the risk. A family history of schizophrenia did not explain or affect the results. Indeed, Mortensen and colleagues (1999) calculated that the population attributable fraction for urban birth was 34.6% (which compared with 9% and 7%, respectively, for having a mother or father who had schizophrenia). Therefore, the effect of urban birth was much larger than the effect of having a parent affected (though we should point out that having an affected parent does not equate with genetic predisposition).

City upbringing

It is important but very difficult to separate place of birth and place of upbringing. Astrup and Odegard (1961) found a stronger effect of city upbringing amongst those who had moved to the city. A recent analysis of the Danish population cohort just described has now addressed this question. Pedersen and Mortensen (2001) used a comprehensive national registration system that accurately recorded every change of residence to show that schizophrenia risk increased with the number of years (between 0 and 20 years of age) that an individual lived in an urbanized area, and with increasing degree of urbanization. Relative risk for those who had spent their entire childhood in the capital was 2.75 (95% CI, 2.31–3.28) compared with those who had always lived in the most rural areas. There was no evidence that urbanicity was particularly toxic for any particular age group. The dose–response relationship found in this study suggests that etiological factors of a pervasive and long-term (either continuous or repeated) nature are operating in urbanized areas.

Social drift and social residue theories

When considering the effect of urbanization, we cannot totally discount the effects of "social drift": people with pre- or prodromal schizophrenia move into urban areas. However, this effect cannot account for the results of recent studies that looked at place of birth and upbringing. For example, Dauncey and colleagues (1993) investigated where patients had lived 5 years before their first admission in Nottingham, UK and were unable to find evidence for systematic geographic drift. Furthermore, it is unlikely that the drift occurred in the previous parental generation, as the magnitude of this movement would need to have been extremely high to explain the findings. For example, in the Danish study, Mortensen and colleagues (1999) calculated that nearly 50 000 children born in the capital and its suburbs needed to have a parent who transmitted a genetic risk equal to that transmitted by a parent with diagnosed schizophrenia to account for the urban excess. Furthermore, a family history of schizophrenia did not explain or effect the urban–rural difference in this and other studies (van Os *et al.*, 2002). This is also relevant for the social residue theory (that those at greater risk are left behind in an area as it becomes less desirable because they do not have the resources to move out).

Possible explanations

No adequate explanation has been found for the urban excess of schizophrenia. Infectious agents were once considered likely etiological factors but they are unlikely to account for much of the risk-increasing effect, given the fact that the urban environment is not only associated with increased rates of schizophrenia but also with increases in much more prevalent expressions of non-clinical psychotic experiences (van Os *et al.*, 2001). Other physical factors associated with city living such as lead pollution require further investigation. However, while there is no direct evidence that the urban excess is caused by social factors, the fact that its effect is so widespread across the population is compatible with the notion that part of the excess risk represents a psychological reaction to factors in the wider social environment. Certainly some of the major differences between urban and rural areas are to do with social cohesion and social support. For example, it has been shown that the physical and mental health of children growing up in an urban environment is adversely influenced by low levels of social cohesion in the neighborhood (Drukker *et al.*, 2003), and within the city, the incidence of schizophrenia has been shown to vary as a function of the social neighborhood environment (van Os *et al.*, 2000).

Although the evidence for an early effect is strong, there may also be an effect of urbanization around the time of onset for non-early-onset schizophrenia and there is evidence of a cumulative effect of urban exposure throughout childhood (Castle *et al.*, 1993). As we will see below, social isolation, deprivation, and adverse life events are associated with increased risk of psychosis. As individuals in big cities may be more likely to be exposed to these factors (Takano and Nakamura, 2001), it is possible that some of the urban excess might be attributed to such factors. However, it is likely that the social factors that increase the risk do not act independently of genetic risk, and a recent report suggested that the urban environment acts by increasing the likelihood that schizophrenia is expressed in those who carry genetic susceptibility (van Os *et al.*, 2003).

Social isolation

During childhood

Numerous reports from Bleuler onwards have shown that children destined to develop schizophrenia tend to be solitary, lack friends, and indeed often prefer to be alone. For example, the British 1946 cohort study of Jones *et al.* (1994), described above, found that preference for solitary play at age 4 and 6 was associated with later schizophrenia (OR, 2.1 and 2.5, respectively). Self-reported anxiety at age 13 and teacher-rated anxiety at age 15 both showed linear associations with later risk for schizophrenia (Jones *et al.*, 1994).

Moving schools in adolescence

A fascinating finding to emerge from the Danish study of Pedersen and Mortensen (2001), discussed above, was that change in municipality (and, therefore, school) increased risk of schizophrenia whereas change of address during childhood within the municipality (usually, therefore, without changing school) was not associated with increased risk. Moves during early teenage years appeared to have the greatest effect, and the more the moves, the greater was the risk. It is possible that the social stress of having to seek out and join a new peer group, or perhaps not being able to join a peer group, adversely affected the childrens' social development.

In young adult life

The Swedish conscript study also looked at the role of premorbid personality at a later stage of development. This study examined a cohort of 50 087 army conscripts (approximately 98% of the entire male population born in Sweden 1949 to 1950). The investigators adjusted for family history of psychiatric illness, intelligence quotient (IQ), city upbringing and diagnosis of non-psychotic disorder at conscription. There was a significantly increased risk of later developing schizophrenia in young men who felt they were more sensitive than their peers, had fewer than two close friends, preferred small groups, and did not have a girl friend (OR, 2.38, 1.7, 2.05, and 3.48, respectively); there was also a risk, to a lesser extent, for other psychoses (Malmberg *et al.*, 1998). Once again, this raises the question of whether these are an expression of a schizoid or schizotypal personality or whether they are in themselves independent risk factors. Until proven otherwise, it is wise to consider that both may be true: individuals with a schizoid or schizotypal personality may be less able to make social relationships, and then the social isolation itself may propel them further toward frank psychosis.

At time of onset

Hare (1956) reported that social isolation, as measured by proportion of single person households in a geographical area, was associated with increased rates of schizophrenia. The findings were not accounted for by movement of people with, or developing, schizophrenia into the area. There has been a recent resurgence of interest in these findings. Thornicroft *et al.* (1993) noted that clustering of individuals with schizophrenia in deprived areas occurs only in urban areas and suggested that social isolation is an important mediator of this. However, it is difficult to distinguish between cause and effect in this context. Related to these ideas is the theory that disruption of social networks decreases an individual's capacity to cope with psychosocial stress and increases the risk of schizophrenia.

Van Os *et al.* (2000) found that people who were single had a slightly higher risk of developing psychosis if they lived in a neighborhood with fewer single people compared with a neighborhood with many other single people. The authors suggested that single status might give rise to perceived (or actual) social isolation if most other people are living with a partner. The question of whether social isolation may increase risk of schizophrenia (or whether a close relationship may be protective) is also raised by Jablensky and Cole (1997), who showed that marriage had a protective effect and that this was not simply a consequence of better adjusted males being able to marry.

Migration and ethnic minority status

As early as 1932, Ødegård (1932) showed that Norwegian migrants to the USA had an increased risk of psychosis. One early interpretation was that this resulted from selective migration; those at risk, less connected with their families, are more likely to leave their homeland. An alternative was that the crucial factor was the alienation and suspicion engendered in the migrant by their unfamiliar surroundings. Ødegård (1932) wrote:

Everywhere you are surrounded by people with strange and unfamiliar ways. . . . They do not seem to be as friendly as the people at home and many of them do their best to profit by your lack of experience. Even if you have not had any disagreeable experiences yourself, your imagination is stirred by all the stories you have heard about how crooked and dangerous they may be. You notice that your own appearance, clothing and language points you out to everyone as a greenhorn.

Studies from different countries and continents have now shown that the incidence of psychosis is high amongst many migrant groups (Castle *et al.*, 1991;

Harrison *et al.*, 1988, 1997; King *et al.*, 1994; Murphy, 1977; Selten and Sijben, 1994; Selten *et al.*, 1998, 2001; Thomas *et al.*, 1993; van Os *et al.*, 1996a,b). Even when migration between very similar cultures is considered, there is still evidence of an increased risk. For example, Bruxner *et al.* (1997) found higher rates of hospital admission with psychosis in British, Irish and southern European migrants to West. Australia; the risk persisted many years after migration.

Methodological issues

There are many methodological pitfalls in migration and minority group research, for example the "category fallacy" (that the categories of mental illness used in one culture cannot be applied to another), misdiagnosis (whether psychiatrists in the host country may wrongly diagnose schizophrenia in migrants because of prejudice or a lack of understanding of their cultural norms), or inaccurate estimation of the denominator (migrants may be under-represented in general population data). However, studies that have overcome these problems have still found an excess of psychosis among migrant groups (Hickling *et al.*, 1999; Mortensen *et al.*, 1997; Sharpley *et al.*, 2001; van Os *et al.*, 1996a,b; Wessely *et al.*, 1991).

Increased rates of schizophrenia amongst migrants and ethnic minorities might also be attributed (at least in part) to the urban effect, as most migrants live in cities and often in the most deprived areas. However, Malzberg (1969) found that controlling for urbanicity reduced but did not explain the excess of psychosis amongst migrants to the USA, and similar findings were reported more recently in the Netherlands (van Os *et al.*, 2001)

African-Caribbeans in the UK

Most work has investigated the increased rates of psychosis in the African-Caribbeans in the UK and the Netherlands. Genetic predisposition cannot be the sole explanation since the increased risk is not shared by the population of origin in the Caribbean (Bhugra *et al.*, 1997; Mahy *et al.*, 1999); in addition the morbid risk for second-generation siblings is much higher than for their first-generation equivalents (Hutchinson *et al.*, 1996; Sugarman and Crawford, 1994). Selective migration has also been largely ruled out. For example, Selten *et al.* (2002) found that, even if the entire Surinamese population had migrated to the Netherlands, this still would not account for the absolute number of cases amongst Surinam migrants unless the incidence had increased. Increased exposure, or susceptibility, to neurodevelopmental insult such as obstetric complications (Glover, 1989; Hutchinson *et al.*, 1997) and viral infections (Selten *et al.*, 1998) have largely been excluded as possible explanations. McGuire *et al.* (1995) found no difference in drug abuse between their white and African- Caribbean patients in South London. Similarly, Selten *et al.* (1997) found that consumption of cannabis was lower amongst

Caribbean migrants to the Netherlands than amongst the native population, but their incidence rate of schizophrenia was higher.

The second generation

There are now several studies showing higher rates of schizophrenia in the children of migrants. This phenomenon has been described when the migration took place in very different circumstances. Children born in Greenland to Danish mothers, in the study described above, had a relative risk of 3.71 for schizophrenia (Mortensen et al., 1999). Malzberg (1969) found that English-born migrants to the USA had lower rates than the native USA-born individuals but the second generation (i.e. children of English-born migrants) had higher rates than both the native born and their own parents. Some studies suggest that second-generation (i.e. children of) migrants from the Caribbean to the UK seem to have higher rates than the first generation (Harrison et al., 1988).

A natural experiment occurred when the entire population of Yemenite Jews migrated to Israel as they were in danger in the Yemen and they believed the Messianic Era had begun. The adults did not integrate into Israeli society and their lifestyle was considered primitive. Weingarten and Orren, 1983 found a high prevalence of schizophrenia among their offspring. Children who had been born in the Yemen and those who were born in Israel both seem to have been at higher risk. Since the entire population moved to Israel, selective migration cannot account for the findings. This study was small and there might have been an element of social residue (i.e. the more able might have moved out of the area studied). There is no satisfactory explanation as to why there are higher rates of psychosis in children of migrants, but the range of countries and circumstances in which this phenomenon has been described is suggestive of a socially induced phenomenon.

Discrimination

The combination of more affective symptoms and a less-deteriorated course has led to the idea that factors in the social environment might cause psychosis in those migrants predisposed but who might not otherwise develop the disease (McKenzie et al., 1995). Racism (overt and institutionalized), social isolation, and reduced social networks are among the factors that some consider may contribute (Hutchinson et al., 1999). Boydell et al. (2001) have found that incidence rates of schizophrenia increased in ethnic minorities as the proportion of ethnic minorities in the locality fell, suggesting social experience (perhaps of isolation or discrimination) contributes to the development of the disorder.

Janssen et al. (2003) measured subjective experience of discrimination and subsequent development of psychotic illness 3 years later. Experience of discrimination strongly predicted for the development of delusional ideation (OR, 2.3; 95% CI,

1.2–4.2). In another analysis in the same sample, it was shown that the effect of ethnic minority status on psychosis was no longer significant when controlling for experience of discrimination (Janssen *et al.*, 2002). Karlsen and Nazroo (2002) studied the experience of racial harassment and perception of discrimination among a UK representative sample of 5000 people from ethnic minorities. They found significantly increased OR values for a number of health problems but particularly psychosis (experience of verbal abuse OR, 2.86 [95% CI, 1.69–4.83] experience of physical attack OR, 4.77 [95% CI, 2.32–9.8]).

Some people may be more susceptible to the deleterious effects of such events than others because they are less able to derive support from those around them (Sharpley *et al.*, 2001). Mallett *et al.* (1998) demonstrated that one of the main distinguishing features of first-onset patients of Caribbean origin with psychosis in London was that they lived alone and additionally had been separated from their mother at an early age.

Unemployment

Bhugra *et al.* (1997) found that unemployment was particularly high amongst people of Caribbean origin first presenting with schizophrenia in the UK. They then went on to compare the unemployment rates in African-Carribean people presenting with their first episode in London and Trinidad, relative to local unemployment rates. In London, the rate was much higher amongst the patients than in the local population, but this was not the case in Trinidad (Bhugra *et al.*, 2000). It is possible, therefore, that the high unemployment rate amongst African-Caribbeans in London (and subsequent social isolation and stigmatization) might have etiological relevance. Alternatively, the social milieu in Trinidad might be more sympathetic to those at risk of developing schizophrenia.

Life events

The first study to find an association between schizophrenia and life events reported an excess of events limited to 3 weeks before onset (Brown and Birley, 1968). Prospective studies have also found an association between life events and relapse of psychosis (Malla *et al.*, 1990; Ventura *et al.*, 1989). Bebbington (2000) carried out a comprehensive case–control study in London and found a significant excess of events and, importantly, independent life events in the 3 months prior to onset of schizophrenia. Not all studies have concurred however (Chung *et al.*, 1986; Jacobs and Myers, 1976).

There is evidence that the kinds of stress that affect individuals with schizophrenia vulnerability are not so much the major life events but rather the hassles and stress that individuals experience in the flow of daily life (Malla *et al.*, 1990). Studies using intensive field methods to examine subjective experience of stress in the flow of daily life have found that individuals with schizophrenia, and individuals with genetic susceptibility to schizophrenia, display greater levels of emotional reactivity to small daily life stressors than do control subjects (Myin-Germeys *et al.*, 2001). Individuals with schizophrenia may be more sensitive to such stressors than individuals with affective disorder (Myin-Germeys *et al.*, 2003a). In addition, part of the sensitivity to daily life stressors may be determined by prior exposure to major life events (Myin-Germeys *et al.*, 2003b), suggesting synergistic environment–environment interactions.

Other research suggests that some individuals carry traits that make them more likely to experience life events, such as the personality trait neuroticism (van Os and Jones, 1999). This finding appears to be relevant to schizophrenia, as several studies have demonstrated that neuroticism is a risk factor for schizophrenia (Krabbendam *et al.*, 2002; van Os and Jones, 2001) and is more prevalent in the first-degree relatives of patients with schizophrenia (Maier *et al.*, 1994). Therefore, the role of life events and daily life hassles as a risk factor for schizophrenia is complex. Stress may be generated in part by underlying personality traits, whose genetic contribution may overlap with that of schizophrenia. Alternatively, individuals with vulnerability to schizophrenia may be more sensitive to the effects of stress, while sensitivity to stress is also determined by the degree of prior exposure to stress, possibly including stress in early life (Janssen *et al.*, 2004).

Socioeconomic factors, deprivation, and inequality

Several studies have found a relationship (not necessarily linear) between deprivation and incidence rates of psychosis (Croudace, 2000), prevalence rates of schizophrenia (Moser, 2001) and admission rates for schizophrenia (Boardman *et al.*, 1997; Harrison *et al.*, 1995; Koppel and McGuffin, 1999). The influence of economic deprivation might be exerted via biological mechanisms such as diet or overcrowding, but recent work has suggested that inequality may also have an effect. Boydell *et al.* (2003) found that the incidence rate of schizophrenia as defined by Research Diagnostic Criteria in deprived (but not in affluent) areas in London increased as inequality within the local area increased (incidence rate ratio, 3.79) after adjusting for age, sex, absolute deprivation, and ethnicity.

Interaction between social and other etiological factors

Gene–environment interaction

There is an apparent paradox in that schizophrenia appears highly heritable and yet, as discussed above, many environmental and social factors, appear to play a role. The predictive power of each of these environmental factors, however, is low (i.e. most people exposed to each of the risk factors remain well and never develop the illness). A unifying explanation seems to be that the environmental factors operate upon genetic risk. There are many forms that this interaction could take: synergistic, additive, multiplicative (van Os and Sham, 2003). We have reviewed evidence from the Finnish and Danish adoption studies and the Israeli High Risk Study that the social environment can operate on genetic factors to increase risk of schizophrenia. Genes might also influence the likelihood of exposure to some social risk factors. According to the model proposed by van Os and Marcelis (1998), individuals vary in their sensitivity to adverse environmental circumstances, and genetically sensitive individuals are more likely to develop psychiatric illness when exposed to certain environments than those without genetic predisposition. In the case of schizophrenia, being different in some way from one's neighbors, and/or experiencing discrimination seem to be important factors.

Social factors and cognitive processing

An important implication of any social theory is that the effects of social factors may operate by impacting not only on brain development but also on psychological processes that may contribute to the symptoms of schizophrenia. The development of cognitive theories of psychosis in general and delusion formation in particular has been a major advance in the understanding of schizophrenia. Detailed discussion of this topic (reviewed by Blackwood et al., 2001) is outside the scope of this chapter, but abnormal cognitive processing could be the mechanism by which a range of social factors exerts an effect. People with persecutory delusions selectively attend to threatening information, tend to jump to conclusions, attribute negative events to external personal causes, and have difficulty in understanding others' intentions, motivations, and states of mind (Blackwood et al., 2001). It is plausible that people with this cognitive style would be even more likely to develop delusions when subjected to social adversity, than if they lived in a more benign social milieu. Attributional style, in particular, has been identified as a pathway through which discrimination and racial harassment could lead to psychosis (Sharpley et al., 2001).

Social causation versus social selection

Any discussion of a possible causal role of social factors needs to be considered within the old debate on social selection versus social causation. There has been ongoing debate as to whether social factors influence the development of schizophrenia (causation) or whether individuals at risk choose adverse social environments (selection). This has been a theme running throughout this chapter; a number of the studies reviewed have produced findings that cannot be accounted for by social selection. The question has now been largely superseded by discussion of more complex interaction but we include it for completeness. The most influential paper to address the causation/selection issue investigated the relative effects of social status and ethnicity on risk for schizophrenia amongst Israeli-born people of north African descent. Social status had a greater effect, leading the authors to conclude that social selection is the more important factor (Dohrenwend *et al.*, 1992). However, the rates were low in this study and so ethnicity might not have been associated with a causal etiological agent whereas it might elsewhere. At the ecological level, Boydell *et al.* (2001) found non-white ethnic minorities to be at higher risk when they were in a smaller minority even though they lived in an area of higher social status. Hence it is likely that opposite results would have been found had the study been carried out in London.

Conclusions

A range of social factors have been reported to be implicated in the etiology of schizophrenia, but the evidence for many of them remains scanty. Even for those where the evidence is more substantial (e.g. urban living, social isolation, and discrimination), it is unclear how these factors contribute to the risk. Indeed, it is likely that more than one mechanism operates, and there may be many different interactions with pre-existing genetic/neurodevelopmental vulnerabilities. It is now clear, however, that, in order to understand the causes of schizophrenia, the role of the social environment cannot continue to be ignored. In saying this, we are not proposing an oppositional social instead of biological approach, which we consider as futile as arguing whether poverty or mycobateria cause tuberculosis! Rather, we suggest that both social and biological factors need to be studied as well as their interaction.

We need to recognize that (i) social factors can impact on brain development, (ii) some social factors give rise to psychological vulnerabilities, and (iii) many social factors act over the life course, creating developmental liabilities. We have presented evidence that early social adversity can affect brain development. For example, structural abnormalities can be demonstrated in adult life in individuals with a history of childhood abuse (Anderson *et al.*, 2002; Bremner *et al.*, 1997; Stein *et al.*, 1997). Now that evidence is emerging that childhood abuse may contribute to schizophrenia risk, it is attractive to speculate that some of the neuroimaging findings associated with abuse are relevant to schizophrenia; for example, decreased hippocampal volume has been reported in both. It is possible that the social environment creates psychological vulnerabilities that act additively to the risk function in combination with genetic or non-genetic neurodevelopmental impairments. For example, chronic exposure to discrimination may give rise to a psychological vulnerability to delusion formation, which in individuals with additional neurodevelopmental impairment may result in overt psychotic disorder. Finally, it is also plausible that the social environment and neurodevelopmental impairments reinforce each other over the life course, creating enduring vulnerabilities. For example, a child who is poorly coordinated may not join in at playtime and so forms fewer friends. This pattern may be exacerbated in those who also have schizotypal traits, leading to the developing adolescent becoming increasingly isolated and, later, through his lack of social support in adult life, more susceptible to the effects of social adversity and formation of early psychosis-like experiences.

The challenge for schizophrenia researchers in the coming decade is first to distinguish those candidate social factors that do contribute to schizophrenia risk from those that do not and, second, to identify the interplay between these factors, genetic susceptibility, and their respective effects on, and interactions with, brain development.

REFERENCES

Agid, O., Shapira, B., Zislin, J., *et al.* (1999). Environment and vulnerability to major psychiatric illness: a case–control study of early parental loss in major depression, bipolar disorder and schizophrenia. *Mol Psychiatry* **4**: 163–172.

Allardyce, J., Boydell, J., van Os, J., *et al.* (2001). A comparison of the incidence of schizophrenia in rural Dumfries and Galloway and urban Camberwell **179**: 335–340.

American Psychiatric Association (1987). *Diagnostic and Statistical Manual III–Revised.* Washington, DC: American Psychiatric Press.

Anderson, C. M., Teicher, M. H., Polcari, A., *et al.* (2002). Abnormal T_2 relaxation time in the cerebellar vermis of adults sexually abused in childhood: potential role of the vermis in stress-enhanced risk for drug abuse. *Psychoneuroendocrinology* **27**: 231–244.

Astrup C, Odegard, O. (1961). Internal migration and mental illness in Norway. *Psychiatr Q* **34**: 116–130.

Bateson, G., Jackson, D., Haley, J., *et al.* (1956). Toward a theory of schizophrenia. *Behav Sci* **1**: 251–264.

Bebbington, P. (2003). In Schizophrenia – not just biological. In *Proceedings of Conference held at the Institute of Psychiatry.* London: Institute of Psychiatry, p. 2.

Beckett, C., Bredenkamp, D., Castle, J., *et al.* (2002). Behavior patterns associated with institutional deprivation: a study of children adopted from Romania. *J Dev Behav Pediatr* **23**: 297–303.

Berenbaum, H. (1999). Peculiarity and reported childhood maltreatment. *Psychiatry* **62**: 21–35.

Bhugra, D., Leff, J., Mallett, R., *et al.* (1997). Incidence and outcome of schizophrenia in Whites, African Caribbeans and Asians in London. *Psychol Med* **27**: 791–798.

Bhugra, D., Hilwig, M., Mallett, R., *et al.* (2000). Factors in the onset of schizophrenia: a comparison between London and Trinidad samples. *Acta Psychiatr Scand* **101**: 135–141.

Blackwood, N., Howard, R., Bentall, R., *et al.* (2001). Cognitive neuropsychiatric models of persecutory delusions. *Am J Psychiatry* **158**: 527–539.

Boardman, A., Hodgson, R., Lewis, M., *et al.* (1997). Social indicators and the prediction of psychiatric admission in different diagnostic groups. *Br J Psychiatry* **171**: 457–462.

Boydell, J., van Os, J., McKenzie, K., *et al.* (2001). Incidence of schizophrenia in ethnic minorities in London: ecological study into interactions with environment. *Br Med J* **7325**: 1336–1338.

Boydell, J., van Os, J., McKenzie, K., Murray, R. (2003). The influence of inequality on the incidence of schizophrenia: an ecological study. *Schizophr Bull* **60**: Suppl. 33.

Bremner, J. D., Randall, P., Vermetten, E., *et al.* (1997). Magnetic resonance imaging-based measurement of hippocampal volume in posttraumatic stress disorder related to childhood physical and sexual abuse: a preliminary report. *Bio Psychiatry* **41**: 23–32.

Brown, G. W., Birley, J. L. (1968). Crises and life changes and the onset of schizophrenia. *J Health Soc Behav* **9**: 203–214.

Bruxner, G., Burvill, P., Fazio, S., *et al.* (1997). Aspects of psychiatric admissions of migrants to hospitals in Perth. *West Aust N Z J Psychiatry* **31**: 532–542.

Bryer, J. B., Nelson, B. A., Miller, J. B., *et al.* (1987). Childhood sexual and physical abuse as factors in adult psychiatric illness. *Am J Psychiatry* **144**: 1426–1430.

Butler, R. W., Mueser, K. T., Sprock, J., *et al.* (1996). Positive symptoms of psychosis in posttraumatic stress disorder. *Biol Psychiatry* **39**: 839–844.

Cannon, M., Caspi, A., Moffitt, T., *et al.* (2002). Evidence for early-childhood, pan-developmental impairment specific to schizophreniform disorder. *Arch Gen Psychiatry* **59**: 449–456.

Castle, D., Wessley, S., Der, G., Murray, R. M. (1991). The incidence of operationally defined schizophrenia in Camberwell, 1965–1984. *Br J Psychiatry* **159**: 790–794.

Castle, D. J., Scott, K., Wessely, S., *et al.* (1993). Does social deprivation during gestation and early life predispose to later schizophrenia? *Soc Psychiatry Psychiatr Epidemiol* **28**: 1–4.

Chung, R. K., Langeluddecke, P., Tennant, C., *et al.* (1986). Threatening life events in the onset of schizophrenia, schizophreniform psychosis and hypomania. *Br J Psychiatry* **148**: 680–685.

Croudace, T. J., Kayne, R., Jones, P. B., *et al.* (2000). Non-linear relationship between an index of social deprivation, psychiatric admission prevalence and the incidence of psychosis. *Psychol Med* **30**: 177–185.

Dauncey, K., Giggs, J., Baker, K., *et al.* (1993). Schizophrenia in Nottingham: lifelong residential mobility of a cohort. *Br J Psychiatry* **163**: 613–619.

DiPietro, J. A. (2000). Baby and the brain: advances in child development. *Annu Rev Publ Health* **21**: 455–471.

Dohrenwend, B. P., Levav, I., Shrout, P. E., *et al.* (1992). Socioeconomic status psychiatric disorders the causation-selection issue. *Science* **255**: 946–952.

Drukker, M., Kaplan, C. D., Feron, F. J. M., *et al.* (2003). Children's health-related quality of life, neighbourhood socio-economic deprivation and social capital. A contextual analysis. *Soc Sci Med* **57**: 825–841.

Eisenberg, L. (1995). The social construction of the human brain. *Am J Psychiatry* **152**: 1563–1575.

Ellason, J. W., Ross, C. A. (1997). Childhood trauma and psychiatric symptoms. *Psychol Rep* **80**: 447–450.

Farris, R., Dunham, H. (1939). *Mental Disorders in Urban Areas*. Chicago, IL: University of Chicago Press.

Fishbein, D. (2000). The importance of neurobiological research to the prevention of psychopathology. *Prev Sci* **1**: 89–106.

Garety, P. A., Kuipers, E., Fowler, D., *et al.* (2001). A cognitive model of the positive symptoms of psychosis. *Psychol Med* **31**: 189–195.

Glover, G. (1989). Why is there a high rate of schizophrenia in British Caribbeans? *Br J Hosp Med* **42**: 48–51.

Hammersley, P., Dias, A., Todd, G., *et al.* (2003). Childhood trauma and hallucinations in bipolar affective disorder: a preliminary investigation. *Br J Psychiatry* **182**: 543–547.

Hare, E. (1956). Mental illness and social conditions in Bristol. *J Ment Sci* **102**: 349–357.

Harrison, G., Owens, D., Holten, A., *et al.* (1988). A prospective study of severe mental disorder in Afro-Caribbean patients. *Psychol Med* **18**: 643–657.

Harrison, G., Glazebrook, C., Brewin, J., *et al.* (1997). Increased incidence of psychotic disorders in migrants from the Caribbean to the United Kingdom. *Psychol Med* **27**: 799–806. [See comments in *Psychol Med* (1998). **28**: 496–497.]

Harrison, J., Barrow, S., Creed, F., *et al.* (1995). Social deprivation and psychiatric admission rates among different diagnostic groups. *Br J Psychiatry* **167**: 456–462.

Heidbreder, C. A., Foxton, R., Cilia, J., *et al.* (2001). Increased responsiveness of dopamine to atypical but not typical antipsychotics in the medial pre-frontal cortex of rats reared in isolation. *Psychopharmacology* **156**: 338–351.

Heins, T., Gray, A., Tennant, M., *et al.* (1990). Persisting hallucinations following childhood sexual abuse. *Aust N Z J Psychiatry* **24**: 561–565.

Hickling, W., McKenzie, K., Mullen, R., *et al.* (1999). A Jamaican psychiatrist evaluates diagnoses at a London hospital. *Br J Psychiatry* **175**: 283–285.

Hirsch, S. R., Leff, J. P. (1975). *Maudsley Monograph No. 22. Abnormalities in Parents of Schizophrenics.* London: Oxford University Press.

Hutchinson, G., Takei, N., Fahy, T. A., *et al.* (1996). Morbid risk of schizophrenia in first-degree relatives of white and African-Caribbean patients with psychosis. *Br J Psychiatry* **169**: 776–780.

Hutchinson, G., Takei, N., Bhugra, T., *et al.* (1997). Increased rate of psychosis among African-Caribbeans in Britain is not due to an excess of pregnancy and birth complications. *Br J Psychiatry* **171**: 145–147.

Hutchinson, G., Mallett, R., Fletcher, H., *et al.* (1999). Are the increased rates of psychosis reported for the population of Caribbean origin in Britain an urban effect? *Int Rev Psychiatry* **11**: 122–128.

Jablensky, A., Cole, S. W. (1997). Is the earlier age at onset of schizophrenia in males a confounded finding? Results from a cross-cultural investigation. *Br J Psychiatry* **170**: 234–240.

Jacobs, S., Myers, J. (1976). Recent life events and acute schizophrenic psychosis: a controlled study. *J Nerv Ment Dis* **162**: 75–87.

Janssen, I., Hanssen, M., Bak, M., *et al.* (2002). Evidence that ethnic group effects on psychosis risk are confounded by experiences of discrimination. *Schizophr Res* **53**: 34.

Janssen, I., Hansen, M., Bak, M., *et al.* (2003). Discrimination and delusional ideation. *Br J Psychiatry* **182**: 71–76.

Janssen, I., Krabbendam, L., Bak, M., *et al.* (2004). Childhood abuse as a risk factor for psychotic experience. *Acta Psychiatr Scand* in press.

Johns, L. C., van Os, J. (2001). The continuity of psychotic experiences in the general population. *Clin Psychol Rev* **21**: 1125–1141.

Jones, P., Rodgers, B., Murray, R., *et al.* (1994). Child developmental risk factors for adult schizophrenia in the British 1946 birth cohort. *Lancet* **344**: 1398–1402.

Johnstone, E. C., Crow, T. J., Frith, C. D., *et al.* (1976). Cerebral ventricular size and cognitive impairment in chronic schizophrenia. *Lancet*, ii: 924–926.

Karlsen, S., Nazroo, J. (2002). Relation between racial discrimination and health among ethnic minority groups. *Am J Publ Health* **92**: 624–631.

King, M., Coker, E., Leavey, G. *et al.* (1994). Incidence of psychotic illness in London: a comparison of ethnic groups. *Br Med J* **309**: 1115–1119.

Koppel, S., McGuffin, P. (1999). Socioeconomic factors that predict psychiatric admissions. *Psychol Med* **29**: 1235–1241.

Krabbendam, L., Janssen, I., Bak, M., *et al.* (2002). Neuroticism and low self-esteem as risk factors for psychosis. *Soc Psychiatry Psychiatr Epidemiol* **37**: 1–6.

Kubicka, L., Matejcek, Z., David, H.P., *et al.* (1995). Children from unwanted pregnancies in Prague, Czech Republic revisted at age 30. *Acta Psychiatr Scand* **91**: 361–369.

Lewis, G., David, A., Andreasson, S., *et al.* (1992). Schizophrenia and city life. *Lancet* **340**: 137–140.

Lidz, T. (1958). Schizophrenia and the family. *Psychiatry* **21**: 21–27.

Lyons, D. M., Afarian, H., Schatzberg, A. F., *et al.* (2002). Experience-dependent asymmetric variation in primate prefrontal morphology. *Behav Brain Res* **136**: 51–59.

Mahy, G., Mallett, R., Leff, J., Bhugra, D. (1999). First-contact incidence rate of schizophrenia on Barbados. *Br J Psychiatry* **175**: 28–33.

Maier, W., Minges, J., Lichtermann, D., *et al.* (1994). Personality variations in healthy relatives of schizophrenics. *Schizophr Res* **12**: 81–88.

Malla, A. K., Cortese, L., Shaw, T. S., *et al.* (1990). Life events and relapse in schizophrenia. A one year prospective study. *Soc Psychiatry Psychiatr Epidemiol* **25**: 221–224.

Mallett, R., Hutchinson, G., Leff, J., *et al.* (1998). Social conditions and schizophrenia in African-Caribbeans: Edward Hare revisited. In *Proceedings of Winter Meeting 39 of the Royal College of Psychiatrists.* London: Royal College of Psychiatrists.

Mallett, R., Leff, J., Bhugra, D., Pang, D., Zhao, J. (2002). Social environment, ethnicity and schizophrenia. A case-control study. *Soc Psychiatry Psychiatr Epidemiol* **37**: 329–335.

Malmberg, A., Lewis, G., David, A., *et al.* (1998). Premorbid adjustment and personality in people with schizophrenia. *Br J Psychiatry* **172**: 308–313.

Malzberg, B. (1969). Are immigrants psychologically disturbed? In *Changing Perspectives in Mental illness*, ed. S. Plog, R. Edgerton. New York: Holt, Rinehart and Winston, pp. 395–421.

Marcelis, M., Navarro-Mateu, F., Murray, R., *et al.* (1998). Urbanization and psychosis: a study of 1942–1978 birth cohorts in the Netherlands. *Psychol Med* **28**: 871–879.

Marcelis, M., Takei, N., van Os, J., *et al.* (1999). Urbanization and risk for schizophrenia: does the effect operate before or around the time of illness onset? *Psychol Med* **29**: 1197–1203.

Matthews, M. K., Dalleny, J. W., Matthews, C., *et al.* (2001). Periodic maternal separation of neonatal rats produces region- and genetic-specific effects on bioamine content in post-mortem adult brain. *Synapse* **40**: 1–10

McGuire, P., Jones, P., Harvey, M., *et al.* (1995). Morbid risk of schizophrenia in relatives of patients with cannabis-associated psychosis. *Schizophr Res* **15**: 277–281.

McKenzie, K., van Os, J., Fahy, T., *et al.* (1995). Psychosis with good prognosis in Afro-Caribbean people now living in the United Kingdom. [See comments] *Br Med J* **311**: 1325–1328.

Mednick, S.A., Parnas, J., Schulsinger, F., *et al.* (1987). The Copenhagen High Risk Project 1962–1986. *Schizophr Bull* **133**: 485–495.

Mirsky, A. F., Silberman, E. K., Latz, A., *et al.* (1985). Adult outcomes of high-risk children: differential effects of town and kibbutz rearing. *Schizophr Bull* **11**: 150–156.

Mortensen, P. B., Cantor-Graae, E., McNeil, T. F., *et al.* (1997). Increased rates of schizophrenia among immigrants: some methodological concerns raised by Danish findings. *Psychol Med* **274**: 813–820.

Mortensen, P., Pedersen, C., Westergaard, T., *et al.* (1999). Effects of family history and place and season of birth on the risk of schizophrenia. *N Eng J Med* **340**: 603–608. [Sec correspondence in *N Engl J Med* (1999) **341**: 370–372].

Moser, K. (2001). Inequalities in treated heart disease and mental illness in England and Wales 1994–1998. *Br J Gen Pract* **51**: 438–444.

Murphy, H. B. (1977). Migration, culture and mental health. *Psychol Med* **7**: 677–684.

Murray, R., Fearon, P. (1999). The developmental "risk factor" model of schizophrenia. *J Psychiatr Res* **33**: 497–499.

Murray, R. M., O'Callaghan, E., Castle, D. J., *et al.* (1992). A neurodevelopmental approach to the classification of schizophrenia. *Schizophr Bull* **18**: 319–332.

Myhrman, A. (1992). Unwanted pregnancy, its occurrence and significance for the family and the child. *Acta Univ Ouluen Ser* **249**: 1–46.

Myhrman, A., Rantakallio, P., Isohanni, M., *et al.* (1996). Unwantedness of pregnancy and schizophrenia in the Child. *Br J Psychiatry* **169**: 637–640.

Myin-Germeys, I., van Os, J., Schwartz, J. E., *et al.* (2001). Emotional reactivity to daily life stress in psychosis. *Arch Gen Psychiatry* **58**: 1137–1144.

Myin-Germeys, I., Peeters, F., Havermans, R., *et al.* (2003a). Emotional reactivity to daily life stress in psychosis and affective disorder: an experience sampling study. *Acta Psychiatr Scand* **107**: 124–131.

Myin-Germeys, I., Krabbendam, L., Delespaul, P. A., *et al.* (2003b). Do life events have their effect on psychosis by influencing the emotional reactivity to daily life stress? *Psychol Med* **33**: 327–333.

Ødegård, O. (1932). Emigration and insanity: a study of mental disease among Norwegian born population in Minnesota. *Acta Psychiatr Neurol Scand* **7**(Suppl. 4): 1–206.

Ovtscharoff, Jr., W., Braun, K. (2001). Maternal separation and social isolation modulate the postnatal development of synaptic composition in the infralimbic cortex of Octodon degus. *Neuroscience* **104**: 33–40.

Pedersen, C. B., Mortensen, P. B. (2001). Evidence of a dose–response relationship between urbanicity during upbringing and schizophrenia risk. *Arch Gen Psychiatry* **58**: 1039–1046.

Putnam, F. W., Guroff, J. J., Silberman, E. K., *et al.* (1986). The clinical phenomenology of multiple personality disorder: review of 100 recent cases. *J Clin Psychiatry* **47**: 285–293.

Read, J., Argyle, N. (1999). Hallucinations, delusions, and thought disorder among adult psychiatric inpatients with a history of child abuse. *Psychiatr Serv* **50**: 1467–1472.

Read, J., Perry, B. D., Moskowitz, A., *et al.* (2001). The contribution of early traumatic events to schizophrenia in some patients: a traumagenic neurodevelopmental model. *Psychiatry* **64**: 319–345.

Read, J., Agar, K., Argyle, N., *et al.* (2003). Sexual and physical abuse during childhood and adulthood as predictors of hallucinations, delusions and thought disorder. *Psychol Psychother Theory Res Pract* **76**: 1–22.

Rosenthal, D., Wender, P., Kety, S., *et al.* (1971). The adopted-away offspring of schizophrenics. *Am J Psychiatry* **128**: 307–311.

Ross, C. A., Joshi, S. (1992). Schneiderian symptoms and childhood trauma in the general population. *Compr Psychiatry* **33**: 269–273.

Ross, C. A., Norton, G. R., *et al.* (1989). Multiple personality disorder: an analysis of 236 cases. *Can J Psychiatry Rev Can Psychiatry* **34**: 413–418.

Ross, C. A., Anderson, G., Clark, P., Wozney, K. (1994). Childhood abuse and the positive symptoms of schizophrenia. *Hosp Community Psychiatry* **45**: 489–491.

Sanchez, M. M., Ladd, C. O., Plotsky, P. M. (2001). Early adverse experience as a developmental risk factor for later psychopathology: evidence from rodent and primate models. *Dev Psychopathol* **13**: 419–449.

Sansonnet-Hayden, H., Haley, G., Marriage, K., *et al.* (1987). Sexual abuse and psychopathology in hospitalized adolescents. *J Am Acad Child Adolesc Psychiatry* **26**: 753–757.

Selten, J. P., Sijben, N. (1994). First admission rate for schizophrenia in immigrants to the Netherlands: the Dutch National Register. *Soc Psychiatry Psychiatr Epidemiol* **29**: 71–72.

Selten, J. P., Slaets, J. P., Kahn, R. S., *et al.* (1997). Schizophrenia in Surinamese and Dutch Antillean immigrants to the Netherlands: evidence of an increased incidence. *Psychol Med* **27**: 807–811.

(1998). Prenatal exposure to influenza and schizophrenia in Surinamese and Dutch Antillean immigrants to the Netherlands. *Schizophr Res* **30**: 101–103.

Selten, J. P., Veen, N., Feller, W., *et al.* (2001). Incidence of psychotic disorders in immigrant groups to the Netherlands. *Br J Psychiatry* **178**: 1–7.

Selten, J. P., Cantor-Graae, E., Slaets, J., *et al.* (2002). Ødegårds selection hypothesis revisited: schizophrenia in Surinamese immigrants to the Netherlands. *Am J Psychiatry* **159**: 669–671.

Sharpley, M., Hutchinson, G., McKenzie, K., *et al.* (2001). Understanding the excess of psychosis among the African-Caribbean population in England. Review of current hypotheses. *Br J Psychiatry* **178**(Suppl. 40): 60–68.

Startup, M. (1999). Schizotypy, dissociative experiences and childhood abuse: relationships among self-report measures. *Br J Clin Psychol* **38**: 333–344.

Stein, M. B., Koverola, C., Hanna, C., *et al.* (1997). Hippocampal volume in women victimized by childhood sexual abuse. *Psychol Med* **27**: 951–959.

Sugarman, P., Crawford, D. (1994). Schizophrenia in the Afro-Caribbean community. *Br J Psychiatry* **164**: 474–480.

Swett, Jr., C., Surrey, J., Cohen, C., *et al.* (1990). Sexual and physical abuse histories and psychiatric symptoms among male psychiatric outpatients. *Am J Psychiatry* **147**: 632–636.

Takano, T., Nakamura, K. (2001). An analysis of health levels and various indicators of urban environments for healthy cities projects. *J Epidemiol Community Health* **55**: 263–270.

Thomas, C. S., Stone, K., Osborn, M., *et al.* (1993). Psychiatric morbidity and compulsory admission among UK born Europeans, Afro-Caribbeans and Asians in central Manchester. *Br J Psychiatry* **163**: 91–99.

Thornicroft, G., Bisoffi, G., De Salva, D., *et al.* (1993). Urban–rural differences in the associations between social deprivation and psychiatric service utilization in schizophrenia and all diagnoses: a case-register study in Northern Italy. *Psychol Med* **23**: 487–496.

Tienari, P. (1991). Interaction between genetic vulnerability and family environment: The Finnish adoptive family study of schizophrenia. *Acta Psychiatrica Scand* **84**: 460–465.

Tienari, P., Wynne, L., Laksy, K., *et al.* (2000). Finnish Adoptive Family Study. *Acta Psychiatr Scand* **101** 433–443.

van Os, J., Jones, P. B. (1999). Early risk factors and adult person–environment relationships in affective disorder. *Psychol Med* **29**: 1055–1067.

    (2001). Neuroticism as a risk factor for schizophrenia. *Psychol Med* **31**: 1129–1134.

van Os, J., Marcelis, M. (1998). The ecogenetics of schizophrenia: a review. *Schizophr Res* **32**: 127–135.

van Os, J., Sham, P. (2003). Gene–environment correlation and interaction in schizophrenia. In *The Epidemiology of Schizophrenia*, ed. R. Murray, P. Jones, E. Susser, J. van Os, M. Cannon. Cambridge, UK: Cambridge. University Press.

van Os, J., Castle, D. J., Takei, N., *et al.* (1996a). Psychotic illness in ethnic minorities: clarification from the 1991 census. *Psychol Med* **26**: 203–208.

van Os, J., Takei, N., Castle, D. J., *et al.* (1996b). The incidence of mania: time trends in relation to gender and ethnicity. *Soc Psychiatry Psychiatr Epidemiol* **31**: 129–136.

van Os, J., Driessen, G., Gunther, N., *et al.* (2000). Neighbourhood variation in incidence of schizophrenia. Evidence for person–environment interaction. *Br J Psychiatry* **176**: 243–248.

van Os, J., Hanssen, M., Bijl, R. V., *et al.* (2001). Prevalence of psychotic disorder and community level of psychotic symptoms: an urban–rural comparison. *Arch Gen Psychiatry* **58**: 663–668.

van Os, J., Hanssen, M., de Graaf, R., *et al.* (2002). Does the urban environment independently increase the risk for both negative and positive features of psychosis? *Soc Psychiatry Psychiatr Epidemiol* **37**: 460–464.

van Os, J., Hanssen, M., Bak, M., *et al.* (2003). Do urbanicity and familial liability coparticipate in causing psychosis? *Am J Psychiatry* **160**: 477–482.

Vaughn, C. E., Leff, J. P. (1976). The influence of family and social factors on the course of psychiatric illness. *Br J Psychiatry* **129**: 125–137.

    (1982). Patterns of emotional responses in the relatives of schizophrenic patients. *Schizophr Bull* **7**: 43–44.

Ventura, J., Nuechterlein, K. H., Lukoff, D., *et al.* (1989). A prospective study of stressful life events and schizophrenic relapse. *J Abnorm Psychol* **98**: 407–411.

Wahlberg, K. E., Wynne, L., Oja, H., *et al.* (1997). Gene–environment interaction in vulnerability to schizophrenia: findings from the Finnish Adoptive Family Study of Schizophrenia. *Am J Psychiatry* **154**: 355–362.

Wahlberg, K. E., Wynne, L., Oja, H., *et al.* (2000). Thought disorder index of Finnish adoptees and communication deviance of their adoptive parents. *Psychol Med* **30**: 127–136.

Weingarten, M. A., Orron, D. E. (1983). Schizophrenia in a Yemenite immigrant town in Israel. *Int J Soc Psychiatry* **29**: 249–254.

Wessely, S., Castle, D., Der, R., *et al.* (1991). Schizophrenia and Afro-Caribbeans. A case-control study. *Br J Psychiatry* **159**: 795–801.

Whitaker-Azmitia, P., Zhou, F., Hobin, J., *et al.* (2000). Isolation rearing of rats produces deficits as adults in the serotonergic innervation of hippocampus. *Peptides* **21**: 1755–1759.

Wiesel, T. N., Hubel, D. H. (1974). Ordered arrangement of orientation columns in monkeys lacking visual experience. *J Comp Neurol* **158**: 307–318.

Wing, J. K. (1978). The social context of schizophrenia. *Am J Psychiatry* **135**: 1333–1339.

World Health Organization (1967). *Manual of International Statistical Classification of Diseases, Injuries and Causes of Death, 8th edn.* Geneva: World Health Organization.

Wynne, L., Ryckoff, I., Day, J., *et al.* (1958). Pseudo-mutuality in the family relations of schizophrenics. *Psychiatry* **21**: 205–220.

14

How does drug abuse interact with familial and developmental factors in the etiology of schizophrenia?

Chih-Ken Chen[1] and Robin M. Murray[2]

[1] Chang Gung Memorial Hospital, Keelung, Taiwan
[2] Institute of Psychiatry, King's College, London, UK

Schizophrenia is frequently described as a neurodevelopmental disease with a strong genetic component (Tsuang *et al.*, 2001). While it may be an exaggeration to call schizophrenia a neurodevelopmental disease, it is clear that it has a major developmental component. Furthermore, family, twin, and adoption studies suggest that 65–85% of the liability to schizophrenia can be attributed to genes (Cannon *et al.*, 1998; Cardno *et al.*, 1999; Kendler and Diehl, 1993). As outlined elsewhere in this volume (see Ch. 11), the environmental risk factors for schizophrenia can be summarized as operating either early in life or later nearer the onset of frank psychosis. In this chapter, we focus on the role of drug abuse as one of the later factors, and on how it interacts with familial and developmental factors.

Association of drug abuse and psychosis

Numerous studies have found that those with psychosis commonly use drugs. In the USA, a study from the Eastern Pennsylvania Psychiatric Institute (Muesser *et al.*, 1990) reported that, among schizophrenia patients, 47% used alcohol, 42% used cannabis, 25% used stimulants, 18% used hallucinogens, 7% used sedatives, and 4% used narcotics. A Veterans Administration inpatient study reported that 60% of those admitted with schizophrenia had a current or past history of drug abuse (Selzer and Lieberman, 1993). A meta-analysis concluded that substance-use disorders occur in approximately 40–50% of schizophrenia individuals in the USA. These rates are much higher than those for the general population. For example, in the US Epidemiologic Catchment Area Study, the rate of lifetime substance-use disorder in the general population was 17%, but it was 48% among persons with schizophrenia (Regier *et al.*, 1990).

Neurodevelopment and Schizophrenia, ed. Matcheri S. Keshavan *et al.* Published by Cambridge University Press. © Cambridge University Press 2004.

Elsewhere in the world, rates of substance abuse are generally lower, but again consumption is more frequent in those with psychosis than in the rest of the population. In the UK, in South London, the 1-year prevalence rate among patients with psychotic illnesses was found to be 36.3% for any substance problem and 15.8% for drug problems (Menezes *et al.*, 1996). A more recent study from Scotland (McCreadie, 2002) revealed that problem use of drugs by people with schizophrenia was greater than in the general population for both the previous year (7% versus 2%) and at any time previously (20% versus 6%). Cantwell *et al.* (1999) examined 168 subjects with first-episode psychosis in the UK and reported that 37% of the sample met criteria for drug use, drug misuse, or alcohol misuse; 8.4% of the subjects received a primary diagnosis of substance-related psychotic disorder. The rates of substance use among individuals with schizophrenia in Continental Europe are similar to this and rarely as high as those reported in US studies (Cassano *et al.*, 1998; Modestin *et al.*, 1997; Soyka *et al.*, 1993; Verdoux *et al.*, 1996a).

Direction of the association

The associations between use of certain drugs and schizophrenia are generally not disputed. However, there are several possible explanations for these observed associations (Blanchard *et al.*, 2000; Murray *et al.*, 2003; Thornicroft, 1990).

Self-medication

A long-standing notion has been that substance abuse is often the product of psychopathology, resulting from the patient's attempt to "self-medicate" dysphoric symptoms (Khantzian, 1985). Patients suffering from schizophrenia are postulated to use substances either to improve their negative, depressive, or anxiety symptoms (DeQuardo *et al.*, 1994; Dixon *et al.*, 1991; Mueser *et al.*, 1998; Schneier and Siris, 1987) or to alleviate the side effects of antipsychotic drugs (Dixon *et al.*, 1991; Lopez and Jeste, 1997). For example, small amounts of cannabis are said to attenuate anxiety, depression, and negative symptoms in schizophrenia (Linszen *et al.*, 1994; Peralta and Cuesta, 1992). However, empirical studies (Fischman and Schuster, 1982; Griffith *et al.*, 1972) on the effects of cannabis and stimulants have often failed to produce any evidence to substantiate the self-medication hypothesis.

Common factor hypothesis

The common factor hypothesis proposes that substance abuse and schizophrenia share common etiological factors, which may include low socioeconomic status, certain personality traits (Mueser *et al.*, 1998), or genetic vulnerability (Blanchard *et al.*, 2000). Mueser *et al.* (1998) speculate that antisocial personality may underlie both schizophrenia and substance misuse, but this argument has not been supported by cohort studies (Jones *et al.*, 1994). So far there is little evidence for a common genetic vulnerability for schizophrenia and drug abuse.

Vulnerability hypothesis

As with other common chronic diseases such as diabetes and coronary artery disease, many consider that the appropriate etiological model (Murray and Fearon, 1999) for schizophrenia is one involving multiple genes and environmental risk factors. As discussed elsewhere in this book, genetic and/or early environmental factors are postulated to cause the development of anomalous neural networks, which interact in the growing child with inherited schizotypal traits to establish a trajectory towards an increasingly solitary and deviant lifestyle. The vulnerablity hypothesis postulates that stressors, including the use of drugs, then precipitate the individual across the threshold for expression of psychosis (e.g. Bebbington *et al.*, 1993; Jones, *et al.*, 1994; Tsuang *et al.*, 2001; Verdoux *et al.*, 1996b).

Drug abuse as a cause of psychosis

Breakey *et al.* (1974) suggested that taking certain drugs (amphetamines, cannabis, or hallucinogens) might play a precipitating role in the onset of schizophrenia, bringing the disorder on earlier and increasing its likelihood in patients who otherwise seemed somewhat less-constitutionally vulnerable than the average psychotic individual. Obviously, different drugs may have different associations with psychosis because of their varying actions on the brain. In this review, we will concentrate on drugs that have been shown to have a clear association with schizophrenia, namely the psychostimulants cocaine, amphetamine, and methamphetamine, as well as cannabis and phenyclidine (PCP).

Amphetamine-induced psychosis

Amphetamine psychosis is a reaction that usually occurs following chronic use of amphetamines, though it can occur after only a short period of amphetamine consumption. Patients with amphetamine psychosis show a picture very similar to paranoid schizophrenia (Bell, 1965; Connell, 1958). Indeed, amphetamine psychosis so closely resembles schizophrenia, especially the paranoid type, that it has been viewed as a model of schizophrenia (Crow *et al.*, 1976; Snyder, 1973).

Connell (1958) and Bell (1965) originally conceptualized amphetamine psychosis as lasting no more than 1 week after the urine becomes negative for amphetamines. However, the psychosis does not always remit so readily, and use of methamphetamine has been reported in several studies to result in psychotic symptoms lasting several months or more (Iwanami *et al.*, 1994; Nakatani *et al.*, 1989; Sato *et al.*, 1983; Tatetsu *et al.*, 1956). Methamphetamine is a derivative of amphetamine, with similar but more pronounced psychotropic properties (National Institute on Drug Abuse, 1998). Methamphetamine comes in many forms and can be smoked, snorted, orally ingested, or injected. In the Pacific region, especially Japan and Taiwan, abuse of methamphetamine and the resultant psychosis are common (Chou *et al.*, 1999; Suwaki *et al.*, 1997). Tatetsu (1963) reported that a substantial minority of patients with methamphetamine psychosis did not recover within the first month but rather went on to develop a chronic schizophrenic-like state. Almost 15% of Japanese patients with methamphetamine psychosis since 1945 took 5 or more years to recover in the absence of ongoing methamphetamine use (Konuma, 1994). Such prolonged psychotic symptoms are hypothesized by some investigators to represent a triggering or unmasking of vulnerability to psychosis by the amphetamine abuse (Bell, 1973; Flaum and Schultz, 1996; Gold and Bowers, 1978).

In Connell's original report (1958) 9 of 42 subjects developed psychosis after a single dose of amphetamine. Connell considered amphetamine to be a true hallucinogen that was directly related to the syndrome and he, therefore, regarded amphetamine psychosis as a distinct disorder. Several prospective studies, in which amphetamine psychosis was experimentally induced in non-schizophrenia drug abusers, indicated that amphetamine does not simply activate latent schizophrenia since the psychosis can be produced in apparently normal subjects (Angrist and Gershon, 1970; Bell, 1973; Griffith *et al.*, 1969).

Cannabis-induced psychosis:

Of the plant-based drugs, the illicit consumption of cannabis is most widespread (United Nations International Drug Control Programme, 1997). Many studies (Dixon *et al.*, 1991; Linszen, *et al.*, 1994; Longhurst, 1997; Mathers *et al.*, 1991; Rolfe *et al.*, 1993; Schneier and Siris, 1987) have reported a positive association between cannabis use and psychosis. Furthermore, in a prospective cohort study of psychotic patients, Linszen *et al.* (1994) found that significantly more and earlier relapses occurred in the cannabis-abusing group. In all but one of their subjects, cannabis abuse preceded the onset of the first psychotic symptoms by at least 1 year. The authors, therefore, concluded that cannabis abuse, and particularly heavy abuse, can elicit relapse in patients with schizophrenia and related disorders, and it may possibly precipitate the initial psychosis.

Thornicroft (1990), in a review of the evidence for an association between cannabis and psychosis, concluded that there is no convincing support for a separate clinical diagnosis of "cannabis psychosis." A retrospective study of 272 psychotic inpatients (70 with cannabis-related psychosis) also failed to find any consistent pattern of symptoms associated with cannabis use (Imade and Ebie, 1991). However, arguments against the use of this particular diagnostic label should not be confused with arguments against any association between the drug and psychosis

(Thomas, 1993). Chronic psychosis following prolonged cannabis abuse may reflect the precipitation of schizophreniform disorder or schizophrenia in a vulnerable individual, rather than a separate diagnosis of cannabis psychosis (Thornicroft, 1990). To establish conclusively whether cannabis consumption actually causes the onset of schizophrenia, one must obtain prospective data and establish whether there is evidence of a dose–response relationship between the amount consumed and the risk of psychosis.

The first prospective cohort study was reported in 1987. Andreasson *et al.* (1987) followed up almost 50 000 individuals conscripted into the Swedish Army and reported the relative risk of developing schizophrenia was 2.4 for cannabis users compared with non-users, rising to 6.0 for heavy users. An extension of this Swedish Conscript Study has recently been carried out (Zammit *et al.*, 2002). Consistent with previous findings, this showed that "heavy cannabis users" by the age of 18 years were 6.7 times more likely than non-users to be diagnosed with schizophrenia in the ensuing 27 years. The risk was reduced but remained significant after controlling for other potential confounding factors such as disturbed behavior, low intelligence quotient score, growing up in a city, cigarette smoking, other drug use, and poor social integration.

However, this study was largely ignored for 15 years. Then, in the Netherlands, van Os and his colleagues (2002) examined the effect of cannabis use on psychotic symptoms among the general population, assessing 4045 subjects at baseline and again 3 years later. Compared with non-users, individuals using cannabis at baseline were nearly three times more likely to manifest psychotic symptoms at follow-up. This risk remained significant after statistical adjustment for a range of confounders. There was a dose–response relationship with the highest risk (odds ratio, 6.81) being observed for the highest level of cannabis use. Further analysis revealed that lifetime history of cannabis use at baseline, as opposed to use of cannabis at follow-up, was a stronger predictor of psychosis 3 years later than cannabis use at the later point. This suggests that the association between cannabis use and psychosis was not merely a short-term effect of cannabis use leading to an acute psychotic episode.

The Swedish and Dutch studies were open to criticism on a number of points (Johnson *et al.*, 1988; Negrete, 1989), notably that both the cannabis use and the schizophrenia may have been related to an underlying predisposing factor such as premorbid personality. This criticism has been at least partly overcome in a study from New Zealand, which followed-up a general population birth cohort of 1037 individuals born in Dunedin, New Zealand in 1972–1973 (96% follow-up rate at age 26). Although much smaller, this study has information on self-reported psychotic symptoms at age 11 years (i.e. before the likely onset of cannabis use) and then information on cannabis use (self-reports) at 15 and 18 years. Thus, it allows the age of onset of cannabis use to be examined in relation to later psychiatric outcome.

Results showed that both cannabis users by age 15 and cannabis users by age 18 had elevated schizophrenia symptoms at age 26, which remained significant after controlling for psychotic symptoms predating the onset of cannabis use (Arseneault *et al.*, 2002). The effect was much stronger with earlier use, and onset of cannabis use by age 15 was associated with an increased likelihood of meeting diagnostic criteria for schizophreniform disorder at age 26. Indeed, 10.3% of those using cannabis at age 15 in this cohort were diagnosed with schizophreniform disorder at age 26, as opposed to 3% of the controls.

Phencyclidine-induced psychosis

PCP is a dissociative anesthetic originally employed in human anesthesia in the late 1950s. It can produce hallucinations, relaxation, feeling of dissociation from the environment, and sometimes intense euphoria (Jacobs *et al.*, 1987). Further characterization of the psychomimetic actions of PCP was facilitated by the epidemic of PCP abuse that occurred in the USA during the late 1960s and 1970s. Although hallucinations, agitation, and paranoid delusions occur after PCP administration, the most striking and consistent behavioral effects of PCP are alterations in body image, disorganization of thought, negativism, and apathy (Javitt and Zukin, 1991). Javitt and Zukin (1991) suggested that the symptoms induced by PCP are similar to the "four A's" proposed by Bleuler as the primary symptoms of schizophrenia: affective blunting, ambivalence, autism, and disturbance of association. They also suggested that PCP psychosis may provide a neurochemical model corresponding uniquely to the Bleulerian conception of schizophrenia.

PCP interacts selectively with a specific binding site (PCP receptor) that is associated with the N-methyl-D-aspartate (NMDA)-type excitatory amino acid receptor. Occupation of its receptor by PCP induces non-competitive inhibition of NMDA receptor-mediated neurotransmission (Snell *et al.*, 1988). Primary dysfunction of NMDA receptor functioning could potentially account for the deficit in cognitive functioning associated with schizophrenia, as well as for the dopaminergic hyperactivity and dysregulation associated with acute schizophrenia (Kleinman *et al.*, 1988).

In short, PCP psychosis has been an attractive fashionable model for psychosis. Unfortunately, there have been few studies of its role in precipitating long-lasting schizophrenia-like psychoses in real life.

Lysergic acid diethylamide-induced psychosis

Hallucinogens, by comparison, do not generally create psychoses that truly simulate schizophrenia. Drugs like lysergic acid diethylamide (LSD) and mescaline evoke chemical psychosis with characteristic hallucinogenic distortions of perception such as synesthesia (a condensation of two sensations); for instance, a person will "taste" green, "smell" grey or "see" music (Jacobs *et al.*, 1987; Slaby, 1991). However, the picture in some patients remains sufficiently complex to render LSD psychosis very difficult to distinguish from acute schizophrenia (Vardy and Kay, 1983). Many believe that LSD alone does not produce an enduring psychosis but rather precipitates schizophrenia in predisposed personalities (Slaby, 1991). Strassman (1984) suggested that the development of chronic LSD psychosis is multifactorial in origin and that premorbid factors such as family history and personality characteristics, as well as exposure to a multitude of drugs, play important roles.

Individual differences in liability to developing drug-related psychosis

It is clear that a number of drugs in different classes can cause, or increase the susceptibility for, a state of chronic psychosis. Why do some individuals develop psychotic symptoms after taking a specific drug, while others use regularly over long periods and remain unscathed? There is a striking paucity of studies that have examined the predisposing factors systematically. It is obvious that the drug abuse, which is at least partly genetically determined, plays a critical role in substance-induced psychosis. Nevertheless, in addition to factors related to drug consumption, a series of variables relating to a patient's personality and genetic predisposition seem crucial in determining the response to a given agent (Post, 1975).

In short, the risk for developing a substance-abuse problem is not equally distributed in the general population. Freud (1885) was cognizant of the importance of predisposing characterisitics in relation to cocaine's effects, stating:

I could not fail to note, however, that the individual disposition plays a major role in the effects of cocaine, perhaps a more important role than with other alkaloids. The subjective phenomena after ingestion of cocaine differ from person to person, and only a few persons experience, like myself, a pure euphoria without alteration. Others already experience slight intoxication, hyperkinesia and talkativeness after the same amount of cocaine, while still others have no subjective symptoms of the effects of cocaine at all.

Genetic determinants of response to stimulants are also highlighted by the demonstration of significant differences in response to amphetamine in animals, for example, hyperthymic responses in different strains of mice (Jori and Garattini, 1973). Again, the effects of an acute systemic injection of methamphetamine on motor behavior (stereotypy, locomotor activity, and rearing) and extracellular dopamine in the ventral striatum are different in two different strains of rats (Camp *et al.*, 1994).

Childhood development and personality

Tsuang *et al.* (1982) studied premorbid schizoid/paranoid personality and family psychiatric history of drug abusers with psychosis. They compared hospital records for four groups: (i) 72 drug abusers with psychosis lasting less than 6 months before admission, (ii) drug abusers with psychosis of a longer duration, (iii) drug abusers without psychosis, and (iv) patients with schizophrenia and atypical schizophrenia without drug abuse. Their study examined the role of premorbid personality, family, and genetic factors by comparison of multiple subgroups, and thus it provides a good model for studying predisposing factors to substance-induced psychosis. They reported that more drug abusers with prolonged psychosis have schizoid or paranoid premorbid personality than drug abusers without psychosis and those with short-term psychosis.

Vardy and Kay (1983) compared family history, manifest symptoms, premorbid adjustment, and profiles on an extensive test battery between patients with LSD psychosis and those with matched first-episode schizophrenia. The two groups were distinguished on some clinical features but were equivalent in premorbid adjustment and in number of subsequent rehospitalizations. The authors, therefore, suggested that in most respects the patients with LSD psychosis were fundamentally similar to those with schizophrenia in geneology, phenomenology, and course of illness, and the study supported a model of LSD psychosis as a drug-induced schizophreniform reaction in persons vulnerable to psychosis (Vardy and Kay, 1983).

Schizotypy is related genetically to schizophrenia and is often considered to represent a phenotypic expression of familial–genetic liability to schizophrenia (Battaglia *et al.*, 1997). A few investigators have reported correlations of drug abuse and schizotypal personality traits in non-clinical individuals (Dumas *et al.*, 2002; Kwapil, 1996; Williams *et al.*, 1996). Dumas *et al.* (2002) reported that cannabis users exhibit more psychotic-like schizotypal traits compared with never-users, regardless of their anxiety or depression dimension levels. Verdoux *et al.* (2002) found in a non-clinical population that the acute effects of cannabis were modified by the subject's level of psychosis-proneness. Those with low vulnerability for psychosis experienced enhanced feelings of pleasure after taking cannabis, while those with high vulnerability for psychosis were more likely to respond with increased hostility and suspiciousness (Verdoux *et al.*, 2002).

We compared childhood premorbid characteristics between 88 methamphetamine users with a lifetime diagnosis of methamphetamine psychosis and 116 methamphetamine users without psychosis by interviewing their parents with the Premorbid Schizoid and Schizotypal Traits (PSST) schedule. Subjects with experience of psychotic symptoms before their first use of methamphetamine were

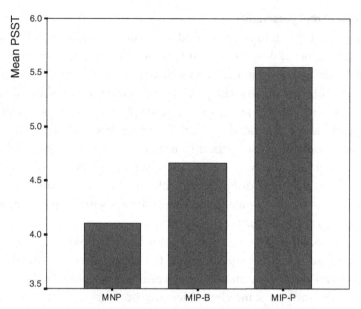

Fig. 14.1.   Premorbid schizoid/schizotypal traits between methamphetamine users with and without psychosis. MNP, methamphetamine users with no experience of psychotic symptom; MIP-B, subjects with brief methamphetamine psychosis; MIP-P, subjects with prolonged methamphetamine psychosis; PSST, score of Premorbid Schizoid and Schizotypal Traits.

excluded. Compared with their non-psychotic counterparts, those with methamphetamine psychosis had a significantly higher mean PSST score (Chen *et al.*, 2003). Indeed, we found a linear correlation between premorbid schizoid/schizotypal personality traits and liability to psychosis after methamphetamine abuse (Fig. 14.1). If schizotypy is one phenotypic expression of the familial–genetic liability to schizophrenia or other psychotic disorders, a hypothesis can be proposed that a continuum of vulnerability to psychosis accounts, at least to a certain degree, for individual differences in liability to drug-induced psychosis. In addition, it is reasonable to speculate that the patients with drug-induced psychosis, particularly if prolonged, may share some common vulnerability with schizophrenia.

Of course, one must remember that childhood problem behaviors may also precede substance abuse (Tarter *et al.*, 1990). Boyle *et al.* (1992) concluded that conduct disorder significantly predicts later abuse of marijuana and hard drugs. Many other studies have reported a link between childhood conduct disorder and antisocial behaviors on the one hand and later substance abuse on the other. However, no such link with childhood conduct disorder has been reported for schizophrenia, and the deviations that precede substance abuse appear different from those that precede psychotic disorders. Indeed, there is some evidence that individuals with schizophrenia and comorbid substance abuse have better premorbid adjustment levels than those with schizophrenia only (Arndt *et al.*, 1992).

A possible explanation for the latter finding is that those schizophrenia patients with marked childhood impairment are less likely to have acquired the social skills and initiative necessary first to expose themselves to drug use and then to be able to afford the cost of prolonged consumption of drugs, which are usually expensive. Alternatively, it could be that those with little or no neurodevelopmental impairment are likely to need more precipitating stressors such as drug abuse before becoming psychotic, while those with significant premorbid deviation require little or no additional stress to develop frank psychosis.

Familial predisposition

There have been only a few competent studies of the relationship between familial risk of psychosis and the occurrence and duration of drug-related psychoses. Tsuang *et al.* (1982) revealed that the familial risks of schizophrenia and affective disorder were greater in drug abusers with prolonged psychosis than those without psychosis or with psychosis of short duration. McGuire *et al.* (1995) compared the lifetime morbid risk of psychiatric disorder among the first-degree relatives of patients admitted with acute psychosis who were cannabis positive on urinary screening with that of psychotic controls who screened negatively for all substances. Patients with cannabis-associated psychosis had a significantly increased familial morbid risk for schizophrenia. This might be taken to imply that cannabis abuse acts on genetic predisposition to trigger psychosis.

In an early study, Tatetsu *et al.* (1956) reported that the prevalence of schizophrenia in the families of methamphetamine psychotics (4.7% for siblings, 3.4% for parents) was lower than that for schizophrenia patients (13.1% for siblings, 10.1% for parents) but higher than that for normal controls (0.6% for siblings, 0.25 for parents). Their interpretation was that methamphetamine psychosis is not genetically identical to schizophrenia, and that the higher prevalence of schizophrenia in families of patients with methamphetamine psychosis than in families of normal controls may have resulted from a small number of schizophrenia patients being included in the group of methamphetamine psychotics. An alternative formulation is that the psychosis predisposition of methamphetamine psychotics falls between that of schizophrenia patients and that of the normal population.

We assessed 445 methamphetamine users with the Diagnostic Interview for Genetic Studies and the Family Interview for Genetic Study. Familial morbid risk for psychotic disorders and other mental illnesses of first-degree relatives was compared after age correction between the methamphetamine users with a lifetime diagnosis of methamphetamine psychosis and those without. This study obtained psychiatric information for 1983 first-degree relatives of the methamphetamine users. The relatives of those with methamphetamine psychosis had higher morbid risks for schizophrenia than those of methamphetamine abusers without psychosis (3.1% versus 0.6%). The familial morbid risk for schizophrenia was even higher (6.5%) among those with prolonged methamphetamine psychosis.

Therefore, it appears that familial loading is an important factor in determining not only the occurrence of psychosis associated with drug abuse but also its duration. Furthermore, these findings are consistent with the notion of an underlying continuum of genetic liability that has schizophrenia as only one of its possible outcomes (Tsuang *et al.*, 2001; van Os *et al.*, 1998).

Molecular genetic studies of substance-associated psychosis

Dopamine receptor genes

Numerous studies have looked for genes associated with schizophrenia, and many others for possible associations with substance-use disorders, but until recently no unambiguous findings had been found (but see Harrison and Owen, 2003). Dopamine receptor (DRD) genes have been much studied in both conditions.

Dopamine D_2 receptor gene

Persico *et al.* (1996) reported that polysubstance users with histories of heavy daily preferential psychostimulant use more often displayed one or two copies of the *TaqI* A1 and B1 markers at the dopamine D_2 receptor (*DRD2*) locus. Ralph *et al.* (1999) reported that *DRD2* is essential for the disruption of prepulse inhibition produced by amphetamine in mice. Similar disruptions in prepulse inhibition have, of course, also been reported in schizophrenia (Braff *et al.*, 1992).

Dopamine D_3 receptor gene

DRD3 is reported to control the expression of sensitization to drugs of abuse (Guillin *et al.*, 2001) and to modulate drug-cue controlled cocaine-seeking behavior (Pilla *et al.*, 1999). Staley and Mash (1996) reported that elevated levels of DRD3 in the reward circuitry of the brain are associated with chronic cocaine abuse. *DRD3* expression is controlled by brain-derived neurotropic factor (Guillin *et al.*, 2001), and interestingly, elevated levels of this factor have been found in the anterior cingulate cortex and the hippocampus of patients with schizophrenia (Takahashi *et al.*, 2000). There are isolated reports of an association of *DRD3* polymorphism with substance abuse in schizophrenia (Krebs *et al.*, 1998) and with opiate dependence (Duaux *et al.*, 1998).

Dopamine D_4 receptor gene

Substance abuse is associated with novelty seeking, a heritable human personality trait that has been reported as associated with the seven-repeat variant of the *DRD4* variable number of tandem repeats (VNTR) (Ebstein *et al.*, 1996). Kotler *et al.*

(1997), therefore, analysed the *DRD4* VNTR in opiate-dependent subjects from Israel and found a significant excess of the seven-repeat allele. Other studies have failed to replicate the association of *DRD4* with substance abuse (Franke *et al.*, 2000; Li *et al.*, 2000); however, recently, we have found marginally significant differences in the *DRD4* exon III VNTR (C. K. Chen *et al.*, unpublished data) between 445 methamphetamine abusers and 416 normal controls.

Other genes

In the sample of 445 methamphetamine abusers, an association was noted between methampthetamine abuse and the allele giving rise to a valine or methionine at one position in catechol-*O*-methyltransferase (COMT) (T. Li *et al.*, unpublished data). This is interesting as individuals with the Val/Val genotype break down dopamine in the frontal cortex more rapidly than those with the Met/Met genotype, and there is experimental evidence that those with the former genotype experience fewer adverse reactions to amphetamine than those with the latter. One might, therefore, speculate that, among individuals who try methamphetamine, those with the Met/Met genotype may be more likely to experience adverse reactions and, therefore, not persist in taking the drug.

We did not find genetic differences between methamphetamine abusers with and without psychosis: indeed, this is the general finding so far. However, Kikuchi *et al.* (2001) found significant differences in both the *DRD1* and the *DRD5* locus in 107 methamphetamine users (96 with methamphetamine psychosis) compared with 192 healthy controls; it is not clear whether these polymorphisms are associated with liability to psychosis or to methamphetamine abuse. Using the same sample, Ujike *et al.* (2003) genotyped four types of dopamine transporter gene polymorphism. There were no significant differences in these four polymorphisms between methamphetamine users and controls. However, patients with prolonged methamphetamine psychosis (lasting more than 1 month after therapy) showed significant excess in the non-10-repeat alleles of the VNTR in the 3′ untranslated region of the dopamine transporter gene compared with those with brief methamphetamine psychosis.

Cubells *et al.* (2000) found an association of cocaine-induced paranoia and a haplotype associated with low dopamine β-hydroxylase activity, while low levels of dopamine β-hydroxylase protein in plasma or cerebrospinal fluid were previously reported to be associated with greater vulnerability to positive psychotic symptoms in several psychiatric disorders (Ewing *et al.*, 1977; Meltzer *et al.*, 1976; Meyers *et al.*, 1999).

Summary

All the molecular genetic study results discussed above are preliminary; both the positive and the negative findings need replication in larger samples. Nevertheless, rapid advances in molecular techniques will certainly promote progress in the search for the candidate genes of these disorders. It is likely that certain drugs change the expressions of genes related to neurotransmitter systems such as dopamine or glutamic acid and also for transcription factors, cell proliferation, apoptosis, cell adhesion, and the synapse (Ito, 2002). Hopefully, identifying these alterable gene expressions may facilitate the discovery of the genes that underlie the development of drug-associated psychosis.

Animal models of the interaction of drugs with perinatal brain damage

Patients with schizophrenia have been consistently shown to have experienced more pregnancy and labour complications than have normal controls (Cantor-Graae et al., 1994; Geddes and Lawrie, 1995; Lewis and Murray, 1987; O'Callaghan et al., 1992); such complications are associated with damage to the hippocampus and amygdala (Stefanis et al., 1999). Animal researchers have attempted to model such effects. In one of the best known models, Lipska and her colleagues (1992) showed that rats with neonatal damage of the ventral hippocampus display in adulthood a variety of abnormalities said also to occur in schizophrenia; for example, they show exaggerated behavioral response to amphetamine compared with controls. This provides an animal model of the interaction of drugs and perinatal insults in developing psychosis. Lipska and her colleagues (2002) concluded that transient loss of ventral hippocampal function during a critical time in maturation of intracortical connections permanently changes the development of neural circuits mediating certain dopamine- and NMDA-related behaviors.

Other studies have revealed that animals who were subject to Cesarean section birth (Vaillancourt and Boksa, 1998, 2000) or perinatal anoxia (Brake et al., 1997) are more prone to develop a sensitized response to amphetamine. Moreover, Berger et al. (2000) demonstrated the interaction of genetic predisposition, birth compli-cations, and amphetamine-induced locomotion by revealing different patterns of association between Cesarean section birth and amphetamine-induced locomotor activity in strains of rats differing in their genetic constitution.

Dopamine sensitization

Behavioral sensitization is a phenomenon whereby exposure to a given stimu-lus such as a drug or a stressor results in an enhanced response at subsequent exposures (Wolf et al., 1993). Repeated cocaine use leads to progressive sensitiza-tion, with short-term psychotic symptoms triggered more rapidly and after smaller amounts of cocaine (Bartlett et al., 1997). The process of sensitization does not necessarily require subsequent exposures to exactly the same stimulus that induced the process. For example, Gorriti et al. (1999) showed that chronic treatment with

$(-)$-Δ^9-tetrahydrocannabinol, the active ingredient of cannabis, resulted in sensitization to the effects of D-amphetamine on locomotion, exploration and stereotypies in rats. In an analogous manner, methamphetamine psychosis shows a marked tendency toward recurrence, which can be provoked by methamphetamine re-use at low dose or a wide variety of stressors, even after long-term abstinence (Sato et al., 1983). Interestingly, patients with schizophrenia are particularly sensitive to the psychosis-inducing effects of amphetamine in doses that are subpsychotogenic in normals (Lieberman et al., 1987), and they show an exaggerated release of dopamine in the ventral striatum following amphetamine challenge (Breier et al., 1997; Laruelle, 2000).

It seems likely that dopamine plays a modulatory role on corticoventrostriatal circuits, and that the psychotomimetic actions of dopaminergic agents and PCP may result from interference with these circuits (Carlsson, 1988). Positron emission tomography studies have suggested that dopamine transporter density in the caudate/putamen is reduced in methamphetamine users (McCann et al., 1998; Sekine et al., 2001; Volkow et al., 2001). Sekine et al. (2001) showed that the reduction of dopamine transporter may be long lasting, even if methamphetamine use ceases, and that persistent psychiatric symptoms in methamphetamine users, including psychotic symptoms, may be attributable to the reduction of dopamine transporter density.

Dopamine sensitization has been proposed to play a critical role in the disease process in schizophrenia. For example, Lieberman and his colleagues (1997) postulated that the symptoms of schizophrenia may be caused by deficits in neural regulation resulting in a pathological condition of neurochemical sensitization analogous to the preclinical model of pharmacologically induced behavioral sensitization. Dopamine sensitization may also explain the association between schizophrenia and abuse of psychostimulants and cannabis. It seems likely that familial predisposition to psychosis and perinatal insult increase the vulnerability to, dopamine sensitization, and that individuals with these predispositions may be more sensitive to the psychosis-inducing effects of certain drugs.

Conclusions

It is generally not disputed that the use of certain drugs, particularly cannabis and psychostimulants, which have major effects on dopamine is associated with schizophrenia. We regard the vulnerability hypothesis as the most likely explanation for this association. Early environmental insults often compound the genotype for psychosis to produce developmental deviance, but this is in itself sometimes not sufficient to produce a psychotic illness. Later environmental factors, such as drug abuse, then act on the underlying predisposition to precipitate frank psychosis.

Recent research suggests that dopamine sensitization may underlie both craving and the onset of drug-associated psychosis. Whether an individual develops psychosis after drug abuse may be determined by various factors, such as drug-use patterns, premorbid mental health, and the individual's place on a continuum of psychosis proneness. The liability for psychosis of each individual falls within a normal distribution. A drug abuser with low liability to psychosis may use psychostimulant drugs regularly for long periods without developing psychosis or, at worst may have just brief psychotic symptoms. By comparison, an individual with heavy liability may develop psychosis after using drugs only a few times and may have a prolonged psychosis in spite of subsequently remaining abstinent from the drug.

REFERENCES

Andreasson, S., Alleback, A., Engstrom, A., Rydberg, U. (1987). Cannabis and schizophrenia: a longitudinal study of Swedish conscripts. *Lancet i*: 1483–1485.

Angrist, B. M., Gershon, S. (1970). The phenomenology of experimentally induced amphetamine psychosis: preliminary observations. *Biol Psychiatry* 2: 95–107.

Arndt, S., Tyrrell, G., Flaum, M., Andreasen, N. C. (1992). Comorbidity of substance abuse and schizophrenia: the role of premorbid adjustment. *Psychol Med* 22: 379–388.

Arseneault, L., Cannon, M., Poulton, R., *et al.* (2002). Cannabis use in adolescence and risk for adult psychosis: longitudinal prospective study. *Br Med J* 325: 1212–1213.

Bartlett, E., Hallin, A., Chapman, B., Angrist, B. (1997). Selective sensitization to the psychosis-inducing effects of cocaine: a possible marker for addiction relapse vulnerability? *Neuropsychopharmacology* 16: 77–82.

Battaglia, M., Cavallini, M. C., Macciardi, F., Bellodi, L. (1997). The structure of DSM-III-R schizotypal personality disorder diagnosed by direct interviews. *Schizophr Bull* 23: 83–92.

Bebbington, P., Wilkins, S., Jones, P., *et al.* (1993). Life events and psychosis. Initial results from the Camberwell Collaborative Psychosis Study. *Br J Psychiatry* 162: 72–79.

Bell, D. S. (1965) Comparison of amphetamine psychosis and schizophrenia. *Br J Psychiatry* III: 701–707.

(1973). The experimental reproduction of amphetamine psychosis. *Arch Gen Psychiatry* 29: 35–40.

Berger, N., Vaillancourt, C., Boksa, P. (2000). Genetic factors modulate effects of C-section birth on dopaminergic function in the rat. *Neuroreport* 11: 639–643.

Blanchard, J. J., Brown, S. A., Horan, W. P., Sherwood, A. R. (2000). Substance use disorders in schizophrenia: review, integration, and a proposed model. *Clin Psychol Rev* 20: 207–234.

Boyle, M. H., Offord, D. R., Racine, Y. A., *et al.* (1992). Predicting substance use in late adolescence: results from the Ontario child health study follow-up. *Am J Psychiatry* 149: 761–767.

Braff, D. L., Grillon, C., Geyer, M. A. (1992). Gating and habituation of the startle reflex in schizophrenic patients. *Arch Gen Psychiatry* 49: 206–215.

Brake, W. G., Boksa, P., Gratton, A. (1997). Effects of perinatal anoxia on the acute locomotor response to repeated amphetamine administration in adult rats. *Psychopharmacology* **133**: 389–395.

Breakey, W. R., Goodell, H., Lorenz, P. C., McHugh, P. R. (1974). Hallucinogenic drugs as precipitants of schizophrenia. *Psychol Med* **4**: 255–261.

Breier, A., Su, T. P., Saunders, R., *et al.* (1997). Schizophrenia is associated with elevated amphetamine-induced synaptic dopamine concentrations: evidence from a novel positron emission tomography method. *Proc Natl Acad Sci USA* **94**: 2569–2574.

Camp, D. M., Browman, K. E., Robinson, T. E. (1994). The effects of methamphetamine and cocaine on motor behavior and extracellular dopamine in the ventral striatum of Lewis versus Fischer 344 rats. *Brain Res* **668**: 180–193.

Cannon, T. D., Kaprio, J., Lonnqvist, J., Huttunen, M., Koskenvuo, M. (1998). The genetic epidemiology of schizophrenia in a Finnish twin cohort. A population-based modeling study. *Arch Gen Psychiatry* **55**: 67–74.

Cantor-Graae, E., McNeil, T. F., Sjostrom, K., Nordstrom, L. G., Rosenlund, T. (1994). Obstetric complications and their relationship to other etiological risk factors in schizophrenia. A case–control study. *J Nerv Ment Dis* **182**: 645–650.

Cantwell, R., Brewin, J., Glazebrook, C., *et al.* (1999). Prevalence of substance misuse in first-episode psychosis. *Br J Psychiatry* **174**: 150–153.

Cardno, A. G., Marshall, E. J., Coid, B., *et al.* (1999). Heritability estimates for psychotic disorders: the Maudsley twin psychosis series. *Arch of Gen Psychiatry* **56**: 162–168.

Carlsson, A. (1988). The current status of the dopamine hypothesis of schizophrenia. *Neuropsychopharmacology* **1**: 179–186.

Cassano, G. B., Pini, S., Saettoni, M., Rucci, P., Dell'Osso, L. (1998). Occurrence and clinical correlates of psychiatric comorbidity in patients with psychotic disorders. *J Clin Psychiatry* **59**: 60–68.

Chen, C. K., Lin, S. K., Sham, P., *et al.* (2003). Premorbid characteristics and comorbidity of methamphetamine users with and without psychosis. *Psychol Med* **33**: 1407–1414.

Chou, P., Liou, M. Y., Lai, M. Y., Hsiao, M. L., Chang, H. J. (1999). Time trend of substance use among adolescent students in Taiwan, 1991–1996. *J Formos Med Assoc* **98**: 827–831.

Connell, P. H. (1958). *Amphetamine Psychosis* London: Chapman, Hall.

Crow, T. J., Johnstone, E. C., Deakin, J. F., Longden, A. (1976). Dopamine and schizophrenia. *Lancet* **ii**: 563–566.

Cubells, J. F., Kranzler, H. R., McCance-Katz, E., *et al.* (2000). A haplotype at the DBH locus, associated with low plasma dopamine beta-hydroxylase activity, also associates with cocaine-induced paranoia. *Mol Psychiatry* **5**: 56–63.

DeQuardo, J. R., Carpenter, C. F., Tandon, R. (1994). Patterns of substance abuse in schizophrenia: nature and significance. *J Psychiatr Res* **28**: 267–275.

Dixon, L., Haas, G., Weiden, P. J., Sweeney, J., Frances, A. J. (1991). Drug abuse in schizophrenic patients: clinical correlates and reasons for use. *Am J Psychiatry* **148**: 224–230.

Duaux, E., Gorwood, P., Griffon, N., *et al.* (1998). Homozygosity at the dopamine D_3 receptor gene is associated with opiate dependence. *Mol Psychiatry* **3**: 333–336.

Dumas, P., Saoud, M., Bouafia, S., *et al.* (2002). Cannabis use correlates with schizotypal personality traits in healthy students. *Psychiatry Res* **109**: 27–35.

Ebstein, R. P., Novick, O., Umansky, R., *et al.* (1996). Dopamine D_4 receptor (D4DR) exon III polymorphism associated with the human personality trait of novelty seeking. *Nat Genet* **12**: 78–80.

Ewing, J. A., Mueller, R. A., Rouse, B. A., Silver, D. (1977). Low levels of dopamine beta-hydroxylase and psychosis. *Am J Psychiatry* **134**: 927–928.

Fischman, M. W., Schuster, C. R. (1982). Cocaine self-administration in humans. *Fed Proc* **41**: 241–246.

Flaum, M., Schultz, S. K. (1996). When does amphetamine-induced psychosis become schizophrenia? [Clinical conference] *Am J Psychiatry* **153**: 812–815.

Franke, P., Nothen, M. M., Wang, T., *et al.* (2000). DRD4 exon III VNTR polymorphism-susceptibility factor for heroin dependence? Results of a case–control and a family-based association approach. *Mol Psychiatry* **5**: 101–104.

Freud, S. (1885). On the general effects of cocaine. [Lecture before Psychiatric Union, 5 March, 1885. Translated to English.] *Drug Depend* **5**: 15–17.

Geddes, J. R., Lawrie, S. M. (1995). Obstetric complications and schizophrenia: a meta-analysis. *Br J Psychiatry* **167**: 786–793.

Gold, M. S., Bowers, Jr. M. B. (1978). Neurobiological vulnerability to low-dose amphetamine psychosis. *Am J Psychiatry* **135**: 1546–1548.

Gorriti, M. A., de Rodriguez, F., Navarro, M., Palomo, T. (1999). Chronic (−)-delta9-tetrahydrocannabinol treatment induces sensitization to the psychomotor effects of amphetamine in rats. *Eur J Pharmacol* **365**: 133–142.

Griffith, J. D., Cavanaugh, J., Oates, J. A. (1969). Schizophreniform psychosis induced by large-dose administration of D-amphetamine. *J Psychedel Drugs* **2**: 42–48.

Griffith, J. D., Cavanaugh, J., Held, J., Oates, J. A. (1972). Dextroamphetamine. Evaluation of psychomimetic properties in man. *Arch Gen Psychiatry* **26**: 97–100.

Guillin, O., Diaz, J., Carroll, P., *et al.* (2001). BDNF controls dopamine D_3 receptor expression and triggers behavioral sensitization. *Nature* **411**: 86–89.

Harrison, P. J., Owen, M. J. (2003). Genes for schizophrenia? Recent findings and their pathophysiological implications. *Lancet* **361**: 417–419.

Imade, A. G. T., Ebie, J. C. (1991). A retrospective study of symptom patterns of cannabis-induced psychosis. *Acta Psychiatr Scand* **83**: 134–136.

Ito, C. (2002). Analysis of overall gene expression induced by amphetamine and phencyclidine: novel targets for the treatment of drug psychosis and schizophrenia. *Curr Pharm Des* **8**: 147–153.

Iwanami, A., Suga, I., Kaneko, T., Sugiyama, A., Nakatani, Y. (1994). P300 component of event-related potentials in methamphetamine psychosis and schizophrenia. *Prog Neuropsychopharmacol Biol Psychiatry* **18**: 465–475.

Jacobs, M. R., Fehr, K. O., Cox, T. C., *et al.* (1987). *Drugs and Drug Abuse. A Reference Text.* Toronto: Addiction Research Foundation.

Javitt, D. C., Zukin, S. Z. (1991). Recent advances in the phencyclidine model of schizophrenia. *Am J Psychiatry* **148**: 1301–1308.

Johnson, B. A., Smith, B. L., Taylor, P. (1988). Cannabis and schizophrenia. *Lancet* i: 593.

Jones, P., Rodgers, B., Murray, R., Marmot, M. (1994). Child developmental risk factors for adult schizophrenia in the British 1946 birth cohort. *Lancet* **344**: 1398–1402.

Jori, A., Garattini, S. (1973). Catecholamine metabolism and amphetamine effects on sensitive and insensitive mice. In *Frontiers in Catecholamine Research*, ed. E. Usdin, S. H. Snyder. New York: Pergamon Press, pp. 939–941.

Kendler, K. S., Diehl, S. R. (1993). The genetics of schizophrenia: a current, genetic-epidemiologic perspective. *Schizophr Bull* **19**: 261–285.

Khantzian, E. J. (1985). The self-medication hypothesis of addictive disorders: focus on heroin and cocaine dependence. *Am J Psychiatry* **142**: 1259–1264.

Kikuchi, K., Inada, T., Iijima, Y., *et al.* (2001). Association between dopamine D_1 receptor family (DRD1, DRD5) gene polymorphisms and methamphetamine psychosis. In *Proceedings of the International College of Neuro-Psychopharmacology Regional Meeting*, Hiroshima, p. 398.

Kleinman, J. E., Casanova, F. M., Jaskiv, G. E. (1988). The neuropathology of schizophrenia. *Schizophrenia Bulletin* **14**: 209–216.

Konuma, K. (1994). Use and abuse of amphetamines in Japan. In *Amphetamine and its Analogs* pp. 415–435.

Kotler, M., Cohen, H., Segman, R., *et al.* (1997). Excess dopamine D4 receptor (D4DR) exon III seven repeat allele in opioid-dependent subjects. *Mol Psychiatry* **2**: 251–254.

Krebs, M. O., Sautel, F., Bourdel, M. C., *et al.* (1998). Dopamine D3 receptor gene variants and substance abuse in schizophrenia. *Mol Psychiatry* **3**: 337–341.

Kwapil, T. R. (1996). A longitudinal study of drug and alcohol use by psychosis-prone and impulsive-nonconforming individuals. *J Abnorm Psychol* **105**: 114–123.

Laruelle, M. (2000). The role of endogenous sensitization in the pathophysiology of schizophrenia: implications from recent brain imaging studies. *Brain Res Brain Res Rev* **31**: 371–384.

Lewis, S. W., Murray, R. M. (1987). Obstetric complications, neurodevelopmental deviance, and risk of schizophrenia. *J Psychiatr Res* **21**: 413–421.

Li, T., Zhu, Z. H., Liu, X., *et al.* (2000). Association analysis of polymorphisms in the *DRD4* gene and heroin abuse in Chinese subjects. *Am J Med Genet* **96**: 616–621.

Lieberman, J. A., Kane, J. M., Alvir, J. (1987). Provocative tests with psychostimulant drugs in schizophrenia. *Psychopharmacology* **91**: 415–433.

Lieberman, J. A., Sheitman, B. B., Kinon, B. J. (1997). Neurochemical sensitization in the pathophysiology of schizophrenia: deficits and dysfunction in neuronal regulation and plasticity. *Neuropsychopharmacology* **17**: 205–229.

Linszen, D. H., Dingemans, P. M., Lenior, M. E. (1994). Cannabis abuse and the course of recent-onset schizophrenic disorders. *Arch of Gen Psychiatry* **51**: 273–279.

Lipska, B. K., Jaskiw, G. E., Chrapusta, S., Karoum, F., Weinberger, D. R. (1992). Ibotenic acid lesion of the ventral hippocampus differentially affects dopamine and its metabolites in the nucleus accumbens and prefrontal cortex in the rat. *Brain Res* **585**: 1–6.

Lipska, B. K., Halim, N. D., Segal, P. N., Weinberger, D. R. (2002). Effects of reversible inactivation of the neonatal ventral hippocampus on behavior in the adult rat. *J Neurosci* **22**: 2835–2842.

Longhurst, J. G. (1997). Cannabis and schizophrenia. *Br J Psychiatry* **171**: 584–585.

Lopez, W., Jeste, D. V. (1997). Movement disorders and substance abuse. *Psychiatr Serv* **48**: 634–636.

Mathers, D. C., Ghodse, A. H., Caan, A. W., Scott, S. A. (1991). Cannabis use in a large sample of acute psychiatric admissions. *Br J Addict* **86**: 779–784.

McCann, U. D., Wong, D. F., Yokoi, F., *et al.* (1998). Reduced striatal dopamine transporter density in abstinent methamphetamine and methcathinone users: evidence from positron emission tomography studies with [^{11}C]WIN-35,428. *J Neurosci* **18**: 8417–8422.

McCreadie, R. G. (2002). Use of drugs, alcohol and tobacco by people with schizophrenia: case–control study. *Br J Psychiatry* **181**: 321–325.

McGuire, P. K., Jones, P., Harvey, I., *et al.* (1995). Morbid risk of schizophrenia for relatives of patients with cannabis-associated psychosis. *Schizophr Res* **15**: 277–281.

Meltzer, H. Y., Cho, H. W., Carroll, B. J., Russo, P. (1976). Serum dopamine-beta-hydroxylase activity in the affective psychoses and schizophrenia. Decreased activity in unipolar psychotically depressed patients. *Arch of Gen Psychiatry* **33**: 585–591.

Menezes, P. R., Johnson, S., Thornicroft, G., *et al.* (1996). Drug and alcohol problems among individuals with severe mental illness in south London. *Br J Psychiatry* **168**: 612–619.

Meyers, B. S., Alexopoulos, G. S., Kakuma, T., *et al.* (1999). Decreased dopamine beta-hydroxylase activity in unipolar geriatric delusional depression. *Biol Psychiatry*, **45**: 448–452.

Modestin, J., Nussbaumer, C., Angst, K., Scheidegger, P., Hell, D. (1997). Use of potentially abusive psychotropic substances in psychiatric inpatients. *Eur Arch Psychiatry Clin Neurosci* **247**: 146–153.

Mueser, K. T., Yarnold, P. R., Levinson, D. F., *et al.* (1990). Prevalence of substance abuse in schizophrenia, demographic and clinical correlates. *Schizophr Bull* **6**: 10–41.

Mueser, K. T., Drake, R. E., Wallach, M. A. (1998). Dual diagnosis: a review of etiological theories. *Addict Behav* **23**: 717–734.

Murray, R. M., Fearon, P. (1999). The developmental "risk factor" model of schizophrenia. *J Psychiatr Res* **33**: 497–499.

Murray, R. M., Grech, A., Phillips, P., Johnson, S. (2003). What is the relationship between substance abuse and schizophrenia? In *The Epidemiology of Schizophrenia*, ed. R. M. Murray, P. Jones, E. Susser, J. van Os, M. Cannon. Cambridge, UK: Cambridge University Press, pp. 317–342.

Nakatani, Y., Yoshizawa, F., Yamada, H., *et al.* (1989). Methamphetamine psychosis in Japan: a survey. *Br J Addict* **84**: 1548–1549.

National Institute on Drug Abuse (1998). *Methamphetamine abuse and addiction.* (*Publication 98–4210*). Bethesda, MD: National Institutes of Health.

Negrete, J. C. (1989). Cannabis and schizophrenia. *Br J Addiction* **84**: 349–351.

O'Callaghan, E., Gibson, T., Colohan, H. A., *et al.* (1992). Risk of schizophrenia in adults born after obstetric complications and their association with early onset of illness: a controlled study. *Br Med J* **305**: 1256–1259.

Peralta, V., Cuesta, M. J. (1992). Influence of cannabis abuse on schizophrenic psychopathology. *Acta Psychiatr Scand* **85**: 127–130.

Persico, A. M., Bird, G., Gabbay, F. H., Uhl, G. R. (1996) D_2 dopamine receptor gene *TaqI* A1 and B1 restriction fragment length polymorphisms: enhanced frequencies in psychostimulant-preferring polysubstance abusers. *Biol Psychiatry* **40**: 776–784.

Pilla, M., Perachon, S., Sautel, F., *et al.* (1999). Selective inhibition of cocaine-seeking behavior by a partial dopamine D_3 receptor agonist. *Nature* **400**: 371–375.

Post, R. M. (1975). Cocaine psychosis: a continuum model. *Am J Psychiatry* **132**: 225–231.

Ralph, R. J., Varty, G. B., Kelly, M. A., *et al.* (1999). The dopamine D_2, but not D_3 or D_4, receptor subtype is essential for the disruption of prepulse inhibition produced by amphetamine in mice. *J Neurosci* **19**: 4627–4633.

Regier, D. A., Farmer, M. E., Rae, D. S., *et al.* (1990). Comorbidity of mental disorders with alcohol and other drug abuse. Results from the Epidemiologic Catchment Area (ECA) Study. *J Am Med Assoc* **264**: 2511–2518.

Rolfe, M., Tang, C. M., Sabally, S., *et al.* (1993). Psychosis and cannabis abuse in The Gambia. A case–control study. *Br J Psychiatry* **163**: 798–801.

Sato, M., Chen, C. C., Akiyama, K., Otsuki, S. (1983). Acute exacerbation of paranoid psychotic state after long-term abstinence in patients with previous methamphetamine psychosis. *Biol Psychiatry* **18**: 429–440.

Schneier, F. R., Siris, S. G. (1987). A review of psychoactive substance use and abuse in schizophrenia. Patterns of drug choice. *J Nerv Ment Dis* **175**: 641–652.

Sekine, Y., Iyo, M., Ouchi, Y., *et al.* (2001). Methamphetamine-related psychiatric symptoms and reduced brain dopamine transporters studied with PET. *Am J Psychiatry* **158**: 1206–1214.

Selzer, J. A., Lieberman, J. A. (1993). Schizophrenia and substance abuse. *Psychiatr Clin North Am* **16**: 401–412.

Slaby, A. E. (1991). Dual diagnosis: fact or fiction? In *Dual Diagnosis in Substance Abuse*, ed. M. S. Gold, A. E. Slaby. New York: Marcel Dekker, pp. 3–28.

Snell, L. D., Yi, S.-J., Johnson, K. M. (1988). Comparison of the effects of MK-801 and phencyclidine on catecholamine uptake and NMDA-induced norepinephrine release. *Eur J Pharmacol* **145**: 223–226.

Snyder, S. H. (1973). Amphetamine psychosis: a "model" schizophrenia mediated by catecholamines. *Am J Psychiatry* **130**: 61–67.

Soyka, M., Albus, M., Kathmann, N., *et al.* (1993). Prevalence of alcohol and drug abuse in schizophrenic inpatients. *Eur Arch Psychiatry Clin Neurosci* **242**: 362–372.

Staley, J. K., Mash, D. C. (1996). Adaptive increase in D_3 dopamine receptors in the brain reward circuits of human cocaine fatalities. *J Neurosci* **16**: 6100–6106.

Stefanis, N., Frangou, S., Yakeley, J., *et al.* (1999). Hippocampal volume reduction in schizophrenia: effects of genetic risk and pregnancy and birth complications. *Biol Psychiatry* **46**: 697–702.

Strassman, R. J. (1984). Adverse reactions to psychedelic drugs. A review of the literature. *J Nerv Ment Dis* **172**: 577–595.

Suwaki, H., Fukui, S., Konuma, K. (1997) Methamphetamine abuse in Japan: its 45 year history and the current situation. In *Amphetamine Misuse: International Perspective on Current Trends*, ed. H. Klee. Amsterdam: Harwood Academic, pp. 199–214.

Takahashi, M., Shirakawa, O., Toyooka, K., *et al.* (2000). Abnormal expression of brain-derived neurotrophic factor and its receptor in the corticolimbic system of schizophrenic patients. *Mol Psychiatry* **5**: 293–300.

Tarter, R. E., Laird, S. B., Kabene, M., Bukstein, O., Kaminer, Y. (1990). Drug abuse severity in adolescents is associated with magnitude of deviation in temperament traits. *Br J Addiction* **85**: 1501–1504.

Tatetsu, S. (1963). Methamphetamine. *Folia Psychiatr Neurol Jap Suppl* **7**: 377–380.

Tatetsu, S., Goto, A., Fujiwara, T. (1956). *The Methamphetamine Psychosis*. Tokyo: Igakushoin.

Thomas, H. (1993). Psychiatric symptoms in cannabis users. *Br J Psychiatry* **163**: 141–149.

Thornicroft, G. (1990). Cannabis and psychosis: is there epidemiological evidence for an association? *Br J Psychiatry* **157**: 25–33.

Tsuang, M. T., Simpson, J. C., Kronfol, Z. (1982). Subtypes of drug abuse with psychosis. Demographic characteristics, clinical features, and family history. *Arch Gen Psychiatry* **39**: 141–147.

Tsuang, M. T., Stone, W. S., Faraone, S. V. (2001). Genes, environment and schizophrenia. *Br J Psychiatry* **178**: 18–24.

Ujike, H., Harano, M., Inada, T., *et al.* (2003). Nine- or fewer repeat alleles in VNTR polymorphism of the dopamine transporter gene is a strong risk factor for prolonged methamphetamine psychosis. *Pharmacogenom J* **3**: 242–247.

United Nations International Drug Control Programme (1997). *World Drug Report*. New York: Oxford University Press.

Vaillancourt, C., Boksa, P. (1998). Caesarean section birth with general anesthesia increases dopamine-mediated behavior in the adult rat. *Neuroreport* **9**: 2953–2959.

(2000). Birth insult alters dopamine-mediated behavior in a precocial species, the guinea pig. Implications for schizophrenia. *Neuropsychopharmacology* **23**: 654–666.

van Os, J., Jones, P., Sham, P., Bebbington, P., Murray, R. M. (1998). Risk factors for onset and persistence of psychosis. *Soc Psychiatry Psychiatr Epidemiol* **33**: 596–605.

van Os, J., Bak, M., Hanssen, M., *et al.* (2002). Cannabis use and psychosis: a longitudinal population-based study. *Am J Epidemiol* **156**: 319–327.

Vardy, M. M., Kay, S. R. (1983). LSD psychosis or LSD-induced schizophrenia? A multimethod inquiry. *Arch Gen Psychiatry* **40**: 877–883.

Verdoux, H., Mury, M., Besancon, G., Bourgeois, M. (1996a). [Comparative study of substance dependence comorbidity in bipolar, schizophrenic and schizoaffective disorders.] *Encephale* **22**: 95–101.

Verdoux, H., van Os, J., Sham, P., *et al.* (1996b). Does familiality predispose to both emergence and persistence of psychosis? A follow-up study. *Br J Psychiatry* **168**: 620–626. [Published erratum appears in *Br J Psychiatry* (1996). **169**: 116].

Verdoux, H., Gindre, C., Sorbara, F., Tournier, M., Swendsen, J. D. (2002). Cannabis use and the expression of psychosis vulnerability in daily life. *Schizophr Res* **53** (Suppl.): 225.

Volkow, N. D., Chang, L., Wang, G. J., *et al.* (2001). Association of dopamine transporter reduction with psychomotor impairment in methamphetamine abusers. *Am J Psychiatry* **158**: 377–382.

Williams, J. H., Wellman, N. A., Rawlins, J. N. (1996). Cannabis use correlates with schizotypy in healthy people. *Addiction* **91**: 869–877.

Wolf, M. E., White, F. J., Nassar, R., Brooderson, R. J., Khansa, M. R. (1993). Differential development of autoreceptor subsensitivity and enhanced dopamine release during amphetamine sensitization. *J Pharmacol Exp Ther* **264**: 249–255.

Zammit, S., Allebeck, P., Andreasson, S., Lundberg, I., Lewis, G. (2002). Self reported cannabis use as a risk factor for schizophrenia in Swedish conscripts of 1969: historical cohort study. *Br Med J* **325**: 1199.

Part III

Pathophysiology

15

Developmental dysregulation of the dopamine system and the pathophysiology of schizophrenia

Anthony A. Grace

University of Pittsburgh, Pittsburgh, USA

Evidence suggests that the dopamine (DA) system plays a key role in the pathophysiology and treatment of schizophrenia. Therefore, drugs that increase DA transmission are known to exacerbate this disorder and mimic paranoid psychosis in normal individuals (Angrist *et al.*, 1974, 1980), and drugs that are effective antipsychotic agents all have DA receptor-blocking properties in common (Creese *et al.*, 1976; Grace *et al.*, 1997; Seeman, 1987). However, despite substantial effort, there has been little direct evidence for a pathology within at least the subcortical DA system (Beuger *et al.*, 1996; Post *et al.*, 1975; Van Kammen *et al.*, 1986). Nonetheless, schizophrenia patients show significantly higher levels of DA release in the striatum in response to low doses of amphetamine, particularly in patients in whom the amphetamine leads to an exacerbation of their psychosis (Laruelle, 2000; Laruelle and Abi-Dargham, 1999). This has led to the suggestion that the DA system may be abnormally regulated in the brains of schizophrenia patients, leading to the psychopathological state. One system in particular that has attracted attention as a potential source of this dysregulatory influence is the cortical glutamatergic system. This is based on evidence that drugs that interfere with glutamate transmission exert a symptom-specific exacerbation of schizophrenia in susceptible patients and will mimic the entire spectrum of schizophrenia symptoms in some normal individuals (Goff and Coyle, 2001; Jentsch and Roth, 1999; Olney and Farber, 1995). There is also evidence for a pathology within the limbic cortex of schizophrenia patients (Weinberger, 1999).

Substantial evidence exists to suggest that the pathological processes contributing to schizophrenia occur early in life, supporting the contention that schizophrenia is a developmental disorder. Thus, the incidence of schizophrenia is higher in individuals with a genetic predisposition to the disorder, with the rate of occurrence

Neurodevelopment and Schizophrenia, ed. Matcheri S. Keshavan *et al.* Published by Cambridge University Press. © Cambridge University Press 2004.

being proportional to the relative amount of shared genetic background. However, unlike true genetic diseases such as Huntington's disease, schizophrenia does not appear to be completely genetically determined. Even in identical twins, which should have identical genetic make-up, the concordance rate for schizophrenia is only 50% (Kendler, 1983). This is approximately 50 times higher than that found in the general population but still is not supportive of a fully expressed genotype. In addition, it is known that birth insults will often correlate with higher incidence of schizophrenia in the offspring. For example, there is a significantly higher incidence of births of individuals who later develop schizophrenia where the mother was exposed to areas of famine or severe influenza infections during the second trimester (McDonald and Murray, 2000; Pilowsky et al., 1993; Susser et al., 1996). Moreover, the incidence of birth of schizophrenia patients is higher during spring months, which corresponds to the sensitive second trimester occurring during the winter months when illness is more common (Torrey et al., 1997). Together, this evidence suggests that an insult during the second trimester, which is a time when limbic cortices are developing, combined with a genetic susceptibility may lead to a predisposition for schizophrenia illness (Bayer et al., 1999; Lewis and Levitt, 2002; Weinberger, 1996).

The prefrontal cortex

Role in the pathophysiology of schizophrenia

One question that has been difficult to fit into a pathological model of schizophrenia relates to the age of onset of symptoms. From the above, it appears that the trigger for the illness is present during gestation. However, although the prodromal state may be present for variable intervals prior to the onset of psychosis, the first episode of psychotic symptoms typically occurs during late adolescence or early adulthood (DeLisi, 1992). One possibility is that the developmental insult causes the limbic system to reorganize in a type of temporary compensatory manner, which subsequently fails to perform when the subject reaches adolescence (Grace and Moore, 1998). One focus for a source of this delayed development is the prefrontal cortex, based in part on the protracted development of this region, which extends well into adolescence (Lewis, 1997). Subjects at high risk for the development of schizophrenia as well as first-degree relatives of schizophrenia patients often show disturbed performance in tasks that measure prefrontal cortical activity, typically referred to as tests of executive function or working memory (Cohen and Servan-Schreiber, 1992; Goldman-Rakic, 1999). Performance of working memory tasks are associated with activation of the prefrontal cortex (Goldman-Rakic, 1995). Moreover, working memory within the prefrontal cortex is believed to depend on its DA innervation (Goldman-Rakic, 1996), which has been shown to be pathologically decreased by as much as 33% in this structure in the brains of schizophrenia patients (Akil *et al.*, 1999). Together, these data suggest that pathology within the prefrontal cortex may be an etiological factor in the onset of schizophrenia. However, although prefrontal cortical lesions in adults may mimic some of the negative symptoms of schizophrenia, there is little evidence that such an insult will lead to psychosis.

Role in stress and emotional reactivity

A deficit in prefrontal cortical function would be expected to produce several specific disturbances in brain function. In particular, our studies have shown that the prefrontal cortex exerts an important suppressive role on the basolateral amygdala (Rosenkranz and Grace, 1999, 2001), a structure known to be important in the expression of emotion (LeDoux, 2000). Stimulation of the prefrontal cortex was found to activate interneurons preferentially within the basolateral amygdala; as a consequence, it exerted a suppressive effect over excitatory afferents arising from the sensory association cortex (Rosenkranz and Grace, 2001, 2002a). One interpretation of this finding is that the prefrontal cortex will suppress emotional responses to stimuli that experience has determined to be benign or non-threatening in nature. The prefrontal cortex was also found to suppress conditioned responses to noxious stimuli at the cellular level (Rosenkranz and Grace, 2002b). The amygdala also appears to play a role in the reaction to chronic stressors. Via the projections from the central nucleus of the amygdala to the hypothalamus (Pitkanen *et al.*, 1997), the amygdala is positioned to exert influence over the hypothalamic–pituitary–adrenal (HPA) axis, which among other things would provide a link between stress-induced emotional responses and release of stress hormones such as glucocorticoids. Indeed, it is likely that the amygdala is involved in a variety of psychiatric disorders ranging from depression to attention-deficit hyperactivity disorder (Breier *et al.*, 1992; Drevets, 1999; Goddard and Charney, 1997; Grace, 2000; Lawrie and Abukmeil, 1998; Ninan, 1999; Tebartz van Elst *et al.*, 1999). This structure is also capable of showing plasticity in response to stress, including conditioned associations (McKernan and Shinnick-Gallagher, 1997; Ono *et al.*, 1995; Pare and Collins, 2000; Rogan *et al.*, 1997; Rosenkranz and Grace, 2002b).

Exposure to stress is known to activate several central systems, principally the noradrenergic system of the locus coeruleus. Upon presentation of a stressor, there is an increase in locus coeruleus neuron firing (Abercrombie and Jacobs, 1987), norepinephrine levels and metabolites at postsynaptic sites (Abercrombie *et al.*, 1988; Shanks *et al.*, 1991; Thierry *et al.*, 1968), and the capacity to synthesize norepinephrine (Chang *et al.*, 2000; Sabban and Kvetnansky, 2001; Serova *et al.*, 1999). Corticotropin-releasing hormone (CRH) is the primary regulator of adrenocorticotropic hormone release from the pituitary during stress (Vale *et al.*, 1981), although evidence has demonstrated a prominent extrahypothalamic role for CRH as well (Valentino *et al.*, 1993). Therefore, intraventricular injection of CRH is known to elicit numerous stress-like behaviors (Dunn and Berridge, 1987; Kalin, 1985; Sherman and Kalin, 1986), and studies have shown that CRH injected intraventricularly or into the locus coeruleus will activate noradrenergic neuron firing and norepinephrine release (Curtis *et al.*, 1997; Finlay *et al.*, 1997; Page and Abercrombie, 1999; Smagin *et al.*, 1995; Valentino and Foote, 1986; Valentino *et al.*, 1983, 1993). In addition, administration of CRH antagonists will attenuate stress-evoked increases in locus coeruleus neuronal activity and norepinephrine release (Emoto *et al.*, 1993; Lechner *et al.*, 1997; Smagin *et al.*, 1997; Valentino and Wehby, 1988; Valentino *et al.*, 1991) and behavioral responses (Smagin *et al.*, 1996) to select stressors.

The amygdala is known to provide a CRH input to the locus coeruleus, both directly and indirectly, which synapses preferentially in the pericoerulear region, an area that contains dendritic processes of locus coeruleus neurons (Van Bockstaele *et al.*, 1996, 1998, 1999). This region is also the recipient zone for the afferents from the prefrontal cortex to the locus coeruleus (Ennis *et al.*, 1998; Zhu and Aston-Jones, 1996). Based on this anatomical arrangement, it has been suggested that direct CRH and glutamate inputs to the locus coeruleus proper from regions such as the perigigantocelluaris region and Barrington's nucleus (Aston-Jones *et al.*, 1986; Valentino *et al.*, 1996) act to convey messages that are of immediate physiological survival value (i.e. the "systemic" stressors; (Herman and Cullinan, 1997), whereas inputs to the pericoerulear region, which would contact major dendrites of locus coeruleus neurons (Ennis *et al.*, 1998), would act more in a modulatory role (Herman and Cullinan, 1997). In this way, inputs to the dendrites could, in turn, modulate the response of locus coeruleus neurons to the afferents that carry physiological information (e.g., the perigigantocelluaris) onto processes more proximal to the locus coeruleus somata. Such a modulatory function would be expected to subserve the types of emotion or cognition activity associated with psychopathology or exposure to chronic stress or drug abuse.

Our studies show that rats exposed to chronic cold stress exhibit increased responses to acute stressors within the basolateral amygdala (Correll *et al.*, 2001) and the locus coeruleus (Jedema and Grace, 2003; Mana and Grace, 1997; Ramsooksingh *et al.*, 2002). In addition, following chronic stress exposure, the prefrontal cortex has less inhibitory action over the locus coeruleus (Ramsooksingh *et al.*, 2001). When considered in the light of the role of the prefrontal cortex in suppressing amygdala responses (Rosenkranz and Grace, 1999, 2001), it is clear that the prefrontal cortex plays an essential role in regulating emotional expression, and that disruption of this prefrontal cortical influence would be expected to result in a pathological increase in emotional responsivity of the subject. The prefrontal cortex has also been reported to play a role in other aspects of the response to stress. Studies have shown that exposure to a stressor leads to increased DA release in the prefrontal cortex, with substantially smaller increases in DA within subcortical structures (Abercrombie *et al.*, 1989; Imperato *et al.*, 1989). However, if the DA innervation of the prefrontal cortex is disrupted, two consequences are noted. First, there is a decrease in the spontaneous activity of ventral tegmental DA neurons (Harden *et al.*, 1998); second, there is an increase in the stress-induced DA response within subcortical limbic structures such as the nucleus accumbens (King *et al.*, 1997).

Together, these studies suggest that, in the absence of a normally functioning prefrontal cortex, the system would over-react to potentially anxiogenic stimuli, resulting in increased levels of stress. Indeed, such a model is consistent with observations of high-risk individuals by E. C. Johnstone (personal communication), who found that those adolescents who eventually go on to develop schizophrenia typically show a higher reactivity to stress compared with those who do not develop psychosis. What consequence would such an increase in stress produce? One region that may be of particular significance in this regard is the ventral hippocampus.

One pathological finding that has been reported with some consistency is a decrease in ventral hippocampal volume in schizophrenia patients, particularly when comparing afflicted versus normal monozygotic twins (Suddath *et al.*, 1990). A focus on the ventral hippocampus is also supported by prospective studies, in which an increase in hippocampal volume is observed in high-risk individuals prior to the onset of psychosis (Pantelis *et al.*, 2003; Phillips *et al.*, 2002). Such a condition suggests that the ventral hippocampus may undergo some type of pathological alteration during the first episode that would lead to the expression of psychosis. A potential etiological factor involving developmental disruption of the ventral hippocampus or limbic cortex has been exploited in the advancement of animal models of this disorder.

Developmental models of schizophrenia

An impediment to advancing our understanding of the relationship between limbic pathophysiology and the etiology of schizophrenia is the lack of an appropriate animal model for this disorder. Because schizophrenia is a uniquely human affliction, it is difficult to approximate its complex psychological and cognitive components. Furthermore, neuroanatomical studies of schizophrenia brains have failed to yield concrete pathological correlates of this disorder. Instead, pathological changes are reported to be rather variable and diffuse, involving mainly limbic and frontal cortical regions (Harrison, 1999). However, as reviewed above, several epidemiological results suggest that gestational factors may contribute to schizophrenia. This has led to the suggestion that it may arise from an interaction between a genetic predisposition combined with a developmental insult (Bayer *et al.*, 1999; Weinberger, 1996).

Recent studies have suggested the presence of an early disruption in cortical development in schizophrenia (Jones, 1997; Weinberger and Lipska, 1995). Such a pathology is thought to lead to the widespread but subtle pathological changes in the cerebral cortex in schizophrenia, which include a decrease in cortical thickness (Harrison, 1999; McCarley *et al.*, 1999) with no significant alteration in total neuron number (Thune and Pakkenberg, 2000) and the absence of evidence for neurodegeneration (Arnold *et al.*, 1998). This is consistent with the reported increase in neuronal density accompanied by reduced neuropil (e.g. Harrison, 1999; Selemon *et al.*, 1995). Studies have also reported decreases in structures related to synaptic transmission (Eastwood *et al.*, 2000; Garey *et al.*, 1998; Glantz and Lewis, 1997; Mirnics *et al.*, 2000). Such alterations are most commonly reported to be present in medial temporal and frontal cortices (Harrison, 1999; McCarley *et al.*, 1999). Moreover, the behavioral symptoms associated with schizophrenia are most often correlated with pathology within limbic regions of the frontal lobes and their associated target structures (Arnold, 1997; Bilder *et al.*, 1995; Liddle *et al.*, 1992; Tamminga *et al.*, 1992). Studies have also shown that the mesolimbic DA system is hyperreactive in schizophrenia (Laruelle, 2000; Laruelle and Abi-Dargham, 1999), a state that has been proposed to be secondary to pathology within limbic cortex (Bertolino *et al.*, 1999; Grace, 1991; Weinberger and Lipska, 1995).

One approach to examining the consequences of developmentally related pathological alterations in an animal model was proposed by Lipska and Weinberger (Lipska *et al.*, 1993; Weinberger and Lipska, 1995). These investigators showed that lesions created in the ventral subiculum of the hippocampus in neonatal rats led to behaviors in the adult animal consistent with hyperactivation within the mesolimbic DA system (Lipska *et al.*, 1993). Similarly, in primates, early temporal lobe lesions were found to result in alterations in metabolism in the prefrontal cortex and consequent abnormalities in striatal DA that are analogous to the changes observed in the rat (Lipska and Weinberger, 2000; Saunders *et al.*, 1998). These studies showed that an alteration in a specific neuronal circuit in the neonatal animal could lead to pathology within limbic circuits in the adult that is consistent with what would be expected in schizophrenia; however, the pathology produced by this manipulation was markedly dissimilar from the more subtle anatomical alterations observed in the brain of the schizophrenia patient (Harrison, 1999), which presumably was the result of genetically derived pathological brain development.

It is unclear how one may be able to duplicate a human genetically based alteration in brain development using an animal model. However, we have found that administration of a developmental mitotoxin methyl azoxymethanol acetate (MAM) (Nagata and Matsumoto, 1969) to pregnant dams may approximate this condition. Administration of MAM to the pregnant dam at gestational day 17, which is when the proliferation and migration of neurons within the limbic cortex is occurring (Bayer and Altman, 1991), disrupted the normal development of these limbic circuits. The resultant adult offspring demonstrated a number of the anatomical and behavioral characteristics that would be predicted for an animal model of this disorder. Anatomically, there is a selective decrease (10–30%) in the thickness of the paralimbic and limbic cortical regions but no change in anterior sensorimotor cortex or subcortical regions (Moore and Grace, 1997; Moore et al., 2001a), which is in concert with that described in schizophrenia, allowing, of course, for the anatomical differences between cortical regions when determining homologies between rat and human brain. Behaviorally, these rats showed spontaneously occurring orofacial dyskinesias and a hyperresponsiveness to novelty (Ghajarnia et al., 1998; Moore et al., 2001a); such behaviors are typically associated with lesions of the frontal lobes (Edwards, 1970; Gunne et al., 1982; Waddington, 1990) or administration of glutamate antagonists to the ventral striatum (Kelley and Delfs, 1994; Kelley and Swanson, 1997). There was also an increased response to phenyclidine and to amphetamine, and the rats also showed deficits in prepulse inhibition of the startle response (Ghajarnia et al., 1998): a characteristic that has been found in human schizophrenia subjects (Braff et al., 1992).

In physiological studies, the MAM-treated rats exhibited a loss of hippocampal-driven bistable activity in the nucleus accumbens. As a result, the hippocampus no longer exerted its normal gating influence over the accumbens (O'Donnell and Grace, 1995). Moreover, we have found that the modulatory actions of DA in the prefrontal cortex of MAM-treated rats is significantly attenuated (Lavin and Grace, 1997). As a consequence, the amygdala exhibited an abnormally large influence within the accumbens. Such a condition suggests that, in this animal model, emotion plays a much greater role in guiding behavior when compared with goal-directed (prefrontal cortex) or context-dependent (hippocampal) cues (Grace and Moore, 1998).

Possible origins of the delayed onset of schizophrenia

One issue that remains to be considered is why a genetically or developmentally based pathology would not be present at birth, but instead show an onset that is delayed for several decades. One possibility is that the delayed pathology in the hippocampus, as suggested by imaging studies (Pantelis et al., 2003; Phillips et al., 2002), may be related to the changes in stress placed upon the system secondary to prefrontal cortical disruption. So, some studies have shown that the hippocampus is particularly susceptible to damage as a result of stress (Sapolsky et al., 1985). Moreover, the hippocampus is involved in modulating the actions of the

HPA axis in response to glucocorticoids (Sapolsky et. al. 1990), which are released in response to stress (Cullinan *et al.*, 1995). Indeed, in an animal model of this disorder, Lipska *et al.* (1993) have shown that rats with neonatal damage to the hippocampus exhibit hyperresponsiveness to stress. This interaction between stress and hippocampal damage has been proposed as a model for delayed onset of disorders such as schizophrenia (Walker and Diforio, 1997). In addition, a pathology of prefrontal cortex function may also place increased demand on the hippocampus. It has been suggested that some of the higher-order functions that are mediated by specific cortical regions in the adult, such as the prefrontal cortex, may be mediated by subcortical regions during developmental periods prior to the maturation of the cortex under question (Goldman and Rosvold, 1972). Specifically, it has been proposed that, early in life, the hippocampus may subsume some of the working memory functions of the individual while the prefrontal cortex is developing during early life (Diamond, 1990), with this responsibility being off-loaded to the prefrontal cortex as it reaches functional maturity. One consequence of a prefrontal pathology would be that this region may not be capable of taking over such functions from the hippocampus. Indeed, this is supported by data showing that some working memory functions in the schizophrenia patient are mediated by the hippocampus (Meyer-Lindenberg *et al.*, 2001; Weinberger *et al.*, 1993). Therefore, at a time when stress may be taking an increasing toll on the hippocampus, it will also be placed under abnormally high functional demand because of the increased working memory load placed upon it. Indeed, the increased hippocampal volume prior to the first episode of psychotic symptoms (Pantelis *et al.*, 2003; Phillips *et al.*, 2002) may be an indicator of such a pathological condition.

The result is that maturation-related stressors could trigger a cascade whereby prefrontal dysfunction interrupts coping mechanisms for stress at the level of the amygdala, which, via projections from the central nucleus of the amygdala to the hypothalamus, could augment stress hormone release. The hyperactivated subcortical DA system could serve to overwhelm the system further with a flooding of sensory input, thus increasing the stress-induced responses of the system. As reviewed above, the glucocorticoids released in response to stress are known to damage the hippocampus (Sapolsky *et al.*, 1985), and it is known that the hippocampus is involved in modulating the glucocorticoid response to stress (Hoschl and Hajek, 2001; McEwen, 1998; Sapolsky, 1992; Sapolsky *et al.*, 1990). Therefore, the multiple systems that contribute to an augmented stress response and the stress-induced release of glucocorticoids, when combined with increased functional demand placed on the hippocampus, could lead to hippocampal damage, which would reduce the hippocampal modulation of the stress response, thus leading to further heightened response to stress and more hippocampal damage in a positive feedback system. Such an interaction could explain the delayed onset of

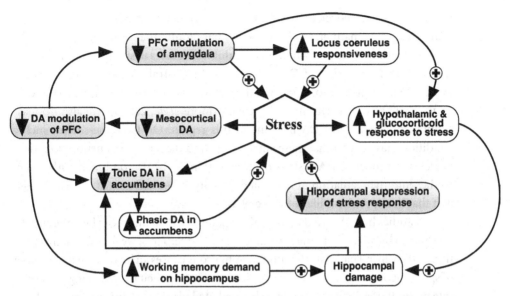

Fig. 15.1.   A model of the developmental pathophysiology of schizophrenia. This model consists of a series of interconnected loops, with the common endpoint being a disruption in the regulation of phasic dopamine (DA) release. One feature of this model is that the positive feedback loop could be initiated from a number of starting points. For example, a perinatal deficit in DA in the prefrontal cortex (PFC) is proposed to result in (i) disruption of tonic DA regulation in the nucleus accumbens; (ii) removal of regulation of affective responses within the basolateral amygdala; and (iii) a failure to offload working memory demand from the hippocampus during maturation. This would lead to abnormally potentiated stress responses, which would drive hippocampal pathology and DA imbalance further. Similarly, an initiation within the hippocampal system would also be expected to exacerbate the stress response, ultimately leading to disruption of PFC regulation and subcortical DA system responsivity. Note that each of these feedback pathways loops through the stress response. Thus, one potential means to alter the course of this pathological process would be to treat the exacerbated stress response prior to the initiation of the damaging positive feedback cascade that is proposed to lead to irreversible system damage and psychosis.

this pathology (Fig. 15.1). This is likely to have important implications for how it ultimately affects DA system function.

Pathophysiological impact on dopamine transmission

A triumvirate of pathophysiology is proposed to take place: (i) decreased prefrontal cortical function as a result of an extant loss of DA modulation or in response to stress; (ii) increased subcortical stress response secondary to the loss of prefrontal cortical modulatory influences; and (iii) stress-induced damage to the hippocampus. Moreover, each of these processes is known to affect DA system function in a specific manner. For example, we have found that rats with lesions of the DA innervation of the prefrontal cortex exhibit decreases in spontaneous firing and increases in burst firing of DA neurons in the ventral tegmental area (Harden et al., 1998). Furthermore, inactivation of the ventral hippocampus (Floresco et al., 2001) as well as chronic cold stress (Moore et al., 2001b) will also decrease spontaneous activity of DA neurons in this region. On first assessment, such a condition may suggest that these antecedents would decrease DA neuron function; however, a model of DA system regulation (Grace, 1991) combined with recent studies into the regulation of DA system activity (Floresca et al., 2003) would suggest that the opposite is likely to take place.

Our studies have shown that the activity states of DA neurons can be differentially modulated by afferents to the ventral tegmental area. Thus, we found that inactivation of the ventral pallidal afferents to DA neurons causes an increase in the number of spontaneously active DA neurons without affecting their overall firing pattern or rate of discharge. This is thought to be mediated via the fast-firing ventral pallidal gamma-aminobutyric acid (GABA)-ergic afferents to DA neurons (Chrobak and Napier, 1993; Yang and Mogenson, 1985), which we predict holds a subset of neurons in a hyperpolarized, non-firing state (Floresco et al., 2001). However, when ventral pallidal firing is inactivated via local microinjection of the GABA $_{A/B}$ agonists muscimol and baclofen, these non-firing neurons are released from inhibition. In contrast, activation of the pedunculopontine cholinergic/glutamatergic afferents to the ventral tegmental area had no effect on the number of spontaneously firing DA neurons; instead, it only caused an increase in burst firing. Since burst firing is believed to be mediated via N-methyl-D-aspartate (NMDA) receptors, this suggests that activation of NMDA receptors on spontaneously firing DA neurons would cause them to begin burst firing. In contrast, the neurons that are being held in a hyperpolarized state by the ventral pallidal GABAergic afferents would not be activated by NMDA as a result of voltage-dependent magnesium block of this ionotropic receptor site (Mayer et al., 1984). As a consequence, we found that we could separately regulate DA neuron population activity and firing pattern via manipulation of these afferents (Floresco et al., 2001, 2003).

Being able to regulate activity states of the ventral tegmental DA neurons independently enabled us to examine the impact of changes in activity states on DA release in the nucleus accumbens. When the ventral pallidum was inactivated (to increase the number of spontaneously active DA neurons), we observed a 50% increase in extracellular DA in the accumbens. In contrast, when the pedunculopontine tegmentum was activated (to increase burst firing), there was no detectable change in extracellular DA. However, by using microdialysis measures, we were measuring overflow of DA from the synapse rather than DA release per se. For this reason, we tested the effects of blockade of DA uptake on accumbens DA levels. Administration of the DA uptake blocker nomifensine locally through the microdialysis probe caused a 10-fold increase in baseline levels of extracellular DA. Under these conditions, increasing DA population activity (via ventral pallidal inactivation) still caused a 50% increase in extracellular DA over baseline levels. However, in marked contrast, activation of burst firing (via pedunculopontine activation) now caused a greater than 300% increase in extracellular DA in the accumbens (Floresco *et al.*, 2003).

These data suggest that extracellular DA levels are regulated primarily by the number of DA neurons firing. We have defined this previously as "tonic" DA levels (Grace, 1991), since this appears to be the low-level, constant amount of DA present in the extrasynaptic space. Levels of DA in this region are quite low (estimated to be approximately 5–40 nM); such levels are clearly too low to impact directly on postsynaptic DA receptors within the synapse, which are believed to be exposed to many times higher concentrations (Wightman and Robinson, 2002). However, this level is sufficient to stimulate presynaptic receptors (Richfield *et al.*, 1989), such as the inhibitory presynaptic DA autoreceptors present on the DA terminal. As a consequence, tonic DA levels are proposed to downregulate DA released by spike activity (Fig. 15.2B).

In contrast, the DA released by burst firing appears to be confined to the vicinity of the synapse by the reuptake process, which is consistent with the location of the dopamine transporters at the borders of the synaptic junction (Nirenberg *et al.*, 1997) where they can most effectively limit diffusion of DA out of the synapse. This "phasic" (Grace, 1991) DA level is proposed to be the actual DA signal that mediates behaviorally relevant DA transmission, which is consistent with the burst activation reported to occur during behavioral tasks (Schultz, 1998). In addition to being high in amplitude, this DA signal is also brief in duration, as it is rapidly inactivated via reuptake into the DA terminal before it can leave the synaptic space (Fig.15.2A). Phasic DA is proposed to be modulated by tonic DA, in which stimulation of presynaptic DA autoreceptors by tonic DA will downmodulate burst firing-induced phasic DA release (Fig. 15.2C).

Consequently, a decrease in DA neuron population activity produced by disruption of the hippocampus, by repeated stress, or by lesion of the prefrontal cortex DA innervation will result in attenuation of tonic DA release. As a result, stimuli that cause burst firing-mediated phasic DA release would be expected to release much more DA than would occur normally, owing to this loss of tonic downregulation. This would be accentuated by the increased burst firing noted as a consequence of prefrontal cortical DA lesions. Therefore, one consequence of stress-related pathological changes within the prefrontal–amygdala–hippocampal–HPA axis would be hyperactivation of the DA system in response to stimuli, analogous to that reported

A Phasic DA transmission

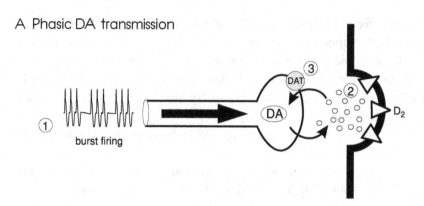

B Tonic DA transmission

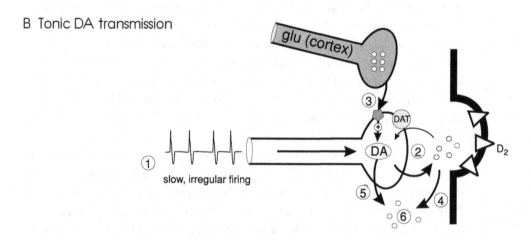

C Tonic modulates phasic

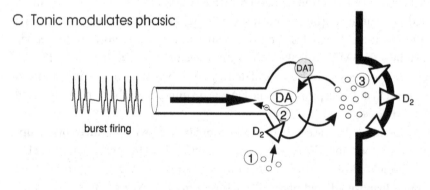

Fig. 15.2.   The dopamine (DA) system is under a complex set of regulatory influences. (A) In response
to a behaviorally salient stimulus, the DA neuron emits bursts of action potentials (1), leading
to a massive release of DA (in micro- to millimolar concentrations) into the synaptic cleft,
where it can stimulate postsynaptic receptors (2). The DA that is released is then rapidly taken
back up into the terminal by the dopamine transporter (DAT; 3) before it can escape the
synaptic cleft. The DAT achieves this because it is located at the periphery of the synaptic cleft

to take place in schizophrenia patients (Laruelle, 2000; Laruelle and Abi-Dargham, 1999).

Conclusions

I have presented a model whereby stress is proposed to interact with an existing pathology within the limbic system to cause the delayed emergence of the positive symptoms of schizophrenia. The involvement of stress is demonstrated by the finding that, of the children at risk for developing schizophrenia, those that do go on to show the pathology exhibit higher levels of anxiety and stress premorbidly (E. C. Johnstone, personal communication). Moreover, stress is known to exacerbate the symptoms of schizophrenia and lead to a relapse in patients under remission (Birley and Brown, 1970; Norman and Malla, 1993a,b). One implication of this model is that, given that the DA system does not appear to be abnormal prior to the first episode of psychotic symptoms, prophylactic treatment with antipsychotic drugs may not be an effective course of action for preventing the ultimate transition to schizophrenia. In contrast, drugs that act to reduce indices of stress or anxiety may be more effective at preventing the triggering of the cascade of events that eventually lead to the development of schizophrenia.

Acknowledgements

This work was supported by USPHS MH01055, MH57440, and MH45156. I thank Stan Floresco for his help in producing the figures used in this manuscript.

(Nirenberg *et al.*, 1997), where it can effectively limit diffusion of released transmitter. (B) In contrast, slow, irregular firing of DA neurons (1) leads to substantially lower levels of DA release into the synaptic cleft; this DA release is not as potently affected by the DAT (2) but is modulated by glutamatergic (glu) afferents that synapse in the vicinity of the DA terminal (3). As a result, a small amount of DA will escape the synaptic cleft (4) or be released from non-synaptic sites on the terminal (5). This low (approximately 20 nM) concentration of tonic DA (6) is then free to diffuse away from the synaptic terminal. (C) Although the levels of tonic DA (1) are too low to stimulate postsynaptic receptors, this concentration is sufficient to activate D_2 autoreceptors on the DA terminal, which would cause an attenuation of burst firing-dependent phasic DA release (2). As a result, there is a tonic inhibition in the amplitude of the phasic DA release (3). Systems that will attenuate tonic DA release, either decreasing tonic DA neuron activity (i.e. less DA neurons active) or a pathological decrease in cortical glutamatergic drive, would thereby remove tonic inhibition of phasic DA release (Grace, 1991).

REFERENCES

Abercrombie, E. D., Jacobs, B. L. (1987). Single-unit response of noradrenergic neurons in the locus coeruleus of freely moving cats. I. Acutely presented stressful and nonstressful stimuli. *J Neurosci* 7: 2837–2843.

Abercrombie, E. D., Keller, Jr., R. W., Zigmond, M. J. (1988). Characterization of hippocampal norepinephrine release as measured by microdialysis perfusion: pharmacological and behavioral studies. *Neuroscience* 27: 897–904.

Abercrombie, E. D., Keefe, K. A., DiFrischia, D. S., Zigmond, M. J., (1989). Differential effect of stress on in vivo dopamine release in striatum, nucleus accumbens, and medial frontal cortex. *J Neurochem* 52: 1655–1658.

Akil, M., Pierri, J. N., Whitehead, R. E., *et al.* (1999). Lamina-specific alterations in the dopamine innervation of the prefrontal cortex in schizophrenic subjects. *Am J Psychatry* 156: 1580–1589.

Angrist, B., Santhananthan, G., Wilk, S., Gershon, S. (1974). Amphetamine psychosis: behavioral and biochemical aspects. *J. Psychiatr Res* 11: 13–23.

Angrist, B., Rotrosen, J., Gershon, S. (1980). Differential effects of amphetamine and neuroleptics on negative vs. positive symptoms in schizophrenia. *Psychopharmacology* 72: 17–19.

Arnold, S. E. (1997). The medial temporal lobe in schizophrenia. *J Neuropsychiatry Clin Neurosci* 9: 460–470.

Arnold, S. E., Trojanowski, J. Q., Gur, R. E., *et al.* (1998). Absence of neurodegeneration and neural injury in the cerebral cortex in a sample of elderly patients with schizophrenia. *Arch Gen Psychiatry* 55: 225–232.

Aston-Jones, G., Ennis, M., Pieribone, V. A., Nickell, W. T., Shipley, M. T. (1986). The brain nucleus locus coeruleus: restricted afferent control of a broad efferent network. *Science* 234: 734–737.

Bayer, S. A., Altman, J. (1991). *Neocortical Development.* New York: Raven Press.

Bayer, T. A., Falkai, P., Maier, W. (1999). Genetic and non-genetic vulnerability factors in schizophrenia: the basis of the "two hit hypothesis". *J Psychiatr Res* 33: 543–548.

Bertolino, A., Knable M. B., Saunders R. C., *et al.* (1999). The relationship between dorsolateral prefrontal *N*-acetylaspartate measures and striatal dopamine activity in schizophrenia. *Biol Psychiatry* 45: 660–667.

Beuger, M., van Kammen, D. P., Kelley, M. E., Yao, J. (1996). Dopamine turnover in schizophrenia before and after haloperidol withdrawal. CSF, plasma, and urine studies, *Neuropsychopharmacology* 15: 75–86.

Bilder, R. M., Bogerts, B., Ashtari, M., *et al.* (1995). Anterior hippocampal volume reductions predict frontal lobe dysfunction in first episode schizophrenia. *Schizophr Res* 17: 47–58.

Birley, J., Brown, G. W. (1970). Crisis and life changes preceding the onset or relapse of acute schizophrenia: clinical aspects. *Br J Psychiatry* 16: 327–333.

Braff, D. L., Grillon, C., Geyer, M. A. (1992). Gating and habituation of the startle reflex in schizophrenic patients. *Arch Gen Psychiatry* 49: 206–215.

Breier, A., Buchanan, R. W., Elkashef, A., *et al.* (1992). Brain morphology and schizophrenia. A magnetic resonance imaging study of limbic, prefrontal cortex, and caudate structures. *Arch Gen Psychiatry* 49: 921–926.

Chang, M. S., Sved, A. F., Zigmond, M. J., Austin, M. C. (2000). Increased transcription of the tyrosine hydroxylase gene in individual locus coeruleus neurons following footshock stress. *Neuroscience* **101**: 131–139.

Chrobak, J. J., Napier, T. C. (1993). Opioid and GABA modulation of accumbens-evoked ventral pallidal activity. *J Neur Transm Gen Sect* **93**: 123–143.

Cohen, J. D., Servan-Schreiber, D. (1992). Context, cortex and dopamine: a connectionist approach to behavior and biology in schizophrenia. *Psychol Rev* **99**: 45–77.

Correll, C. J., Rosenkranz, J. A., Grace, A. A. (2001). Chronic cold stress alters basal neuronal firing rate and response to acute stressors of basolateral amygdala neurons in rats. *Soc Neurosci Abstr* **27**: 2540.

Creese, I., Burt, D. R., Snyder, S. H. (1976). Dopamine receptor binding predicts clinical and pharmacological potencies of antischizophrenic drugs. *Science* **192**: 596–598.

Cullinan, W. E., Herman, J. P., Helmreich, D. L., Watson, Jr., S. J. (1995). A neuroanatomy of stress. In *Neurobiological and Clinical Consequences of Stress: From Normal Adaptation to PTSD*, ed. M. J. Friedman, D. S. Charney, A. Y. Deutch. Philadelphia, PA: Lippincott, pp. 3–25.

Curtis, A. L., Lechner, S. M., Pavcovich, L. A., Valentino, R. J. (1997). Activation of the locus coeruleus noradrenergic system by intracoerulear microinfusion of corticotropin-releasing factor: effects on discharge rate, cortical norepinephrine levels and cortical electroencephalographic activity. *J Pharmacol Exp Ther* **281**: 163–172.

DeLisi, L. E. (1992). The significance of age of onset for schizophrenia. *Schizophr Bull* **18**: 209–215.

Diamond, A. (1990). The development and neural bases of memory functions as indexed by the AB and delayed response tasks in human infants and infant monkeys. *Ann NY Acad Sci* **608**: 267–309. [Discussion 309–317.]

Drevets, W. C. (1999). Prefrontal cortical–amygdalar metabolism in major depression. *Ann N Y Acad Sci* **877**: 614–637.

Dunn, A. J., Berridge, C. W. (1987). Corticotropin-releasing factor administration elicits a stress-like activation of cerebral catecholaminergic systems. *Pharmacol Biochem Behav* **27**: 685–691.

Eastwood, S. L., Cairns, N. J., Harrison, P. J. (2000). Synaptophysin gene expression in schizophrenia. Investigation of synaptic pathology in the cerebral cortex. *Br J Psychiatry* **176**: 236–242.

Edwards, H. (1970). The significance of brain damage in persistent oral dyskinesia. *Br J Psychiatry* **116**: 271–275.

Emoto, H., Koga, C., Ishii, H., *et al.* (1993). A CRF antagonist attenuates stress-induced increases in NA turnover in extended brain regions in rats. *Brain Res* **627**: 171–176.

Ennis, M., Shipley, M. T., Aston-Jones, G., Williams, J. T. (1998). Afferent control of nucleus locus ceruleus: differential regulation by "shell" and "core" inputs. *Adv Pharmacol* **42**: 767–771.

Finlay J. M., Jedema H. P., Rabinovic, A. D., *et al.* (1997). Impact of corticotropin-releasing hormone on extracellular norepinephrine in prefrontal cortex after chronic cold stress. *J Neurochem* **69**: 144–150.

Floresco, S. B., Todd, C. L., Grace, A. A. (2001). Glutamatergic afferents from the hippocampus to the nucleus accumbens regulate activity of ventral tegmental area dopamine neurons. *J Neurosci* **21**: 4915–4922.

Floresco, S. B., West, A. R., Ash, B., Moore, H., Grace, A. A. (2003). Afferent modulation of dopamine neuron firing differentially regulates tonic and phasic dopamine transmission. *Nat Neurosci* **6**: 968–973.

Garey, L. J., Ong, W. Y., Patel, T. S., *et al.* (1998). Reduced dendritic spine density on cerebral cortical pyramidal neurons in schizophrenia. *J Neurol Neurosurg Psychiatry* **65**: 446–453.

Ghajarnia, M., Moore, H., Grace, A. A. (1998). Enhanced behavioral effects of phencyclidine (PCP) in rats with developmental abnormalities of the temporal lobe. *Soc Neurosci Abstr* **24**: 2177.

Glantz, L. A., Lewis, D. A. (1997). Reduction of synaptophysin immunoreactivity in the prefrontal cortex of subjects with schizophrenia. Regional and diagnostic specificity. *Arch Gen Psychiatry* **54**: 943–952.

Goddard, A. W., Charney, D. S. (1997). Toward an integrated neurobiology of panic disorder. *J Clin Psychiatry* **58**(Suppl. 2): 4–11.

Goff, D. C., Coyle, J. T. (2001). The emerging role of glutamate in the pathophysiology and treatment of schizophrenia. *Am J Psychiatry* **158**: 1367–1377.

Goldman, P. S., Rosvold, H. E. (1972). The effects of selective caudate lesions in infant and juvenile rhesus monkeys. *Brain Res* **43**: 53–66.

Goldman-Rakic, P. S. (1995). Cellular basis of working memory. *Neuron* **14**: 477–485.

(1996). Regional and cellular fractionation of working memory. *Proc Natl Acad Sci USA* **93**: 13473–13480.

(1999). The physiological approach: functional architecture of working memory and disordered cognition in schizophrenia. *Biol Psychiatry* **46**: 650–661.

Grace, A. A. (1991). Phasic versus tonic dopamine release and the modulation of dopamine system responsivity: a hypothesis for the etiology of schizophrenia. *Neuroscience* **41**: 1–24.

(2000). Gating of information flow within the limbic system and the pathophysiology of schizophrenia. [In *Proceedings from the Nobel Symposium – Schizophrenia: Pathophysiological Mechanisms*.] *Brain Res Rev* **31**: 330–361. Online at *Brain Research Interactive: http://www.elsevier.nl/gej-ng/29/19/30/26/43/article.html.*

Grace, A. A., Moore, H. (1998). Regulation of information flow in the accumbens: a model for the pathophysiology of schizophrenia. In *Origins and Development of Schizophrenia: Advances in Experimental Psychopathology*, ed. M. F. Lenzenweger, R. H. Dworkin. Washington, DC: American Psychological Association Press, pp. 123–157.

Grace, A. A., Bunney, B. S., Moore, H., Todd. C. L. (1997). Dopamine cell depolarization block as a model for the therapeutic actions of antipsychotic drugs. *Trends Neurosci* **20**: 31–37.

Gunne, L. M., Growdon, J., Glaeser, B. (1982). Oral dyskinesia in rats following brain lesions and neuroleptic drug administration. *Psychopharmacology* **77**: 134–139.

Harden, D. G., King, D., Finlay, J., Grace, A. A. (1998). Depletion of dopamine in the prefrontal cortex decreases the basal electrophysiological activity of mesolimbic dopamine neurons. *Brain Res* **794**: 96–102.

Harrison, P. J. (1999). The neuropathology of schizophrenia. A critical review of the data and their interpretation. *Brain* **122**: 593–624.

Herman, J. P., Cullinan, W. E. (1997). Neurocircuitry of stress: central control of the hypothalamo–pituitary–adrenocortical axis. *Trends Neurosci* **20**: 78–84.

Hoschl, C., Hajek, T. (2001). Hippocampal damage mediated by corticosteroids: a neuropsychiatric research challenge. *Eur Arch Psychiatry Clin Neurosci* **251**(Suppl. 2): 81–88.

Imperato, A., Puglisi-Allegra, S., Casolini, P., Zocchi, A., Angelucci, L. (1989). Stress-induced enhancement of dopamine and acetylcholine release in limbic structures: role of corticosterone. *Eur J Pharmacol* **165**: 337–338.

Jedema, H. P., Grace, A. A. (2003). Chronic exposure to cold stress alters electrophysiological properties of locus coeruleus neurons recorded in vitro. *Neuropsychopharmacology* **28**: 63–72.

Jentsch, J. D., Roth, R. H. (1999). The neuropsychopharmacology of phencyclidine: from NMDA receptor hypofunction to the dopamine hypothesis of schizophrenia. *Neuropsychopharmacology* **20**: 201–225.

Jones, E. G. (1997). Cortical development and thalamic pathology in schizophrenia. *Schizophr Bull* **23**: 483–501.

Kalin, N. H. (1985). Behavioral effects of ovine corticotropin-releasing factor administered to rhesus monkeys. *Fed Proc* **44**: 249–253.

Kelley, A. E., Delfs, J. M. (1994). Excitatory amino acid receptors mediate the orofacial stereotypy elicited by dopaminergic stimulation of the ventrolateral striatum. *Neuroscience* **60**: 85–95.

Kelley, A. E., Swanson, C. J. (1997). Feeding induced by blockade of AMPA and kainate receptors within the ventral striatum: a microinfusion mapping study. *Behav Brain Res* **89**: 107–113.

Kendler, K. (1983). Overview: a current perspective on twin studies of schizophrenia. *Am J Psychiatry* **140**: 1413–1425.

King, D., Zigmond, M. J., Finlay, J. M. (1997). Effects of dopamine depletion in the medial prefrontal cortex on the stress-induced increase in extracellular dopamine in the nucleus accumbens core and shell. *Neuroscience* **77**: 141–153.

Laruelle, M. (2000). The role of endogenous sensitization in the pathophysiology of schizophrenia: implications from recent brain imaging studies. *Brain Res Rev* **31**: 371–384.

Laruelle, M., Abi-Dargham, A. (1999). Dopamine as the wind of the psychotic fire: new evidence from brain imaging studies. *J Psychopharmacol* **13**: 358–371.

Lavin, A., Grace, A. A. (1997). Effects of afferent stimulation and DA application on prefrontal cortical cells recorded intracellularly *in vivo*: comparisons between intact rats and rats with pharmacologically-induced disruption of cortical development. *Soc Neurosci Abstr* **23**: 2080.

Lawrie, S. M., Abukmeil, S. S. (1998). Brain abnormality in schizophrenia. A systematic and quantitative review of volumetric magnetic resonance imaging studies. *Br J Psychiatry* **172**: 110–120.

Lechner, S. M., Curtis, A. L., Brons, R., Valentino, R. J. (1997). Locus coeruleus activation by colon distention: role of corticotropin-releasing factor and excitatory amino acids. *Brain Res* **756**: 114–124.

LeDoux, J. E. (2000). Emotion circuits in the brain. *Annu Rev of Neurosci* **23**: 155–184.

Lewis, D. A. (1997). Development of the prefrontal cortex during adolescence: insights into vulnerable neural circuits in schizophrenia. *Neuropsychopharmacology* **16**: 385–398.

Lewis, D. A., Levitt, P. (2002). Schizophrenia as a disorder of neurodevelopment. *Annu Rev Neurosci* **25**: 409–432.

Liddle, P. F., Friston, K. J., Frith, C. D., Frackowiak, R. S. (1992). Cerebral blood flow and mental processes in schizophrenia. *J Roy Soc Med* **85**: 224–227.

Lipska, B. K., Weinberger, D. R. (2000). To model a psychiatric disorder in animals: schizophrenia as a reality test. *Neuropsychopharmacology* **23**: 223–239.

Lipska, B. K., Jaskiw, G. E., Weinberger, D. (1993). Postpubertal emergence of hyperresponsiveness to stress and to amphetamine after neonatal hippocampal damage: a potential animal model of schizophrenia. *Neuropsychopharmacology* **9**: 67–75.

Mana, M. J., Grace, A. A. (1997). Chronic cold stress alters the basal and evoked electrophysiological activity of rat locus coeruleus neurons. *Neuroscience* **81**: 1055–1064.

Mayer, M. L., Westbrook, G. L., Guthrie, P. B. (1984). Voltage-dependent block by Mg^{2+} of NMDA responses in spinal cord neurones. *Nature* **309**: 261–263.

McCarley, R. W., Wible, C. G., Frumin, M., *et al.* (1999). MRI anatomy of schizophrenia. *Biol Psychiatry* **45**: 1099–1119.

McDonald, C., Murray, R. M. (2000). Early and late environmental risk factors for schizophrenia. *Brain Res Rev* **31**: 130–137.

McEwen, B. S. (1998). Protective and damaging effects of stress mediators. *N Engl J Med* **338**: 171–179.

McKernan, M. G., Shinnick-Gallagher, P. (1997). Fear conditioning induces a lasting potentiation of synaptic currents in vitro. *Nature* **390**: 607–611.

Meyer-Lindenberg, A., Poline, J. B., Kohn, P. D., *et al.* (2001). Evidence for abnormal cortical functional connectivity during working memory in schizophrenia. *Am J Psychiatry* **158**: 1809–1817.

Mirnics, K., Middleton, F. A., Marquez. A., Lewis, D. A., Levitt, P. (2000). Molecular characterization of schizophrenia viewed by microarray analysis of gene expression in prefrontal cortex. *Neuron* **28**: 53–67.

Moore, H., Grace, A. A. (1997). Anatomical changes in limbic structures produced by methylazoxymethanol acetate (MAM) during brain development are associated with changes in physiological interactions among afferents to the nucleus accumbens. *Soc Neurosci Abstr* **23**: 2378.

Moore, H., Ghajarnia, M., Geyer, M., Jentsch, J. D., Grace, A. A. (2001a). Selective disruption of prefrontal and limbic corticostriatal circuits by prenatal exposure to the DNA methylation agent methylazoxymethanol acetate (MAM): anatomical, neurophysiological and behavioral studies. *Schizophr Res* **49**(Suppl. 1–2): 48.

Moore, H., Rose, H. J., Grace, A. A. (2001b). Chronic cold stress reduces the spontaneous activity of ventral tegmental dopamine neurons. *Neuropsychopharmacology* **24**: 410–419.

Nagata, Y., Matsumoto, H. (1969). Studies on methylazoxymethanol: methylation of nucleic acids in the fetal rat brain. *Proc Soc Exp Biol Med* **132**: 383–385.

Ninan, P. T. (1999). The functional anatomy, neurochemistry, and pharmacology of anxiety. *J Clin Psychiatry* **60**(Suppl. 22): 12–17.

Nirenberg, M. J., Chan, J., Pohorille, A., *et al.* (1997). The dopamine transporter: comparative ultrastructure of dopaminergic axons in limbic and motor compartments of the nucleus accumbens. *J Neurosci* **17**: 6899–6907.

Norman, R. M., Malla, A. K. (1993a). Stressful life events and schizophrenia: I. A review of the research. *Br J Psychiatry* **162**: 161–166.

(1993b). Stressful life events and schizophrenia: II. Conceptual and methodological issues. *Br J Psychiatry* **162**: 166–174.

O'Donnell, P., Grace, A. A. (1995). Synaptic interactions among excitatory afferents to nucleus accumbens neurons: hippocampal gating of prefrontal cortical input. *J Neurosci* **15**: 3622–3639.

Olney, J. W., Farber, N. B. (1995). NMDA antagonists as neurotherapeutic drugs, psychotogens, neurotoxins, and research tools for studying schizophrenia. *Neuropsychopharmacology* **13**: 335–345.

Ono, T., Nishijo, H., Uwano, T. (1995). Amygdala role in conditioned associative learning. *Prog Neurobiol* **46**: 401–423.

Page, M. E., Abercrombie, E. D. (1999). Discrete local application of corticotropin-releasing factor increases locus coeruleus discharge and extracellular norepinephrine in rat hippocampus. *Synapse* **33**: 304–313.

Pantelis, C., Velakoulis, D., McGorry, P. D., *et al.* (2003). Neuroanatomical abnormalities before and after onset of psychosis: a cross-sectional and longitudinal MRI comparison. *Lancet* **361**: 281–288.

Pare, D., Collins, D. R. (2000). Neuronal correlates of fear in the lateral amygdala: multiple extracellular recordings in conscious rats. *J Neurosci* **20**: 2701–2710.

Phillips, L. J., Velakoulis, D., Pantelis, C., *et al.* (2002). Non-reduction in hippocampal volume is associated with higher risk of psychosis. *Schizophr Res* **58**: 145–158.

Pilowsky, L. S., Kerwin, R. W., Murray, R. M. (1993). Schizophrenia: a neurodevelopmental perspective. *Neuropsychopharmacology* **9**: 83–91.

Pitkanen, A., Savander, V., LeDoux, J. E. (1997). Organization of intra-amygdaloid circuitries in the rat: an emerging framework for understanding functions of the amygdala. *Trends Neurosci* **20**: 517–523.

Post, R. M., Fink, E., Carpenter, W. T., Goodwin, F. K. (1975). Cerebrospinal fluid amine metabolites in acute schizophrenia. *Arch Gen Psychiatry* **32**: 1063–1069.

Ramsooksingh M. D., Jedema, H. P., Moore, H., Sved, A. F., Grace, A. A. (2001). The effects of chronic stress on the regulation of locus coeruleus neurons by peripheral, limbic, and prefrontal cortical inputs. *Soc Neurosci Abstr* **27**: 1961.

Ramsooksingh, M. D., Jedema, H. P., Moore, H., Sved, A. F., Grace, A. A. (2002). Chronic cold stress leads to persistent changes in the behavioral response to footshock with coincident changes in evoked spike activity in the locus coeruleus. *Soc Neurosci Abstr* **28**: [Program No.] 669.4.

Richfield, E. K., Penney, J. B., Young, A. B. (1989). Anatomical and affinity state comparisons between dopamine D_1 and D_2 receptors in the rat central nervous system. *Neuroscience* **30**: 767–777.

Rogan, M. T., Stauble, U. V., LeDoux, J. E. (1997). Fear conditioning induces associative long-term potentiation in the amygdala. *Nature* **390**: 604–607.

Rosenkranz, J. A., Grace, A. A. (1999). Modulation of basolateral amygdala neuronal firing and afferent drive by dopamine receptor activation in vivo. *J Neurosci* **19**: 11027–11039.

(2001). Dopamine attenuates prefrontal cortical suppression of sensory inputs to the basolateral amygdala of rats. *J Neurosci* **21**: 4090–4103.

(2002a). Cellular mechanisms of infralimbic and prelimbic prefrontal cortical inhibition and dopaminergic modulation of basolateral amygdala neurons in vivo. *J Neurosci* **22**: 324–337.

(2002b). Dopamine-mediated modulation of odour-evoked amygdala potentials during Pavlovian conditioning. *Nature* **417**: 282–287.

Sabban, E. L., Kvetnansky, R. (2001). Stress-triggered activation of gene expression in catecholaminergic systems: dynamics of transcriptional events. *Trends Neurosci* **24**: 91–98.

Sapolsky, R. (1992). *Stress, The Aging Brain, and the Mechanisms of Neuron Death*. Cambridge, MA: MIT Press.

Sapolsky, R., Krey, L., McEwen, B. (1985). Prolonged glucocorticoid exposure reduces hippocampal neural number: Implications for aging. *J Neurosci* **5**: 1221–1224.

Sapolsky, R. M., Armanini, M. P., Packan, D. R., Sutton, W. S., Plotsky, P. M. (1990). Glucocorticoid feedback inhibition of adrenocorticotropic hormone secretagogue release. *Neuroendocrinology* **51**: 328–336.

Saunders R. C., Kolachana, B. S., Bachevalier, J., Weinberger, D. R. (1998). Neonatal lesions of the medial temporal lobe disrupt prefrontal cortical regulation of striatal dopamine. *Nature* **393**: 169–171.

Seeman, P. (1987). Dopamine receptors and the dopamine hypothesis of schizophrenia. *Synapse* **1**: 133–152.

Schultz, W. (1998). Predictive reward signal of dopamine neurons. *J Neurophysiol* **80**: 1–27.

Selemon, L. D., Rajkowska, G., Goldman-Rakic, P. S. (1995). Abnormally high neuronal density in the schizophrenic cortex. A morphometric analysis of prefrontal area 9 and occipital area 17. *Arch Gen Psychiatry* **52**: 805–818.

Serova, L. I., Nankova, B. B., Feng, Z., *et al.* (1999). Heightened transcription for enzymes involved in norepinephrine biosynthesis in the rat locus coeruleus by immobilization stress. *Biol Psychiatry* **45**: 853–862.

Shanks, N., Zalcman, S., Zacharko, R. M., Anisman, H. (1991). Alterations of central norepinephrine, dopamine and serotonin in several strains of mice following acute stressor exposure. *Pharmacol Biochem Behav* **38**: 69–75.

Sherman, J. E., Kalin, N. H. (1986). ICV–CRH potently affects behavior without altering antinociceptive responding. *Life Sci* **39**: 433–441.

Smagin, G. N., Swiergiel. A. H., Dunn, A. J. (1995). Corticotropin-releasing factor administered into the locus coeruleus, but not the parabrachial nucleus, stimulates norepinephrine release in the prefrontal cortex. *Brain Res Bull* **36**: 71–76.

Smagin, G. N., Harris, R. B., Ryan, D. H. (1996). Corticotropin-releasing factor receptor antagonist infused into the locus coeruleus attenuates immobilization stress-induced defensive withdrawal in rats. *Neurosci Lett* **220**: 167–170.

Smagin, G. N., Zhou, J., Harris, R. B., Ryan, D. H. (1997). CRF receptor antagonist attenuates immobilization stress-induced norepinephrine release in the prefrontal cortex in rats. *Brain Res Bull* **42**: 431–434.

Suddath, R. L., Christison, G. W., Torrey, E. F., Casanova, M. F., Weinberger, D. R. (1990). Anatomical abnormalities in the brains of monozygotic twins discordant for schizophrenia. *N Engl J Med* **322**: 789–794.

Susser, E., Neugebauer, R., Hoek, H. W., *et al.* (1996). Schizophrenia after prenatal famine. *Arch Gen Psychiatry* **53**: 25–31.

Tamminga, C. A., Thaker, G. K., Buchanan, R., *et al.* (1992). Limbic system abnormalities identified in schizophrenia using positron emission tomography with fluorodeoxyglucose and neocortical alterations with deficit syndrome. *Arch Gen Psychiatry* **49**: 522–530.

Tebartz van Elst, L., Woermann, F. G., Lemieux, L., Trimble, M. R. (1999). Amygdala enlargement in dysthymia: a volumetric study of patients with temporal lobe epilepsy. *Biol Psychiatry* **46**: 1614–1623.

Thierry, A. M., Javoy. F., Glowinski, J., Kety, S. S. (1968). Effects of stress on the metabolism of norepinephrine, dopamine and serotonin in the central nervous system of the rat. I. Modifications of norepinephrine turnover. *J Pharmacol Exp Ther* **163**: 163–171.

Thune, J. J., Pakkenberg, B. (2000). Stereological studies of the schizophrenic brain. *Brain Res Rev* **31**: 200–204.

Torrey, E. F., Miller, J., Rawlings, R., Yolken R. H. (1997). Seasonality of births in schizophrenia and bipolar disorder: a review of the literature. *Schizophr Res* **28**: 1–38.

Vale, W., Spiess, J., Rivier, C., Rivier, J. (1981). Characterization of a 41-residue ovine hypothalamic peptide that stimulates secretion of corticotropin and beta-endorphin. *Science* **213**: 1394–1397.

Valentino, R. J., Foote, S. L. (1986). Brain noradrenergic neurons, corticotropin-releasing factor, and stress. In: *Neural and Endocrine Peptides and Receptors*, ed. T. W. Moody. New York: Plenum Press, pp. 101–120.

Valentino, R. J., Wehby, R. G. (1988). Corticotropin-releasing factor: evidence for a neurotransmitter role in the locus ceruleus during hemodynamic stress. *Neuroendocrinology* **48**: 674–677.

Valentino, R. J., Foote S. L., Aston-Jones G (1983). Corticotropin-releasing factor activates noradrenergic neurons of the locus coeruleus. *Brain Res* **270**: 363–367.

Valentino, R. J., Page, M. E., Curtis, A. L. (1991). Activation of noradrenergic locus coeruleus neurons by hemodynamic stress is due to local release of corticotropin-releasing factor. *Brain Res* **555**: 25–34.

Valentino, R. J., Foote, S. L., Page, M. E. (1993). The locus coeruleus as a site for integrating corticotropin-releasing factor and noradrenergic mediation of stress responses. *Ann NY Acad Sci* **697**: 173–188.

Valentino, R. J., Chen, S., Zhu, Y., Aston-Jones, G. (1996). Evidence for divergent projections to the brain noradrenergic system and the spinal parasympathetic system from Barrington's nucleus. *Brain Res* **732**: 1–15.

Van Bockstaele, E. J., Colago, E. E., Valentino, R. J. (1996). Corticotropin-releasing factor-containing axon terminals synapse onto catecholamine dendrites and may presynaptically modulate other afferents in the rostral pole of the nucleus locus coeruleus in the rat brain. *J Comp Neurol* **364**: 523–534.

(1998). Amygdaloid corticotropin-releasing factor targets locus coeruleus dendrites: substrate for the co-ordination of emotional and cognitive limbs of the stress response. *J Neuroendocrinol* **10**: 743–757.

Van Bockstaele, E. J., Peoples, J., Valentino, R. J. (1999). A. E. Bennett Research Award. Anatomic basis for differential regulation of the rostrolateral peri-locus coeruleus region by limbic afferents. *Biol Psychiatry* **46**: 1352–1363.

Van Kammen, D. P., Bok van Kammen, W., Mann, L. S., Seppala, T., Linnoila, M. (1986). Dopamine metabolism in the cerebrospinal fluid of drug-free schizophrenic patients with and without cortical atrophy. *Arch Gen Psychiatry* **43**: 978–983.

Waddington, J. L. (1990). Spontaneous orofacial movements induced in rodents by very long-term neuroleptic drug administration: phenomenology, pathophysiology and putative relationship to tardive dyskinesia. [See comments] *Psychopharmacology* **101**: 431–447.

Walker, E. F., Diforio, D. (1997). Schizophrenia: a neural diathesis-stress model. *Psychol Rev* **104**: 667–685.

Weinberger, D. R. (1996). On the plausibility of "the neurodevelopmental hypothesis" of schizophrenia. *Neuropsychopharmacology* **14**(Suppl. 3): 1S–11S.

(1999). Cell biology of the hippocampal formation in schizophrenia. *Biol Psychiatry* **45**: 395–402.

Weinberger, D. R., Lipska, B. K. (1995). Cortical maldevelopment, anti-psychotic drugs, and schizophrenia: a search for common ground. *Schizophr Res* **16**: 87–110.

Weinberger, D. R., Berman, K. F., Ostrem, J. L., Abi-Dargham, A., Torrey, E. F. (1993). Disorganization of prefrontal-hippocampal connectivity in schizophrenia: a PET study of discordant MZ twins. *Soc Neurosci Abstr* **19**: 7.

Wightman, R. M., Robinson, D. L. (2002). Transient changes in mesolimbic dopamine and their association with 'reward.' *J Neurochem* **82**: 721–735.

Yang, C. R., Mogenson, G. J. (1985). An electrophysiological study of the neural projection from the hippocampus to the ventral pallidum and subpallidal areas by way of the nucleus accumbens. *Neuroscience* **15**: 1015–1024.

Zhu, Y., Aston-Jones, G. (1996). The medial prefrontal cortex prominently innervates a peri-locus coeruleus zone in rat. *Soc Neurosci Abstr* **22**: 601.

16

The development of "mis-wired" limbic lobe circuitry in schizophrenia and bipolar disorder

Francine M. Benes

McLean Hospital, Belmont and Harvard Medical School, Boston, USA

Since the early 1980s, neuroscience studies have begun to define the pathophysiology of schizophrenia and bipolar disorder by using a combination of highly selective molecular probes and quantitative microscopy. It is now possible to define how neural circuits have been altered in psychosis in terms of an evolving set of neurobiological principles (Benes, 2000). In patients with schizophrenia, and more recently bipolar disorder, a variety of anomalies have been detected in the limbic lobe, a phylogenetically old portion of the cerebral cortex that includes the anterior cingulate region and hippocampal formation (Fig. 16.1). In addition, the basolateral subdivision of the amygdala (not shown), another component of the limbic lobe, has been implicated in the pathophysiology of psychotic disorders, in part because it sends important inputs to the cingulate cortex and hippocampus. It now seems likely that the three major components of the limbic lobe play a central role in generating disturbances in motivation, attention, emotion, and social interactions in schizophrenia and bipolar disorder (Benes, 1993). The discussion below describes studies in both human and rodent brains that have contributed to our understanding of how this complex circuitry may be altered during development, leading to the appearance of psychotic disorders during late adolescence and early adulthood. A clear understanding of how the brain is normally changing during the postnatal period is an essential ingredient in building plausible models for what may be happening during the prodrome of psychotic disorders.

Postmortem findings in schizophrenia and bipolar disorder

Postmortem studies of the brains of schizophrenia patients have examined many different neuronal and glial markers and it is virtually impossible to review all of them here. Instead, this discussion will focus on two particular neurotransmitters,

Neurodevelopment and Schizophrenia, ed. Matcheri S. Keshavan *et al.* Published by Cambridge University Press. © Cambridge University Press 2004.

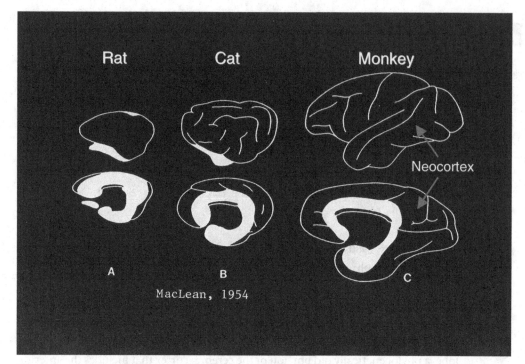

Fig. 16.1.   The limbic lobe is shown on the midsagittal surface of the brains of a rat, cat, and monkey. There is a remarkable degree of preservation of this structure across mammalian species. In contrast, the surrounding neocortex show a marked expansion in primates when compared with that in rodents. (Adapted from McLean, 1954.)

gamma-aminobutyric acid (GABA) and dopamine, that have been implicated in both the pathophysiology of psychosis and its treatment with antipsychotic medications.

The gamma-aminobutyric acid system

The neurotransmitter GABA has long been considered the most important inhibitory molecule in the mammalian brain (Jones, 1993) and recent evidence has consistently pointed to a defect of this system in schizophrenia and bipolar disorder (Benes, 2000). For example, a preferential decrease in the density of non-pyramidal cells has been reported in the anterior cingulate and prefrontal cortex (Benes *et al.*, 1991, 2001), as well as in the hippocampal formation (Benes *et al.*, 1998). The non-pyramidal cells are local circuit neurons, or interneurons, that are largely GABAergic in nature. Although this particular finding has been the subject of considerable controversy (Selemon *et al.*, 2002), a number of studies have suggested that a dysfunction of this system might occur in schizophrenia (Benes *et al.*, 1992a, 1996a) based on markers such as the GABA$_A$ receptor; terminals showing

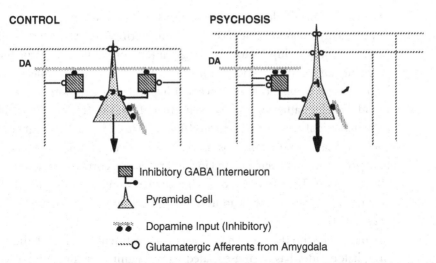

CONTROL   PSYCHOSIS

DA   DA

▨ Inhibitory GABA Interneuron

△ Pyramidal Cell

•• Dopamine Input (Inhibitory)

···O Glutamatergic Afferents from Amygdala

Fig. 16.2.   A schematic diagram depicting a "mis-wired" circuit within layer II of the anterior cingulate cortex of a normal control (left) and psychotic (right) subject. A pyramidal neuron in the psychotic circuit is receiving a reduced inhibition from both dopaminergic (DA) and gamma-aminobutyric acid (GABA)-ergic inputs, while the GABA cell is receiving increased inputs from the mutually antagonistic amygdalar (excitatory) and dopaminergic (inhibitory) fibers. The release of DA might prevent the GABA cell from responding to increased excitatory inflow from the amygdala. Overall, the circuit associated with psychotic disorders has too much excitation, too little inhibition, and would result in abnormal information processing and possibly apoptotic changes. Antipsychotic drugs would ameliorate the effect of stress by blocking DA receptors on GABA cells and allowing the GABA cells to inhibit the firing of pyramidal neurons.

immunoreactivity for glutamate decarboxylase (GAD) 65 kDa isoform (GAD_{65}) (Todtenkopf and Benes, 1998) mRNA for GAD_{67} (Guidotti *et al.*, 2000; Heckers *et al.*, 2002; Volk *et al.*, 2000), and GAD_{65} (Heckers *et al.*, 2002); the GABA transporter (Pierri *et al.*, 1999; Volk *et al.*, 2001; Woo *et al.*, 1998); and several peptides, including parvalbumin (Beasley and Reynolds, 1997; Zhang and Reynolds, 2002), calbindin (Daviss and Lewis, 1995; Iritani *et al.*, 1999), and reelin (Fatemi *et al.*, 1999; Guidotti *et al.*, 2000; Impagnatiello *et al.*, 1998). Most studies have pointed to a decrease of GABAergic activity. As depicted in Fig. 16.2, the postmortem changes detected in the anterior cingulate cortex include a decrease of GABAergic modulation in the anterior cingulate region, a change that could give rise to abnormal information processing (see below).

The dopamine system

All models of schizophrenia must take into account the dopamine system because neuroleptic drugs block dopamine receptors. To explore this issue, we evaluated the distribution of dopamine projections in the anterior cingulate cortex and unexpectedly obtained evidence for a "mis-wiring" of these fibers (Benes et al., 1997). Dopamine inputs to GABAergic interneurons in layer II of the anterior cingulate cortex may be increased, while those to the main projection cells may be decreased. Using a careful process of hypothesis generation and testing, it was found that this pattern was most likely attributable to a trophic shift of fibers away from pyramidal cells to interneurons (Benes, 1998) (Fig. 16.2). A change of this type could be related to pre- and postnatal stress, since an increase of dopamine inputs to interneurons has been induced in adult rats using corticosterone administration (Benes, 1997). The net effect of such a change would be a decline of GABAergic activity, as dopamine exerts an inhibitory effect on the interneurons (Penit-Soria et al., 1989).

Consistent with the above model, chronic treatment of rats with the neuroleptic drug haloperidol has been associated with a significant sprouting of GABAergic terminals in the medial prefrontal cortex (equivalent to the anterior cingulate of human brain), a change that could help to compensate for such circuitry defects (Vincent et al., 1994). Taken together, there is accumulating evidence suggesting that a "mis-wiring" of dopaminergic inputs to GABA cells may be a potential target for antipsychotic medications to exert their therapeutic action. More recent studies (Benes et al., 2000; Heckers et al., 2002) have suggested that a GABA defect may be a feature not only of schizophrenia but also of bipolar disorder. This could also help to explain why neuroleptic drugs and GABA-mimetic mood-stabilizing anti-convulsants are used to treat both disorders, although the latter are more effective in patients with bipolar disorder. Therefore the GABAergic neuron, together with its dopaminergic inputs, may be a final common factor in the pathophysiology of psychotic disorders and a target for treatment.

The role of the amygdala in limbic lobe changes

It is relevant to consider whether changes in the GABA and dopamine systems may be related to one another or whether they are induced by a third system that interacts with both. Several of our studies have pointed to changes in glutamatergic fibers in the anterior cingulate region playing a role in schizophrenia, which is particularly intriguing because this neurotransmitter has been associated with excitotoxic injury to neurons (Coyle and Puttfarcken, 1993). In the mid-1980s, we observed an increase of axons with a vertical, but not horizontal, orientation in superficial layers of the anterior cingulate cortex in schizophrenia (Benes et al., 1987). This finding was later replicated using a more specific technique that visualized glutamatergic axons (Benes et al., 1992b). Based on the orientation and location, it was postulated that these vertical axons might be incoming excitatory fibers from another region. Although there were several candidate regions, the amygdala seemed to be a particularly likely source because an increase of glutamatergic axons was also observed in the entorhinal cortex, which receives a significant projection from the basolateral subdivision of the amygdala (Longson *et al.*, 1996) (Fig. 16.2). In contrast, the dorsolateral prefrontal area, which does not receive an appreciable input from the amygdala, did not show this axonal change in schizophrenia patients (Benes *et al.*, 1992b), providing further support for this hypothesis. It is noteworthy that the basolateral nuclear complex sends a massive projection to layer II of the anterior cingulate cortex (Amaral and Price, 1984; Cunningham *et al.*, 2002; Van Hoesen *et al.*, 1993), as well as to sectors CA2/3 of the hippocampal formation (Berretta *et al.*, 2001; Pitkanen *et al.*, 2000), the two sites where we have observed a preponderance of microscopic changes in our postmortem studies. As shown in Fig. 16.2, the working model predicts that there might be excessive excitatory inputs to both pyramidal cells and GABAergic interneurons in patients with schizophrenia, although the former would be vulnerable to excitotoxicity.

In order to test the hypothesis that amygdalar projections may play a role in a decompensation of GABA cells, we have developed a "partial" rodent model to mimic a defect of GABAergic transmission. In this model, a local infusion of the $GABA_A$ receptor antagonist picrotoxin is made into the basolateral nucleus (Fig. 16.3). As a result, a selective reduction of GABAergic terminals was observed in sectors CA3 and CA2 of the hippocampus (Berretta *et al.*, 2001), a pattern that is remarkably similar to the one observed in our postmortem studies (Todtenkopf and Benes, 1998). Overall, these findings suggest that the defect of GABAergic cells seen in schizophrenia and bipolar disorder may involve, at least in part, an increased flow of excitatory activity from the amygdala to the hippocampus and anterior cingulate cortex.

Postnatal maturation of limbic lobe circuitry

A relevant question to ask regarding the model circuit shown in Fig. 16.2 is when during development might these changes have appeared in schizophrenia: this disorder has a characteristic age of onset between 16 and 25 years and it is possible that alterations in layer II of the anterior cingulate cortex or sectors CA3/2 of the hippocampus might have been present from birth and/or were induced at the time the illness presents. Since the development of the brain is now known to continue well into the postnatal period, it is possible that there are normal maturation changes that may "trigger" the start of the schizophrenia syndrome.

The development of the gamma-aminobutyric acid system

Extensive neurochemical studies of the development of the rodent brain suggest that the maturation of the cortex continues well into the postnatal period (reviewed by Johnston, 1988). For example, GABA-accumulating cells show a progressive

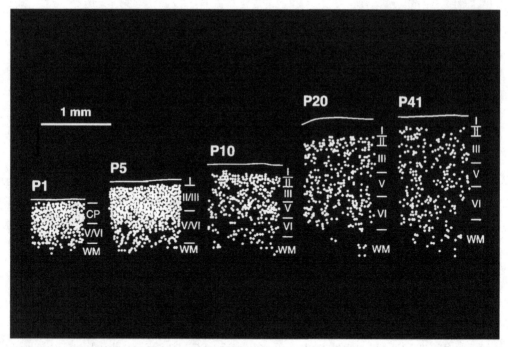

Fig. 16.3.   The distribution of gamma-aminobutyric acid (GABA)-ergic cells in the medial prefrontal cortex of rat brain during the postnatal period. Between day 1 (P1) and day 10 (P10), the density of cells is much greater than that seen at days 20 to 41 (P20 to P41), the postweanling period that is considered to be the equivalent in rats of human adolescence. Although the overall number of cells at day 41 is identical to that found at day 5, the packing density decreases dramatically as the cortical mantle increases its thickness. The GABAergic cells are surrounded by neuropil, where axons and dendrites occupy most of the space.

increase in numerical density until postnatal day II (Chronwall and Wolff, 1980). In contrast, the concentration of GABA and the specific activity of GAD (Coyle and Enna, 1976), as well as the binding activity of the GABA receptor (Coyle and Enna, 1976; Palacios *et al.*, 1979) and its mRNA (Gambarana *et al.*, 1990), all increase until the third postnatal week.

As shown in Fig. 16.3, the numerical density of GABA-immunoreactive neurons in the anterior cingulate cortex of the rat reaches a peak at approximately postnatal day 5 and then diminishes until day 20, when the thickness of the cortical mantle is maximal (Vincent *et al.*, 1995). During this same period, the relative amount of neuropil surrounding all cell bodies in this region is expanding as dendritic and axonal fibers are increasing. GABAergic cell bodies not only show a gradual increase in their size, but by postnatal days 20 to 40, primary, secondary, and tertiary branches of their dendritic tree can also be visualized. The expansion of neuropil in rat medial prefrontal cortex probably involves an increase of both dendritic branches

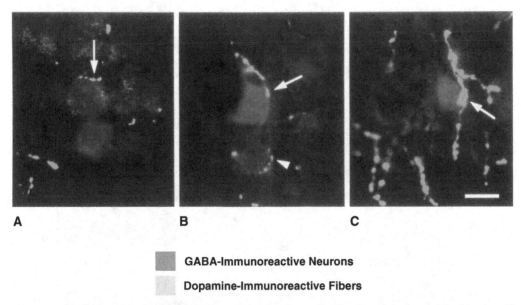

GABA-Immunoreactive Neurons

Dopamine-Immunoreactive Fibers

Fig. 16.4.   A series of confocal photomicrographs showing colocalization of gamma-aminobutyric acid (GABA) neurons (green) and dopamine fibers (yellow) in rat medial prefrontal cortex before (A) and after (B) weaning and in the early adult period (C). There is an apparent increase in the number of dopamine fibers and they appear to form increased contacts with GABA neurons. For a colour version of this figure, see www.cambridge.org/9780521126595.

and terminals of GABAergic neurons, a process that continues in the superficial layers until day 25 (Vincent *et al.*, 1995) when the efficacy of GABAergic synaptic transmission also becomes optimal (Luhmann and Prince, 1991). In general terms, the maturation of the GABA system in rats continues for approximately 2–3 weeks postnatally. Presumably, then, the dendritic branches of GABAergic interneurons will await ingrowing dopamine fibers to target them for the formation of functional interactions.

Late maturation of dopamine projections

Dopaminergic projections to rat medial prefrontal cortex increase progressively beyond the weanling stage until the early adult period (Kalsbeek *et al.*, 1988; Verney *et al.*, 1982). During the first 2 weeks of postnatal life, the distribution of dopaminergic varicose fibers in medial prefrontal cortex is quite low but with the highest density in deeper laminae. During the third postnatal week, however, the density of such fibers clearly increases and this pattern continues until adulthood (Fig. 16.4). The increase of fiber density occurs to a proportionate degree across layers VI–II and does not progress in a distinct "inside-out" manner. For sections in which single immunoperoxidase-processing is combined with

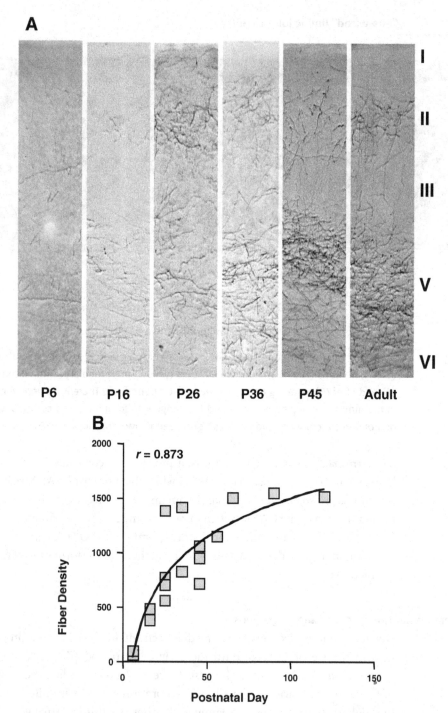

Fig. 16.5. Amygdala projections to the anterior cingulate cortex after birth in rats. (A) Amygdalar fibers visualized with anterograde tracing show a marked increase in layers II and V during the postnatal period. (B) The increase in fiber density shows a highly significant curvilinear rise between birth (postnatal day 0) and adulthood (postnatal day 120) in layer II.
For a colour version of this figure, see www.cambridge.org/9780521126595.

cresyl violet staining, DA-containing varicose fibers can be observed throughout the neuropil, but very commonly, such fibers course toward neuronal cell bodies.

These postnatal increases in the density of dopaminergic projections to rat medial prefrontal cortex are paralleled by an increase in the binding activity of D_2 receptors, which begins prenatally (Bruinink et al., 1983) and continues until the fourth postnatal week (Deskin et al., 1981). Interestingly, administration of 6-hydroxydopamine prevents this increase in D_2 receptor binding, an effect that is associated with dystrophic changes in the basal dendrites of pyramidal neurons (Kalsbeek et al., 1989). Lesions induced in the prefrontal cortex of adult monkeys using 6-hydroxydopamine result in impaired performance of the spatial delayed alternation task (Brozoski et al., 1979) and it seems likely that this functional deficit could be associated with changes in the D_2 receptor on pyramidal neurons. It is noteworthy that dopamine fibers show non-random interactions with cortical neurons that are probably of functional significance (Benes et al., 1993). As shown in Fig. 16.4, as the cortical dopamine system actively grows into the anterior cingulate cortex during the equivalent of adolescence in rats, its fibers contact GABAergic neurons (Benes et al., 1996b). These contacts continue to form until the early adult period. At this point, there is an overall increase of 150% compared with the period before weaning (which would correspond to childhood in humans). As discussed above, the formation of GABA terminals in the cortex reaches a plateau at approximately the fourth postnatal week and the development of the GABA system seems to precede that of the dopamine system. Accordingly, GABA cells may act as passive targets for the reception of functional dopaminergic inputs during the equivalent of late adolescence and early adulthood. If this interpretation is correct, it could have far-reaching implications for our understanding of psychotic disorders.

The ingrowth of amygdalar fibers into the anterior cingulate cortex

If dopamine fibers show such late developmental changes, is it possible that there might be analogous changes occurring in other projection systems, such as that from the basolateral amygdala? As shown in Fig. 16.5, using anterograde tracing, amygdalar projections to the anterior cingulate cortex do show significant increases during the postnatal period, as they form synaptic connections with both the spines and shafts of dendrites (Cunningham et al., 2002). A significant proportion of these fibers form increased connections with GABAergic neurons (Cunningham et al., 2002), an observation that is consistent with electrophysiological studies, which have suggested that these latter cells may be a pivotal target of amygdalar activation (Perez-Jananay and Vives, 1991). In addition, a recent study has demonstrated a marked increase in the frequency with which amygdalar fibers form contacts on GABAergic cells in rat cingulate cortex (Cunningham et al., 2002). Since the amygdalar projections and dopamine fibers show extensive overlap in layer V

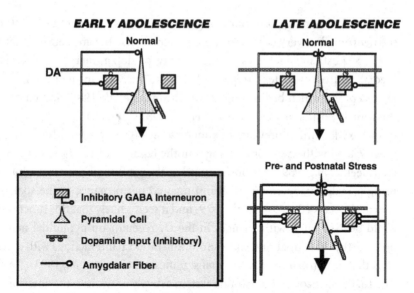

Fig. 16.6.   A set of schematic diagrams depicting the normal development of an intrinsic circuit in the anterior cingulate cortex during early and late adolescence. Gamma-aminobutyric acid (GABA) cell development is probably relatively complete by early adolescence while that of dopamine fibers and amygdalar projections continues into late adolescence and early adulthood. By late adolescence, the neural response to emotionally stressful situations may be relatively complete in normal individuals. However, individuals exposed to stress early in life may be sensitized to the effects of stress later. During late adolescence, the stressed circuit could theoretically develop excessive dopaminergic and amygdalar inputs. Such changes may be associated with a decompensation of the circuit if GABAergic cells are unable to provide sufficient inhibitory modulation.

of the cingulate cortex, it will be relevant to know whether these two systems may actually interact with one another through a presynaptic mechanism.

A model for how a "mis-wired" circuit might lead to decompensation

The findings described above indicate that dopamine and amygdalar fibers seem to be increasing in number and converging on individual GABAergic cells at a stage when schizophrenia is beginning. According to the working model shown in Fig. 16.6, amygdalar fibers would provide increased excitatory drive (McDonald *et al.*, 1989) while dopamine fibers would provide increased inhibitory modulation (Retaux *et al.*, 1991). Under stressful conditions when the release of dopamine is markedly increased (Roth *et al.*, 1988), the target GABA cell could fail to provide adequate amounts of inhibitory modulation to pyramidal neurons. In this setting, these latter cells could fire excessively, particularly since excitatory activity from the amygdala is probably increasing at the same time. This proposed mechanism could theoretically result in oxidative stress to pyramidal cells and/or GABA neurons and lead to further dysfunction or perhaps even decompensation of the circuit. As observed clinically, neuroleptic drugs produce prompt remission of psychotic symptoms in the early stages of a psychotic illness, possibly by blocking dopamine receptors on these GABA cells. The net effect of dopamine receptor blockade would be the release of GABA cells to fire more optimally.

Overall, the studies and model discussed above have suggested the importance of viewing psychotic disorders from the standpoint of the development of integrated circuitry involving the amygdala, anterior cingulate cortex, and hippocampus. Changes in the activity level of convergent inputs to GABA cells in one or all of these regions during adolescence may serve as "triggers" for the onset of psychosis in susceptible individuals. A more detailed understanding of how such developmental changes could interplay with defective neurons may eventually suggest novel treatment strategies that can be applied early in the course of the illness to offset the deterioration in functioning that often occurs in individuals with a chronic psychotic disorder.

Acknowledgements

This work has been supported by grants from the National Institutes of Health (MH00423, MH31862, MH31154), the Stanley Foundation, the Carmella and Menachem Abraham Fund and the Taplin Fund.

REFERENCES

Amaral, D. G., Price, J. L. (1984). Amygdalo-cortical projections in the monkey (macaca fascicularis). *J Comp Neurol* **230**: 465–496.

Beasley, C. L., Reynolds, G. P. (1997). Parvalbumin-immunoreactive neurons are reduced in the prefrontal cortex of schizophrenics. *Schizophr Res* **24**: 349–355.

Benes, F. M. (1993). Neurobiological investigations in cingulate cortex of schizophrenic brain. *Schizophr Bull* **19**: 537–549.

(1997). The role of stress and dopamine–GABA interactions in the vulnerability for schizophrenia. *J Psychiatr Res* **31**: 257–275.

(1998). Model generation and testing to probe neural circuitry in the cingulate cortex of postmortem schizophrenic brain. *Schizophr Bull* **24**: 219–230.

(2000). Emerging principles of altered neural circuitry in schizophrenia. *Brain Res Brain Res Rev* **31**: 251–269.

Benes, F. M., Majocha, R., Bird, E. D., Marotta, C. A. (1987). Increased vertical axon numbers in cingulate cortex of schizophrenics. *Arch Gen Psychiatry* **44**: 1017–1021.

Benes, F. M., McSparren, J., Bird, E. D., SanGiovanni, J. P., Vincent, S. L. (1991). Deficits in small interneurons in prefrontal and cingulate cortices of schizophrenic and schizoaffective patients. *Arch Gen Psychiatry* **48**: 996–1001.

Benes, F. M., Vincent, S. L., Alsterberg, G., Bird, E. D., SanGiovanni, J. P. (1992a). Increased GABA$_A$ receptor binding in superficial layers of cingulate cortex in schizophrenics. *J Neurosci* **12**: 924–929.

Benes, F. M., Sorensen, I., Vincent, S. L., Bird, E. D., Sathi, M. (1992b). Increased density of glutamate-immunoreactive vertical processes in superficial laminae in cingulate cortex of schizophrenic brain. *Cereb Cortex* **2**: 503–512.

Benes, F. M., Vincent, S. L., Molloy, R. (1993). Dopamine-immunoreactive axon varicosities form nonrandom contacts with GABA-immunoreactive neurons of rat medial prefrontal cortex. *Synapse* **15**: 285–295.

Benes, F. M., Khan, Y., Vincent, S. L., Wickramasinghe, R. (1996a). Differences in the subregional and cellular distribution of GABA$_A$ receptor binding in the hippocampal formation of schizophrenic brain. *Synapse* **22**: 338–349.

Benes, F. M., Vincent, S. L., Molloy, R., Khan, Y. (1996b). Increased interaction of dopamine-immunoreactive varicosities with GABA neurons of rat medial prefrontal cortex occurs during the postweanling period. *Synapse* **23**: 237–245.

Benes, F. M., Todtenkopf, M. S., Taylor, J. B. (1997). Differential distribution of tyrosine hydroxylase fibers on small and large neurons in layer II of anterior cingulate cortex of schizophrenic brain. *Synapse* **25**: 80–92.

Benes, F. M., Kwok, E. W., Vincent, S. L., Todtenkopf, M. S. (1998). A reduction of nonpyramidal cells in sector CA2 of schizophrenics and manic depressives. [See comments] *Biol Psychiatry* **44**: 88–97.

Benes, F. M., Todtenkopf, M. S., Logiotatos, P., Williams, M. (2000). Glutamate decarboxylase(65)-immunoreactive terminals in cingulate and prefrontal cortices of schizophrenic and bipolar brain. *J Chem Neuroanat* **20**: 259–269.

Benes, F. M., Vincent, S. L., Todtenkopf, M. S. (2001). The density of pyramidal and nonpyramidal neurons in anterior cingulate cortex of schizophrenic and bipolar subjects. *Biol Psychiatry* **50**: 395–406.

Berretta, S., Munno, D. W., Benes, F. M. (2001). Amygdalar activation alters the hippocampal GABA system: "partial" modelling for postmortem changes in schizophrenia. *J Comp Neurol* **431**: 129–138.

Brozoski, T., Brown, R. M., Rosvold, H. E., Goldman, P. S. (1979). Cognitive deficit caused by depletion of dopamine in prefrontal cortex of rhesus monkey. *Science* **205**: 929–931.

Bruinink, A., Lichtensteiner, W., Schlumpf, M. (1983). Pre- and postnatal ontogeny and characterization of dopaminergic D2, serotonergic S2, and spirodecanone binding sites in rat forebrain. *J Neurochem* **40**: 1227–1237.

Chronwall, B., Wolff, J. R. (1980). Prenatal and postnatal development of GABA-accumulating cells in the occipital neocortex of rat. *J Comp Neurol* **190**: 187–208.

Coyle, J. T., Enna, S. (1976). Neurochemical aspects of the ontogenesis of GABAnergic neurons in the rat brain. *Brain Res* **111**: 119–133.

Coyle, J. T., Puttfarcken, P. (1993). Oxidative stress, glutamate, and neurodegenerative disorders. [Review] *Science* **262**: 689–695.

Cunningham, M. G., Bhattacharyya, S., Benes, F. M. (2002). Amygdalo-cortical sprouting continues into early adulthood: Implications for the development of normal and abnormal function during adolescence. *J Comp Neurol* **453**: 116–130.

Daviss, S. R., Lewis, D. A. (1995). Local circuit neurons of the prefrontal cortex in schizophrenia: selective increase in the density of calbindin-immunoreactive neurons. *Psychiatry Res* **59**: 81–96.

Deskin, R., Seidler, F. J., Whitmore, W. L., Slotkin, T. A. (1981). Development of α-noradrenergic and dopaminergic receptor systems depends on maturation of their presynaptic nerve terminals in the rat brain. *J Neurochem* **36**: 1683–1690.

Fatemi, S. H., Emamian, E. S., Kist, D., *et al.* (1999). Defective corticogenesis and reduction in Reelin immunoreactivity in cortex and hippocampus of prenatally infected neonatal mice. *Mol Psychiatry* **4**: 145–154.

Gambarana, C., Pittman, R., Siegel, R. E. (1990). Development expression of the GABA-A receptor $\gamma 1$ subunit mRNA in the rat brain. *J Neurobiol* **21**: 1169–1179.

Guidotti, A., Auta, J., Davis, J. M., *et al.* (2000). Decrease in Reelin and glutamate acid decarboxylase$_{67}$ (GAD$_{67}$) expression in schizophrenia and bipolar disorder. *Arch Gen Psychiatry* **57**: 1061–1069.

Heckers, S., Stone, D., Walsh, J., *et al.* (2002). Differential hippocampal expression of glutamic acid decarboxylase 65 and 67 messenger RNA in bipolar disorder and schizophrenia. *Arch Gen Psychiatry* **59**: 521–529.

Impagnatiello, F., Guidotti, A. R., Pesold, C., *et al.* (1998). A decrease of reelin expression as a putative vulnerability factor in schizophrenia. *Proc Natl Acad Sci USA* **95**: 15718–15723.

Iritani, S., Kuroki, N., Ikeda, K., Kazamatsuri, H. (1999). Calbindin immunoreactivity in the hippocampal formation and neocortex of schizophrenics. *Prog Neuropsychopharmacol Biol Psychiatry* **23**: 409–421.

Johnston, M. V. (1988). Biochemistry of neurotransmitters in cortical development. In *Cerebral Cortex*, ed. E. G. Jones. New York: Plenum Press, pp. 211–236.

Jones, E. G. (1993). GABAergic neurons and their role in cortical plasticity in primates. *Cereb Cortex* **3**: 361–372.

Kalsbeek, A., Voorn, P., Buijs, R. M., Pool, C. W., Uylings, H. B. (1988). Development of the dopaminergic innervation in the prefrontal cortex of the rat. *J Comp Neurol* **269**: 58–72.

Kalsbeek, A., Matthijssen, M. A., Uylings, H. B. (1989). Morphometric analysis of prefrontal cortical development following neonatal lesioning of the dopaminergic mesocortical projection. *Exp Brain Res* **78**: 279–289.

Longson, D., Deakin, J. F., Benes, F. M. (1996). Increased density of entorhinal glutamate-immunoreactive vertical fibers in schizophrenia. *J Neur Transm* **103**: 503–507.

Luhmann, H. J., Prince, D. A. (1991). Postnatal maturation of the GABAergic system in rat neocortex. *J Neurophysiol* **65**: 247–263.

McDonald, A. J., Beitz, A. J., Larson, A. A., *et al.* (1989). Co-localization of glutamate and tubulin in putative excitatory neurons of the hippocampus and amygdala: an immunohistochemical study using monoclonal antibodies. *Neuroscience* **30**: 405–421.

McLean, P. D. (1954). Studies on limbic system (visceral brain) and their bearing on psychosomatic problems. In *Recent Developments in Psychosomatic Medicine*, ed. E. Wittkower, R. Cleghorn. Philadelphia, PA: Lippincott, p. 106.

Palacios, J. M., Niehoff, D. L., Kuhar, M. J. (1979). Ontogeny of GABA and benzodiazepine receptors: effects of Triton X-100, bromide and muscimol. *Brain Res* **179**: 390–395.

Penit-Soria, J., Retaux, S., Maurin, Y. (1989). Effets de la stimulation des recepteurs D_1 et D_2 dopaminergiques sur la liberation d'acide γ-[^{3}H] aminobutyrique induite electriquement dans le cortex prefrontal du rat. *C R Acad Sci Paris* **309**: 441–446.

Perez-Jananay, J. M., Vives, F. (1991). Electrophysiological study of the response of medical prefrontal cortex neurons to stimulation of the basolateral nucleus of the amygdala in the rat. *Brain Res* **564**: 97–101.

Pierri, J. N., Chaudry, A. S., Woo, T. U., Lewis, D. A. (1999). Alterations in chandelier neuron axon terminals in the prefrontal cortex of schizophrenic subjects. *Am J Psychiatry* **156**: 1709–1719.

Pitkanen, A., Pikkarainen, M., Nurminen, N., Ylinen, A. (2000). Reciprocal connections between the amygdala and the hippocampal formation, perirhinal cortex, and postrhinal cortex in rat. A review. *Ann N Y Acad Sci* **911**: 369–391.

Retaux, S., Besson, M. J., Penit-Soria, J. (1991). Opposing effects of dopamine D2 receptor stimulation on the spontaneous and the electrically evoked release of [^{3}H] GABA on rat prefrontal cortex slices. *Neuroscience* **42**: 61–71.

Roth, R. H., Tam, S. Y., Ida, Y., Yang, J. X., Deutch, A. Y. (1988). Stress and the mesocorticolimbic dopamine systems. *Ann N Y Acad Sci* **537**: 138–147.

Selemon, L. D., Goldman, Rakic, P., Rajkowska, G. (2002). 2D versus 3D cell counting. *Biol Psychiatry* **51**: 838–840.

Todtenkopf, M. S., Benes, F. M. (1998). Distribution of glutamate decarboxylase65 immunoreactive puncta on pyramidal and nonpyramidal neurons in hippocampus of schizophrenic brain. *Synapse* **29**: 323–332.

Van Hoesen, G. W., Morecraft, R. J., Vogt, B. A. (1993). Connections of the monkey cingulate cortex. In *Neurobiology of Cingulate Cortex and Limbic Thalamus*, ed. M. Gabriel. Boston, MA: Birkhauser, pp. 249–284.

Verney, C., Berger, B., Adrien, J., Vigny, A., Gay, M. (1982). Development of the dopaminergic innervation of the rat cerebral cortex. A light microscopic immunocytochemical study using anti-tyrosine hydroxylase antibodies. *Brain Res* **281**: 41–52.

Vincent, S. L., Adamec, E., Sorensen, I., Benes, F. M. (1994). The effects of chronic haloperidol administration on GABA-immunoreactive axon terminals in rat medial prefrontal cortex. *Synapse* **17**: 26–35.

Vincent, S. L., Pabreza, L., Benes, F. M. (1995). Postnatal maturation of GABA-immunoreactive neurons of rat medial prefrontal cortex. *J Comp Neurol* **355**: 81–92.

Volk, D. W., Austin, M. C., Pierri, J. N., Sampson, A. R., Lewis, D. A. (2000). Decreased glutamic acid decarboxylase67 messenger RNA expression in a subset of prefrontal cortical gamma-aminobutyric acid neurons in subjects with schizophrenia. *Arch Gen Psychiatry* **57**: 237–245.

(2001). GABA transporter-1 mRNA in the prefrontal cortex in schizophrenia: decreased expression in a subset of neurons. *Am J Psychiatry* **158**: 256–265.

Woo, T. U., Whitehead, R. E., Melchitzky, D. S., Lewis, D. A. (1998). A subclass of prefrontal gamma-aminobutyric acid axon terminals are selectively altered in schizophrenia. *Proc Natl Acad Sci USA* **95**: 5341–5346.

Zhang, Z. J., Reynolds, G. P. (2002). A selective decrease in the relative density of parvalbumin-immunoreactive neurons in the hippocampus in schizophrenia. *Schizophr Res* **55**: 1–10.

17

Development of thalamocortical circuitry and the pathophysiology of schizophrenia

Darlene S. Melchitzky[1] and David A. Lewis[2]

[1] Mercyhurst College, Erie, USA
[2] University of Pittsburgh, Pittsburgh, USA

Schizophrenia is clearly a multithetic disorder in which the diverse signs and symptoms of the illness arise as a result of dysfunction in a number of brain regions. Of these clinical features, a growing body of literature indicates that core features of the illness are represented by disturbances in certain cognitive functions, such as those mediated by neural circuits that include components of the dorsolateral prefrontal cortex (DLPFC) and the mediodorsal nucleus (MDN) of the thalamus (Elvevåg and Goldberg, 2000). The specific causal factors that give rise to these brain abnormalities remain enigmatic, with a number of genes and a range of environmental events identified as potential risk factors for schizophrenia (Lewis and Lieberman, 2000). In addition, developmental processes appear to play a central role in the translation of these etiological factors into the appearance of the clinical features of the illness (Lewis and Levitt, 2002). Consequently, understanding the structural and functional maturation of the intrinsic and extrinsic circuitry of the DLPFC and MDN is essential for understanding the pathophysiological basis for the cognitive deficits in schizophrenia.

Function and development of the circuitry of the mediodorsal nucleus and dorsolateral prefrontal cortex

Individuals with schizophrenia perform poorly on cognitive tasks that require the use of working memory: the ability to maintain information "on line" in order to guide behavior (Goldman-Rakic, 1994). For example, subjects with schizophrenia are impaired on oculomotor delayed-response tasks (Park and Holzman, 1992), a cognitive paradigm on which non-human primates with structural or reversible cooling lesions of the DLPFC also perform poorly (Fuster, 1997). Consistent with these observations, many subjects with schizophrenia fail to show normal activation

Neurodevelopment and Schizophrenia, ed. Matcheri S. Keshavan *et al.* Published by Cambridge University Press. © Cambridge University Press 2004.

of the DLPFC when attempting to perform tasks that tap working memory (Weinberger *et al.*, 1986).

The DLPFC maintains reciprocal excitatory connections with specific subdivisions of the MDN, the principal source of thalamic inputs to the DLPFC (Barbas *et al.*, 1991; Giguere and Goldman-Rakic, 1988; Goldman-Rakic and Porrino, 1985). Like the DLPFC, the MDN has been implicated as a site of dysfunction in schizophrenia (Lewis, 2000), and it also appears to play a critical role in working memory functioning. For example, destruction of some or all of the MDN produces deficits in working memory performance (Isseroff *et al.*, 1982). Furthermore, during the delay period of delayed-response tasks, neurons in both the DLPFC (Funahashi *et al.*, 1989) and the MDN (Fuster and Alexander, 1971) exhibit sustained activity, which, at least in the DLPFC, has been proposed to be the neural substrate for working memory (Fuster, 1997; Goldman-Rakic, 1995).

The ability to perform delayed-response tasks first appears between 2 and 4 months of age in monkeys (Goldman-Rakic, 1987) and around 1 year of age in humans (Diamond, 1985). Performance on these tasks then continues to improve (as evidenced by the ability to withstand longer delay periods) at a slower rate until adult functional competence is achieved after puberty in both monkeys (Alexander and Goldman, 1978) and humans (Casey *et al.*, 2000; Diamond, 2002). Although the contributions of the MDN are less well studied, studies in humans clearly indicate that changes in the frontal cortex between the ages of 12 and 19 years contribute to the maturation of cognitive control (Bunge *et al.*, 2002).

Studies in monkeys also suggest that DLPFC neural circuitry is increasingly involved in the mediation of these improvements in cognitive performance during postnatal development. That is, the emergence of the ability to perform delayed-response tasks during infancy does not appear to depend upon the integrity of the DLPFC but appears to be mediated by subcortical structures like the MDN. For example, ablation of the DLPFC in infant monkeys does not produce the same degree of impairment on spatial delayed-response tasks that is observed in adult animals with such lesions (Alexander and Goldman, 1978). In contrast, during the first year of life, performance of oculomotor delayed-response tasks do appear to depend upon the integrity of the MDN (Alexander and Goldman, 1978). Furthermore, during postnatal development, the percentage of DLPFC neurons exhibiting delay period activity doubles between 12 and 36 months of age (Alexander, 1982). In contrast, the MDN does not exhibit this type of developmental increase in the number of delay-activated neurons (Alexander, 1982). Together, these findings suggest that postnatal development is associated with an increasing dependence upon the DLPFC for the mediation of delayed-response behavior, such that the maturation of the DLPFC enhances the function of brain regions like the MDN, which appear to subserve these tasks earlier in life (Alexander and Goldman, 1978).

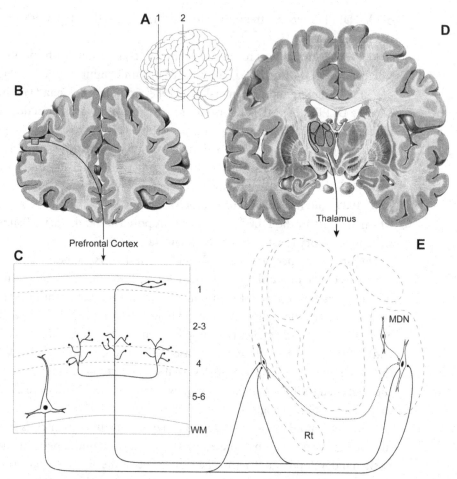

Fig. 17.1.   Connections between the human prefrontal cortex and the mediodorsal nucleus (MDN) of the thalamus. (A) Schematic view of the lateral surface of the human brain. (B) Coronal section of the prefrontal cortex, taken at the level of vertical line 1 in (A). (C) Expanded schematic drawing of the box in (A). Pyramidal neurons in layer 6 send projections to the MDN as well as to the reticular nucleus of the thalamus (Rt). (D) Coronal section through the thalamus, taken at the level of vertical line 2 in (A). The individual thalamic nuclei are outlined. (E) Expanded view of the outline of the thalamus shown in (D). Neurons in the MDN send axons to the prefrontal cortex that arborize primarily in deep layers 3 and 4 but also extend into layer 1 (C). MDN neurons also send axon collaterals to the inhibitory neurons of the Rt. Large cortically projecting excitatory neurons in the MDN receive inhibitory input from smaller GABA neurons located in the MDN and Rt.

Organization of thalamocortical circuitry

In both rodent and primate brains, retrograde tracing studies have demonstrated that projection neurons in the MDN are topographically organized such that different MDN subdivisions project to specific areas of the frontal lobe (Barbas *et al.*, 1991; Goldman-Rakic and Porrino, 1985). In general, the magnocellular MDN subdivision is connected primarily with medial and orbital prefrontal regions, whereas the parvocellular subdivision projects to the DLPFC (Barbas *et al.*, 1991; Giguere and Goldman-Rakic, 1988; Goldman-Rakic and Porrino, 1985). However, the three-dimensional topography of these connections is complex and parvocellular MDN projections are not restricted to the DLPFC. For example, a recent study demonstrated that portions of the parvocellular subdivision may be more extensively connected with more caudal areas of frontal cortex, such as areas 8 (frontal eye fields) and 6 (premotor cortex), than with the DLPFC proper (Erickson and Lewis, 2000).

Within the DLPFC, MDN thalamic axons terminate primarily in deep layers 3 and 4 (Giguere and Goldman-Rakic, 1988), although other cortical layers do contain thalamic axons (Fig. 17.1C). For example, MDN thalamic axons have been observed in layers 1, 2, and superficial 3, although these axons are not as branched and they exhibit a lower density of boutons compared with those in deep layers 3 and 4 (Erickson and Lewis, 2000). Axons arising from a given location within the MDN also exhibit both global and local discontinuities in their cortical terminal fields. However, the relationship between clusters of thalamic axon terminals and the columnar organization of the intrinsic circuitry of the DLPFC (see below) has not been directly examined.

The majority of the axon terminals arising from the MDN form asymmetric synaptic contacts onto the dendritic spines of DLPFC pyramidal neurons, at least in the rodent (Kuroda *et al.*, 1998). In addition, several studies have demonstrated that the calcium-binding protein parvalbumin (PV) is present in axon terminals arising from thalamic nuclei (DeFelipe and Jones, 1991). More specifically, in deep layers 3 and 4 of monkey DLPFC, PV-immunoreactive axon terminals with the morphological features of thalamic axons form asymmetric synapses onto the dendritic spines of pyramidal neurons (Fig. 17.2A) (Melchitzky *et al.*, 1999). Although most axon terminals arising from thalamic nuclei contact the dendritic spines of pyramidal neurons, the dendrites of gamma-aminobutyric acid (GABA)-ergic cells are also targets of thalamic axons. For example, dendritic shafts of PV-containing GABA neurons in the DLPFC receive asymmetric synapses from PV-immunoreactive axon terminals, which most likely arise from the MDN (Melchitzky *et al.*, 1999).

In the DLPFC, spines on the basilar dendrites of layer 3 pyramidal neurons are among the targets of afferents from the MDN. Layer 3 pyramidal neurons play a central role in the flow of information both between and within cortical regions.

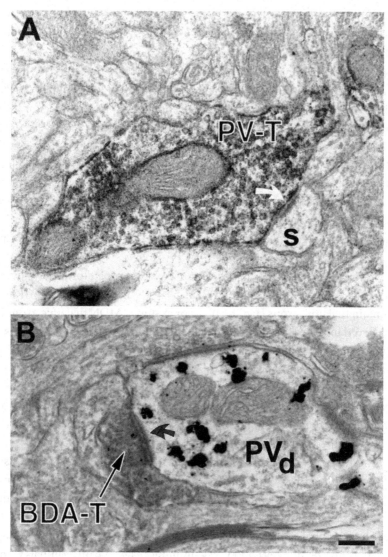

Fig. 17.2.   Axon terminals in the dorsolateral prefrontal cortex (DLPFC). (A) Electron micrograph of a
parvalbumin-immunoreactive thalamic axon terminal (PV-T) in layer 4 of the DLPFC forming
an asymmetric, excitatory synapse onto a dendritic spine(s). (B) Electron micrograph of a
biotinylated dextran amine-labeled intrinsic axon terminal (BDA-T) in DLPFC layer 3 forming
an asymmetric synapse onto a parvalbumin-containing dendritic shaft (PV$_d$). (Adapted from
Melchitzky *et al.*, 1999 (A) and 2001 (B).)

In addition to furnishing projections through the white matter to other cortical regions (Fig. 17.3B), these neurons have long-range intrinsic axon collaterals that travel horizontally through the gray matter and give rise to stripe-like clusters of axon terminals in layers 1–3 (Fig. 17.3A) (Levitt *et al.*, 1993; Pucak *et al.*, 1996). The dendritic spines of other pyramidal neurons constitute the postsynaptic targets of almost all (95%) of both the white matter and the long-range intrinsic projections of these neurons (Melchitzky *et al.*, 1998). These findings suggest that specific groups of pyramidal neurons, clustered as stripes that are reciprocally interconnected by long-range axon collaterals, form functional modules that may serve to recruit and/or coordinate the activity of specific, spatially segregated populations of DLPFC pyramidal neurons (Fig. 17.3C, D).

Layer 3 pyramidal neurons also provide local axon collaterals that arborize and terminate near (within 300 μm) the parent cell body, thus contributing to the regulation of the neuronal activity of a given DLPFC stripe. In contrast to the long-range axons, the targets of the local axon terminals are equally divided between dendritic shafts and dendritic spines (Melchitzky *et al.*, 2001). Furthermore, the PV-containing subclass of GABAergic neurons (Fig. 17.2B) are the primary target of these local inputs to dendritic shafts (Melchitzky and Lewis, 2003). Given the potent inhibitory inputs that PV-containing cells provide to the soma and the axon initial segment (AIS) of pyramidal neurons (Condé *et al.*, 1994), these data suggest, at least within the middle layers of the monkey DLPFC, that the connectivity of PV-containing neurons enables them to serve a critical role in feedback inhibition, constraining the propagation of pyramidal cell excitation both locally and at a distance.

The dendritic spines of layer 4 pyramidal neurons may also be targets of afferents from the MDN. Such contacts would result in a complementary activation of the DLPFC compared with that resulting from the MDN inputs to layer 3 pyramidal neurons. For example, unlike the horizontally oriented axon collaterals of layer 3 pyramidal neurons (Fig. 17.3C), axons emanating from layer 4 pyramidal cells have a distinct and restricted vertical orientation, projecting to other cortical layers in the same column (Levitt *et al.*, 1993). Thus, MDN inputs to layer 4 pyramidal neurons result in the propagation of excitation within a column of the DLPFC, whereas those to layer 3 pyramidal cells produces a more widespread excitation to a spatially distributed network of stripes (see Fig. 17.3D).

The last link in MDN–DLPFC circuitry involves the reciprocal excitatory projections from DLPFC back to MDN (Fig. 17.1). The majority of MDN-projecting cells are small pyramidal neurons located in superficial layer 6, with small pyramidal cells in deep layer 6 and large pyramidal cells in layer 5 making up the remainder (Erickson and Lewis, 2000; Giguere and Goldman-Rakic, 1988). The corticothalamic axons target both the projection neurons of the MDN and the GABAergic

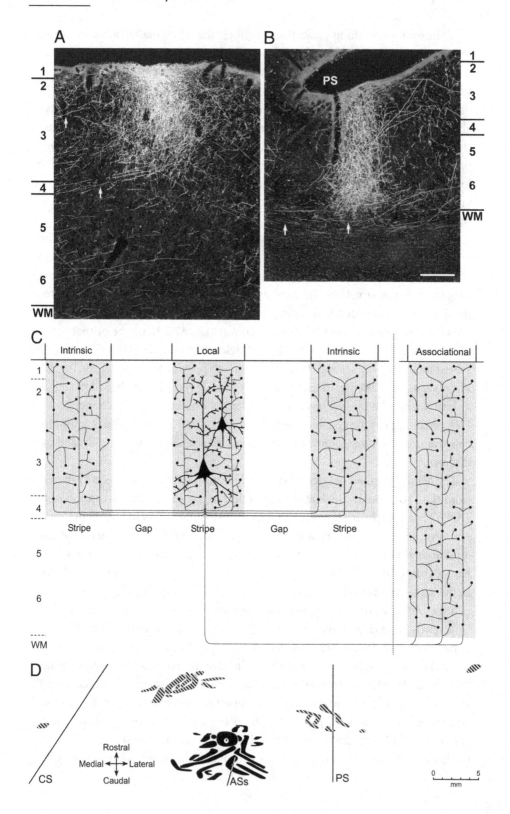

neurons of the reticular thalamic nucleus, which, in turn, provide inhibitory regulation of MDN projection neurons (Fig. 17.1E).

Unfortunately, attempts to explore the functional properties of the circuitry between the MDN and DLPFC face certain limitations. First, because they lack direct connections with the periphery, it is very difficult to manipulate the inputs to or intrinsic components of MDN–DLPFC circuitry; therefore, most of our knowledge base involves inferences from sensory thalamocortical systems. For example, in contrast to the deprivation or manipulation of visual inputs that have been used to study the functional properties of lateral geniculate thalamus and primary visual cortex circuitry, such manipulations cannot be made to study the connections between the MDN and the DLPFC. Second, the majority of studies investigating thalamo-corticothalamic circuitry have been performed in non-primates, such as rodents and cats. Given the apparent differences in DLPFC circuitry between rodents and primates (Lewis, 2002), extrapolation of rodent data to primate systems can only be made with a number of caveats.

Development of thalamocortical circuitry

Our knowledge of the development of the connections between the MDN and DLPFC are subject to the same limitations: most studies are performed in rodents and focus on the sensory thalamic systems. Therefore, the following account of the

Fig. 17.3.   Neuron circuits in the dorsolateral prefrontal cortex (DLPFC). (A, B) Darkfield photomicro-graphs of biotinylated dextran amine (BDA)-labeled axons resulting from an injection site in layer 3 of monkey DLPFC. Horizontally oriented, long-range intrinsic axon collaterals of layer 3 pyramidal neurons travel through the gray matter (A: arrows) and form a stripe-like cluster of labeled axons and terminals confined to layers 1–3 (A). The labeled associational axons from the same injection site travel through the white matter (B: arrows) and form a dense cluster that extends across all cortical layers (B). PS indicates principal sulcus. (Scale bar = 100 m.) (C) Schematic diagram illustrating the spatial distribution of the three types of axon terminal furnished by layer 3 pyramidal neurons in monkey DLPFC. BDA-labeled axons of pyramidal neurons terminate nearby (local) or after traveling horizontally through the gray matter (intrinsic) or through the white matter (associational) to form stripes of labeled terminals. (D) Tangential reconstruction of all stripe-like clusters of retrogradely labeled neurons arising from a single injection in monkey DLPFC. On this unfolded map, the PS is oriented as a vertical line, and all labeled structures and other sulci are shown relative to the PS. The location of the injection site is indicated by asterisk. Intrinsic stripes are shaded in black, and associational stripes are cross-hatched. Note that the associational projections form several distinct groups of stripes located at varying distances from the intrinsic stripes. ASs, superior ramus of arcuate sulcus; CS, cingulate sulcus. (Adapted from Melchitzky et al., 1998 (A, B) and 2001 (C) and Pucak et al., 1996 (D).)

development of the connections between MDN and DLPFC has been extrapolated from data from primary sensory regions in primates and rodents. In primates, the growth of thalamic axons towards the cortical plate (a dense sheet of immature neurons that, with differentiation, acquire the characteristic laminated appearance of the mature cortex) occurs relatively early in the gestation period of 165 days for macaque monkeys. For example, axons from the lateral geniculate nucleus begin to approach the area of the primary visual cortex by embryonic day 78 (Rakic, 1977). Although the thalamic axons begin their journey towards the developing cerebral cortex early, they appear to "wait" for an extended time in the subplate (composed of loosely packed neurons located below and born prior to those that form the cortical plate) before invading the cortical plate. During this "waiting period," thalamic axons appear to form transient, synapse-like structures with subplate neurons, and such contacts appear to be critical for the subsequent formation of proper connections between thalamic axons and cortical neurons. For example, following lesions of the subplate, axons from the lateral geniculate nucleus continue to grow past the visual cortex, suggesting that subplate neurons are required for these thalamic axons to recognize their appropriate cortical target (Ghosh et al., 1990). After this "waiting period," thalamic axons make a second growth spurt to enter the cortical plate, such that, in the monkey, thalamic axons enter the visual cortex by embryonic day 124. This foray of thalamic axons into the cortical plate is somewhat diffuse. For example, in monkey visual cortex, the presence of ocular dominance columns is not apparent initially and segregation of fibers into these columns begins to appear 3 weeks before birth (Rakic, 1977). Therefore, the formation of thalamocorticothalamic circuitry could be affected by adverse events occurring over a broad period of prenatal development.

During postnatal development, substantial changes transpire in the developmental trajectory for synaptic density in monkey DLPFC observed via electron microscopy (Bourgeois et al., 1994). The number of asymmetric, excitatory synapses on dendritic spines increases rapidly between birth and 2 months of age; it then remains at this relatively high level until adolescence, when the number declines to adult levels (Fig. 17.4A). A similar process of synaptic overproduction and elimination also occurs in human DLPFC (Huttenlocher, 1979). In addition, imaging studies of the DLPFC in children and young adults demonstrate a similar pattern of initial gray matter growth in childhood followed by gray matter reduction starting in adolescence (Giedd, 1999; Sowell et al., 2001).

Developmental changes in markers of synaptic inputs to the pyramidal neurons that participate in thalamocorticothalamic connections occur in a similar fashion. For example, dendritic spines are the primary sites of excitatory synaptic inputs to pyramidal cells, and changes in spine number appear to reflect parallel alterations in excitatory inputs to these neurons (Lund and Holbach, 1991). In monkey DLPFC,

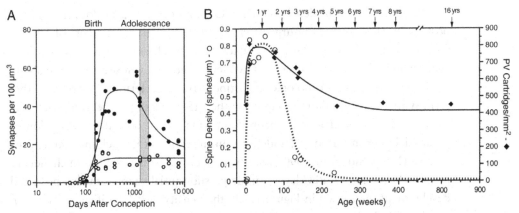

Fig. 17.4.   Age-related changes. (A) Changes during development in the densities of asymmetric excitatory (•) and symmetric inhibitory (○) synapses in area 46 of monkey dorsolateral prefrontal
cortex (DLPFC). (B) Age-related changes in the mean densities of spines on the dendrites of
layer 3 pyramidal neurons (♦) and of parvalbumin (PV)-containing chandelier neuron axon
cartridges (○) in layer 3 of monkey DLPFC. Note the parallel time course of developmental
changes in these markers of excitatory and inhibitory inputs to layer 3 pyramidal neurons.
(Adapted from Bourgeois *et al.*, 1994 (A) and Anderson *et al.*, 1995 (B).)

the density of dendritic spines on layer 3 pyramidal neurons undergoes substantial
changes during postnatal development (Fig. 17.4B) (Anderson *et al.*, 1995). The
number of spines rapidly increases between birth and 2–3 months of age and this
high density of spines, approximately 50% higher than at birth, is maintained until
about 18 months of age. Layer 3 pyramidal neurons undergo spine attrition, again by
approximately 50%, until adult levels are achieved by 5 years of age. Although spines
exhibit remarkably rapid changes under certain conditions, recent in vivo two-
photon imaging studies in transgenic mice expressing yellow fluorescent protein
demonstrate that the vast majority of dendritic spines are stable in adult animals
(Grutzendler *et al.*, 2002).

   As described above, the axons of DLPFC layer 3 pyramidal neurons are a major
source of inputs to the dendritic spines of other layer 3 pyramidal cells. Interestingly, limited data suggest that pruning of the long-range intrinsic collaterals
may make a greater contribution to the adolescence-related reduction in excitatory
inputs to dendritic spines than do associational projections. For example, the densities of varicosities and axonal branch points (measures of the relative number of
synapses and degree of arborization, respectively) decreased by approximately half
for long-range intrinsic collaterals during adolescence (Woo *et al.*, 1997). Interestingly, computational model approaches support the idea that excessive pruning of
such intrinsic connections may contribute to the symptomatology of schizophrenia
(Siekmeier and Hoffman, 2002).

Although the overall density of DLPFC inhibitory synapses does not change postnatally (Fig. 17.4A) (Bourgeois *et al.*, 1994), functional markers of DLPFC GABA circuits exhibit substantial postnatal changes. These changes are particularly prominent in the chandelier class of GABAergic neurons, whose axon terminals are vertically aligned as morphologically distinct structures (termed "cartridges") that form symmetric, inhibitory synapses on the AIS of pyramidal neurons (DeFelipe *et al.*, 1985). Thus, chandelier neurons provide potent inhibitory regulation of pyramidal neuron output. Chandelier neurons express the calcium-binding protein PV (Lewis and Lund, 1990), and PV-containing axon cartridges of chandelier neurons located in DLPFC layer 3 undergo substantial changes during postnatal development. As shown in Figure 17.4B, the density of PV-positive cartridges in monkey DLPFC increases rapidly during the first 3 months of postnatal development, undergoes a plateau period that lasts until at least 1.5 years of age, and then declines during the peripubertal age range to stable adult values (Anderson *et al.*, 1995). The close temporal match between the developmental changes in spine density on layer 3 pyramidal neurons and that of PV-containing chandelier neuron axon cartridges, reflecting a coordination between excitatory and inhibitory inputs, could be achieved via the synaptic contacts of the axon collaterals of layer 3 pyramidal cells onto the dendrites of PV-containing chandelier neurons (Melchitzky and Lewis, 2003).

Both pre- and postsynaptic markers of GABA neurotransmission at the AIS of pyramidal neurons also undergo postnatal developmental changes. Like PV, antibodies against the GABA membrane transporter (GAT-1) label the axon cartridges of chandelier cells. The density of GAT-1-positive cartridges rapidly increases from birth to 3 months of age, when maximal levels are achieved (Cruz *et al.*, 2003). GAT-1-positive cartridge density is maintained at these high levels until adolescence, after which a rapid decline brings the density to adult levels. In contrast, immunoreactivity for the GABA$_A$ α_2-receptor at postsynaptic AIS is greatest at birth, after which the density of GABA$_A$ α_2-receptor-immunoreactive AIS steadily decreases to adult levels (Cruz *et al.*, 2003).

The specificity of these postnatal developmental changes in chandelier neuron inputs to pyramidal cells is illustrated by comparison with the development of the axon terminals of another subclass of PV-expressing GABA cells, the wide-arbor neuron. For example, the density of PV-positive axon terminals arising from wide-arbor cells is low at birth in monkeys and then increases 10-fold, reaching adult levels approximately 3–4 years of age (Erickson and Lewis, 2002). Because changes in activity level are associated with corresponding changes in PV content (Heizmann, 1984), these findings suggest that chandelier neurons provide intra-columnar inhibition at early postnatal ages, whereas wide-arbor cells supply inter-columnar inhibition later during postnatal development (Erickson and Lewis,

2002). This gradual shift from intra- to intercolumnar inhibition may be related to the late emergence of mature functional properties in the DLPFC, such as spatially tuned delay-period activity between adjacent GABA and pyramidal neurons (Rao *et al.*, 1999).

Dysfunction of thalamocortical circuitry in schizophrenia

Both imaging and postmortem studies have revealed abnormalities in the thalamus of subjects with schizophrenia. For example, a recent meta-analysis examining 15 magnetic resonance studies of thalamic volume found significant reductions (composite effect size of −0.29) in schizophrenia (Konick and Friedman, 2001). Furthermore, a correlation between thalamic volumes and prefrontal white matter has been reported in individuals with schizophrenia but not in normal subjects (Portas *et al.*, 1998), suggesting that reductions in thalamocortical projection neurons may contribute to the decrease in DLPFC volume. In addition, two recent imaging studies that subdivided the thalamus support a selective reduction in MDN volume (Byne *et al.*, 2001; Gilbert *et al.*, 2001). Reductions in thalamic volume have also been reported in postmortem studies (Byne *et al.*, 2002; Pakkenberg, 1990; Popken *et al.*, 2000), and these changes may be localized to MDN and related association relay nuclei (e.g. anterior nucleus and pulvinar) while sparing the sensory- and motor-related thalamic nuclei.

These reductions in MDN volume have been associated with a decreased number of MDN neurons in schizophrenia (Fig. 17.5) (Byne *et al.*, 2002; Pakkenberg, 1990; Popken *et al.*, 2000; Young *et al.*, 2000). Furthermore, reduced neuronal numbers in the parvocellular and densocellular portions of the MDN, which furnish projections to the DLPFC, have been reported, whereas neuronal number was unchanged in the magnocellular region, which is connected with the medial and orbital prefrontal regions (Popken *et al.*, 2000). In addition, decreased somal volume in the MDN has also been reported (Byne *et al.*, 2002). However, these postmortem studies have generally involved older individuals with schizophrenia, making it difficult to determine whether the reductions in MDN neuron number are a cause or a consequence of MDN–DLPFC circuitry dysfunction.

Neuroimaging studies have revealed a 3–5% reduction in cerebral gray matter in subjects with schizophrenia (Pearlson and Marsh, 1999), with areas such as the DLPFC having the largest reductions (McCarley *et al.*, 1999). Such reductions in gray matter may reflect decreases in synaptic connections in the DLPFC (Selemon and Goldman-Rakic, 1999). This abnormal synaptic connectivity may involve disturbances in afferent projections to the DLPFC as well as in excitatory and/or inhibitory neurons within the DLPFC.

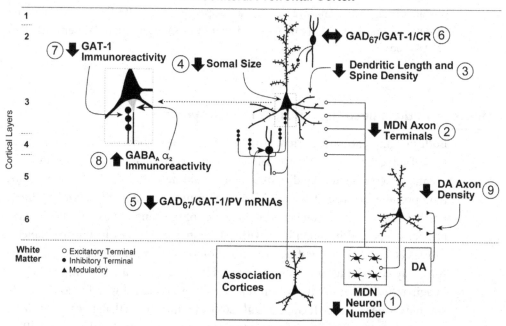

Dorsolateral Prefrontal Cortex

Fig. 17.5.   Schematic diagram summarizing the findings from postmortem studies showing alterations in mediodorsal nucleus of the thalamus (MDN) and dorsolateral prefrontal cortex (DLPFC) connectivity in schizophrenia. (1) The MDN exhibits a 30–35% reduction in neuron number and (2) axon terminals from the MDN are reduced by 25% in the thalamic recipient layers in the DLPFC. (3) Dendritic spine density is decreased by 25% on pyramidal neurons in deep layer 3 of DLPFC, and (4) the somal size of pyramidal neurons is reduced by 10%. (5) A subpopulation of gamma-aminobutyric acid (GABA)-ergic neurons exhibit decreased glutamic acid decarboxylase isoform of 67 kDa (GAD_{67}), GABA membrane transporter 1 (GAT-1) and parvalbumin (PV) mRNAs, whereas (6) calretinin (CR) mRNA levels are unchanged. Therefore, the affected subclass of GABA cells is likely to be the PV-containing chandelier neuron and not the CR-containing double bouquet cell, an interpretation supported by (7) the decreased density of GAT1-containing axon cartridges and (8) the increased density of $GABA_A\ \alpha_2$-receptor-immunoreactive pyramidal neuron axon initial segments. (9) In layer 6, the location of the pyramidal neurons that project to MDN, the density of dopamine (DA)-containing axons is decreased. (Adapted from Lewis and Lieberman, 2000.)

Evidence for abnormalities in MDN to DLPFC projections includes reductions of both pre- and postsynaptic markers for these axons. For example, the density of a marker of axonal varicosities, presumably originating from the MDN, is reduced only in thalamic recipient layers (deep layers 3 and 4) in the DLPFC (Fig. 17.5) (Lewis *et al.*, 2001). Furthermore, because dendritic spine integrity depends on intact presynaptic inputs (see above), reductions in MDN axon projections may also cause reduced dendritic spine density in the thalamic recipient layers in the DLPFC. Indeed, in schizophrenia, spine density is decreased on the basilar dendrites of DLPFC layer 3 pyramidal cells (Glantz and Lewis, 2000). Furthermore, the largest reduction in spine density was for those pyramidal cells whose basilar dendrites extend through the thalamic recipient zone. In addition, the somal size of deep layer 3 pyramidal neurons is reduced in the DLPFC of schizophrenia subjects (Fig. 17.5) (Pierri *et al.*, 2001; Rajkowska *et al.*, 1998), a finding that may reflect deafferentation. However, only a subpopulation of deep layer 3 pyramidal neurons appear to be reduced in somal size (Pierri *et al.*, 2003), making it unlikely that a reduction in thalamic inputs accounts for this observation.

The presence of reciprocal excitatory connections between the DLPFC and MDN raises the question of whether corticothalamic projections are also compromised. Although one study reported a decreased neuronal density in layer 6 of the DLPFC (Benes *et al.*, 1986), the primary site of origin of corticothalamic projections, other studies of neuronal size and number have not revealed any changes in this layer (Rajkowska *et al.*, 1998). These findings suggest that abnormalities in DLPFC efferent projection neurons do not contribute significantly to abnormalities in MDN–DLPFC connectivity. However, the density of dopamine-containing projections to the DLPFC, which principally target pyramidal cells, is reduced in layer 6 in subjects with schizophrenia (Fig. 17.5) (Akil *et al.*, 1999). Therefore, although layer 6 pyramidal cells appear to be unaffected structurally in schizophrenia, more subtle disturbances in afferents that could affect the function of these neurons may be present in schizophrenia.

A number of findings consistent with functional anomalies in DLPFC GABA interneurons have been reported in schizophrenia, and recent studies have revealed that a subset of these neurons, the chandelier class, may be preferentially affected (Volk and Lewis, 2003). Abnormal function of DLPFC chandelier cells in schizophrenia is suggested by the finding that reductions in the mRNA level of the 67 kDa isoform of glutamic acid decarboxylase (GAD_{67}) (Akbarian *et al.*, 1995; Guidotti *et al.*, 2000), an enzyme involved in GABA synthesis, are present in a subset of GABA neurons found in the same cortical layers in which the chandelier cells are distributed (Fig. 17.5) (Volk *et al.*, 2000, 2001). In addition, decreased GAT-1 mRNA in a subset of GABA neurons is paralleled by an apparent reduction in GAT-1 protein in the axon cartridges of chandelier cells (Fig. 17.5) (Volk *et al.*, 2001). Finally, GAD_{67} mRNA appears to be selectively decreased in PV-containing GABA neurons and not in neurons that contain another calcium-binding protein, calretinin, which is not found in chandelier neurons (Fig. 17.5) (Hashimoto *et al.*, 2003).

If these reductions in the expression of mRNAs and proteins reflect a deficit in synaptic GABA, one would expect compensatory upregulation of postsynaptic receptors. As noted above, immunoreactivity for the α_2-subunit of the $GABA_A$

receptor is preferentially localized to pyramidal AIS. Accordingly, a recent study found an increased density of $GABA_A$ α_2-receptor immunoreactive AIS in the DLPFC of subjects with schizophrenia (Fig. 17.5)(Volk et al., 2002) that was inversely related to GAT-1-positive cartridges in the same subjects.

Studies of the primate visual system have revealed that decreased input from thalamic afferents results in reduced markers of cortical GABA neuron activity. It has been hypothesized that DLPFC GABAergic connectivity may be altered as a result of changes in afferent input from the MDN (Harrison and Lewis, 2003). Interestingly, in monkey DLPFC, both the local axon collaterals of layer 3 pyramidal neurons and a portion of the thalamic axon terminals form synapses onto the dendrites of PV-containing GABA cells (Melchitzky et al., 2001), which include the chandelier neuron subclass. Thus, a reduction in the projections from nearby pyramidal cells and/or the thalamus could produce the observed reductions in GABA neurotransmission in chandelier cells. However, large excitotoxic lesions of the MDN in adult rats did not result in a reduction of prefrontal GAD_{67} mRNA (Volk and Lewis, 2003). The failure of the MDN lesions to produce alterations in a marker of GABA neurotransmission may reflect the age of the animal. Given that the age of onset of schizophrenia is in adolescence, the cortical effects of MDN lesions may only occur in young animals with immature thalamocortical connections. In addition, a functional alteration in, rather than a loss of, thalamocortical projections may be necessary to produce a change in GABA neurotransmission in the cortex. For example, preventing visual input from reaching the lateral geniculate nucleus by enucleation results in decreased cortical GAD_{67} mRNA levels, whereas lesions of the thalamus do not (Jones et al., 1994). Despite these caveats, no available data directly support the hypothesis that abnormalities in the MDN produce the DLPFC GABA abnormalities in schizophrenia.

Conclusions and future directions

The findings reviewed above suggest that alterations in MDN–DLPFC circuitry play a critical role in the pathophysiology of cognitive dysfunction in schizophrenia (see Fig. 17.5). In addition, given the protracted postnatal maturation of this circuitry in the primate brain, normal development processes, or disturbances in them, may be essential for these cognitive disturbances to become manifest. However, there are substantial gaps in our knowledge of the functional architecture and development of MDN–DLPFC circuitry. For example, as noted above, relatively few studies have examined details of the organization of MDN–DLPFC circuitry in primates, and much of our understanding of the functional attributes of this circuitry represents reasonable but speculative extrapolation from studies of sensory thalamic systems. Furthermore, the findings implicating disturbances in

MDN–DLPFC circuitry in schizophrenia have not yet adequately addressed a number of critical issues, including the potential influence of confounds such as pharmacological treatments, substance abuse, disease duration, etc. Finally, as in other areas of schizophrenia research, our understanding of the mechanisms that give rise to these cognitive disturbances awaits the implementation of model systems that incorporate potential pathogenetic processes in the context of the protracted maturation of primate MDN–DLPFC circuitry.

REFERENCES

Akbarian, S., Kim, J. J., Potkin, S. G., *et al.* (1995). Gene expression for glutamic acid decarboxylase is reduced without loss of neurons in prefrontal cortex of schizophrenics. *Arch Gen Psychiatry* **52**: 258–266.

Akil, M., Pierri, J. N., Whitehead, R. E., *et al.* (1999). Lamina-specific alteration in the dopamine innervation of the prefrontal cortex in schizophrenic subjects. *Am J Psychiatry* **156**: 1580–1589.

Alexander, G. E. (1982). Functional development of frontal association cortex in monkeys: behavioral and electrophysiological studies. *Neurosci Res Prog Bull* **20**: 471–479.

Alexander, G. E., Goldman, P. S. (1978). Functional development of the dorsolateral prefrontal cortex: an analysis utilizing reversible cryogenic depression. *Brain Res* **143**: 233–249.

Anderson, S. A., Classey, J. D., Condé, F., Lund, J. S., Lewis, D. A. (1995). Synchronous development of pyramidal neuron dendritic spines and parvalbumin-immunoreactive chandelier neuron axon terminals in layer III of monkey prefrontal cortex. *Neuroscience* **67**: 7–22.

Barbas, H., Haswell Henion, T. H., Dermon, C. R. (1991). Diverse thalamic projections to the prefrontal cortex in the rhesus monkey. *J Comp Neurol* **313**: 65–94.

Benes, F. M., Davidson, J., Bird, E. D. (1986). Quantitative cytoarchitectural studies of the cerebral cortex of schizophrenics. *Arch Gen Psychiatry* **43**: 31–35.

Bourgeois, J.-P., Goldman-Rakic, P. S., Rakic, P. (1994). Synaptogenesis in the prefrontal cortex of rhesus monkeys. *Cereb Cortex* **4**: 78–96.

Bunge, S. A., Dudukovic, N. M., Thomason, M. E., Vaidya, C. J., Gabrieli, J. D. E. (2002). Immature frontal lobe contributions to cognitive control in children: Evidence from MRI. *Neuron* **33**: 311.

Byne, W., Buchsbaum, M. S., Kemether, E., *et al.* (2001). Magnetic resonance imaging of the thalamic mediodorsal nucleus and pulvinar in schizophrenia and schizotypal personality disorder. *Arch Gen Psychiatry* **58**: 133–140.

Byne, W., Buchsbaum, M. S., Mattiace, L. A., *et al.* (2002). Postmortem assessment of thalamic nuclear volumes in subjects with schizophrenia. *Am J Psychiatry* **159**: 59–65.

Casey, B. J., Giedd, J. N., Thomas, K. M. (2000). Structural and functional brain development and its relation to cognitive development. *Biol Psychol* **54**: 241–257.

Condé, F., Lund, J. S., Jacobowitz, D. M., Baimbridge, K. G., Lewis, D. A. (1994). Local circuit neurons immunoreactive for calretinin, calbindin D-28k, or parvalbumin in monkey prefrontal cortex: distribution and morphology. *J Comp Neurol* **341**: 95–116.

Cruz, D. A., Eggan, S. M., Lewis, D. A. (2003). Postnatal development of pre- and post-synaptic GABA markers at chandelier cell inputs to pyramidal neurons in monkey prefrontal cortex. *J Comp Neurol* **465**: 385–400.

DeFelipe, J., Jones, E. G. (1991). Parvalbumin immunoreactivity reveals layer IV of monkey cerebral cortex as a mosaic of microzones of thalamic afferent terminations. *Brain Res* **562**: 39–47.

DeFelipe, J., Hendry, S. H. C., Jones, E. G., Schmechel, D. (1985). Variability in the terminations of GABAergic chandelier cell axons on initial segments of pyramidal cell axons in the monkey sensory-motor cortex. *J Comp Neurol* **231**: 364–384.

Diamond, A. (1985). Development of the ability to use recall to guide action, as indicated by infants' performances on AB. *Child Devel* **56**: 868–883.

(2002). Normal development of prefrontal cortex from birth to young adulthood: cognitive functions, anatomy, and biochemistry. In *Principles of Frontal Lobe Function*, ed. D. T. Stuss, R. T. Knight. London: Oxford University Press, pp. 466–503.

Elvevåg, B., Goldberg, T. E. (2000). Cognitive impairment in schizophrenia is the core of the disorder. *Crit Rev Neurobiol* **14**: 1–21.

Erickson, S. L., Lewis, D. A. (2000). Prefrontal cortical inputs to monkey mediodorsal thalamus. *Soc Neurosci Abstr* **26**: 1237.

(2002). Postnatal development of parvalbumin- and GABA transporter-immunoreactive axon terminals in monkey prefrontal cortex. *J Comp Neurol* **448**: 186–202.

Funahashi, S., Bruce, C. J., Goldman-Rakic, P. S. (1989). Mnemonic coding of visual space in the monkey's dorsolateral prefrontal cortex. *J Neurophysiol* **61**: 331–349.

Fuster, J. M. (1997). *The Prefrontal Cortex: Anatomy, Physiology, and Neuropsychology of the Frontal Lobe*. Philadelphia, PA: Lippincott-Raven.

Fuster, J. J., Alexander, G. E. (1971). Neuron activity related to short-term memory. *Science* **173**: 652–654.

Ghosh, A., Antonini, A., McConnell, S. K., Shatz, C. J. (1990). Requirement for subplate neurons in the formation of thalamocortical connections. *Nature* **347**: 179–181.

Giedd, J. N. (1999). Brain development during childhood and adolescence: a longitudinal MRI study. *Nat Neurosci* **2**: 861–863.

Giguere, M., Goldman-Rakic, P. S. (1988). Mediodorsal nucleus: areal, laminar, and tangential distribution of afferents and efferents in the frontal lobe of rhesus monkeys. *J Comp Neurol* **277**: 195–213.

Gilbert, A. R., Rosenberg, D. R., Harenski, K., *et al.* (2001). Thalamic volumes in patients with first-episode schizophrenia. *Am J Psychiatry* **158**: 618–624.

Glantz, L. A., Lewis, D. A. (2000). Decreased dendritic spine density on prefrontal cortical pyramidal neurons in schizophrenia. *Arch Gen Psychiatry* **57**: 65–73.

Goldman-Rakic, P. S. (1987). Development of cortical circuitry and cognitive function. *Child Devel* **58**: 601–622.

(1994). Working memory dysfunction in schizophrenia. *J Neuropsychiatry* **6**: 348–357.

(1995). Cellular basis of working memory. *Neuron* **14**: 477–485.

Goldman-Rakic, P. S., Porrino, L. J. (1985). The primate mediodorsal (MD) nucleus and its projection to the frontal lobe. *J Comp Neurol* **242**: 535–560.

Grutzendler, J., Kasthuri, N., Gan, W. B. (2002). Long-term dendritic spine stability in the adult cortex. *Nature* **420**: 812–816.

Guidotti, A., Auta, J., Davis, J. M., *et al.* (2000). Decrease in reelin and glutamic acid decarboxylase$_{67}$ (GAD$_{67}$) expression in schizophrenia and bipolar disorder. *Arch Gen Psychiatry* **57**: 1061–1069.

Harrison, P. J., Lewis, D. A. (2003). Neuropathology in schizophrenia. In *Schizophrenia*, 2nd edn, ed. S. Hirsch, D. R. Weinberger. Oxford: Blackwell Science, Oxford University Press, pp. 310–325.

Hashimoto, T., Volk, D. W., Eggan, S. M., *et al.* (2003). Gene expression deficits in a subclass of GABA neurons in the prefrontal cortex of subjects with schizophrenia. *J Neurosci* **23**: 6315–6326.

Heizmann, C. W. (1984). Parvalbumin an intracellular calcium-binding protein. Distribution properties and possible roles in mammalian cells. *Experientia* **40**: 910–921.

Huttenlocher, P. R. (1979). Synaptic density in human frontal cortex: developmental changes and effects of aging. *Brain Res* **163**: 195–205.

Isseroff, A., Rosvold, H. E., Galkin, T. W., Goldman-Rakic, P. S. (1982). Spatial memory impairments following damage to the mediodorsal nucleus of the thalamus in rhesus monkeys. *Brain Res* **232**: 97–113.

Jones, E. G., Hendry, S. H. C., DeFelipe, J., Benson, D. L. (1994). GABA neurons and their role in activity-dependent plasticity of adult primate visual cortex. In *Cerebral Cortex*, Vol. 10: *Primary Visual Cortex in Primates*, ed. A. Peters, K. S. Rockland. New York: Plenum Press, pp. 61–140.

Konick, L. C., Friedman, L. (2001). Meta-analysis of thalamic size in schizophrenia. *Biol Psychiatry* **49**: 28–38.

Kuroda, M., Yokofujita, J., Murakami, K. (1998). An ultrastructural study of the neural circuit between the prefrontal cortex and the mediodorsal nucleus of the thalamus. *Prog Neurobiol* **54**: 417–458.

Levitt, J. B., Lewis, D. A., Yoshioka, T., Lund, J. S. (1993). Topography of pyramidal neuron intrinsic connections in macaque monkey prefrontal cortex (areas 9 and 46). *J Comp Neurol* **338**: 360–376.

Lewis, D. A. (2000). Is there a neuropathology of schizophrenia? *The Neuroscientist* **6**: 208–218.
    (2002). Neural circuitry approaches to understanding the pathophysiology of schizophrenia. In *Neuropsychopharmacology: The Fifth Generation of Progress*, ed. K. L. Davis, D. S. Charney, J. T. Coyle, C. B. Nemeroff. Philadelphia, PA: Lippincott Williams and Wilkins, pp. 729–743.

Lewis, D. A., Levitt, P. (2002). Schizophrenia as a disorder of neurodevelopment. *Annu Rev Neurosci* **25**: 409–432.

Lewis, D. A., Lieberman, J. A. (2000). Catching up on schizophrenia: natural history and neurobiology. *Neuron* **28**: 325–334.

Lewis, D. A., Lund, J. S. (1990). Heterogeneity of chandelier neurons in monkey neocortex: corticotropin-releasing factor and parvalbumin immunoreactive populations. *J Comp Neurol* **293**: 599–615.

Lewis, D. A., Cruz, D. A., Melchitzky, D. S., Pierri, J. N. (2001). Lamina-specific reductions in parvalbumin-immunoreactive axon terminals in the prefrontal cortex of subjects with schizophrenia: evidence for decreased projections from the thalamus. *Am J Psychiatry* **158**: 1411–1422.

Lund, J. S., Holbach, S. (1991). Postnatal development of thalamic recipient neurons in monkey striate cortex: I. A comparison of spine acquisition and dendritic growth of layer 4C alpha and beta spiny stellate neurons. *J Comp Neurol* **309**: 115–128.

McCarley, R. W., Wible, C. G., Frumin, M., *et al.* (1999). MRI anatomy of schizophrenia. *Biol Psychiatry* **45**: 1099–1119.

Melchitzky, D. S., Lewis, D. A. (2003). Preferential targeting of parvalbumin interneurons by local axon terminals of supragranular pyramidal neurons in monkey prefrontal cortex. *Cereb Cortex* **13**: 452–460.

Melchitzky, D. S., Sesack, S. R., Pucak, M. L., Lewis, D. A. (1998). Synaptic targets of pyramidal neurons providing intrinsic horizontal connections in monkey prefrontal cortex. *J Comp Neurol* **390**: 211–224.

Melchitzky, D. S., Sesack, S. R., Lewis, D. A. (1999). Parvalbumin-immunoreactive axon terminals in monkey and human prefrontal cortex: Laminar, regional and target specificity of type I and type II synapses. *J Comp Neurol* **408**: 11–22.

Melchitzky, D. S., Gonzalez-Burgos, G., Barrionuevo, G., Lewis, D. A. (2001). Synaptic targets of the intrinsic axon collaterals of supragranular pyramidal neurons in monkey prefrontal cortex. *J Comp Neurol* **430**: 209–221.

Pakkenberg, B. (1990). Pronounced reduction of total neuron number in mediodorsal thalamic nucleus and nucleus accumbens in schizophrenics. *Arch Gen Psychiatry* **47**: 1023–1028.

Park, S., Holzman, P. S. (1992). Schizophrenics show spatial working memory deficits. *Arch Gen Psychiatry* **49**: 975–982.

Pearlson, G. D., Marsh, L. (1999). Structural brain imaging in schizophrenia: a selective review. *Biol Psychiatry* **46**: 627–649.

Pierri, J. N., Volk, C. L. E., Auh, S., Sampson, A., Lewis, D. A. (2001). Decreased somal size of deep layer 3 pyramidal neurons in the prefrontal cortex in subjects with schizophrenia. *Arch Gen Psychiatry* **58**: 466–473.

(2003). Somal size of prefrontal cortical pyramidal neurons in schizophrenia: differential effects across neuronal subpopulations. *Biol Psychiatry* **54**: 111–120.

Popken, G. J., Bunney, Jr W. E., Potkin, S. G., Jones, E. G. (2000). Subnucleus-specific loss of neurons in medial thalamus of schizophrenics. *Proc Natl Acad Sci USA* **97**: 9276–9280.

Portas, C. M., Goldstein, J. M., Shenton, M. E., *et al.* (1998). Volumetric evaluation of the thalamus in schizophrenic male patients using magnetic resonance imaging. *Biol Psychiatry* **43**: 649–659.

Pucak, M. L., Levitt, J. B., Lund, J. S., Lewis, D. A. (1996). Patterns of intrinsic and associational circuitry in monkey prefrontal cortex. *J Comp Neurol* **376**: 614–630.

Rajkowska, G., Selemon, L. D., Goldman-Rakic, P. S. (1998). Neuronal and glial somal size in the prefrontal cortex: a postmortem morphometric study of schizophrenia and Huntington disease. *Arch Gen Psychiatry* **55**: 215–224.

Rakic, P. (1977). Prenatal development of the visual system in rhesus monkey. *Philos Trans R Soc Lond Ser B* **278**: 245–260.

Rao, S. G., Williams, G. V., Goldman-Rakic, P. S. (1999). Isodirectional tuning of adjacent interneurons and pyramidal cells during working memory: evidence for microcolumnar organization in PFC. *J Neurophysiol* **81**: 1903–1916.

Selemon, L. D., Goldman-Rakic, P. S. (1999). The reduced neuropil hypothesis: a circuit based model of schizophrenia. *Biol Psychiatry* **45**: 17–25.

Siekmeier, P. J., Hoffman, R. E. (2002). Enhanced semantic priming in schizophrenia: a computer model based on excessive pruning of local connections in association cortex. *Br J Psychiatry* **180**: 345–350.

Sowell, E. R., Thompson, P. M., Tessner, K. D., Toga, A. W. (2001). Mapping continued brain growth and gray matter density reduction in dorsal frontal cortex: inverse relationships during postadolescent brain maturation. *J Neurosci* **21**: 8819–8829.

Volk, D. W., Lewis, D. A. (2003). Effects of a mediodorsal thalamus lesion on prefrontal inhibitory circuitry: implications for schizophrenia. *Biol Psychiatry* **53**: 385–389.

Volk, D. W., Austin, M. C., Pierri, J. N., Sampson, A. R., Lewis, D. A. (2000). Decreased GAD_{67} mRNA expression in a subset of prefrontal cortical GABA neurons in subjects with schizophrenia. *Arch Gen Psychiatry* **57**: 237–245.

(2001). GABA transporter-1 mRNA in the prefrontal cortex in schizophrenia: decreased expression in a subset of neurons. *Am J Psychiatry* **158**: 256–265.

Volk, D. W., Pierri, J. N., Fritschy, J.-M., Auh, S., Sampson, A. R., Lewis, D. A. (2002). Reciprocal alterations in pre- and postsynaptic inhibitory markers at chandelier cell inputs to pyramidal neurons in schizophrenia. *Cereb Cortex* **12**: 1063–1070.

Weinberger, D. R., Berman, K. F., Zec, R. F. (1986). Physiologic dysfunction of dorsolateral prefrontal cortex in schizophrenia. I. Regional cerebral blood flow evidence. *Arch Gen Psychiatry* **43**: 114–124.

Woo, T.-U., Pucak, M. L., Kye, C. H., Matus, C. V., Lewis, D. A. (1997). Peripubertal refinement of the intrinsic and associational circuitry in monkey prefrontal cortex. *Neuroscience* **80**: 1149–1158.

Young, K. A., Manaye, K. F., Liang, C.-L., Hicks, P. B., German, D. C. (2000). Reduced number of mediodorsal and anterior thalamic neurons in schizophrenia. *Biol Psychiatry* **47**: 944–953.

18

X chromosome, estrogen, and brain development: implications for schizophrenia

Michael Craig, William Cutter, Ray Norbury, and Declan Murphy

Institute of Psychiatry, King's College, London, UK

The "neurodevelopmental theory" is now regarded by many psychiatrists as the dominant explanatory model of schizophrenia (O'Connell *et al.*, 1997). In order to evaluate this model critically, it is important to understand how the normal brain develops and changes across the lifespan. Nonetheless, there are relatively few studies by schizophrenia researchers on the biological factors affecting maturation of brain regions implicated in psychosis. The determinants of normal neurodevelopment, and hence brain function, are most likely multifactorial and include both genetic and environmental factors. For example, recent work has examined the role of the gene for the catechol-*O*-methyltransferase (COMT) (Egan *et al.*, 2001) and a polymorphism of the promoter region of the gene for the serotonin 5-hydroxytryptamine (5-HT) transporter (5-HTTLPR) (Hariri *et al.*, 2002) in normal brain function (e.g. amygdala function during processing of facial emotion), and the effect of deletions at q11 chromosome 22 on the anatomy of prefrontal and medial temporal regions (van Amelsvoort *et al.*, 2001a). Other important factors, to be reviewed in this chapter, include the sex chromosomes and sex steroids. We do not suggest that schizophrenia is an X-linked disorder, or that sex steroids cause schizophrenia (just as schizophrenia is unlikely to be explained solely by variations in the COMT gene or the serotonin transporter promoter polymorphism). Rather, we will offer evidence that sex chromosomes and sex steroids (in particular estrogen) significantly modulate the structure and function of normal brain, and this needs to be considered when forming developmental theories of schizophrenia, when attempting to explain sex differences in schizophrenia, and when considering the role of sex steroids in the genesis and treatment of schizophrenia.

Neurodevelopment and Schizophrenia, ed. Matcheri S. Keshavan *et al.* Published by Cambridge University Press. © Cambridge University Press 2004.

Sex differences in epidemiology and clinical features of schizophrenia

There is a significantly greater male to female ratio in schizophrenia when "restrictive" (e.g. Feighner) diagnostic criteria are used (Castle *et al.*, 1993) and in patients who have an onset over the age of 40 years (late-onset) (Howard *et al.*, 2000). However, the male to female ratio approaches unity when less restrictive criteria are used (e.g. Research Diagnostic Criteria; Spitzer *et al.*, 1978).

There may also be gender differences in age of onset. A later age of onset of schizophrenia amongst women has been a consistent finding across many studies. Females are generally reported as having a mean age of onset that is approximately 3–4 years later than males, regardless of the definition applied (Hafner *et al.*, 1993, 1994, 1998a,b). Also, men are reported to have a peak in illness onset between 15 and 25 years of age, with a steady decline after 30 years. In contrast, women have a broader onset peak between 15 and 30 years, with a second peak between 45 and 49 years, and perhaps a third peak amongst women over 75 years of age. These findings have been replicated across a variety of cultures, and in both rural and urban settings (Castle and Murray, 1993; Jablensky *et al.*, 1992).

There is a high degree of overlap in the clinical symptoms between the genders; however, women are generally reported to present with a less-severe form of schizophrenia, with more affective symptoms, but fewer negative symptoms and hospitalizations (Leung and Chue, 2000).

Anatomical differences between men and women with schizophrenia

Studies on sex differences in the brain anatomy of patients with schizophrenia have reported that males have a significantly smaller temporal lobe volume than females (Shenton *et al.*, 1992) but a greater ventricular–brain ratio (Andreasen *et al.*, 1986, 1990a,b; Flaum *et al.*, 1990; Harvey *et al.*, 1990; Nopoulos *et al.*, 1997; Shelton *et al.*, 1988; Williams *et al.*, 1985) and right–left ventricular asymmetry (Haas *et al.*, 1989, 1991). However, most of these studies were relatively small and some have not been replicated; for example, ventricular dilatation has been reported to be significantly more common in women than men in some studies (Andreasen *et al.*, 1982; Gur *et al.*, 1994; Nasrallah *et al.*, 1990; Vazquez-Barquero *et al.*, 1995) but not others (Lauriello *et al.*, 1997). Moreover, studies of gender differences in neuropathology, or symptoms, need to take account of *normal* gender differences in the brain. For example, postmortem studies suggested that early onset and negative symptoms in schizophrenia are associated with a thickened corpus callosum (Coger and Serafetinides, 1990). This would predict that women with schizophrenia have a thinner corpus callosum than men with schizophrenia because women generally have fewer negative symptoms and a later illness onset than men. However, there is no consistent evidence for gender differences in callosal thickness in schizophrenia (Salem and Kring, 1998). Moreover, there are significant gender differences in development and aging of many brain regions (including hippocampus and frontal lobe; see below), and this needs to be controlled for in studies of schizophrenia.

Normal brain development and aging

Myelination starts near the end of the second trimester of fetal development and in some brain regions (e.g. hippocampus) may continue until the sixth decade or beyond (Benes *et al.*, 1994). Myelination progresses from inferior to superior and posterior to anterior and the brainstem and cerebellar regions are myelinated prior to the cerebral hemispheres, and the frontal lobes and hippocampus are myelinated last. This suggests that humans, unlike other primates, have non-synchronous development of the cerebral cortex (i.e. different areas of the cortex develop at different times). Furthermore, females have been reported to have greater myelination than males during adolescence in areas such as the superior medullary lamina (Benes *et al.*, 1994). It has been suggested that earlier myelination in females may contribute to their greater early achievement in language skills and reading. Similarly, later myelination in males may contribute to their increased vulnerability to various forms of psychopathology (Benes, 1998).

Non-synchronous development of the cerebral cortex has recently been confirmed by longitudinal magnetic resonance imaging (MRI) studies, and there is preliminary evidence for gender differences in maturation of brain regions implicated in schizophrenia. For example, in healthy populations, the volume of the frontal and temporal lobes peaks at about 12 years and 16 years, respectively, whereas the occipital lobe continues to develop into the twenties (Giedd *et al.*, 1999). Furthermore, during childhood and adolescence, volume of frontal gray matter peaks approximately 1 year earlier in females than males: the left amygdala increases significantly only in males but the right hippocampus increases significantly only in females (Giedd *et al.*, 1996). In the age range 7–17 years, males also show a significantly greater *loss* of cerebral gray matter volume and *increase* in white matter volume and corpus callosal area compared with females (De Bellis *et al.*, 2001).

There are also significant gender differences in brain maturation in mid-life and later years. Studies using MRI have reported that age-related volume loss is significantly greater in the hippocampus and parietal lobes in women compared with men, whereas age-related volume loss in men is greater in the frontal and temporal lobes (Murphy *et al.*, 1996). A positron electron tomography (PET) study of 120 healthy people reported that women have a greater age-related metabolic decline in the hippocampus and thalamus than men, and that age-related decline in brain metabolism is asymmetric in males but symmetric in females (Murphy *et al.*, 1996). Consequently, there is now substantial evidence for gender differences in the development and aging of brain regions implicated in schizophrenia (see Ch. 2 for a further discussion). It has, therefore, been suggested that this may modify symptom expression (Murphy *et al.*, 1996) and that the earlier age of onset and increase in severity of schizophrenia in males may be attributable to an accelerated rate of pruning in male gray matter volume during the adolescent period (De Bellis *et al.*, 2001).

Development and aging of the serotonergic and dopaminergic systems

In all mammals, the highest functional status of the serotonin system is reached earliest in development: and adult levels of the system are much lower than in the younger animal (Goldman-Rakic and Brown, 1982; Lidow *et al.*, 1991). In human brain, serotonergic neurons are first evident by 5 weeks of gestation (Sundstrom *et al.*, 1993) and increase rapidly through the tenth week (Levallois *et al.*, 1997). By 15 weeks of gestation, the typical organization of serotonin cell bodies into the raphe nucleus can be seen (Takahashi *et al.*, 1986). In humans, there are higher levels of the serotonin metabolite 5-Hydroxyindolacetic acid in children than in adults; serotonin levels increase throughout the first 2 years of life and then decline to adult levels by 5 years of age (Hedner *et al.*, 1986; Seifert *et al.*, 1980).

Serotonin acts as a trophic or differentiation factor in addition to its role as a neurotransmitter, and alteration of serotonin during brain development alters neuronal differentiation (reviewed by Whitaker-Azmitia, 2001). For example, serotonin plays a role in modulation of synaptogenesis in sensory cortices postnatally in the rat (Cases *et al.*, 1995; D'Amato *et al.*, 1987), and this may represent transient expression of the high-affinity serotonin transporter and vesicular monoamine transporter by glutamatergic thalamocortical neurons (Bennett-Clarke *et al.*, 1996; Lebrand *et al.*, 1996). Decreased or increased brain serotonin during this period of development results in disruption of brain development (Bennett-Clarke *et al.*, 1994; Cases *et al.*, 1995, 1996). For example, depletion of serotonin delays the development (Blue *et al.*, 1991) and decreases the size (Bennett-Clarke *et al.*, 1994) of barrel fields in rat somatosensory cortex; it prolongs cell division and increases neuronal cell numbers in hippocampus, superior colliculus, and several thalamic nuclei (Lauder and Krebs, 1978); and it decreases the number of hippocampal dendritic spines (Yan *et al.*, 1997). In contrast, increased serotonin during development results in increased tangential arborization of somatosensory axons and blurring of the boundaries of the cortical barrels (Cases *et al.*, 1996).

Later life is associated with a reduction in serotonergic responsivity to neuroendocrine probes (e.g. prolactin response to fenfluramine), and this decline is more pronounced in women (Lerer *et al.*, 1999). Also there are age-related reductions in the number of cortical serotonin receptors 5-HT$_{1A}$, 5-HT$_{1B\delta}$: and 5-HT$_{2A}$ in the frontal and occipital lobes and the hippocampus (Meltzer *et al.*, 1998).

Dopaminergic neurons begin to develop by 6–8 weeks of gestation in humans (Sundstrom *et al.*, 1993), and development begins earlier in females than in males (Herlenius and Lagercrantz, 2001). Interestingly, with the onset of puberty, dopaminergic activity (unlike serotoninergic) increases in some cortical regions, especially the frontal cortex (Spear, 2000). It has been hypothesized that the increased risk for the onset of psychosis during adolescence/early adulthood may be linked to the elevation in dopaminergic activity (Walker, 1994).

PET studies of age-related differences in the dopaminergic system reported a reduction in dopamine D$_2$ receptor concentration of the caudate nuclei and the frontal lobes in both men and women (Wong *et al.*, 1984). Furthermore, this decline is more pronounced in women than in men (Wong *et al.*, 1988).

In summary, therefore, there are age and gender differences in the maturation of brain regions and neurochemical systems implicated in schizophrenia. What then is the evidence that gender differences in the brain are caused by sex steroids or sex chromosomes?

The role of estrogen in brain development and aging

Development

There is increasing evidence that estrogen modulates sexual differentiation of the brain and affects neuronal development both directly and indirectly. For example, receptors for estrogen and neurotrophins (such as nerve growth factor [NGF]) are located on the same neurons in rodent basal forebrain, hippocampus, and cerebral cortex, and this colocalization may be important for the long-term survival of neurons (Toran-Allerand, 1996).

Traditionally, sexual differentiation of brain has been explained in terms of the presence or absence of testosterone during the perinatal period (Phoenix *et al.*, 1959). Development of the female brain was perceived as a passive process occurring by default in the absence of testosterone. However, the current view is that this process may be more complex for two main reasons. First, in many brain regions testosterone is converted (by the enzyme aromatase) to estradiol and, therefore, "masculinization" is primarily attributable to the action of estrogen at estrogen receptors. Females avoid masculinization in utero from high circulating levels of maternal estrogen because α-fetoprotein binds to circulating estrogen and prevents it from entering the neuron. Second, animal studies suggest that ovarian estrogen may have an effect independent of testosterone on corpus callosum size once circulating α-fetoprotein has been "switched off" (Fitch and Denenberg, 1998). In vitro studies suggest that filopodial outgrowth (an important part of neurotrophism because filopodia act as an early support for dendritic spine maturation) occurs within minutes of exposure to 17β-estradiol (Brinton, 1993). The mechanism by which estrogen initiates filopodial outgrowth is most likely direct activation of the Rac1B G-protein, a member of the Rho family of GTPases involved in actin organization (Dumontier *et al.*, 2000). Further development of dendritic spines appears to be mediated by estrogen activation of a Src tyrosine kinase that phosphorylates the glutamate *N*-methyl-D-aspartate (NMDA) receptor (Yu *et al.*, 1997). For example, in cortical and hippocampal neurons without synaptic contacts, 17β-estradiol induces a significant increase in the outgrowth of both macro- and micromorphological features, which is blocked by a NMDA receptor antagonist. Activation of these intracellular signaling cascades appears to be dependent on the subtype of estrogen receptor present: neuroblastoma cells with the α-subtype, for example, are dependent on the Rac1B G-protein, whereas mechanisms appear independent of Rac1B where the β-subtype occurs (Brinton, 2001).

These findings have been confirmed by in vivo studies. In the adult female rat, the densities of dendritic spines and synapses on hippocampal CA1 pyramidal cells fluctuate across the menstrual cycle with natural fluctuations in ovarian steroid estradiol levels. Furthermore, these estradiol-induced dendritic changes are blocked by treatment with an NMDA receptor antagonist (Woolley and McEwen, 1994).

In addition to direct effects on neurons, estrogen also acts with neurotrophins (such as NGF) to stimulate nerve cell growth indirectly. NGF is essential for early neuronal development and influences neuron differentiation and growth. Other important neurotrophins are brain-derived neurotrophic factor (BDNF) and neurotrophins 3 and 4/5 (NT-3 and NT-4/5). Binding of NGF and neurotrophins to their cognate receptors results in the activation of mechanisms necessary for growth and survival of neurites, as well as in stimulation of functions related to neurotransmitter production and release. Importantly, receptors for estrogen and neurotrophins are located on the same neurons in rodent basal forebrain, hippocampus, and cerebral cortex (Toran-Allerand, 1996). This colocalization of estrogen and neurotrophin receptors suggests that they act synergistically on the same neuron to regulate expression of specific genes enhancing neuronal survival, differentiation, and plasticity (Toran-Allerand, 1996).

Cognition and aging

The most robust effect of estrogen on cognitive function is most likely on verbal memory. Prospective randomized studies of hormone replacement therapy (HRT) versus placebo following total abdominal hysterectomy and bilateral salpingoophorectomy report a significant positive effect of estrogens on verbal memory (Phillips and Sherwin, 1992; Sherwin, 1988). Performance in some cognitive tasks also varies as a function of menstrual cycle in healthy premenopausal women. During the luteal phase (characterized by high levels of estrogen and progesterone), verbal articulation is improved whereas spatial ability is decreased (Hampson, 1990), a pattern that is reversed during the follicular phase (when there is relatively low estrogen and progesterone). A similar pattern of cognitive performance is also observed if subjects are tested during the preovulatory estradiol surge (to control for the potential effects of progesterone on cognitive performance), suggesting that estrogen rather than progesterone is responsible for the observed cognitive effects.

Functional imaging techniques have also been employed to assess the effects of estrogen on networks subserving various aspects of cognitive function (reviewed by Maki and Resnick, 2001). A recent randomized placebo-controlled crossover study using functional MRI (Shaywitz et al., 1999) found estrogen-induced alterations in brain activation patterns during encoding and retrieval of both verbal and nonverbal stimuli. More recently, Maki and Resnick (2000) used PET and oxygen-15 to examine longitudinal changes in regional cerebral blood flow over a 2 year interval in women on and off HRT (both with and without adjuvant progesterone therapy). Significant differences were found in right hippocampus, parahippocampal gyrus, and left middle temporal gyrus. We recently reported that estrogen reduces age-related differences in neuronal membrane breakdown (as measured by proton magnetic resonance spectroscopy) in hippocampus and parietal lobe, and this was related to memory function (Robertson et al., 2001) (Fig. 18.1). Therefore, there is increasing evidence from in vivo brain imaging studies that estrogen modulates cognitive function, cerebral blood flow, and membrane breakdown. However, further prospective randomized studies are required.

Estrogen replacement therapy may also modulate aging of the serotonergic system. For example, van Amelsvoort et al. (2001b) reported that postmenopausal women who use estrogen replacement therapy have a significant reduction in age-related differences in serotonergic responsivity (as measured by prolactin response to a fenfluaramine challenge) (Fig. 18.2). Also both PET (Moses et al., 2000) and single-photon PET studies (Travis et al., 1999) found that a short course of estradiol increases cortical 5-HT$_{2A}$ receptor density in healthy postmenopausal women.

Estrogen can also modulate dopaminergic function. In animal studies, estrogen reduces dopamine concentration in the striatum and modulates the sensitivity and number of dopamine receptors (Bedard et al., 1984; Foreman and Porter, 1980; Gordon et al., 1980). In human adults, dopamine D$_2$ receptor concentration reduces with increasing age, especially in frontal and basal ganglia regions (Wong et al., 1984). Also, women exhibit a linear decline in caudate D$_2$ density, whereas

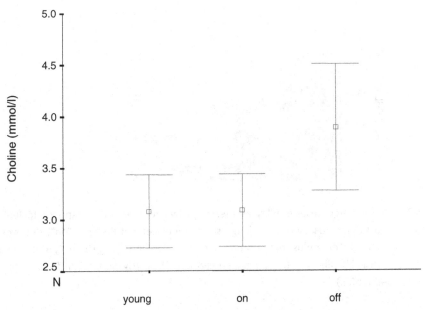

Fig. 18.1.   Mean right hippocampal choline as an indication of neuronal membrane breakdown in postmenopausal women taking estrogen replacement therapy ("on") or never using such therapy ("off") plus that in premenopausal women ("young"). Bars indicate 95% confidence internal. "Off" values versus "young," $p < 0.03$; "off" values versus "on," $p < 0.04$. (From Robertson D. M. W., *et al.*, *Neurology* 2001, **57**(11): 2114–2117.)

men exhibit a decline best represented by a second-degree polynomial regression, with a much steeper fall between 20 and 40 years of age. It has been suggested that the later age of onset of schizophrenia in females than in males reflects a loss of the antidopaminergic effect of estrogen as levels decline in older age. This hypothesis is partially supported by the observation that psychotic symptoms emerge in some females when estrogen levels are low, for example during the perimenopausal (Castle and Murray, 1993; Jablensky *et al.*, 1992) and postpartum periods (Kendell *et al.*, 1987), and during low estrogen phases of the menstrual cycle (Seeman and Lang, 1990). Furthermore, adjunct estrogen treatment has been reported to improve response to antipsychotic medication (Kulkarni *et al.*, 2001).

Therefore, there is evidence that estrogen significantly modulates the development and aging of brain regions and neurochemical systems implicated in schizophrenia. However, there is little evidence that physiological differences in estrogen cause schizophrenia per se; rather, estrogen most likely modifies symptom presentation and/or disease onset in women already at risk for developing schizophrenia.

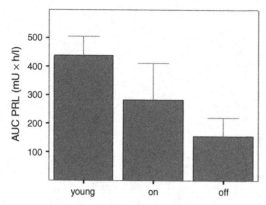

Fig. 18.2.   Serotonergic responsibility as measured by prolactin (PRL) response to fenfluramine in postmenopausal women taking estrogen replacement therapy ("on") or never using such therapy ("off") plus that in premenopausal women ("young"). AUC, area under the curve. Kruskal-Wallis, $p = 0.02$. (van Amelsvoort *et al. Psychoneuroendocrinology* 2001a, **26**: 493–502.)

X chromosome

It has been suggested that a gene(s) for schizophrenia could be X-linked or X–Y linked, with homologous loci on both X and Y chromosomes (DeLisi *et al.*, 1994), but support for this view has been limited and there is currently little evidence that schizophrenia is an X-linked disorder. Nonetheless, it is clear that cognitive functions which are usually highly lateralized (e.g. language) and have gender differences in development are affected in schizophrenia. Also it has been suggested that schizophrenia arises from abnormalities in development of cerebral asymmetry. Consequently, it is of interest to investigate if/how the X chromosome affects hemispheric asymmetry and development/function of brain regions implicated in schizophrenia.

Normally in women, the second X chromosome is randomly inactivated; however, some genes escape inactivation and so may have significant effects on brain. Also, males always receive their X chromosome from their mother whereas "normal" females inherit one X chromosome from each of their parents. Turner syndrome is a genetic disorder in which all or part of one X chromosome is deleted (45X). Individuals with Turner syndrome provide a model where the effect of loss of the second X chromosome and/or mode of inheritance on the brain can be investigated. We reported that loss of the second X chromosome affects the development of anatomical, metabolic, and functional cerebral asymmetry; language; and visuospatial skills (Murphy *et al.*, 1993, 1994, 1997). We suggested that this most likely arises from loss of genes carried on the X chromosome that normally escape inactivation. Recently, it has been suggested that social cognition might be "imprinted" from a genetic locus on the X chromosome (Skuse *et al.*, 1997). The authors examined the association between the parental origin of the X chromosome in women with Turner syndrome and their social cognition. Women with paternally derived X chromosomes were found to be significantly better adjusted, with superior verbal and executive function skills, than those with maternally derived X chromosomes. The authors suggested that there is a locus for social cognition that is imprinted from the paternally derived X chromosome and not expressed from the maternal one, and that this explains why men are more vulnerable to social communication disorders than women.

Another way to examine the effect of the X chromosome on the brain is to study the effect of specific genes and/or gene products, such as trinucleotide triplet repeats. Expanded trinucleotide repeats are associated with several neurological and neuropsychiatric conditions, including Huntington's disease, mytonic dystrophy, spinal and bulbar muscular atrophy, and fragile X syndrome. It has been proposed by some that transmission of schizophrenia may be associated with expanded triplet repeats (Morris *et al.*, 1995; O'Donovan *et al.*, 1995), although this suggestion has not been supported by others. The current genetic model proposes that fragile X syndrome results from having more than 200 cytosine–guanine–guanine (CGG) trinucleotide repeats, with subsequent methylation of the fragile X mental retardation gene (*FMR1*) and loss of production of its protein product FMRP. It was originally thought that premutation expansion of CGGs trinucleotide repeats has no biological effect. FMRP is an RNA-binding protein, required for the normal process of synaptic maturation. Mice with that *Fmr1* gene "knocked out" have abnormal dendritic spines, hyperactivity, and deficits in learning memory; recent studies of *dfxr* mutations in *Drosophila* have demonstrated synaptic alterations and impaired circadian rhythms. Overexpression of *fmr1* homologs in mice and flies produces opposing adverse effects, such as lethargy. People with full mutation fragile X syndrome display variable levels of mental retardation with particular deficits in language, attention, and visuospatial abilities; they also have a high prevalence of neuropsychiatric abnormalities, including deviant language and communication patterns, attention deficit disorder, schizotypal personality disorder, and perhaps psychosis (Freund *et al.*, 1992; Fryns, 1986; Hagerman, 1987). These clinical deficits become more severe as they pass from one generation to another; this phenomenon is known as genetic anticipation and is also reported to occur in families with schizophrenia (McInnis *et al.*, 1993).

However, studies of the biological actions of trinucleotide repeats in people with full mutation fragile X syndrome are confounded by the presence of learning disability. Consequently, we examined the effect of premutation expansion of X chromosome trinucleotide repeats on brain morphometry (using MRI) and regional metabolism (using PET and [^{18}F]-2-fluoro-2-deoxy-D-glucose). Carrier of such a premutation expansion had significant differences in the anatomy and metabolism of hippocampus and temporal regions plus differences in right–left asymmetry of the Wernicke and Broca language areas. Therefore, premutation expansion of X chromosome CGG trinucleotide repeats does affect the development of brain regions implicated in schizophrenia and the right–left symmetry of language areas. This may be of relevance to the general population, since approximately 0.5% are premutation carriers of fragile X syndrome; moreover, intermediate alleles (with CGG repeats over 40) occur in up to 4% of people.

Conclusions

Both estrogen and the X chromosome affect the development of brain regions and neurochemical systems that are both crucial to higher cognitive function and implicated in neuropsychiatric disorders such as schizophrenia.

There are gender differences in schizophrenia and because estrogen has putative antidopaminergic/antipsychotic actions, it has been suggested that estrogen may be responsible in women for the delayed onset of the first incidence peak and that the second peak seen in women may result from the decline in estrogen levels at menopause. There is evidence that estrogen protects the nigrostriatal dopaminergic system against the neurotoxic effects of 1-methyl-a-phenyl-2, 2, 3, 6-tetrahydropyridine in rats (Dluzen et al., 1996). An antipsychotic action of estrogens is supported by clinical studies reporting that women have increased admission rates for psychosis around the menses (Hallonquist et al., 1993) and that psychotic symptomatology varies with the phase of the menstrual cycle (Lindamer et al., 1997). Also, women with schizophrenia may have reduced estradiol levels compared with non-schizophrenia controls (Riecher-Rossler et al., 1994). However, there is currently little evidence to support the therapeutic use of estrogen in schizophrenia. For example, when women with schizophrenia are treated with adjunctive estrogen there is a slight increase in speed of recovery, but no improvement overall compared with antipsychotic medication alone (Kulkarni et al., 2001). Despite the lack of clear evidence for the efficacy of estrogen as an antipsychotic treatment, it remains plausible that estrogen replacement therapy might protect against late-onset schizophrenia in postmenopausal women by reducing age-related changes in brain structure and neurochemistry (e.g. in the hippocampus).

We do not propose that estrogen and the X chromosome are crucial to the development of schizophrenia in most people. Rather, we suggest that they play a modulatory role in brain maturation, and their mechanism of action needs to be understood in order to place the "neurodevelopmental theory" of schizophrenia in context.

REFERENCES

Andreasen, N. C., Smith, M. R., Jacoby, C. G., Dennert, J. W., Olsen, S. A. (1982). Ventricular enlargement in schizophrenia: definition and prevalence. *Am J Psychiatry* **139**: 292–296.

Andreasen, N. C., Nasrallah, H. A., Dunn, *et al.* (1986). Structural abnormalities in the frontal system in schizophrenia: a magnetic resonance imaging study. *Arch Gen Psychiatry* **43**: 136–144.

Andreasen, N. C., Ehrhardt, J. C., Swayze, III, V. W., *et al.* (1990a). Magnetic resonance imaging of the brain in schizophrenia. The pathophysiologic significance of structural abnormalities. *Arch Gen Psychiatry* **47**: 35–44.

Andreasen, N. C., Swayze, III, V. W., Flaum, M., *et al.* (1990b). Ventricular enlargement in schizophrenia evaluated with computed tomographic scanning. Effects of gender, age, and stage of illness. *Arch Gen Psychiatry* **47**: 1008–1015.

Bedard, P. J., Boucher, R., Daigle, M., di Paolo, T. (1984). Similar effect of estradiol and haloperidol on experimental tardive dyskinesia in monkeys. *Psychoneuroendocrinology* **9**: 375–379.

Benes, F. M. (1998). Brain development, VII. Human brain growth spans decades. *Am J Psychiatry* **155**: 1489.

Benes, F. M., Turtle, M., Khan, Y., Farol, P. (1994). Myelination of a key relay zone in the hippocampal formation occurs in the human brain during childhood, adolescence, and adulthood. *Arch Gen Psychiatry* **51**: 477–484.

Bennett-Clarke, C. A., Leslie, M. J., Lane, R. D., Rhoades, R. W. (1994). Effect of serotonin depletion on vibrissa-related patterns of thalamic afferents in the rat's somatosensory cortex. *J Neurosci* **14**: 7594–7607.

Bennett-Clarke, C. A., Chiaia, N. L., Rhoades, R. W. (1996). Thalamocortical afferents in rat transiently express high-affinity serotonin uptake sites. *Brain Res* **733**: 301–306.

Blue, M. E., Erzurumlu, R. S., Jhaveri, S. (1991). A comparison of pattern formation by thalamocortical and serotonergic afferents in the rat barrel field cortex. *Cereb Cortex* **1**: 380–389.

Brinton, R. D. (1993). 17-Estradiol induction of filopodial growth in cultured hippocampal neurons within minutes of exposure. *Mol Cell Neurosci* **4**: 36–46.

(2001). Cellular and molecular mechanisms of estrogen regulation of memory function and neuroprotection against Alzheimer's disease: recent insights and remaining challenges. *Learn Mem* **8**: 121–133.

Cases, O., Seif, I., Grimsby, J., Gaspar, P., *et al.* (1995). Aggressive behavior and altered amounts of brain serotonin and norepinephrine in mice lacking MAOA. *Science* **268**: 1763–1766.

Cases, O., Vitalis, T., Seif, I., *et al.* (1996). Lack of barrels in the somatosensory cortex of monoamine oxidase A-deficient mice: role of a serotonin excess during the critical period. *Neuron* **16**: 297–307.

Castle, D. J., Murray, R. M. (1993). The epidemiology of late-onset schizophrenia. *Schizophr Bull* **19**: 691–700.

Castle, D. J., Wessely, S., Murray, R. M. (1993). Sex and schizophrenia: effects of diagnostic stringency, and associations with and premorbid variables. *Br J Psychiatry* **162**: 658–664.

Coger, R. W., Serafetinides, E. A. (1990). Schizophrenia, corpus callosum, and interhemispheric communication: a review. *Psychiatr Res* **34**: 163–184.

D'Amato, R. J., Blue, M. E., Largent, B. L., *et al.* (1987). Ontogeny of the serotonergic projection to rat neocortex: transient expression of a dense innervation to primary sensory areas. *Proc Natl Acad Sci USA* **84**: 4322–4326.

De Bellis, M. D., Keshavan, M. S., Beers, S. R., *et al.* (2001). Sex differences in brain maturation during childhood and adolescence. *Cereb Cortex* **11**: 552–557.

DeLisi, L. E., Devoto, M., Lofthouse, R., *et al.* (1994). Search for linkage to schizophrenia on the X and Y chromosomes. *Am J Med Genet* **54**: 113–121.

Dluzen, D. E., McDermott, J. L., Liu, B. (1996). Estrogen alters MPTP-induced neurotoxicity in female mice: effects on striatal dopamine concentrations and release. *J Neurochem* **66**: 658–666.

Dumontier, M., Hocht, P., Mintert, U., Faix, J. (2000). Rac1 GTPases control filopodia formation, cell motility, endocytosis, cytokinesis and development in Dictyostelium. *J Cell Sci* **113**: 2253–2265.

Egan, M. F., Goldberg, T. E., Kolachana, B. S., *et al.* (2001). Effect of COMT Val108/158 Met genotype on frontal lobe function and risk for schizophrenia. *Proc Natl Acad Sci USA* **98**: 6917–6922.

Fitch, R. H., Denenberg, V. H. (1998). A role for ovarian hormones in sexual differentiation of the brain. *Behav Brain Sci* **21**: 311–327; discussion 327–352.

Flaum, M., Arndt, S., Andreasen, N. C. (1990). The role of gender in studies of ventricle enlargement in schizophrenia: a predominantly male effect. *Am J Psychiatry* **147**: 1327–1332.

Foreman, M. M., Porter, J. C. (1980). Effects of catechol estrogens and catecholamines on hypothalamic and corpus striatal tyrosine hydroxylase activity. *J Neurochem* **34**: 1175–1183.

Freund, L. S., Reiss, A. L., Hagerman, R., Vinogradov, S. (1992). Chromosome fragility and psychopathology in obligate female carriers of the fragile X syndrome. *Arch Gen Psychiatry* **49**: 54–60.

Fryns, J. P. (1986). The female and the fragile X A study of 144 obligate female carriers. *Am J Med Genet* **23**: 157–169.

Giedd, J. N., Vaituzis, A. C., Hamburger, S. D., *et al.* (1996). Quantitative MRI of the temporal lobe, amygdala, and hippocampus in normal human development: ages 4–18 years. *J Comp Neurol* **366**: 223–230.

Giedd, J. N., Blumenthal, J., Jeffries, N. O., *et al.* (1999). Brain development during childhood and adolescence: a longitudinal MRI study. *Nat Neurosci* **2**: 861–863.

Goldman-Rakic, P. S., Brown, R. M. (1982). Postnatal development of monoamine content and synthesis in the cerebral cortex of rhesus monkeys. *Brain Res* **256**: 339–349.

Gordon, J. H., Borison, R. L., Diamond, B. I. (1980). Modulation of dopamine receptor sensitivity by estrogen. *Biol Psychiatry* **15**: 389–396.

Gur, R. E., Mozley, P. D., Shtasel, D. L., *et al.* (1994). Clinical subtypes of schizophrenia: differences in brain and CSF volume. *Am J Psychiatry* **151**: 343–350.

Haas, G. L., Hien, D. A., Waked, W., *et al.* (1989). Sex differences in schizophrenia. *Schizophr Res* 2: 11.

Haas, G. L., Sweeney, J. A., Hien, D. A., Goldman, D., Deck, M. (1991). Gender differences in schizophrenia. *Schizophr Res* 4: 277.

Hafner, H., Riecher-Rossler, A., Maurer, K., Fatkenheuer, B., Loffler, W. (1993). Generating and testing a causal explanation of the gender difference in age at first onset of schizophrenia. *Psychol Med* 23: 925–940.

Hafner, H., Maurer, K., Loffler, W., *et al.* (1994). The epidemiology of early schizophrenia. Influence of age and gender on onset and early course. *Br J Psychiatry Suppl* 23: 29–38.

Hafner, H., An der Heiden, W., Behrens, S., *et al.* (1998a). Causes and consequences of the gender difference in age at onset of schizophrenia. *Schizophr Bull* 24: 99–113.

Hafner, H., Maurer, K., Loffler, W., *et al.* (1998b). The ABC Schizophrenia Study: a preliminary overview of the results. *Soc Psychiatry Psychiatr Epidemiol* 33: 380–386.

Hagerman, R. J. (1987). Fragile X syndrome. *Curr Probl Pediatr* 17: 627–674.

Hallonquist, J. D., Seeman, M. V., Lang, M., Rector, N. A. (1993). Variation in symptom severity over the menstrual cycle of schizophrenics. *Biol Psychiatry* 33: 207–209.

Hampson, E. (1990). Variations in sex-related cognitive abilities across the menstrual cycle. *Brain Cogn* 14: 26–43.

Hariri, A. R., Mattay, V. S., Tessitore, A., *et al.* (2002). Serotonin transporter genetic variation and the response of the human amygdala. *Science* 297: 400–403.

Harvey, I., Williams, M., Toone, B. K., *et al.* (1990). The ventricular–brain ratio (VBR) in functional psychoses: the relationship of lateral ventricular and total intracranial area. *Psychol Med* 20: 55–62.

Hedner, J., Lundell, K. H., Breese, G. R., Mueller, R. A., Hedner, T. (1986). Developmental variations in CSF monoamine metabolites during childhood. *Biol Neonate* 49: 190–197.

Herlenius, E., Lagercrantz, H. (2001). Neurotransmitters and neuromodulators during early human development. *Early Hum Dev* 65: 21–37.

Howard, R., Rabins, P. V., Seeman, M. V., Jeste, D. V., *et al.* (2000). Late-onset schizophrenia and very-late-onset schizophrenia-like psychosis: an international consensus. *Am J Psychiatry* 157: 172–178.

Jablensky, A., Sartorius, N., Ernberg, G. (1992). Schizophrenia: manifestations, incidence and course in different cultures. A World Health Organization Ten-Country Study. *Psychol Med Monograph* 20.

Kendell, R. E., Chalmers, J. C., Platz, C. (1987). Epidemiology of puerperal psychoses. *Br J Psychiatry* 150: 662–673.

Kulkarni, J., Riedel, A., de Castella, A. R., *et al.* (2001). Estrogen: a potential treatment for schizophrenia. *Schizophr Res* 48: 137–144.

Lauder, J. M., Krebs, H. (1978). Serotonin as a differentiation signal in early neurogenesis. *Dev Neurosci* 1: 15–30.

Lauriello, J., Hoff, A., Wieneke, M. H., *et al.* (1997). Similar extent of brain dysmorphology in severely ill women and men with schizophrenia. *Am J Psychiatry* 154: 819–825.

Lebrand, C., Cases, O., Adelbrecht, C., *et al.* (1996). Transient uptake and storage of serotonin in developing thalamic neurons. *Neuron* 17: 823–835.

Lerer, B., Gelfin, Y., Shapira, B. (1999). Neuroendocrine evidence for age-related decline in central serotonergic function. *Neuropsychopharmacology* **21**: 321–322.

Leung, A., Chue, P. (2000). Sex differences in schizophrenia, a review of the literature. *Acta Psychiatr Scand Suppl* **401**: 3–38.

Levallois, C., Valence, C., Baldet, P., Privat, A. (1997). Morphological and morphometric analysis of serotonin-containing neurons in primary dissociated cultures of human rhombencephalon: a study of development. *Brain Res Dev Brain Res* **99**: 243–252.

Lidow, M. S., Goldman-Rakic, P. S., Rakic, P. (1991). Synchronized overproduction of neurotransmitter receptors in diverse regions of the primate cerebral cortex. *Proc Natl Acad Sci USA* **88**: 10218–10221.

Lindamer, L. A., Lohr, J. B., Harris, M. J., Jeste, D. V. (1997). Gender, estrogen, and schizophrenia. *Psychopharmacol Bull* **33**: 221–228.

Maki, P. M., Resnick, S. M. (2000). Longitudinal effects of estrogen replacement therapy on PET cerebral blood flow and cognition. *Neurobiol Aging* **21**: 373–383.

     (2001). Effects of estrogen on patterns of brain activity at rest and during cognitive activity: A review of neuroimaging studies. *Neuroimage* **14**: 789–801.

McInnis, M. G., McMahon, F. J., Chase, G. A., *et al.* (1993). Anticipation in bipolar affective disorder. *Am J Hum Genet* **53**: 385–390.

Meltzer, C. C., Smith, G., DeKosky, S. T., *et al.* (1998). Serotonin in aging, late-life depression, and Alzheimer's disease: the emerging role of functional imaging. *Neuropsychopharmacology* **18**: 407–430.

Morris, A. G., Gaitonde, E., McKenna, P. J., Mollon, J. D., Hunt, D. M. (1995). CAG repeat expansions and schizophrenia: association with disease in females and with early age-at-onset. *Hum Mol Genet* **4**: 1957–1961.

Moses, E. L., Drevets, W. C., Smith, G., *et al.* (2000). Effects of estradiol and progesterone administration on human serotonin 2A receptor binding: a PET study. *Biol Psychiatry* **48**: 854–860.

Murphy, D. G., DeCarli, C., Daly, E., *et al.* (1993). X-chromosome effects on female brain: a magnetic resonance imaging study of Turner's syndrome. *Lancet* **342**: 1197–1200.

Murphy, D. G., Allen, G., Haxby, J. V., *et al.* (1994). The effects of sex steroids, and the X chromosome, on female brain function: a study of the neuropsychology of adult Turner syndrome. *Neuropsychologia* **32**: 1309–1323.

Murphy, D. G., DeCarli, C., McIntosh, A. R., *et al.* (1996). Sex differences in human brain morphometry and metabolism: an in vivo quantitative magnetic resonance imaging and positron emission tomography study on the effect of aging. *Arch Gen Psychiatry* **53**: 585–594.

Murphy, D. G., Mentis, M. J., Pietrini, P., *et al.* (1997). A PET study of Turner's syndrome: effects of sex steroids and the X chromosome on brain. *Biol Psychiatry* **41**: 285–298.

Nasrallah, H. A., Schwarzkopf, S. B., Olson, S. C., Coffman, J. A. (1990). Gender differences in schizophrenia on MRI brain scans. *Schizophr Bull* **16**: 205–210.

Nopoulos, P., Flaum, M., Andreasen, N. C. (1997). Sex differences in brain morphology in schizophrenia. *Am J Psychiatry* **154**: 1648–1654.

O'Connell, P., Woodruff, P. W. R., Wright, I., Jones, P., Murray, R. M. (1997). Developmental insanity or dementia praecox: was the wrong concept adopted? *Schizophr Res* **23**: 97–106.

O'Donovan, M. C., Guy, C., Craddock, N., *et al.* (1995). Expanded CAG repeats in schizophrenia and bipolar disorder. *Nat Genet* **10**: 380–381.

Phillips, S. M., Sherwin, B. B. (1992). Effects of estrogen on memory function in surgically menopausal women. *Psychoneuroendocrinology* **17**: 485–495.

Phoenix, C. H., Goy, R. W., Gerall, A. A., Young, W. C. (1959). Organizing action of prenatally administered testosterone proprionate on the tissues mediating behavior in the guinea pig. *Endocrinology* **65**: 369–382.

Riecher-Rossler, A., Hafner, H., Dutsch-Strobel, A., *et al.* (1994). Further evidence for a specific role of estradiol in schizophrenia? *Biol Psychiatry* **36**: 492–494.

Robertson, D. M., van Amelsvoort, T., Daly, E., *et al.* (2001). Effects of estrogen replacement therapy on human brain aging: an in vivo ^{1}H MRS study. *Neurology* **57**: 2114–2117.

Salem, J. E., Kring, A. M. (1998). The role of gender differences in the reduction of etiologic heterogeneity in schizophrenia. *Clin Psychol Rev* **18**: 795–819.

Seeman, M. V., Lang, M. (1990). The role of estrogens in schizophrenia gender differences. *Schizophr Bull* **16**: 185–194.

Seifert, Jr., W. E., Foxx, J. L., Butler, I. J. (1980). Age effect on dopamine and serotonin metabolite levels in cerebrospinal fluid. *Ann Neurol* **8**: 38–42.

Shaywitz, S. E., Shaywitz, B. A., Pugh, K. R., *et al.* (1999). Effect of estrogen on brain activation patterns in postmenopausal women during working memory tasks. *J Am Med Assoc* **281**: 1197–1202.

Shelton, R. C., Karson, C. N., Doran, A. R., *et al.* (1988). Cerebral structural pathology in schizophrenia: evidence for a selective prefrontal cortical defect. *Am J Psychiatry* **145**: 154–163.

Shenton, M. E., Kikinis, R., Jolesz, F. A., *et al.* (1992). Abnormalities of the left temporal lobe and thought disorder in schizophrenia. A quantitative magnetic resonance imaging study. *N Engl J Med* **327**: 604–612.

Sherwin, B. B. (1988). Estrogen and/or androgen replacement therapy and cognitive functioning in surgically menopausal women. *Psychoneuroendocrinology* **13**: 345–357.

Skuse, D. H., James, R. S., Bishop, D. V., *et al.* (1997). Evidence from Turner's syndrome of an imprinted X-linked locus affecting cognitive function. *Nature* **387**: 705–708.

Spear, L. P. (2000). The adolescent brain and age-related behavioral manifestations. *Neurosci Biobehav Rev* **24**: 417–463.

Spitzer, R., Endicott, J., Robins, E. (1978). Research Diagnostic Criteria (RDC): rationale and reliability. *Arch Gen Psychiatry* **35**: 773–782.

Sundstrom, E., Kolare, S., Souverbie, F., *et al.* (1993). Neurochemical differentiation of human bulbospinal monoaminergic neurons during the first trimester. *Dev Brain Res* **75**: 1–12.

Takahashi, H., Nakashima, S., Ohama, E., Takeda, S., Ikuta, F. (1986). Distribution of serotonin-containing cell bodies in the brainstem of the human fetus determined with immunohisto-chemistry using antiserotonin serum. *Brain Dev* **8**: 355–365.

Toran-Allerand, C. D. (1996). The estrogen/neurotrophin connection during neural development: is co-localization of estrogen receptors with the neurotrophins and their receptors biologically relevant? *Dev Neurosci* **18**: 36–48.

Travis, M. J., Mulligan, O., Mulligan, R. S., *et al.* (1999). Preliminary investigation of the effect of oestradiol treatment on cortical 5–HT2A receptor binding: a single photon emission tomography (SPET) study using ^{123}I -5-I-R91150. *Neuroimage* **9**: S672.

van Amelsvoort, T. A. M. J., Daly, E. Robertson, D. M. R., *et al.* (2001a). Structural brain abnormalities associated with deletion of chromosome 22qaa: quantitative neuroimaging study of adults with velo-cardio-facial syndrome. *Br J Psychiatry* **178**: 412–419.

van Amelsvoort, T. A. M. J., Abel, K. M., Robertson, D. M. R., *et al.* (2001b). Prolactin response to d-fenfluramine in postmenopausal women on and off ERT: comparison with young women. *Psychoneuroendocrinology* **26**: 493–502.

Vazquez-Barquero, J. L., Cuesta Nunez, M. J., Quintana Pando, F., *et al.* (1995). Structural abnormalities of the brain in schizophrenia: sex differences in the Cantabria First Episode of Schizophrenia Study. *Psychol Med* **25**: 1247–1257.

Walker, E. F. (1994). Developmentally moderated expressions of the neuropathology underlying schizophrenia. *Schizophr Bull* **20**: 453–480.

Whitaker-Azmitia, P. M. (2001). Serotonin and brain development: role in human developmental diseases. *Brain Res Bull* **56**: 479–485.

Williams, A. O., Reveley, M. A., Kolakowska, T., Ardern, M., Mandelbrote, B. M. (1985). Schizophrenia with good and poor outcome. II: Cerebral ventricular size and its clinical significance. *Br J Psychiatry* **146**: 239–246.

Wong, D. F., Wagner, Jr., H. N., Dannals, R. F., *et al.* (1984). Effects of age on dopamine and serotonin receptors measured by positron tomography in the living human brain. *Science* **226**: 1393–1396.

Wong, D. F., Broussolle, E. P., Wand, G., *et al.* (1988). In vivo measurement of dopamine receptors in human brain by positron emission tomography. Age and sex differences. *Ann N Y Acad Sci* **515**: 203–214.

Woolley, C. S., McEwen, B. S. (1994). Estradiol regulates hippocampal dendritic spine density via an N-methyl-D-aspartate receptor-dependent mechanism. *J Neurosci* **14**: 7680–7687.

Yan, W., Wilson, C. C., Haring, J. H. (1997). Effects of neonatal serotonin depletion on the development of rat dentate granule cells. *Brain Res Dev Brain Res* **98**: 177–184.

Yu, X.-M., Askalan, R., Keil, II, G. J., Salter, M. W. (1997). NMDA channel regulation by channel-associated protein tyrosine kinase Src. *Science* **275**: 674–678.

19

Premorbid structural abnormalities in schizophrenia

Stephen M. Lawrie

Royal Edinburgh Hospital, Edinburgh, UK

Hundreds of structural brain imaging studies in groups of patients have demonstrated that there is a neuroanatomy of schizophrenia. When the various abnormalities are first evident, however, remains unknown. This is not merely an academic issue. If all or even some differences are present from early life in people who go on to develop schizophrenia, then very early detection is a possibility; if some findings are only manifest later in development, or around the time of onset, therapeutic opportunities may arise.

Identifying the time course of the structural abnormalities in schizophrenia is a difficult task. Ideally, prospective studies would follow people from early fetal life to the onset of schizophrenia and beyond, but this is impractical for a host of technological, clinical, and epidemiological reasons. The best available compromise is to conduct repeated longitudinal examinations of populations at high risk of developing schizophrenia a relatively short time before onset. Even these studies are expensive, vulnerable to changes in technology, and potentially biased by participant drop-out. Case–control studies are most practical, but generally less reliable; these seek to relate early exposures (e.g. family history, adverse obstetric complications [OCs]) and/or developmental indices (e.g. motor milestones, premorbid adjustment) to imaging findings. These measurements are usually retrospective and often imprecise.

This chapter attempts to review all of the evidence, from these types of imaging study, for premorbid abnormalities in patients with schizophrenia and related populations. Before considering these, it is necessary to highlight the anatomical abnormalities that require explanation.

The neuroanatomy of schizophrenia

Table 19.1 lists the main findings from quantitative systematic reviews of structural imaging studies comparing patients with schizophrenia and healthy controls.

Neurodevelopment and Schizophrenia, ed. Matcheri S. Keshavan *et al.* Published by Cambridge University Press. © Cambridge University Press 2004.

Table 19.1. Systematic reviews of structural brain abnormalities in schizophrenia versus controls

Reference	Type of study	Measures	Main findings
Raz and Raz, 1990	CT	Lateral ventricles	Enlarged (ES, 0.7)
	CT	Third ventricle	Enlarged (ES, 0.66)
	CT	Cortical sulci/fissures	Widened (ES, 0.35)
Van Horn and McManus (1992)	CT/sMRI	Ventricular to brain ratio	Enlarged
Woodruff et al. (1995)	sMRI	Corpus callosum	Reduced area non-significant after control for brain area
Ward et al. (1996)	sMRI/CT/PM	Brain size	Reduced (ES, 0.31)
	sMRI/CT	Intracranial size	Reduced (ES, 0.16)
Nelson et al. (1998)	sMRI	Hippocampus	Reduced (ES, 0.4) by about 4% bilaterally
		Amygdala/hippocampus	Reduced (ES, 0.7) by about 8% bilaterally
		Amygdala	Reduced (ES, 0.3) by about 4% bilaterally
Lawrie and Abukmeil (1998) (amended in Lawrie et al., 2000)	sMRI	Most regions measured in previous studies	Include reductions in whole brain (~3%), frontal and temporal lobes (~5%), and parahippocampal gyrus (10%), and increases in CSF (~15%)
Shapleske et al. (1999)	sMRI	Planum temporale	Possibly reversed asymmetry
Wright et al. (2000)	sMRI	All regions measured in previous studies	Include reductions in gray and white matter (~3%), superior temporal gyrus (~3%) and increases in globus pallidus (~20%)
Konick and Friedman (2001)	sMRI/PM	Thalamus	Reduced (ES, 0.4)
Sommer et al. (2001)	sMRI	All studies of cerebral asymmetry	Reduced asymmetry of posterior superior temporal gyrus (and possibly of Sylvian fissure)

CT, computed tomography; sMRI, structural magnetic resonance imaging; PM, postmortem; ES, effect size; CSF, cerebrospinal fluid.

Computed tomography (CT) demonstrated ventricular enlargement and a generalized loss of brain tissue (Raz and Raz, 1990; van Horn and McManus, 1992), albeit in one composite area measure, the ventricular to brain ratio (VBR), which may have conflated separate disease processes. Magnetic resonance imaging, which now requires a structural prefix (sMRI), has replicated these findings and convincingly shown additional volume deficits in the prefrontal and temporal lobes, as well as further decrements in the medial and superior temporal lobe. The largest percentage differences are in the body of the lateral ventricle, which is approximately 50% enlarged, and the parahippocampal gyrus, which is approximately 10% reduced in volume (Lawrie and Abukmeil, 1998; Wright *et al.*, 2000), although the largest effect size reported is for increases in the globus pallidus, which are probably related to therapeutic dopamine blockade (Wright *et al.*, 2000). The thalamus is also reduced in volume and there are strong suggestions that schizophrenia patients may have reduced or even reversed asymmetry of the usually left-lateralized temporal cortex. None of these reviews have, however, been able to relate these abnormalities to any specific period of brain development or risk factor for schizophrenia.

Most sMRI studies have taken a region of interest (ROI) approach, which requires laborious hand tracings facilitated by varying degrees of semi-automated tissue classification and boundary detection. The alternative is to use entirely automated procedures, such as voxel-based morphometry (VBM), to construct statistical probability maps of the likelihood that a particular brain region has a different tissue density in two or more subject groups. This is more reliable and quicker than ROI tracing but cannot identify global effects, requires correction for multiple hypothesis testing at each image voxel, and is likely to be more able to detect changes at the boundaries of structures than within them. Various VBM studies comparing patients with schizophrenia and healthy controls have replicated the main ROI findings and, in addition, repeatedly suggested that the insula and the medial frontal lobe, including the anterior cingulate, have reduced grey matter density in schizophrenia (e.g. Job *et al.*, 2002; Paillere-Martinot *et al.*, 2001; Sigmundsson *et al.*, 2001).

The consistent demonstration of such structural abnormalities is in striking contrast to the lack of associations found with almost any clinical measure in the patients. By far the best replicated finding is an apparent absence of any relationship with illness duration (Lawrie and Abukmeil, 1998; Lewis, 1990). Together with repeated demonstrations that abnormalities are evident in patients with first-episode schizophrenia (FES) (seemingly to a similar extent as in patients with chronic schizophrenia), this provides strong support for neurodevelopmental models of schizophrenia and suggests that at least some of the findings predate the onset of psychosis. Theories of an essentially "static encephalopathy" are, however, seriously challenged by increasing evidence from prospective studies that some abnormalities may be progressive in the first few years after onset (see Ch. 20). They are also challenged by the preliminary findings from prospective high-risk studies.

Prospective studies of high-risk populations

The first high-risk study to include brain structure measurements was the Copenhagen High Risk Project, but this used CT and the scans were not repeated over time. Indeed, as yet, there are published data from only two longitudinal studies of pre- and perimorbid structural differences in people at elevated risk of schizophrenia. These two studies, which recruited high-risk subjects in entirely different ways, will now be discussed in detail.

Edinburgh High Risk Study

In the Edinburgh High Risk Study, we have examined subjects with at least two close relatives with schizophrenia. Potential participants were identified by reviewing the psychiatric case notes of patients with schizophrenia whose clinicians indicated were likely to have family histories. If the diagnosis and family history were confirmed, we then asked permission to approach their healthy relatives aged 16–24. A total of 229 suitable high-risk subjects were identified: 162 provided some data and 150 had one or more sMRI scans between 1994 and 1999. Groups of similarly aged healthy individuals (controls) and patients with FES were also examined. Most of the high-risk subjects and controls have returned for at least one further scan since 1999 and are likely to do so again before 2004.

Our preliminary ROI findings, in the first 100 high-risk subjects (Lawrie et al., 1999), were that the amygdala–hippocampal complex (AHC) was significantly smaller (by about 4%, with an effect size [ES] of 0.3) than in controls, but about 4% larger (ES, 0.3) than in FES. Reductions in the volume of the thalamus were only evident in comparison of the high-risk group versus the controls. An increase in third ventricular volume in the FES group was not significant after controlling for familial clustering (reduced variance) in the full high-risk sample (Lawrie et al., 2001). The main findings have been replicated by VBM analyses of the same data sets (Job et al., 2002, 2003), which extended them by showing anterior cingulate, medial prefrontal, and parahippocampal reductions in gray matter density with the greatest reductions in FES, then in the high-risk group, and then the controls.

Our finding that the volumes of the AHCs in high-risk subjects were midway between those of the controls and FES (Lawrie et al., 1999, 2001) has important implications. Based on their family histories, we expect that only 10–20% of our high-risk subjects will develop schizophrenia. As there is no obvious subgroup of high-risk subjects with particularly small AHCs (and assuming that those who develop schizophrenia will ultimately have AHCs that approximate to those of FES), the reduced AHC volume may be a trait marker. Prefrontal lobe and thalami volumes, but not those of the AHC, were associated with measures of genetic liability (Lawrie *et al.*, 2001). The apparent absence of a relationship between AHC volume and genetic liability was unexpected and may be attributable to a relatively narrow range of liability in the Edinburgh High Risk Study or that hippocampal volumes particularly are related to OCs (see below). If, however, there are further AHC reductions in those who develop schizophrenia, this might reflect genetic effects on later neurodevelopment (but could also reflect environmental effects or a peri-onset effect on plasticity).

In those with psychotic symptoms at any point in the first 5 years of the study, the whole brain volume at study entry was reduced (after controlling for age, sex, paternal social class, height, and handedness) compared with those did not have psychotic symptoms over this time (Lawrie *et al.*, 2001). Those with psychotic symptoms and two or more sMRI scans had non-significant reductions in whole brain and (left) AHC volume over almost 2 years, but did have significant reductions in the (right) temporal lobes over time (Lawrie *et al.*, 2002). Very preliminary results suggest that relatively large brains (and relatively small thalami in women) predict the early onset of psychosis in high-risk subjects (Johnstone *et al.*, 2002).

At the time of writing, the twentieth person in the Edinburgh High Risk Study has just developed schizophrenia or a related psychosis. We are currently analyzing the possible sMRI predictors of schizophrenia and changes as the illness develops, with both ROI and VBM. Future analyses will include relating pre- and perimorbid brain structure to other risk factors for schizophrenia.

Melbourne High Risk Study

Researchers in the Melbourne High Risk Study have adopted a different but complementary approach. They have examined groups of people at "ultra high risk" (UHR) of psychosis, those with first-episode psychosis (FEP; including about 50% with schizophrenia/schizophreniform psychosis), and a large group of healthy controls. The UHR group consists of people aged 14–30 years and referred with "attenuated" partial (positive) psychotic symptoms several times a week for up to 5 years; transient symptoms of less than 1 week's duration in the past year; and/or both trait and state risk factors for psychosis (a family history and a worsening in mental state or general functioning in the past year). Preliminary ROI results suggested non-significant hippocampal reductions in the UHR group and the subgroup of these patients that developed psychosis (Copolov *et al.*, 2000). An early VBM study of nine who developed psychosis and 12 who remained well did identify significant volume reductions in the hippocampus, entorhinal cortex, and inferior frontal and fusiform gyri during the transition to psychosis (Pantelis et al., 2000).

Phillips et al. (2002) examined the traced whole brain and hippocampal volumes as possible predictors of psychosis. Of the eligible referrals, 75% were scanned between 1995 and 1998; 5% of scans were lost through movement artifact, leaving 60 subjects. Twenty (33%) of those with usable scans developed an acute psychosis (defined as an increase of one or more points in psychotic symptom severity, several times a week, for more than 1 week) within a year. A structured clinical interview identified diagnoses of schizophrenia spectrum disorder (11), affective psychosis (3), bipolar disorder (3), and others (3). The UHR groups who did not develop psychosis included four patients with depression, and 11 with an anxiety state.

The scans were conducted at two sites and there was a weak tendency for the scanners to deliver different whole brain volumes and for more of those who developed psychosis (and of one sex) to be scanned at one site (Phillips et al., 2002). Controlling for a slightly smaller whole brain, the 60 UHR patients had significantly smaller hippocampi (by about 11%; ES, 0.9) than the controls but did not differ from the FEP group. However, the UHR patients were on average 10 years younger and 11 points lower in premorbid intelligence quotient (IQ) scores than the normals. The 20 who became psychotic were much more closely similar in demographics to the 40 who remained non-psychotic but, rather counterintuitively, the (left) hippocampus was *larger* in those who went on to develop a psychosis. These confusing results may be attributable to scanner effects, selection bias, and/or confounding, for example by other diagnoses or gender.

Pantelis et al. (2003) have recently reported on their VBM findings in a slightly extended sample. In 75 people with prodromal symptoms, defined as above, 23 (31%) developed a psychotic disorder (with roughly equal numbers of schizophrenia and affective psychoses). Compared with those who did not develop a psychosis, they had less grey matter in (right) medial temporal, lateral temporal, and inferior frontal cortex, and in bilateral cingulate cortex. Twenty-one subjects had a repeat scan after 1–2 years, 10 of whom had become psychotic (five with schizophrenia). They showed reductions over time in (left) parahippocampal, fusiform, orbitofrontal, and cerebellar grey matter, while those who did not become psychotic only exhibited cerebellar reductions. These are intriguing results that suggest grey matter reductions in the run up to psychosis and immediately after it. There are, however, some important issues outstanding; in particular, whether some of those in the UHR group actually had a psychosis before or at study entry, and why the ROI and VBM studies appear to have such different findings.

Summary

These studies illustrate well the difficulties in conducting this type of research: acquiring a representative sample who will continue to participate in longitudinal studies, maintaining technical control of the scanner(s) over lengthy time intervals, and distinguishing psychotic symptoms from psychosis. The two recruitment strategies used so far have different and complementary strengths. Sampling relatives rather than referrals may provide a population who are more committed to the research, may be more likely to develop schizophrenia than other psychoses, and gives the potential to study gene–environment interactions. The main limitation is the time taken to accumulate enough subjects who develop psychosis, which is likely to be longer than in studies of people presenting with psychotic symptoms. The latter studies also have the greater ability to compare diagnoses. Regardless, the two main studies so far both report reduced medial temporal lobe structures as a trait marker of schizophrenia and suggest further volume losses around the time of onset. Such prospective studies are the only way to establish temporal patterns with any certainty, although very important information can also be obtained from case-control studies that examine the associations between imaging abnormalities and known risk factors for the disorder.

Structural imaging and risk factors for schizophrenia

The strongest known risk factor for schizophrenia is family history, which increases the risk of the disorder by approximately 5–50 times depending on the degree of genetic association (Cannon and Jones, 1996). Other risk factors are comparatively weak, with odds ratios of slightly more than 1–3. Of these, OCs have been most commonly related to imaging abnormalities, but there are also some studies of the structural associations of premorbid adjustment, season of birth, and fetal undernutrition/infection.

Family history

Family history is, of course, a proxy for genetic effects and these might only be expressed later in development. Given, however, the relative importance of genetic as opposed to environmental causation of schizophrenia, and that brain growth is maximal prenatally and for 1–2 years thereafter, it is likely that familial structural abnormalities are at least partly evident at or shortly after birth. The relationship between an elevated genetic risk of schizophrenia and structural abnormalities has been examined by scanning relatives (twins, siblings, offspring, parents), comparing known familial with presumed sporadic cases, and by examining people with genetic variants such as schizotypal personality disorder (SPD).

Computed tomography

In the first CT study, Weinberger *et al.* (1981) compared the VBRs of 10 inpatients with schizophrenia; 12 of their siblings (from seven sibships), and 17 controls. The VBR appeared to be, at least partially, under genetic control (as did some local horn enlargements) and differences were evident: largest in the schizophrenia patients, then in the siblings, and then the controls. Reveley *et al.* (1982) obtained a similar pattern of results in discordant monozygotic (MZ) twins and controls, as have other sibling studies (DeLisi *et al.*, 1986; Mourot *et al.*, 1997; Silverman *et al.*, 1998). Mourot *et al.* (1997) also found the same effect for third ventricle width, and Honer *et al.* (1995) reported larger temporal sulci and sylvian fissures (but not temporal horns) in patients compared with unaffected siblings.

The Copenhagen High Risk Project initially examined 34 offspring of mothers with schizophrenia, 10 of whose fathers also had a spectrum disorder. Widened fissures and sulci were related to genetic risk, while an increased VBR appeared to relate to a gene–environment interaction (see below; Cannon *et al.*, 1989). The results were internally consistent on substantially enlarging the sample (Cannon *et al.*, 1993). Widening the sample to include offspring with schizophrenia, SPD, or other psychiatric disorders demonstrated that global effects were evident in schizophrenia and SPD but only the schizophrenia patients had enlarged ventricles (Cannon *et al.*, 1994). However, a subsequent comparison of 16 "discordant sibling pairs" found that the differences were almost as marked for the sulcal area or the sulcal to brain ratio as for ventricular area or VBR (Zorrilla *et al.*, 1997).

Studies of the VBR in "sporadic versus familial" schizophrenia provide less consensus, as one of the originators of the distinction noted in a review of the early studies (Lewis, 1990). Patients without a family history of schizophrenia have been shown repeatedly to have higher VBRs and more marked ventriculomegaly than patients with a positive family history (e.g. Vita *et al.*, 1994; reviewed by DeQuardo *et al.*, 1996). Some notable large studies ($n > 100$) have failed to find an association between family history and the VBR (Johnstone *et al.*, 1989; Jones *et al.*, 1994), yet several studies do report such an association (e.g. Owens *et al.*, 1985), including those which go some way to supporting the distinction (e.g. Vita *et al.*, 1994; Silverman *et al.*, 1998). It may be that schizophrenia patients without an obvious genetic loading are more likely to have had environmental triggers likely to increase the VBR (see below). However, determining sporadic status is at best difficult, when many healthy relatives are likely to be carrying the gene(s), and the limited resolution of CT increases measurement error. Indeed, sMRI studies that have adopted similar approaches have all reported similar or greater abnormalities in familial cases (Dauphinais *et al.*, 1990; Falkai *et al.*, 2002; Harris *et al.*, 2002; Roy *et al.*, 1994; Sanderson *et al.*, 2001; Schwarzkopf *et al.*, 1991; Seidman *et al.*, 2002), with the exception of McDonald *et al.* (2002), and some suggest specific genetic effects in frontal and temporal lobes, the ventricles, and the basal ganglia.

Structural magnetic resonance studies of twins

Twin studies have the ability to distinguish genetic from environmental effects, although this depends upon including both healthy and discordant MZ and dizygotic (DZ) twin pairs. A genetic role is likely when MZ patients and their twins have similar volumes, but differ from healthy MZ twins, and the finding is more pronounced in MZ than DZ twins. Even then, however, the discordance may still be attributable to differences in gene expression or gene–environment interactions.

Suddath *et al.* (1990) found that the affected individuals in 15 pairs of discordant MZ twins had reduced left temporal lobe grey matter and bilaterally smaller hippocampal volumes, as well as larger ventricular structures, with no such differences in the frontal lobe or in white matter. They did not, however, include DZ pairs or healthy controls. Subsequent reports on 8–13 of these MZ pairs discordant for schizophrenia and 5–10 healthy MZ twin pairs have found no difference in sylvian fissure or planum temporale asymmetry (Bartley *et al.*, 1993); whole brain volume reductions of apparent genetic and environmental cause (Noga *et al.*, 1996); but, in a smaller study, no apparent differences in whole brain or thalamus (Bridle *et al.*, 2002).

In the largest ROI twin study so far, Baare *et al.* (2001) examined 15 MZ and 14 DZ twin pairs discordant for schizophrenia and 29 healthy twin pairs. They found within-pair similarity to be greater in MZ twins for intracranial, whole brain, frontal lobe, and hippocampal volumes (and evidence of a high degree of genetic control on the size of the lateral ventricles in healthy twins only). By comparison the intraclass correlation coefficient for the parahippocampal gyrus and third ventricle was lower in discordant MZ than healthy MZ pairs, suggesting primarily environmental effects. The affected twins had smaller brains, more extracerebral cerebrospinal fluid (CSF) and larger lateral ventricles. Therefore, sMRI ROI (and CT) twin studies suggest that most volumetric reductions represent both genetic and environmental effects, but reductions in whole brain and frontal lobes may be more genetic (cf. Lawrie *et al.*, 2001) and increases in the ventricles (in schizophrenia) more environmental. They disagree about the attribution for hippocampal decrements.

Automated structural magnetic resonance imaging studies in relatives

Cannon *et al.* (2002a) constructed probabilistic cortical surface maps in MZ and DZ discordant twins and control twins. Twin group effects (as MZ > DZ > control twin differences) and intraclass correlation coefficient maps (MZ > DZ) highlighted apparently genetic deficits in the poles of the frontal and temporal lobes, the dorsolateral prefrontal cortex, and Broca's and Wernicke's areas. MZ affected status contrasts, and findings of higher intraclass correlation coefficients in healthy than in diseased pairs, suggested environmental effects in the dorsolateral prefrontal cortex and parts of the temporal lobe (including Heschl's gyrus), which were correlated with symptom severity (especially negative) and cognitive dysfunction (especially on memory tasks). Narr *et al.* (2002) used a similar technique to map hippocampal surface morphology in the same twin groups and found both schizophrenia and genetic liability effects. Overall, these studies are compatible with our own findings of effects in parts of the frontal and temporal lobes that were greatest in schizophrenia patients and intermediate in high-risk subjects, compared with controls (Job *et al.*, 2003), with genetic effects being most evident medially. Ananth *et al.* (2002) have also shown that a family history of schizophrenia is negatively correlated with medial prefrontal gray matter. Meyer-Lindenberg *et al.* (2001) have published preliminary results showing dorsolateral prefrontal cortex differences that were greatest in schizophrenia patients, intermediate in their siblings, and least apparant in controls. They also showed anterior hippocampal reductions in gray matter density in patients compared with their siblings. The emergent picture is, therefore, of familial, probably genetic, effects that are generalized but perhaps most evident frontally and in the medial temporal lobe; these effects are likely to be at least partially evident early in development. Phenotypic and possibly later effects may be relatively greater in the temporal cortex.

Structural magnetic resonance imaging studies of siblings, parents, and offspring

The underlying rationale of examining the first-degree relatives of patients with schizophrenia is that they share approximately 50% of their genome and that common differences versus controls probably reflect genetic factors, while differences between unaffected and affected relatives presumably represent phenotypic effects. It is clear that these studies cannot in themselves distinguish genetic and environmental causation, but as schizophrenia is usually found to reflect mainly genetic factors, with a relatively small unique environmental effect and almost no familial environment involvement (e.g. Cannon *et al.*, 1998a; McGuffin *et al.*, 1994), the commonalities between patients and their relatives are probably genetic.

Most of these relatives studies have examined the volumes of the lateral ventricles and/or the AHCs. Only one study has reported significantly enlarged lateral ventricles in relatives compared with controls (Sharma *et al.*, 1998), although most of the studies in siblings (Cannon *et al.*, 1998b; Seidman *et al.*, 1999; Staal *et al.*, 2000) or offspring (Keshavan *et al.*, 1997, 2002; Lawrie *et al.*, 1999, 2001; Schreiber *et al.*, 1999) indicate such enlargement. The few comparisons of patients and siblings are universally significant (Cannon *et al.*, 1998b; McDonald *et al.*, 2002; Sharma *et al.*, 1998; Staal *et al.*, 2000), as are the twin studies, suggesting stronger environmental and phenotypic effects. Indeed, in older "obligate gene carriers," lateral ventriculomegaly (McDonald *et al.*, 2002; Sharma *et al.*, 1998) has not yet been externally replicated (Steel *et al.*, 2002). The increased VBR seen by CT in relatives may, therefore, primarily reflect a reduction in brain volume, although the results on sMRI are equivocal. While some studies find the brain is smaller in relatives than in controls (Cannon *et al.*, 1998b; Keshavan *et al.*, 1997, 2002), and no patient–relative differences (Cannon *et al.*, 1998b; McDonald *et al.*, 2002; Seidman *et al.*, 2002), many find no differences (McDonald *et al.*, 2002; Seidman *et al.*, 1999, 2002; Sharma *et al.*, 1998; Staal *et al.*, 1998) and one small study did actually find differences between "obligate carriers" and their affected siblings (Steel *et al.*, 2002).

The evidence from studies of relatives is also inconclusive for most other brain regions, in some cases because of insufficient studies and in others because of low power. There are, for example, isolated reports of abnormal cerebral torque (Sharma *et al.*, 1999), but the most consistent abnormalities in patients (Table 19.1) have not been found in relatives (Bartley *et al.*, 1993; Frangou *et al.*, 1997); findings of abnormal sylvian fissure (Honer *et al.*, 1995) and AHC asymmetry (Schreiber *et al.*, 1999) have yet to be replicated (Bartley *et al.*, 1993). There is, however, a fair degree of agreement with the twin and automated studies reviewed above for frontotemporal differences with a pattern of most effect seen in schizophrenia patients compared with controls and intermediate effects in relatives. The main support for this from ROI studies in relatives is a trend from a large study using sophisticated segmentation algorithms (Cannon *et al.*, 1998b), and from studies contrasting patients with their unaffected relatives (McDonald *et al.*, 2002; Staal *et al.*, 2000; Steel *et al.*, 2002). Small (Keshavan *et al.*, 1997, 2002; Schreiber *et al.*, 1999) and large (Lawrie *et al.*, 2001) studies of high-risk offspring have not found such differences, and neither have medium-sized studies that did not control for family membership (Sharma *et al.*, 1998). It appears that the relatively small effects can also be detected with automated approaches and/or control for between-family variance.

The importance of statistical power is again illustrated in studies of the third ventricle and the thalamus (the increase in the former probably relating to reductions in the latter and other surrounding structures). The two studies that did not find changes in the third ventricle (Schreiber *et al.*, 1999) and the thalamus (Keshavan *et al.*, 1997) were the two smallest were offspring studies (15 and 11 patients, respectively). Keshavan *et al.* (2002) found thalamus reductions when they increased the sample size from 11 to 19. Differences have, however, been found with samples as small as six (Seidman *et al.*, 1997) and all of the available literature suggests that third ventricle increases and/or thalamus reductions occur in relatives compared with controls (Keshavan *et al.*, 1997, 2002; Lawrie *et al.*, 2001; McDonald *et al.*, 2002; Seidman *et al.*, 1997, 1999; Staal *et al.*, 1998, 2000). Very few studies have looked at patient–relative differences. Staal *et al.* (1998) found that the thalamus was smaller in patients than in their siblings, while thalamus reductions were related to genetic liability but not psychotic symptoms in the Edinburgh High Risk Study (Lawrie *et al.*, 2001). Third ventricle volumes are consistently reported as trends in patient–relative differences (Lawrie *et al.*, 2001; McDonald *et al.*, 2002; Staal *et al.*, 1998), suggesting that environmental influences on third ventricle increases may be related to disease expression.

The studies of relatives do make clear that reductions in the AHC or its component structures are both genetic and phenotypic. In terms of relative differences, patients are generally found to have smaller AHCs than their unaffected relatives, and relatives are generally found to have smaller AHCs than healthy controls (Table 19.2). In terms of statistical significance, relatives have smaller AHCs than controls (Keshavan *et al.*, 1997, 2002; Lawrie *et al.*, 1999, 2001; Schreiber *et al.*, 1999; Seidman *et al.*, 1997, 1999), and schizophrenia patients have smaller AHCs than relatives (Lawrie *et al.*, 1999, 2001; O'Driscoll *et al.*, 2001; Steel *et al.*, 2002), although there are some negative studies (Staal *et al.*, 2000). There are suggestions that the reductions may be more marked anteriorly (Keshavan *et al.*, 2002; O'Driscoll *et al.*, 2001) and on the left side (Keshavan *et al.*, 2002; Lawrie *et al.*, 2001; but see Schreiber *et al.*, 1999). There is, however, good evidence for hippocampal differences as well (Seidman *et al.*, 2002; Waldo *et al.*, 1994; see also van Erp *et al.*, 2002).

Schizotypal personality disorder

The SPD is widely regarded as a genetic variant of, and a risk factor for, schizophrenia. Imaging abnormalities in SPD could, therefore, identify genetic and premorbid effects, although there are, as yet, comparatively few studies and even fewer replicated results. Two CT studies, from the same research group, found larger VBRs in those with SPD than in those with other personality disorders (Siever *et al.*, 1995) or indeed in unaffected siblings (Silverman *et al.*, 1998). However, studies distinguishing brain and ventricles in SPD suggest that the genetic similarities may arise in reduced whole brain grey matter and increased CSF (Cannon *et al.*, 1994; Dickey *et al.*, 2000), and that only patients with schizophrenia have enlarged lateral ventricles (Buchsbaum *et al.*, 1997; Dickey *et al.*, 2000; Levitt *et al.*, 2002). There are replicated accounts of common reductions in the superior temporal gyrus, which might be related to common features such as "disordered thinking" (Dickey *et al.*, 1999; Downhill *et al.*, 2001), but these studies disagree as to whether other reductions in the temporal lobe, and particularly in medial structures, are evident.

Imaging specific gene effects

By far the best indication of genetic effects is, of course, to relate gene frequency or expression directly to specific regional volumes. This approach is obviously limited

Table 19.2. Region of interest studies of the amygdala–hippocampal complex in patients with schizophrenia, their relatives and/or controls

Reference	Study populations	Differences (%)	
		Relatives versus schizophrenia	Relatives versus controls
Suddath et al. (1990)	15 pairs discordant MZ twins	Left Hipp. +11% Right Hipp. +9%	– –
Waldo et al. (1994)	11 schizophrenia, 20 siblings, 13 controls	Left Amyg. −2% Right Amyg. −2% Left Hipp. +7% Right Hipp. +5%	Left Amyg. −13% Rightt Amyg. +2% Left Hipp. +6% Right Hipp. +2%
Schreiber et al. (1999)	15 adolescent offspring, 15 controls	–	Both AHC −11%
Staal et al. (2000)	16 schizophrenia, 16 siblings, 32 controls	Both Amyg. +15% Both Hipp. +6%	Both Amyg. no change Both Hipp. +1%
Baare et al. (2001)	15 MZ discordant twin pairs (15 DZ discordant twin pairs, 15 controls (matched to well co-twin)	Left AHC +4% Right AHC +2%	Left AHC −8% Right AHC −6%
Lawrie et al. (2001)	34 First-episode schizophrenia, 147 high risk, 36 controls	Left AHC +4% Right AHC +2%	Left AHC −4% Right AHC −2%
O'Driscoll et al. (2001)	20 mixed relatives, 14 controls	– –	Left Ant. AHC −8% Right Ant. AHC −9% Left Post. AHC +4% Right Post. AHC −3%
Harris et al. (2002)	6 schizophrenia, 12 parents, 6 controls	Both Hipp. −2%	Both Hipp. +40%
Keshavan et al. (2002)	17 offspring, 22 controls	– –	Left Ant. AHC −25% Right Ant. AHC −12% Left Post. AHC −12% Right Post. AHC −10%
Seidman et al. (2002)	18 schizophrenia, 18 relatives, 48 controls	Left Hipp. −1% Right Hipp +4%	Left Hipp. −12% Right Hipp. +2%
Steel et al. (2002)	6 schizophrenia, 6 obligate, 6 control siblings	Both AHC +8% Left AHC +8% Right AHC +10%	Both AHC −5% Left AHC −5% Right AHC −4%

MZ, monozygotic; DZ, dizygotic; Hipp., hippocampus; Amyg., amygdala; AHC, amygdala–hippocampal complex; Ant., anterior; Post., posterior.

by our knowledge of the genes that increase the liability to schizophrenia. That being said, a small number of studies have directly examined the associations of some putative genes. With probably the greatest justification, Kunugi et al. (1999) examined the relationship between hippocampal volume and the gene for neurotrophin 3 (NT-3) (A3 allele) in a small number of patients with schizophrenia and bipolar disorder. NT-3 A3 allelic status was associated with smaller volumes only in schizophrenia patients: the absence of an effect in those with bipolar disorder suggesting a possible interaction with other schizophrenia genes or environmental risk factors. Any association between hippocampal volume and apolipoprotein E genotype in schizophrenia is at best unreplicated (Fernandez et al., 1999; Hata et al., 2002). Finally, increased VBR and enlarged CSF spaces have been found to be associated with a linkage marker on chromosome 5p in one large pedigree. This is of note as the imaging findings (presumably reflecting generally reduced brain volumes) were more strongly associated with the gene than with the disorder (Shihabuddin et al., 1996). There is, fortunately, rather stronger evidence for specific environmental effects: particularly with arguably the best replicated risk factor, namely OCs.

Obstetric complications

There is actually quite good evidence that people with family histories of schizophrenia do not suffer a greater number of or any more severe OCs. Rather, they appear to be more sensitive to their effects – perhaps because they already have abnormal brains. There is also an extensive literature on the clinical and imaging abnormalities associated with OCs in neonates; a wide array of adverse events have the potential to cause ventriculomegaly, periventricular leucomalacia, and/or hippocampal damage, with a range of neurodevelopmental outcomes. What specificity there is in any relationship between OCs and brain damage in schizophrenia will, therefore, arise from gene–environment interactions. It is on this basis that a number of studies have examined the association between OCs and enlarged ventricles or reduced hippocampi in schizophrenia patients and related populations.

Ventricles

As with family history, studies of the associations between OCs and CT indices in schizophrenia have produced inconsistent results. The largest CT studies of patients tended to find no association (Johnstone et al., 1989; Jones et al., 1994; Owens et al., 1985). Of 10 studies reviewed by Lewis (1990), five reported an association between OCs and ventriculomegaly and two of these were studies of relatives. Further, although Reveley et al. (1982) found an apparent environmental effect on the VBR in discordant MZ twins and controls, which they attributed to common delivery complications with more severe perinatal brain damage in the schizophrenia twin, they actually found a stronger association between OCs and ventricular size in the controls (Reveley *et al.*, 1984). DeLisi *et al.* (1986) also suggested part genetic and part environmental explanations for ventriculomegaly in their sample and found such an effect for the frontal horns; however, both OCs and a history of head injury in childhood were related to ventricular body enlargement, with no effect attributable to a later diagnosis of schizophrenia.

Data from the Copenhagen High Risk Project strongly suggest a gene–environment interaction. In the 27 high-risk subjects who were scanned initially and whose midwife records were available, birth weight was inversely correlated (0.6) with the VBR. There were weaker correlations with duration of labor and length at birth (Schulsinger *et al.*, 1984). Those with relatively lower weight (and those with signs of prematurity) were more likely to have VBRs above the group median, with stronger correlations in those who had subsequently developed schizophrenia (0.77) than in those who had not (Silverton *et al.*, 1985). On stepwise regression, birth weight accounted for 22% of the variance in VBR in the high-risk group, but 64% in the UHR group with schizotypal fathers (Silverton *et al.*, 1988a). There was no apparent effect of genetic risk alone, maternal illness, or maternal neglect (Silverton *et al.*, 1988b). More sophisticated analysis revealed that an increased VBR (and third ventricle width) was particularly related to an interaction between the level of genetic risk and the severity of delivery complications, with a smaller effect of low birth weight and no significant effect of total pregnancy complications (Cannon *et al.*, 1989). Increasing the sample to 157 subjects, with none, one, or two affected parents, replicated these findings (Cannon *et al.*, 1993).

A history of OCs has also been related to enlarged ventricles on sMRI in schizophrenia patients (Alvir *et al.*, 1999) and in relatives. Following Suddath *et al.* (1990), McNeil *et al.* (2000) examined an extended sample of 22 discordant MZ twin pairs and found that those with schizophrenia and large (right lateral and total) ventricle volumes were more likely to have had labor and neonatal problems, in addition to a prolonged labor, but no more total adverse events throughout the pregnancy. More recently, Cannon *et al.* (2002b) compared 64 patients, 51 of their unaffected siblings, and 54 controls with obstetric records of hypoxia, prematurity, being small for dates and any perinatal complication. Hypoxic complications interacted with genetic risk to reduce whole-brain gray matter volumes, especially in the temporal lobe and in schizophrenia patients, with tendencies to do so for sulcal and ventricular CSF. Prematurity, small for gestational age status, and prenatal infection had similar effects but were not associated with adult schizophrenia and mainly rendered the brain more sensitive to the effects of hypoxia.

Hippocampi

There is also some good evidence that OCs are related to small hippocampi in schizophrenia, possibly through gene–environment interaction. A small study of patients with a positive family history found no differences in limbic areas between those with and without a history of birth complications (DeLisi et al., 1988), while Stefanis and colleagues (1999) found smaller (left) hippocampi in patients with a history of pregnancy and birth complications, but not in patients from multiply affected families without OCs. McNeil et al. (2000) reported that intrapair differences in hippocampal volumes between discordant MZ twins were related to a prolonged labor (rather than neonatal complications). Using original hospital records, and focusing on hypoxic events and "blue babies," van Erp et al. (2002) found that 72 patients had smaller hippocampi than 58 siblings, who, in turn, had smaller volumes than healthy controls, but only schizophrenia patients with documented OCs had smaller hippocampi (siblings with OCs did not). The fact that OC frequency was equal across the groups argues against gene–environment covariation, and the relatively small effect size for hypoxia in the probands (0.24) suggests a sensitivity to the effects of OCs in those destined to develop schizophrenia. Further, the intraclass correlation coefficients for healthy sibling pairs were higher than for discordant pairs, suggesting that genetic influences on hippocampal volume are larger in health than in schizophrenia, and that large genetic variation and/or unique environmental events influence hippocampal volume in schizophrenia patients.

Other obstetric complications

One possible non-shared environmental factor is exposure to infection in utero. This is, however, rare and difficult to verify. Small and so far unreplicated studies have reported associations between reduced intracranial volume in patients with schizophrenia and first-trimester famine (Hulshoff Pol et al., 2000) or congenital rubella (Lim et al., 1995). Sanderson et al. (2001) found that a small number of patients with a history of early meningitis had reduced AHCs. Season of birth was a widely examined proxy for possible in utero infection in previous years, but most studies find no association between the VBR and time of birth (e.g. DeQuardo et al., 1996; Silverton et al., 1988b). By far the largest study did, however, find that patients born between December and April had greater VBRs than those born in other months (Sacchetti et al., 1992). This and the Lim et al. (1995) study are of additional interest as neither found any apparent increases in CSF, as would be expected of an early disruption in brain growth but contrary to what is usually found in schizophrenia (see Table 19.1 and below).

Summary

There is fairly persuasive evidence that OCs, particularly labor complications and proven hypoxia in neonates, interact with genetic risk for schizophrenia to produce larger lateral ventricles and smaller hippocampi. It may be that a genetically small, abnormal brain and other OCs increase the susceptibility to these effects. These effects are likely to be observable at birth, although there is no direct evidence for this. There are, however, indications that animals exposed experimentally to hypoxemia in utero have these types of abnormality around term (e.g. Rees *et al.*, 1999). As during early development the enlarging brain drives intracranial volume expansion, an early developmental disruption should not be associated with increases in cortical CSF (Woods, 1998); yet cortical CSF is known to be enlarged in schizophrenia and appears to be related to genetic effects (see above). The implication is that a small brain in schizophrenia is, at least in part, attributable to postnatal events.

Neurodevelopment and premorbid adjustment

Various neurodevelopmental abnormalities and social difficulties are known both to predate and to increase the risk of schizophrenia (Cannon and Jones, 1996). Although there are a few studies reporting an association between left handedness or neurological "soft signs" and an increased VBR on CT, most of the evidence and the largest studies do not find relationships with early development, academic record, or premorbid social functioning (Johnstone *et al.*, 1989; Jones *et al.*, 1994; Lewis, 1990; Owens *et al.*, 1985), and some studies have even reported better function and adjustment in those with larger VBRs. Associations between these retrospective measures and ROI volumes on sMRI are no more consistent. Correlations have, for example, been reported between premorbid adjustment and overall gray matter volume in women (Gur *et al.*, 1999), hippocampal volume in men (Gur *et al.*, 2000), and ventral frontal cortex volume, but not whole brain, in both sexes (Chemerinski *et al.*, 2002). Fannon *et al.* (2000) reported an association between the severity of various developmental problems and ventricular volumes. There is no knowing how many times similar associations have been examined, found to be negative, and not published.

Prospectively acquired data are likely to be much more reliable and there are two reports of interest. In the Copenhagen High Risk Project, social work ratings of scholastic and occupational adjustment at ages 15, 20, and 25 were worse in those with enlarged ventricles on CT (Erel *et al.*, 1991). Childhood home video ratings of early neuromotor deficits and negative affect were associated with ventricular enlargement on sMRI, while reported externalizing behavioral problems were related to smaller brains (Walker *et al.*, 1996). The lack of consistent correlations with structural measures on both CT and sMRI may, however, suggest that function is more heavily determined by other factors and/or that there are structural changes nearer to the time of psychosis. As the evidence for the latter is increasing, one might expect that likely precipitants for schizophrenia – such as stressful life events and cannabis consumption – have been examined in relation to these findings. This does not appear to have happened as yet, at least in relation to schizophrenia. While there are some studies of the structural effects of cannabis in non-psychotic subjects, they are far from conclusive. There are a number of studies in anxiety and depression suggesting that predisposing and precipitating stressors are associated with reduced volumes of the hippocampus (reviewed by Sapolsky, 2000). Such research is now surely a priority, both to build up a coherent picture of the pathophysiology of schizophrenia and because it may well have therapeutic implications.

Conclusions

The results of sMRI studies of twins and of relatives of patients with schizophrenia strongly suggest that at least some of the neuroanatomical features of the disorder are present before onset and probably for some time. It is likely that reductions in the volumes of the whole brain and frontal lobes are primarily genetically mediated and that this partly accounts for reductions in the amygdala and hippocampus. Increases in ventricular size and further reductions in the hippocampus are likely to occur around the time of labor complications. This does not preclude later developmental changes (some of which could be genetic) or degenerative effects. Relatively little is known about structural brain development in childhood and adolescence, in health and schizophrenia, but inference from the degrees of abnormality found in the above studies suggests that there are further changes in frontal and especially temporal lobes, perhaps particularly in medial structures, shortly before and possibly after the onset of psychosis.

More of the same studies can be justified on the grounds that no finding is as yet conclusive. However, ROI studies should probably have minimum group sizes of about 60 – unless variance is reduced by recruiting within families – if subtle differences in the brain and ventricles are to be examined, and particularly if gene–environment interactions are to be assessed. More specific regional effects are probably best assessed with automated approaches. It should be clear that case–control and prospective cohort studies of those at elevated risk, for both genetic and other reasons, are complementary. There may also be important information gained from studies of early-onset schizophrenia and related neurodevelopmental disorders. Other analyses of sMRI data, such as calculating the gyral folding index, and novel uses of MRI, such as proton spectroscopy and diffusion tensor imaging, could give additional insights (but have not been described in this chapter as there are as yet only interesting suggestions and no replicated findings in relatives).

Perhaps the greatest gains in knowledge will arise from more novel approaches. For example, ultrasound images of fetal and neonatal brains could be used to study the time course of the effects of genetic and environmental risk factors relevant to schizophrenia: although studying demonstrable effects rather than even well-documented risks may be most relevant. Levels of psychosocial stress and cannabis consumption need to be related to brain structure in subjects at high risk. Most importantly, specific genetic abnormalities in schizophrenia (once clearly identified) may have regionally and temporally specific effects. The search for these genes is, of course, informed by the foregoing studies, and both will be informed by advances in the knowledge of the genetics and imaging of normal neurodevelopment.

It will take some time before these developments lead to a sophisticated understanding of the time course of subregional anatomical differences in schizophrenia, but it is not too early to begin to think about therapeutic implications. There is good evidence, for example, that hypothermic treatment of hypoxic brains may reduce the number of adverse neurodevelopmental outcomes. Once specified, structural predictors of psychosis would provide a means of identifying subjects at very high risk of conversion. This might justify early interventions to reduce stress or cannabis use, and perhaps to prescribe antipsychotic or neuroprotective drugs, which might ameliorate or even prevent the devastating effects of schizophrenia.

REFERENCES

Alvir, J. M. J., Woerner, M. G., Gunduz, H., Degreef, G., Lieberman, J. A. (1999). Obstretric complications predict treatment response in first-episode schizophrenia. *Psychol Med* **29**: 621–627.

Ananth, H., Popescu, I., Critchley, H. D., *et al.* (2002). Cortical and subcortical gray matter abnormalities in schizophrenia determined through structural magnetic resonance imaging with optimized volumetric voxel-based morphometry. *Am J Psychiatry* **159**: 1497–1505.

Baare, W. F., van Oel, C. J., Hulshoff Pol, H. E., *et al.* (2001). Volumes of brain structures in twins discordant for schizophrenia. *Arch Gen Psychiatry* **58**: 33–40.

Bartley, A. J., Jones, D. W., Torrey, E. F., Zigun, J. R., Weinberger, D. R. (1993). Sylvian fissure asymmetries in monozygotic twins: a test of laterality in schizophrenia. *Biol Psychiatry* **34**: 853–863.

Bridle, N., Pantelis, C., Wood, S. J., *et al.* (2002). Thalamic and caudate volumes in monozygotic twins discordant for schizophrenia. *Aust N Z J Psychiatry* **36**: 347–354.

Buchsbaum, M. S., Yang, S., Hazlett, E., *et al.* (1997). Ventricular volume and asymmetry in schizotypal personality disorder and schizophrenia assessed with magnetic resonance imaging. *Schizophr Res* **27**: 45–53.

Cannon, M., Jones, P. (1996). Schizophrenia. *J Neurol Neurosurg Psychiatry* **61**: 604–613.

Cannon, T. D., Mednick, S. A., Parnas, J. (1989). Genetic and perinatal determinants of structural brain deficits in schizophrenia. *Arch Gen Psychiatry* **46**: 883–889.

Cannon, T. D., Mednick, S. A., Parnas, J., *et al.* (1993). Developmental brain abnormalities in the offspring of schizophrenic mothers. I. Contributions of genetic and perinatal factors. *Arch Gen Psychiatry* **50**: 551–564.

(1994). Developmental brain abnormalities in the offspring of schizophrenic mothers. II. Structural brain characteristics of schizophrenia and schizotypal personality disorder. *Arch Gen Psychiatry* **51**: 955–962.

Cannon, T. D., Kaprio, J., Lönnqvist, J., Huttunen, M., Koskenvuo, M. (1998a). The genetic epidemiology of schizophrenia in a Finnish twin cohort. *Arch Gen Psychiatry* **55**: 67–74.

Cannon, T. D., van Erp, T. G., Huttunen, M., *et al.* (1998b). Regional gray matter, white matter, and cerebrospinal fluid distributions in schizophrenic patients, their siblings, and controls. *Arch Gen Psychiatry* **55**: 1084–1091.

Cannon, T. D., Thompson, P. M., van Erp, T. G., *et al.* (2002a). Cortex mapping reveals regionally specific patterns of genetic and disease-specific gray-matter deficits in twins discordant for schizophrenia. *Proc Natl Acad Sci USA* **99**: 3228–3233.

Cannon, T. D., van Erp, T. G., Rosso, I. M., *et al.* (2002b). Fetal hypoxia and structural brain abnormalities in schizophrenic patients, their siblings, and controls. *Arch Gen Psychiatry* **59**: 35–41.

Chemerinski, E., Nopoulos, P. C., Crespo-Facorro, B., Andreasen, N. C., Magnotta, V. (2002). Morphology of the ventral frontal cortex in schizophrenia: relationship with social dysfunction. *Biol Psychiatry* **52**: 1–8.

Copolov, D., Velakoulis, D., McGorry, P., *et al.* (2000). Neurobiological findings in early phase schizophrenia. *Brain Res Rev* **31**: 157–165.

Dauphinais, I. D., DeLisi, L. E., Crow, T. J., *et al.* (1990). Reduction in temporal lobe size in siblings with schizophrenia: a magnetic resonance imaging study. *Psychiatry Res* **35**: 137–147.

DeLisi, L. E., Goldin, L. R., Hamovit, J. R., *et al.* (1986). A family study of the association of increased ventricular size with schizophrenia. *Arch Gen Psychiatry* **43**: 148–153.

DeLisi, L. E., Dauphinais, I. D., Gershon, E. S. (1988). Perinatal complications and reduced size of brain limbic structures in familial schizophrenia. *Schizophr Bull* **14**: 185–191.

DeQuardo, J. R., Goldman, M., Tandon, R. (1996). VBR in schizophrenia: relationship to family history of psychosis and season of birth. *Schizophr Res* **20**: 275–285.

Dickey, C. C., McCarley, R. W., Voglmaier, M. M., *et al.* (1999). Schizotypal personality disorder and MRI abnormalities of temporal lobe gray matter. *Biol Psychiatry* **45**: 1393–1402.

Dickey, C. C., Shenton, M. E., Hirayasu, Y., *et al.* (2000). Large CSF volume not attributable to ventricular volume in schizotypal personality disorder. *Am J Psychiatry* **157**: 48–54.

Downhill, J. E., Buchsbaum, M. S., Hazlett, E. A., *et al.* (2001). Temporal lobe volume determined by magnetic resonance imaging in schizotypal personality disorder and schizophrenia. *Schizophr Res* **48**: 187–199.

Erel, O., Cannon, T. D., Hollister, J. M., Mednick, S. A., Parnas, J. (1991). Ventricular enlargement and premorbid deficits in school-occupational attainment in a high risk sample. *Schizophr Res* **4**: 49–52.

Falkai, P., Honer, W. G., Alfter, D., *et al.* (2002). The temporal lobe in schizophrenia from uni- and multiply affected families. *Neurosci Lett* **325**: 25–28.

Fannon, D., Tennakoon, L., Sumich, A., *et al.* (2000). Third ventricle enlargement and developmental delay in first-episode psychosis: preliminary findings. *Br J Psychiatry* **177**: 354–359.

Fernandez, T., Yan, W. L., Hamburger, S., *et al.* (1999). Apolipoprotine E alleles in childhood-onset schizophrenia. *Am J Med Genet* **88**: 211–213.

Frangou, S., Sharma, T., Sigmudsson, T., *et al.* (1997). The Maudsley Family Study 4. Normal planum temporale asymmetry in familial schizophrenia. *Br J Psychiatry* **170**: 328–333.

Gur, R. E., Turetsky, B. I., Bilker, W. B., Gur, R. C. (1999). Reduced gray matter volume in schizophrenia. *Arch Gen Psychiatry* **56**: 905–911.

Gur, R. E., Turetsky, B. I., Cowell, P. E., *et al.* (2000). Temporolimbic volume reductions in schizophrenia. *Arch Gen Psychiatry* **57**: 769–775.

Harris, J. G., Young, D. A., Rojas, D. C., *et al.* (2002). Increased hippocampal volume in schizophrenics' parents with ancestral history of schizophrenia. *Schizophr Res* **55**: 11–17.

Hata, T., Kunugi, H., Nanko, S., Fukuda, R., Kaminaga, T. (2002). Possible effect of the APOE e4 allele on the hippocampal volume and asymmetry in schizophrenia. *Am J Med Genet Neuropsychiatr Genet* **114**: 641–642.

Honer, W. G., Bassett, A. S., Squires-Wheeler, E., *et al.* (1995). The temporal lobes, reversed asymmetry and the genetics of schizophrenia. *Neuroreport* **7**: 221–224.

Hulshoff Pol, H. E., Hoek, H. W., Susser, E., *et al.* (2000). Prenatal exposure to famine and brain morphology in schizophrenia. *Am J Psychiatry* **157**: 1170–1172.

Job, D. E., Whalley, H. C., McConnell, S., *et al.* (2002). Structural gray matter differences between first-episode schizophrenics and normal controls on voxel-based morphometry. *Neuroimage* **17**: 880–889.

Job, D. E., Whalley, H. C., Glabus, M., Johnstone E. C., Lawrie, S. M. (2003). Voxel-based morphometry of grey matter reductions in subjects at high risk of schizophrenia. *Schizophr Res* **64**: 1–13.

Johnstone, E. C., Owens, D. G., Bydder, G. M., *et al.* (1989). The spectrum of structural brain changes in schizophrenia: age of onset as a predictor of cognitive and clinical impairments and their cerebral correlates. *Psychol Med* **19**: 91–103.

Johnstone, E. C., Cosway, R., Lawrie, S. M. (2002). Distinguishing characteristics of subjects with good and poor early outcome in the Edinburgh High Risk Study. *Br J Psychiatry* **181**: S26–S29.

Jones, P. B., Harvey, I., Lewis, S. W., *et al.* (1994). Cerebral ventricle dimensions as risk factors for schizophrenia and affective psychosis: an epidemiological approach to analysis. *Psychol Med* **24**: 995–1011.

Keshavan, M. S., Montrose, D. M., Pierri, J. N., *et al.* (1997). Magnetic resonance imaging and spectroscopy in offspring at risk for schizophrenia: preliminary studies. *Prog Neuropsychopharmacol Biol Psychiatry* **21**: 1285–1295.

Keshavan, M. S., Dick, E., Mankowski, I., *et al.* (2002). Decreased left amygddala and hippocampal volumes in young offspring at risk for schizophrenia. *Schizophr Res* **58**: 173–183.

Konick, L. C., Friedman, L. (2001). Meta-analysis of thalamic size in schizophrenia. *Biol Psychiatry* **49**: 28–38.

Kunugi, H., Hattori, M., Nanko, S., *et al.* (1999). Dinucleotide repeat polymorphism in the neurotrophin-3 gene and hippocampal volume in psychoses. *Schizophr Res* **37**: 271–273.

Lawrie, S. M., Abukmeil, S. S. (1998). Brain abnormality in schizophrenia. A systematic and quantitative review of volumetric magnetic resonance imaging studies. *Br J Psychiatry* **172**: 110–120.

Lawrie, S. M., Whalley, H., Kestelman, J. N., *et al.* (1999). Magnetic resonance imaging of brain in people at high risk of developing schizophrenia. *Lancet* **353**: 30–33.

Lawrie, S. M., Adams, C. E., Thornley, B., Joy, C. (2000). Comprehensiveness of systematic review: update. *Br J Psychiatry* **176**: 396–401.

Lawrie, S. M., Whalley, H. C., Abukmeil, S. S., *et al.* (2001). Brain structure, genetic liability and psychotic symptoms in subjects at high risk of developing schizophrenia. *Biol Psychiatry* **49**: 811–823.

(2002). Temporal lobe volume changes in subjects at high risk of schizophrenia with psychotic symptoms. *Br J Psychiatry* **181**: 138–143.

Levitt, J. J., McCarley, R. W., Dickey, C. C., *et al.* (2002). MRI study of caudate nucleus volume and its cognitive correlates in neuroleptic-naive patients with schizotypal personality disorder. *Am J Psychiatry* **159**: 1190–1197.

Lewis, S. W. (1990). Computerised tomography in schizophrenia 15 years on. *Br J Psychiatry* **157**: 16–24.

Lim, K. O., Beal, D. M., Harvey, Jr., R. L., *et al.* (1995). Brain dysmorphology in adults with congenital rubella plus schizophrenia-like symptoms. *Biol Psychiatry* **37**: 764–776.

McDonald, C., Grech, A., Toulopoulou, T., *et al.* (2002). Brain volumes in familial and non-familial schizophrenic probands and their unaffected relatives. *Am J Med Genet (Neuropsychiatric Genetics)* **114**: 616–625.

McGuffin, P., Asherson, P., Owen, M., Farmer, A. (1994). The strength of the genetic effect. Is there room for an environmental influence in the aetiology of schizophrenia? *Br J Psychiatry* **164**: 593–599.

McNeil, T. F., Cantor-Graae, E., Weinberger, D. R. (2000). Relationship of obstetric complications and differences in size of brain structures in monozygotic twin pairs discordant for schizophrenia. *Am J Psychiatry* **157**: 203–212.

Meyer-Lindenberg, A., Japee, S., Verchinski, B., *et al.* (2001). Structural MRI abnormalities in schizophrenic patients and their unaffected siblings: voxel-based morphometry. *Neuroimage* **13**: S217.

Mourot, A., d'Amato, T., Rochet, T., *et al.* (1997). Cerebral investigation of healthy siblings of schizophrenics. *Eur Psychiatry* **12**: 273–278.

Narr, K. L., van Erp, T. G., Cannon, T. D., *et al.* (2002). A twin study of genetic contributions to hippocampal morphology in schizophrenia. *Neurobiol Dis* **11**: 83–95.

Nelson, M. D., Saykin, A. J., Flashman, L. A., Riordan, H. J. (1998). Hippocampal volume reduction in schizophrenia as assessed by magnetic resonance imaging: a meta-analytic study. *Arch Gen Psychiatry* **55**: 433–440.

Noga, J. T., Bartley, A. J., Jones, D. W., Torrey, E. F., Weinberger, D. R. (1996). Cortical gyral anatomy and gross brain dimensions in monozygotic twins discordant for schizophrenia. *Schizophr Res* **22**: 27–40.

O'Driscoll, G. A., Florencio, P. S., Gagnon, D., *et al.* (2001). Amygdala–hippocampal volume and verbal memory in first-degree relatives of schizophrenic patients. *Psychiatry Res Neuroimaging* **107**: 75–85.

Owens, D. G., Johnstone, E. C., Crow, T. J., *et al.* (1985). Lateral ventricular size in schizophrenia: relationship to the disease process and its clinical manifestations. *Psychol Med* **15**: 27–41.

Paillere-Martinot, M., Caclin, A., Artiges, E., *et al.* (2001). Cerebral gray and white matter reductions and clinical correlates in patients with early onset schizophrenia. *Schizophr Res* **50**: 19–26.

Pantelis, C., Velakoulis, D., Suckling, J., *et al.* (2000). Left medial temporal volume reduction occurs during the transition from high-risk to first-episode psychosis. *Schizophr Res* **41**: 35.

Pantelis, C., Velakoulis, D., McGorry, P. D., *et al.* (2003). Neuroanatomical abnormalities before and after onset of psychosis: a cross-sectional and longitudinal MRI comparison. *Lancet* **361**: 281–288.

Phillips, L. J., Velakoulis, D., Pantelis, C., *et al.* (2002). Non-reduction in hippocampal volume is associated with higher risk of psychosis. *Schizophr Res* **58**: 145–158.

Raz, S., Raz, N. (1990). Structural brain abnormalities in the major psychoses: a quantitative review of the evidence from computerized imaging. *Psychol Bull* **108**: 93–108.

Rees, S., Breen, S., Loeliger, M., McCrabb, G., Harding, R. (1999). Hypoxemia near mid-gestation has long-term effects on fetal brain development. *J Neuropathol Exp Neurol* **58**: 932–945.

Reveley, A. M., Reveley, M. A., Clifford, C. A., Murray, R. M. (1982). Cerebral ventricular size in twins discordant for schizophrenia. *Lancet* **i**: 540–541.

Reveley, A. M., Reveley, M. A., Murray, R. M. (1984). Cerebral ventricular enlargement in non-genetic schizophrenia: a controlled twin study. *Br J Psychiatry* **144**: 89–93.

Roy, M. A., Flaum, M. A., Arndt, S. V., Crowe, R. R., Andreasen, N. C. (1994). Magnetic resonance imaging in familial versus sporadic cases of schizophrenia. *Psychiatry Res* **54**: 25–36.

Sacchetti, E., Calzeroni, A., Vita, A., *et al.* (1992). The brain damage hypothesis of the seasonality of births in schizophrenia and major affective disorders: evidence from computerised tomography. *Br J Psychiatry* **160**: 390–397.

Sanderson, T. L., Doody, G. A., Best, J., Owens, D. G. C., Johnstone, E. C. (2001). Correlations between clinical and historical variables and cerebral structural variables in people with mild intellectual disability and schizophrenia. *J Intellect Disabil Res* **45**: 89–98.

Sapolsky, R. M. (2000). Glucocorticoids and hippocampal atrophy in neuropsychiatric disorders. *Arch Gen Psychiatry* **57**: 925–935.

Schreiber, H., Baur-Seack, K., Kornhuber, H. H., *et al.* (1999). Brain morphology in adolescents at genetic risk for schizophrenia assessed by qualitative and quantitative magnetic resonance imaging. *Schizophr Res* **40**: 81–84.

Schulsinger, F., Parnas, J., Petersen, E. T., *et al.* (1984). Cerebral ventricular size in the offspring of schizophrenic mothers. *Arch Gen Psychiatry* **41**: 602–606.

Schwarzkopf, S. B., Nasrallah, H. A., Olson, S. C., Bogerts, B., McLaughlin, J. A., Mitra, T. (1991). Family history and brain morphology in schizophrenia: an MRI study. *Psychiatry Res* **40**: 49–60.

Seidman, L. J., Faraone, S. V., Goldstein, J. M., *et al.* (1997). Reduced subcortical brain volumes in nonpsychotic siblings of schizophrenic patients: a pilot magnetic resonance imaging study. *Am J Med Genet* **74**: 507–514.

(1999). Thalamic and amygdala-hippocampal volume reductions in first-degree relatives of patients with schizophrenia: an MRI-based morphometric analysis. *Biol Psychiatry* **46**: 941–954.

(2002). Left hippocampal volume as a vulnerability indicator for schizophrenia. *Arch Gen Psychiatry* **59**: 839–849.

Shapleske, J., Rossell, S. L., Woodruff, P. W. R., David, A. S. (1999). The planum temporale: a systematic, quantitative review of its structural, functional and clinical significance. *Brain Res Rev* **29**: 26–49.

Sharma, T., Lancaster, E., Lee, D., *et al.* (1998). Brain changes in schizophrenia. Volumetric MRI study of families multiply affected with schizophrenia: the Maudsley Family Study 5. *Br J Psychiatry* **173**: 132–138.

Sharma, T., Lancaster, E., Sigmundsson, T., *et al.* (1999). Lack of normal pattern of cerebral asymmetry in familial schizophrenic patients and their relatives: The Maudsley Family Study. *Schizophr Res* **40**: 111–120.

Shihabuddin, L., Silverman, J. M., Buchsbaum, M. S., *et al.* (1996). Ventricular enlargement associated with linkage marker for schizophrenia-related disorders in one pedigree. *Mol Psychiatry* **1**: 215–222.

Siever, L. J., Rotter, M., Losonczy, M., *et al.* (1995). Lateral ventricular enlargement in schizotypal personality disorder. *Psychiatry Res* **57**: 109–118.

Sigmundsson, T., Suckling, J., Maier, M., *et al.* (2001). Structural abnormalities in frontal, temporal, and limbic regions and interconnecting white matter tracts in schizophrenic patients with prominent negative symptoms. *Am J Psychiatry* **158**: 234–243.

Silverman, J. M., Smith, C. J., Guo, S. L., *et al.* (1998). Lateral ventricular enlargement in schizophrenic probands and their siblings with schizophrenia-related disorders. *Biol Psychiatry* **43**: 97–106.

Silverton, L., Finello, K. M., Schulsinger, F., Mednick, S. A. (1985). Low birth weight and ventricular enlargement in a high-risk sample. *J Abnorm Psychol* **94**: 405–409.

Silverton, L., Mednick, S. A., Schulsinger, F., Parnas, J., Harrington, M. E. (1988a). Genetic risk for schizophrenia, birthweight, and cerebral ventricular enlargement. *J Abnorm Psychol* **97**: 496–498.

Silverton, L., Mednick, S. A., Harrington, M. E. (1988b). Birthweight, schizophrenia and ventricular enlargement in a high-risk sample. *Psychiatry* **51**: 272–280.

Sommer, I., Aleman, A., Ramsey, N., Bouma, A., Kahn, R. (2001). Handedness, language lateralisation and anatomical asymmetry in schizophrenia. Meta-analysis. *Br J Psychiatry* **178**: 344–351.

Staal, W. G., Hulshoff, Pol, H. E., Schnack, H., van der Schot, A. C., Kahn, R. S. (1998). Partial volume decrease of the thalamus in relatives of patients with schizophrenia. *Am J Psychiatry* **155**: 1784–1786.

Staal, W. G., Hulshoff Pol, H. E., Schnack, H. G., *et al.* (2000). Structural brain abnormalities in patients with schizophrenia and their healthy siblings. *Am J Psychiatry* **157**: 416–421.

Steel, R., Whalley, H., Miller, P., *et al.* (2002). Structural MRI of the brain in presumed carriers of genes for schizophrenia, their affected and unaffected siblings. *J Neurol Neurosurg Psychiatry* **72**: 455–458.

Stefanis, N., Frangou, S., Yakeley, J., *et al.* (1999). Hippocampal volume reduction in schizophrenia: effects of genetic risk and pregnancy and birth complications. *Biol Psychiatry* **46**: 697–702.

Suddath, R. L., Christison, G. W., Torrey, E. F., Casanova, M. F., Weinberger, D. R. (1990). Anatomical abnormalities in the brains of monozygotic twins discordant for schizophrenia. *N Engl J Med* **322**: 789–794.

van Erp, T. G. M., Saleh, P. A., Rosso, I. M., *et al.* (2002). Contributions of genetic risk and fetal hypoxia to hippocampal volume in patients with schizophrenia or schizoaffective disorder, their unaffected siblings, and healthy unrelated volunteers. *Am J Psychiatry* **159**: 1514–1520.

van Horn, J. D., McManus, I. C. (1992). Ventricular enlargement in schizophrenia: a meta-analysis of studies of the ventricle: brain ratio (VBR). *Br J Psychiatry* **160**: 687–697.

Vita, A., Dieci, M., Giobbio, G. M., *et al.* (1994). A reconsideration of the relationship between cerebral structural abnormalities and family history of schizophrenia. *Psychiatry Res* **53**: 41–55.

Waldo, M. C., Cawthra, E., Adler, L. E., *et al.* (1994). Auditory sensory gating, hippocampal volume, and catecholamine metabolism in schizophrenics and their siblings. *Schizophr Res* **12**: 93–106.

Walker, E. F., Lewine, R. R., Neumann, C. (1996). Childhood behavioral characteristics and adult brain morphology in schizophrenia. *Schizophr Res* **22**: 93–101.

Ward, K. E., Friedman, L., Wise, A., Schulz, S. C. (1996). Meta-analysis of brain and cranial size in schizophrenia. *Schizophr Res* **22**: 197–213.

Weinberger, D. R., DeLisi, L. E., Neophytides, A. N., Wyatt, R. J. (1981). Familial aspects of CT scan abnormalities in chronic schizophrenic patients. *Psychiatry Res* **4**: 65–71.

Woodruff, P. W. R., McManus, I. C., David, A. S. (1995). Meta-analysis of corpus callosum size in schizophrenia. *J Neurol Neurosurg Psychiatry* **58**: 457–461.

Woods, B. T. (1998). Is schizophrenia a progressive neurodevelopmental disorder? Toward a unitary pathogenetic mechanism. *Am J Psychiatry* **155**: 1661–1670.

Wright, I. C., Rabe-Hesketh, S., Woodruff, P. W., *et al.* (2000). Meta-analysis of regional brain volumes in schizophrenia. *Am J Psychiatry* **157**: 16–25.

Zorrilla, L. T. E., Cannon, T. D., Kronenberg, S., *et al.* (1997). Structural brain abnormalities in schizophrenia: a family study. *Biol Psychiatry* **42**: 1080–1986.

20

Neurodegenerative models of schizophrenia

L. Fredrik Jarskog, John H. Gilmore, and Jeffrey A. Lieberman
University of North Carolina School of Medicine, Chapel Hill, USA

The concept of schizophrenia as a neurodegenerative disorder has a long and somewhat controversial past. Neurodegenerative aspects of schizophrenia were recognized early in the twentieth century by Kraeplin (1919), who described "dementia praecox" as a progressive illness with a deteriorating clinical course. This hypothesis was originally supported both by Alzheimer, who found evidence of cortical neuron loss, and by Southard, who described cerebral atrophy; however, investigators during the remainder of the twentieth century were largely unable to demonstrate consistent and replicable evidence of neurodegeneration (Pinals and Breier, 1997). The reframing of schizophrenia as a disorder of neurodevelopment was met with considerable interest, given the absence of a clear neuropathological phenotype to support a neurodegenerative hypothesis (Murray and Lewis, 1987; Weinberger, 1987). The neurodevelopmental hypothesis postulates that neurobiological insults can adversely influence the course of early neurodevelopment to yield permanent brain deficits; these ultimately manifest as psychosis during the second or third decades of life. Furthermore, it suggests that the illness runs a heterogeneous course following the onset of clinical symptoms but that no further pathophysiological consequences are incurred beyond those associated with normal maturation, aging, and treatment-related factors (Weinberger, 1987). Clearly, the neurodevelopmental hypothesis has substantially advanced our understanding of schizophrenia vis-à-vis the important role that developmental factors play in the etiology and pathophysiology of the disorder. Nevertheless, the neurodevelopmental perspective fails to account adequately for a number of cardinal features of schizophrenia, including the protracted period of symptomatic dormancy between the putative insult and the emergence of clinical symptoms, the progressive clinical deterioration that affects a significant subgroup of patients, recent evidence for progressive changes in ventricular and cortical brain structures, and the apparent ability of antipsychotic treatment to modify the course of the illness.

Neurodevelopment and Schizophrenia, ed. Matcheri S. Keshavan *et al.* Published by Cambridge University Press. © Cambridge University Press 2004.

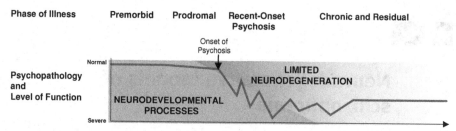

Fig. 20.1.   Model of schizophrenia as a limited neurodegenerative disorder with neurodevelopmental antecedents. The line represents the functional and psychopathological course of
schizophrenia superimposed over the proposed intersection of developmental and degenerative processes. As depicted, the degenerative pathophysiology is most active in the interval
surrounding the onset of psychosis and then attenuates with time.

A neurodegenerative disorder is, by definition, a progressive disease of the nervous system that is initiated by specific biochemical changes which ultimately lead
to a distinct histopathology with associated clinical manifestations (Hardy and
Gwinn-Hardy, 1998). The disorder often has an underlying genetic basis. The timing of the onset of clinical symptoms is usually influenced by the interaction of
the disease process with normal developmental and maturational processes, as well
as with the individual's capacity for adaptive neuroplastic responses. Thus, neurodegenerative disorders may remain clinically dormant until a threshold level of
pathophysiological damage has occurred. The absence of a histopathological phenotype in schizophrenia has been cited as evidence against a neurodegenerative
hypothesis (Weinberger and McClure, 2002). However, studies of schizophrenia
increasingly demonstrate subtle yet consistent histopathological deficits in addition to evidence of progressive clinical and neuroimaging findings. We believe
that schizophrenia can be considered as a limited neurodegenerative disorder with
neurodevelopmental antecedents (Fig. 20.1). Studies from clinical, neurocognitive,
neuroimaging, and neuropathological domains will be reviewed in a critical analysis
of this hypothesis.

Clinical psychopathology and neurocognition

As reviewed elsewhere in this volume, there is substantial evidence that patients in
the premorbid phase of schizophrenia have subtle abnormalities of motor, cognitive,
and social functioning. From this baseline of subtle impairment, most patients with
schizophrenia experience deterioration in overall level of functioning following the
formal onset of illness. This has been convincingly documented for a century by
numerous investigators (Huber *et al.*, 1980; Kraeplin, 1919; Pfohl and Winokur,
1982). Functional deterioration appears to occur mainly in the first 5 years following

the onset of psychosis and then reaches a plateau of stability (McGlashan, 1988). A more recent study suggests that the deterioration is confined to the first year of illness: Mason *et al.* (1996) found that social adjustment deteriorated in the first year of illness, though remained relatively stable over the next 13 years.

While there is general agreement that overall functioning declines in schizophrenia, it is not clear what factors contribute to this functional deterioration. The most parsimonious explanation for this deterioration may be that it is a consequence of the symptoms of schizophrenia itself: positive and negative symptoms, and cognitive dysfunction. Untreated or partially treated positive symptoms would obviously interfere with overall functioning and quality of life, and degeneration or progression of illness would not necessarily be involved. Both Eaton *et al.* (1995) and Mason *et al.* (1996) found that positive symptoms tend to remain stable after the first year of illness. There is evidence that primary negative symptoms or the deficit syndrome does progress in the early years of the illness. In a retrospective chart review study, Fenton and McGlashan (1994) found that primary negative symptoms progressed in severity over the first 5 years of the illness and that the deficit syndrome was associated with poor outcome and long-term disability. Mayerhoff *et al.* (1994) found that first-episode patients had lower rates of the deficit syndrome than more chronic populations, and Eaton *et al.* (1995) found that negative symptoms were stable after the first 2 years of illness. These studies suggest that progression of negative symptoms may be limited to the first few years of illness, though clarification of this issue awaits additional prospective longitudinal studies.

While initial studies reported progressive cognitive impairment in schizophrenia (Abrahamson, 1983; Bilder *et al.*, 1992; Smith, 1964), most of the more recent studies do not indicate a progression of cognitive dysfunction (reviewed by Rund, 1998). While cognitive decline has been described in geriatric, chronically institutionalized patients (Friedman *et al.*, 2002; Harvey *et al.*, 1999), a study of older outpatients found no differences in age-related cognitive decline (Zorrilla *et al.*, 2000). A more recent longitudinal study of neuropsychological deficits in older patients (mean age 47.6 years) with schizophrenia found them to be stable (Heaton *et al.*, 2001). These studies suggest that, if progressive deterioration of cognitive functioning occurs in older patients with schizophrenia, this deterioration is limited to a subset of very severely ill, chronically institutionalized patients. Cross-sectional comparisons of cognitive functioning in patients with first-episode and chronic schizophrenia have found similar degrees of impairment, suggesting that cognitive deficits do not progress (Addington and Addington, 2002; Moritz *et al.*, 2002; Saykin *et al.*, 1994). Longitudinal studies in patients with first-episode schizophrenia found either no progression (Hoff *et al.*, 1999) or even improvement of cognitive impairments (Nopoulos *et al.*, 1994).

Although available evidence suggests that neurocognitive deficits do not progress after the first episode of psychosis, recent data suggest that neurocognitive deterioration may occur during the premorbid and prodromal phases. Children who go on to develop schizophrenia have a variety of cognitive, motor, and social abnormalities in the premorbid stage of their illness (Cannon *et al.*, 2002; Done *et al.*, 1994; Jones *et al.*, 1994; Kremen *et al.*, 1994). In general, the impairment of patients in the premorbid and prodromal phases of the disease appears to be less severe than that documented after the formal onset of symptoms, suggesting that some deterioration has occurred. This is supported by a small study reporting that worsening neuropsychological deficits in prodromal patients tended to predict a transition to psychosis (Hambrecht *et al.*, 2002). The strength of this conclusion is limited by the few studies that have followed prodromal patient cohorts through the transition to psychosis. Nevertheless, the available data suggest that progressive cognitive impairment may occur prior to the first episode. This idea is supported by a recent study showing that children who go on to develop schizophrenia appear to have deterioration on a standardized scholastic test between grades 8 and 11 (Fuller *et al.*, 2002). This deterioration was not related to the age of onset, indicating that the deterioration preceded the first episode. Deterioration late in the premorbid phase, prior to formal onset of the illness, is also suggested in a study by Cannon *et al.* (1999), who found that children who went on to develop schizophrenia often did not attend or complete high school, even though they had normal academic performance in elementary school.

The weight of the evidence indicates that progression of cognitive deficits does occur at some time during the late premorbid, prodromal, or early first-episode phases of schizophrenia. Neurocognitive functioning appears to remain stable subsequent to the first episode, and there is no significant age-related decline in functioning except in very ill, chronically institutionalized patients. Primary negative symptoms appear to worsen during the first few years of the illness and remain stable thereafter. In a similar fashion, overall functional impairment worsens in the first few years of the illness and then stabilizes. If we infer neurodegeneration from the progression of these clinical components of schizophrenia, then the degeneration is limited to the late premorbid/prodromal phase and the first episode of the illness (Fig. 20.1). Thus, a neurodegenerative component would occur in the context of concomitant neurodevelopmental processes that normally operate during adolescence.

Postmortem neuropathology

During the twentieth century, investigations of the postmortem neuropathology of schizophrenia have been most notable for demonstrating the absence of a clear histopathological phenotype (Harrison, 1999). Although Stevens (1982) reported increased periventricular and subependymal gliosis in schizophrenia, subsequent studies have found no evidence of excess gliosis or increased glial fibrillary acidic protein staining (Arnold *et al.*, 1998; Benes *et al.*, 1991; Purohit *et al.*, 1998; Roberts *et al.*, 1986, 1987). The absence of glial proliferation clearly distinguishes the pathophysiology of schizophrenia from that of classic neurodegeneration (e.g. Alzheimer's disease), where gliosis is prominent.

Neuronal cell loss is another potential marker of neurodegeneration. Alzheimer's disease and other classic neurodegenerative disorders are characterized by large-scale neuronal loss, especially during their later stages. In schizophrenia, many studies have not identified reduced numbers of cortical neurons (Akbarian *et al.*, 1995; Pakkenberg, 1993; Selemon *et al.*, 1995, 1998). However, several studies have demonstrated significant yet relatively small layer-specific reductions in the density of pyramidal and non-pyramidal neurons in anterior cingulate cortex in schizophrenia, interpreted to reflect reductions in neuronal number (Benes *et al.*, 1991, 2001). Interestingly, a recent study also suggested that glial density may be reduced in anterior cingulate cortex (Cotter *et al.*, 2001). Furthermore, substantial reductions of neurons have been identified in several subcortical regions including nucleus accumbens (Young *et al.*, 2000) and mediodorsal thalamus (Pakkenberg, 1990). Therefore, while large-scale cortical cell loss is clearly absent in schizophrenia, available data indicate that limited neuronal and/or glial reductions may occur with layer and regional specificity, especially in subcortical areas.

While neuronal cell loss may not be a primary cytoarchitectural deficit in schizophrenia, there is increasing evidence that the cortical neuropathology is characterized by limited atrophy. Several studies indicate that neuronal density is increased in a setting of slight cortical thinning, suggesting that cortical neuropil is reduced (Selemon *et al.*, 1995, 1998). Other studies have found reduced dendritic spines and total dendritic length (Black *et al.*, 2002; Garey *et al.*, 1998; Glantz and Lewis, 2000) as well as reductions of certain synaptic marker proteins (Eastwood and Harrison, 1995; Glantz and Lewis, 1997; Karson *et al.*, 1999; Thompson *et al.*, 1998). Small reductions in somal volume of neurons in prefrontal cortex have also been reported in schizophrenia (Pierri *et al.*, 2001; Rajkowska *et al.*, 1998). Because neuronal size appears to be related to the extent of dendritic and axonal arborization (Harrison and Eastwood, 2001), reduced somal size is consistent with reduced dendrites and synaptic markers in schizophrenia.

In efforts to identify alternative pathophysiological mechanisms that could contribute to the neuropathology of schizophrenia, a role for apoptosis has been increasingly hypothesized (Lewis and Lieberman, 2000; Margolis *et al.*, 1994; Woods, 1998). Although best recognized for its association with rapid cell death, emerging data indicate that apoptosis can also produce non-lethal reductions in cellular viability

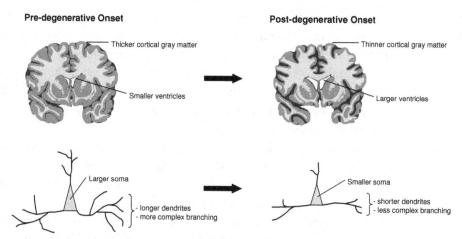

Fig. 20.2.   Model of limited neurodegeneration on structural and histological levels. Longitudinal neuroimaging studies have demonstrated progressive cortical gray matter loss and ventricular enlargement in schizophrenia, especially in childhood-onset and adult new-onset populations. The limited neurodegeneration model proposes that cytopathological correlates of gray matter loss include progressive neuronal atrophy and neuropil loss.

(Ona *et al.*, 1999) and underlies pathological elimination of synapses in a process termed synaptic apoptosis (Mattson *et al.*, 1998). Interestingly, some studies have indicated abnormalities in apoptotic mechanisms, including pro- and antiapoptotic proteins (Jarskog *et al.*, 2000, 2001) and DNA fragmentation profiles (Benes *et al.*, 2003) in postmortem cortical tissue, suggesting that apoptotic pathways may indeed underlie certain neuropathological deficits in schizophrenia.

Therefore, while there is no evidence of classic neurodegenerative lesions in schizophrenia, it is clear that the disorder is characterized by a number of more subtle neuropathological deficits. Unfortunately, these findings in postmortem tissue do not provide a longitudinal perspective and, therefore, offer little insight as to the timing of the events. In other words, limited reductions in glia, dendrites, or neuronal soma could be a consequence of early developmental agenesis or of an atrophic process later in life. Furthermore, these findings must be considered in the context of a number of potential confounding variables, including diagnostic uncertainty, postmortem interval, medication effects, drug abuse, and non-specific effects of chronic illness, to name a few. Nevertheless, we suggest that the emerging picture of subtle dendritic and synaptic deficits in schizophrenia in the context of structural neuroimaging findings and clinical deterioration represents a limited form of neurodegeneration that will become increasingly defined as molecular techniques and genomic/proteomic analyses are applied to the disorder (Fig. 20.2).

Neuroimaging studies

Structural studies

Cross-sectional structural neuroimaging studies have demonstrated a number of consistent brain abnormalities in schizophrenia primarily involving enlargement of the lateral and third ventricles and reduction in cortical gray matter volume, both globally (Gur *et al.*, 1998; Hulshoff Pol *et al.*, 2002; Zipursky *et al.*, 1992) and in cortical subregions including prefrontal (Gur *et al.*, 1998; Hulshoff Pol *et al.*, 2002), temporal (Gur *et al.*, 1998; Schlaepfer *et al.*, 1994), and parietal (Schlaepfer *et al.*, 1994) areas. Since neuropil is a primary component of gray matter, these structural imaging findings provide in vivo support for the postmortem findings of reduced cortical neuropil (Selemon *et al.*, 1995, 1998).

One of the limitations of cross-sectional studies is that they do not adequately address whether a change in brain volume is active or antecedent to the scan. For this reason, a number of longitudinal structural magnetic resonance imaging (sMRI) studies have been conducted to address this issue. Interestingly, progressive brain volume changes have been identified in several different patient cohorts, including in patients with prodromal signs of psychosis, in childhood-onset schizophrenia, in new-onset schizophrenia, and in certain chronic patient populations. In a single small study of prodromal patients judged at high risk of transition to psychosis, a progressive loss of gray matter was found in certain hippocampal and frontal regions only in those patients that developed psychosis (Pantelis *et al.*, 2002). In childhood-onset disease, several progressive volume changes have been reported compared with normal controls, including ventricular enlargement (Rapoport *et al.*, 1997), cortical gray matter loss in frontal and temporal areas (Jacobsen *et al.*, 1998; Rapoport *et al.*, 1999), and cerebellar volume loss (Keller *et al.*, 2003). In new-onset schizophrenia, progressive ventricular enlargement has been identified by several groups (Cahn *et al.*, 2002; DeLisi *et al.*, 1997; Lieberman *et al.*, 2001a) but not others (Gur *et al.*, 1998). Progressive volume loss has been reported in first-episode schizophrenia in cerebral hemispheres bilaterally (DeLisi *et al.*, 1997), total cerebral gray matter (Cahn *et al.*, 2002), frontal cortex (Gur *et al.*, 1998), and in superior temporal gyrus (Kasai *et al.*, 2003), while Lieberman *et al.* (2001a) did not detect cortical volume differences. In adults with chronic schizophrenia, progressive ventricular enlargement has been reported in male patients (Mathalon *et al.*, 2001) and in patients with poor outcome (Davis *et al.*, 1998), also suggested by Nair *et al.* (1997). Mathalon *et al.* (2001) also reported accelerated progression of frontotemporal cortical gray matter loss in males with schizophrenia.

Although the interpretation that progressive brain changes reflect a neurodegenerative process in schizophrenia has been challenged (Weinberger and McClure,

2002), the increasing number of studies that have identified accelerated cortical tissue loss and ventricular enlargement suggest that the pathophysiology of schizophrenia is a dynamic and progressive process, particularly around the onset of psychosis (Lewis and Lieberman, 2000; Fig. 20.2). Longitudinal studies that employ higher-resolution neuroimaging techniques should help to define this process more precisely.

Functional and spectroscopic studies

Reduced metabolic activity in the prefrontal cortex (hypofrontality) in schizophrenia has been demonstrated using positron emission tomography (PET) and functional MRI (fMRI) studies (Andreasen et al., 1997; Weinberger et al., 1986). Since these studies did not follow patients longitudinally, it is not possible to determine whether this metabolic hypofrontality represents a degenerative process. Somewhat more revealing are studies of phosphorus-31 magnetic resonance spectroscopy (MRS) in the prefrontal cortex, which demonstrated decreased phosphomonoesters (Hinsberger et al., 1997; Pettegrew et al., 1991; Stanley et al., 1995) and increased phosphodiesters (Pettegrew et al., 1991; Stanley et al., 1995) in first-episode schizophrenia. A profile of reduced phosphomonoesters and increased phosphodiesters is thought to reflect an accelerated breakdown of membrane phospholipids (Pettegrew et al., 1993). This could indicate an active neurodegenerative process whereby neuronal and/or glial components are undergoing degradation. In addition, several studies using proton MRS have reported reduced N-acetylaspartate levels in temporal and frontal cortex in schizophrenia (Bertolino et al., 1998, Cecil et al., 1999). N-Acetylaspartate is generally considered a measure of neuronal metabolism and reduced levels may, therefore, reflect reduced neuronal viability. Taken together, these functional and spectroscopic studies are only moderately indicative of a limited neurodegenerative process in schizophrenia. Applying longitudinal designs to future functional neuroimaging studies will provide important information regarding progression.

Correlation between neuroimaging data and clinical outcome

There is evidence that a longer duration of untreated initial psychosis is associated with more severe symptoms, poorer treatment response, and more impaired overall level of functioning (reviewed by Lieberman et al., 2001b). This clinical observation has led to the idea that untreated psychosis is neurotoxic (Loebel et al., 1992; Wyatt, 1991) and may cause progression of the underlying neuropathology. However, studies to date have not found correlations between the duration of untreated psychosis and neurostructural abnormalities (Fannon et al., 2000; Ho et al., 2003; Hoff et al., 2000). These studies indicated that the structural abnormalities of the brain observed in first-episode patients precede the onset of formal symptoms and, if they represent progression of the underlying neuropathology, this progression has occurred premorbidly.

There has also been conflicting evidence concerning whether the progression of neurostructural abnormalities observed after the onset of symptoms is associated with worsening clinical symptoms or neurocognitive functioning. In first-episode schizophrenia, greater progression of cerebral gray matter loss and ventricular enlargement appears to correlate with worse functional outcome (Cahn *et al.*, 2002; Lieberman *et al.*, 2001a); frontal cortex loss has been associated with less improvement in negative symptoms but greater improvement in delusions and thought disorder (Gur *et al.*, 1998), while Kasai *et al.* (2003) reported no association between progressive loss of superior temporal gyrus and clinical measures. Gur *et al.* (1998) found cortical volume reductions associated with greater neurocognitive decline in previously treated patients. In males with chronic schizophrenia, Mathalon *et al.* (2001) reported greater clinical severity in patients with accelerated cortical gray matter loss and ventricular enlargement, and Davis *et al.* (1998) found ventricular enlargement in patients with poor outcome. Similarly, in childhood-onset schizophrenia, Jacobsen *et al.* (1998) found progressive decline in right superior temporal gyrus associated with worse clinical outcome.

Therefore, studies to date demonstrate some evidence of correlation between neurostructural progression and clinical/neurocognitive function but these correlations are not found in all studies, across the same brain regions, or in the same clinical symptoms or cognitive domains. One explanation is that the brain has the finite capacity partially to maintain its function in the face of neurostructural progression, and that a number of factors may influence whether a given individual manifests a cognitive decline. Another important variable is the potentially confounding effect of antipsychotic medication, which could explain why cognitive deterioration may be less frequent today than in Kraeplin's era with no neuroleptic drugs. Nevertheless, given that relatively few studies have conducted correlational analyses between structural, clinical, and cognitive variables in carefully defined patient subgroups, it is somewhat difficult to reconcile findings from a number of recent imaging studies reporting structural progression with other studies reporting overall stability of clinical symptoms and cognitive functioning. Further investigation into this important issue is clearly warranted.

Potential mechanisms underlying neurodegeneration

What process underlies the neuropathological progression of schizophrenia? A variety of pathogenic mechanisms have been proposed. These specifically implicate glutamate N-methyl-D-aspartate (NMDA) receptor hypofunction and excitotoxicity (Onley and Farber, 1995), antagonism of NMDA receptors by

N-acetylaspartylglutamate and consequent oxidative stress (Coyle and Puttfarcken, 1993), reduction in gamma-aminobutyric acid (GABA) interneuron-mediated inhibition of pyramidal neurons in the cingulate cortex (Benes, 1995), dopamine-mediated neurochemical sensitization (Lieberman *et al.*, 1997) and neurotoxicity (Wyatt, 1995). Stress has emerged as a potential factor underlying neurostructural changes observed in affective and anxiety disorders. Because glucocorticoids may also play a role in schizophrenia (Arango *et al.*, 2001; Church *et al.*, 2002; see also Ch. 6), stress may be implicated in the progressive elements of schizophrenia, which is generally considered a stress-sensitive illness.

As briefly discussed with the postmortem studies above, abnormal regulation of apoptosis is emerging as a potential mechanism in the pathophysiology of schizophrenia, and one that could be influenced by glutamatergic, GABAergic, and dopaminergic dysfunction. Apoptotic mechanisms can underlie both cell death and non-lethal synaptic apoptosis (Mattson *et al.*, 1998), setting the stage for a process that could potentially produce the type of subtle reduction in neuronal viability seen in schizophrenia. Reduced levels of the antiapoptotic protein Bcl-2 have been shown in postmortem temporal cortex in schizophrenia (Jarskog *et al.*, 2000) as well as elevated ratios of the proapoptotic Bax to Bcl-2 (Jarskog *et al.*, 2001). These findings suggest an increased vulnerability to apoptotic activation in schizophrenic cortex. Yet, caspase 3 (a marker of active apoptosis) was unchanged in schizophrenia versus normal controls, which is consistent with no increase in the rate of single-stranded DNA fragmentation in schizophrenia (Benes *et al.*, 2003). This suggests that apoptosis was not active in schizophrenia at the time of death, although it does not preclude apoptotic activity at other stages of the illness such as the prodromal phase or the first episode of psychosis.

Conclusions

Although the etiology of schizophrenia remains unknown, the current review highlights the complexity of its underlying pathophysiology, appearing to involve both neurodevelopmental and neurodegenerative elements. The histopathology of schizophrenia remains without a defined phenotype; however, increasing evidence is pointing to subtle neuronal atrophy and synaptodendritic reductions in postmortem cortex, which may reflect a limited neurodegenerative process. This conclusion is increasingly supported by neuroimaging studies that find progressive neurostructural changes, especially in gray matter content and ventricle size, and, less convincingly, studies that report limited progression of clinical symptoms and neurocognitive function. Taken as a whole, progressive clinical, neurocognitive, and neuroimaging findings appear most evident in the prodromal phase and the first few years of psychosis, although certain subgroups of chronically ill patients with severe and treatment-refractory schizophrenia may also experience a progression of the illness. However, the longitudinal prodromal cohort findings to date must be considered preliminary given the relatively few studies and the few subjects involved. Future studies utilizing high-resolution neuroimaging and sophisticated neuropsychological testing techniques will undoubtedly provide greater insight on the timing, regionality, and degree of progression in the early stages of schizophrenia.

Given that the strongest evidence for neuroprogressive events in schizophrenia is emerging in the prodromal and first-episode populations, it suggests that any neurodegenerative processes would intersect with normal neuromaturational processes, which include myelination and synaptic pruning during adolescence and early adulthood. Although a number of mechanistic possibilities could be envisaged, this scenario offers the intriguing possibility that apoptotic mechanisms give rise to limited neurodegeneration via perturbations of developmentally regulated synaptic elimination during the prodromal and first-episode phases of schizophrenia. In order to elucidate the mechanisms that underlie the neuropathology of schizophrenia, it will be necessary to gain a much clearer understanding of the mechanisms that guide normal human brain development than is currently available. Such studies will complement those that examine high-risk premorbid and prodromal cohorts to shed more light on the complex interactions of pathophysiology and normal development that underlie schizophrenia.

Acknowledgements

This work was supported in part by the UNC Schizophrenia Research Center, an NIMH Silvio O. Conte Center for the Neuroscience of Mental Disorders (MH064065, JAL), NIMH grant K08 MH-01752 (LFJ), NIMH grant MH-60352 (JHG), and the Foundation of Hope of Raleigh, North Carolina (JAL).

REFERENCES

Abrahamson, D. (1983). Schizophrenia deterioration. *Br J Psychiatry* **143**: 82–83.

Addington, J., Addington, D. (2002). Cognitive functioning in first-episode schizophrenia. *J Psychiatry Neurosci* **27**: 188–192.

Akbarian, S., Kim, J. J., Potkin, S. G., *et al.* (1995). Gene expression for glutamic acid decarboxylase is reduced without loss of neurons in prefrontal cortex of schizophrenics. *Arch Gen Psychiatry* **52**: 258–266.

Andreasen, N. C., O'Leary, D. S., Flaum, M., *et al.* (1997). Hypofrontality in schizophrenia: distributed dysfunctional circuits in neuroleptic-naïve patients. *Lancet* **349**: 1730–1734.

Arango, C., Kirkpatrick, B., Koenig, J. (2001). At issue: stress, hippocampal neuronal turnover, and neuropsychiatric disorders. *Schizophr Bull* **27**: 477–480.

Arnold, S. E., Trojanowski, J. Q., Gur, R. E., *et al.* (1998). Absence of neurodegeneration and neural injury in the cerebral cortex in a sample of elderly patients with schizophrenia. *Arch Gen Psychiatry* **55**: 225–232.

Benes, F. M. (1995). Is there a neuroanatomic basis for schizophrenia? An old question revisited. *Neuroscientist* **1**: 104–115.

Benes, F. M., McSparren, J., Bird, E. D., SanGiovanni, J. P., Vincent, S. L. (1991). Deficits in small interneurons in prefrontal and cingulate cortices of schizophrenic and schizoaffective patients. *Arch Gen Psychiatry* **48**: 996–1001.

Benes, F. M., Vincent, S. L., Todtenkopf, M. (2001). The density of pyramidal and nonpyramidal neurons in anterior cingulate cortex of schizophrenic and bipolar subjects. *Biol Psychiatry* **50**: 395–406.

Benes, F. M., Walsh, J., Bhattacharyya, S., Sheth, A., Berretta, S. (2003). DNA fragmentation is decreased in schizophrenia but not in bipolar disorder. *Arch Gen Psychiatry* **60**: 359–364.

Bertolino, A., Callicott, J. H., Nawroz, S., *et al.* (1998). Reproducibility of proton magnetic resonance spectroscopic imaging in patients with schizophrenia. *Neuropsychopharmacology* **18**: 1–9.

Bilder, R. M., Lipschutz-Broch, R. G., Geisler, S. H., Mayerhoff, D. I., Lieberman, J. A. (1992). Intellectual deficits in first-episode schizophrenia: evidence for progressive deterioration. *Schizophr Bull* **18**: 437–488.

Black, J. E., Klintsova, A. Y., Kodish, I. M., Greenough, W. T., Uranova, N. A. (2002). What is missing in the reduced neuropil of schizophrenic prefrontal cortex? A combined golgi and electron microscopy study. *Biol Psychiatry* **51**: S54.

Cahn, W., Hulshoff Pol, H. E., Lems, E. B. T. E., *et al.* (2002). Brain volume changes in first-episode schizophrenia. *Arch Gen Psychiatry* **59**: 1002–1010.

Cannon, M., Jones, P., Huttunen, M. O., *et al.* (1999). School performance in Finnish children and later development of schizophrenia. *Arch Gen Psychiatry* **56**: 457–463.

Cannon, M., Caspi, A., Moffitt, T. E., *et al.* (2002). Evidence for early-childhood, pan-developmental impairment specific to schizophreniform disorder. Results from a longitudinal birth cohort. *Arch Gen Psychiatry* **59**: 449–456.

Cecil, K. M., Lenkinski, R. E., Gur, R. E., Gur, R. C. (1999). Proton magnetic resonance spectroscopy in the frontal and temporal lobes of neuroleptic naive patients with schizophrenia. *Neuropsychopharmacology* **20**: 131–140.

Church, S. M., Cotter, D., Bramon, E., Murray, R. M. (2002). Does schizophrenia result from developmental or degenerative processes? *J Neural Transm Suppl* **63**: 129–147.

Cotter, D. R., Pariante, C. M., Everall, I. P. (2001). Glial cell abnormalities in major psychiatric disorders: the evidence and implications. *Brain Res Bull* **55**: 585–595.

Coyle, J. T., Puttfarcken, P. (1993). Oxidative stress, glutamate, and neurodegenerative disorders. *Science* **262**: 689–695.

Davis, K. L., Buchsbaum, M. S., Shihabuddin, L., *et al.* (1998). Ventricular enlargement in poor-outcome schizophrenia. *Biol Psychiatry* **43**: 783–793.

DeLisi, L. E., Sakuma, M., Tew, W., *et al.* (1997). Schizophrenia as a chronic active brain process: a study of progressive brain structural change subsequent to the onset of schizophrenia. *Psychiatry Res Neuroimaging* **74**: 129–140.

Done, D. J., Crow, T. J., Johnstone, E. C., Sacker, A. (1994). Childhood antecedents of schizophrenia and affective illness: social adjustment at ages 7 and 11. *Br Med J* **309**: 699–703.

Eastwood, S. L., Harrison, P. J. (1995). Decreased synaptophysin in the medial temporal lobe in schizophrenia demonstrated using immunoautoradiography. *Neuroscience* **69**: 339–343.

Eaton, W. W., Thara, R., Federman, B., Melton, B., Liang, K.-Y. (1995). Structure and course of positive and negative symptoms in schizophrenia, *Arch Gen Psychiatry* **52**: 127–134.

Fannon, D., Chitnis, X., Doku, V., *et al.* (2000). Features of structural brain abnormality in first-episode psychosis. *Am J Psychiatry* **157**: 1829–1834.

Fenton, W. S., McGlashan, T. H. (1994). Antecedents, symptom progression, and long-term outcome of the deficit syndrome in schizophrenia. *Am J Psychiatry* **151**: 351–356.

Friedman, J. I., Harvey, P. D., McGurk, S. R., *et al.* (2002). Correlates of change in functional status of institutionalized geriatric schizophrenic patients: focus on medical comorbidity. *Am J Psychiatry* **159**: 1388–1394.

Fuller, R., Nopoulos, P., Arndt, S., *et al.* (2002). Longitudinal assessment of premorbid cognitive functioning in patients with schizophrenia through examination of standardized scholastic test performance. *Am J Psychiatry* **159**: 1183–1189.

Garey, L. J., Ong, W. Y., Patel, T. S., Kanani, M., Davis, A., Mortimer, A. M., Barnes, T. R. E., Hirsch, S. R. (1998). Reduced dendritic spine density on cerebral cortical pyramidal neurons in schizophrenia. *J Neurol Neurosurg Psychiatry* **65**: 446–453.

Glantz, L. A., Lewis, D. A. (1997). Reduction of synaptophysin immunoreactivity in the prefrontal cortex of subjects with schizophrenia: regional and diagnostic specificity. *Arch Gen Psychiatry* **54**: 943–952.

(2000). Decreased dendritic spine density on prefrontal cortical pyramidal neurons in schizophrenia. *Arch Gen Psychiatry* **57**: 65–73.

Gur, R. E., Cowell, P., Turetsky, B. I., *et al.* (1998). A follow-up magnetic resonance imaging study of schizophrenia. Relationship of neuroanatomical changes to clinical and neurobehavioral measures. *Arch Gen Psychiatry* **55**: 145–152.

Hambrecht, M., Lammertink, M., Klosterkötter, J., Matuschek, E., Pukrop, R. (2002). Subjective and objective neuropsychological abnormalities in a psychosis prodrome clinic. *Br J Psychiatry* **181**(Suppl. 43): S30–S37.

Hardy, J., Gwinn-Hardy, K. (1998). Genetic classification of primary neurodegenerative disease. *Science* **282**: 1075–1079.

Harrison, P. J. (1999). The neuropathology of schizophrenia: a critical review of the data and their interpretation. *Brain* **122**: 593–624.

Harrison, P. J., Eastwood, S. L. (2001). Neuropathological studies of synaptic connectivity in the hippocampal formation in schizophrenia. *Hippocampus* **11**: 508–519.

Harvey, P. D., Silverman, J. M., Mohs, R. C., *et al.* (1999). Cognitive decline in late-life schizophrenia: a longitudinal study of geriatric chronically hospitalized patients. *Biol Psychiatry* **45**: 32–40.

Heaton, R. K., Gladsjo, J. A., Palmer, B. W., *et al.* (2001). Stability and course of neuropsychological deficits in schizophrenia. *Am J Psychiatry* **58**: 24–32.

Hinsberger, A. D., Williamson, P. C., Carr, T. J., Stanley, J. A., Drost, D. J., Densmore, M., MacFabe, G. C., Montemurro, D. G. (1997). Magnetic resonance imaging volumetric and phosphorus 31 magnetic resonance spectroscopy measurements in schizophrenia. *J Psychiatry Neurosci* **22**: 111–117.

Ho, B.-C., Alicata, D., Ward, J., *et al.* (2003). Untreated initial psychosis: relation to cognitive deficits and brain morphology in first-episode schizophrenia. *Am J Psychiatry* **160**: 142–148.

Hoff, A. L., Sakuma, M., Wieneke, M., *et al.* (1999). Longitudinal neuropsychological follow-up study of patients with first-episode schizophrenia. *Am J Psychiatry* **156**: 1336–1341.

Hoff, A. L., Sakuma, M., Razi, K., *et al.* (2000). Lack of association between duration of untreated illness and severity of cognitive and structural brain deficits at the first episode of schizophrenia. *Am J Psychiatry* **157**: 1824–1828.

Huber, G., Gross, G., Shuttler, R., Linz, M. (1980). Longitudinal studies of schizophrenic patients. *Schizophr Bull* **6**: 592–605.

Hulshoff Pol, H. E., Schnack, H. G., Bertens, M. G. B. C., *et al.* (2002). Volume changes in gray matter in patients with schizophrenia. *Am J Psychiatry* **159**: 244–250.

Jacobsen, L. K., Giedd, J., Castellanos, F. X., *et al.* (1998). Progressive reduction of temporal lobe structures in childhood-onset schizophrenia. *Am J Psychiatry* **155**: 678–685.

Jarskog, L. F., Gilmore, J. H., Selinger, E. S., Lieberman, J. A. (2000). Cortical Bcl-2 protein expression and apoptotic regulation in schizophrenia. *Biol Psychiatry* **48**: 641–650.

Jarskog, L. F., Selinger, E. S., Lieberman, J. A., Gilmore, J. H. (2001). Apoptotic regulatory proteins afford reduced neuroprotection in schizophrenia. *Schizophr Res* **49**: 53S.

Jones, P., Rodgers, B., Murray, R., Marmot, M. (1994). Child development risk factors for adult schizophrenia in the British 1946 birth cohort. *Lancet* **344**: 1398–1402.

Karson, C. N., Mrak, R. E., Schluterman, K. O., *et al.* (1999). Alterations in synaptic proteins and their encoding mRNAs in prefrontal cortex in schizophrenia: a possible neurochemical basis for "hypofrontality". *Mol Psychiatry* **4**: 39–45.

Kasai, K., Shenton, M. E., Salisbury, D. F., *et al.* (2003). Progressive decrease of left superior temporal gyrus gray matter volume in patients with first-episode schizophrenia. *Am J Psychiatry* **160**: 156–164.

Keller, A., Castellanos, F. X., Vaituzis, A. C., *et al.* (2003). Progressive loss of cerebellar volume in childhood-onset schizophrenia. *Am J Psychiatry* **160**: 128–133.

Kraeplin E. (1919). *Dementia Praecox and Paraphrenia*, Edinburgh, E and S Livingstone.

Kremen, W. S., Seidman, L. J., Pepple, J. R., *et al.* (1994). Neuropsychological risk indicators for schizophrenia: a review of family studies. *Schizophr Bull* **20**: 103–119.

Lewis, D. A., Lieberman, J. A. (2000). Catching up on schizophrenia: natural history and neurobiology. *Neuron* **28**: 325–334.

Lieberman, J. A., Sheitman, B. B., Kinon, B. J. (1997). Neurochemical sensitization in the pathophysiology of schizophrenia: deficits and dysfunction in neuronal regulation and plasticity. *Neuropsychopharmacology* **17**: 205–229.

Lieberman. J. A., Chakos, M., Wu, H., *et al.* (2001a). Longitudinal study of brain morphology in first episode schizophrenia. *Biol Psychiatry* **49**: 487–499.

Lieberman, J. A., Perkins, D., Belger, A., *et al.* (2001b). The early stages of schizophrenia: speculations on pathogenesis, pathophysiology, and therapeutic approaches. *Biol Psychiatry* **50**: 884–897.

Loebel, A. D., Lieberman, J. A., Alvir, J. M. J., *et al.* (1992). Duration of psychosis and outcome in first-episode schizophrenia. *Am J Psychiatry* **149**: 1183–1188.

Margolis, R. L., Chuang, D. M., Post, R. M. (1994). Programmed cell death: implications for neuropsychiatric disorders. *Biol Psychiatry* **35**: 946–956.

Mason, P., Harrison, G., Glazebrook, C., Medley, I., Croudance, T. (1996). The course of schizophrenia over 13 years. A report from the International Study on Schizophrenia (IsoS) coordinated by the World Health Organization. *Br J Psychiatry* **169**: 580–586.

Mathalon, D. H., Sullivan, E. V., Lim, K. O., Pfefferbaum, A. (2001). Progressive brain volume changes and the clinical course of schizophrenia in men: a longitudinal magnetic resonance imaging study. *Arch Gen Psychiatry* **58**: 148–157.

Mattson, M. P., Keller, J. N., Begley, J. G. (1998). Evidence for synaptic apoptosis. *Exp Neurol* **153**: 35–48.

Mayerhoff, D. I., Loebel, A. D., Alvir, J. M. J., *et al.* (1994). The deficit state in first-episode schizophrenia. *Am J Psychiatry* **151**: 1417–1422.

McGlashan, T. H. (1988). A selective review of recent North American long-term follow-up studies of schizophrenia. *Schizophr Bull* **14**: 515–542.

Moritz, S., Andresen, B., Perro, C., for the PERSIST Study Group (2002). Neurocognitive performance in first-episode and chronic schizophrenic patients. *Eur Arch Psychiatry Clin Neurosci* **252**: 33–37.

Murray, R. M., Lewis, S. W. (1987). Is schizophrenia a neurodevelopmental disorder? *Br Med J* **296**: 681–682.

Nair, T. R., Christensen, J. D., Kingsbury, S. J., *et al.* (1997). Progression of cerebroventricular enlargement and the subtyping of schizophrenia. *Psychiatry Res Neuroimaging* **74**: 141–150.

Nopoulos, P., Flashman, L., Flaum, M., Arndt, S., Andreasen, N. (1994). Stability of cognitive functioning early in the course of schizophrenia. *Schizophr Res* **14**: 29–37.

Ona, V. O., Li, M., Vonsattel, J. P. G., *et al.* (1999). Inhibition of caspase-1 slows disease progression in a mouse model of Huntington's disease. *Nature* **399**: 263–267.

Onley, J. W., Farber, N. B. (1995). Glutamate receptor dysfunction and schizophrenia. *Arch Gen Psychiatry* **52**: 998–1007.

Pakkenberg, B. (1990). Pronounced reduction of total neuron number in mediodorsal thalamic nucleus and nucleus accumbens in schizophrenics. *Arch Gen Psychiatry* **47**: 1023–1028.

(1993). Total nerve cell number in neocortex in chronic schizophrenics and controls estimated using optical disectors. *Biol Psychiatry* **34**: 768–772.

Pantelis, C., Velakoulis, D., McGorry, P. D., *et al.* (2002). Neuroanatomical abnormalities before and after onset of psychosis: a cross-sectional and longitudinal MRI comparison. *Lancet* Accessed 10 December 2002: http://image.thelancet.com/extras/01art9092web.pdf.

Pettegrew, J. W., Keshavan, M. S., Panchalingam, K., *et al.* (1991). Alterations in brain high-energy phosphate and membrane phospholipid metabolism in first-episode, drug-naive schizophrenics: a pilot study of the dorsal prefrontal cortex by in vivo phosphorus 31 nuclear magnetic resonance spectroscopy. *Arch Gen Psychiatry* **48**: 563–568.

Pettegrew, J. W., Keshavan, M. S., Minshew, N. J. (1993). [31]P Nuclear magnetic resonance spectroscopy: neurodevelopment and schizophrenia. *Schizophr Bull* **19**: 35–53.

Pfohl, B., Winokur, G. (1982). The evolution of symptoms in institutionalized hebephrenic/catatonic schizophrenics. *Br J Psychiatry* **141**: 567–572.

Pierri, J. N., Volk, C. L., Auh, S., Sampson, A., Lewis, D. A. (2001). Decreased somal size of deep layer 3 pyramidal neurons in the prefrontal cortex of subjects with schizophrenia. *Arch Gen Psychiatry* **58**: 466–473.

Pinals, D. A., Breier, A. (1997). Schizophrenia. In *Psychiatry*, ed. A. Tasman, J. Kay, J. A. Lieberman. Philadelphia, PA: W. B. Saunders, pp. 927–965.

Purohit, D. P., Perl, D. P., Haroutunian, V., *et al.* (1998). Alzheimer disease and related neurodegenerative diseases in elderly patients with schizophrenia. *Arch Gen Psychiatry* **55**: 205–211.

Rajkowska, G., Selemon, L. D., Goldman-Rakic, P. S. (1998). Neuronal and glial somal size in the prefrontal cortex: a postmortem morphometric study of schizophrenia and Huntington disease. *Arch Gen Psychiatry* **55**: 215–224.

Rapoport, J. L., Giedd, J., Kumra, S., *et al.* (1997). Childhood-onset schizophrenia: progressive ventricular change during adolescence. *Arch Gen Psychiatry* **54**: 897–903.

Rapoport, J. L., Giedd, J. N., Blumenthal, J., *et al.* (1999). Progressive cortical change during adolescence in childhood-onset schizophrenia: a longitudinal magnetic resonance imaging study. *Arch Gen Psychiatry* **56**: 649–654.

Roberts, G. W., Colter, N., Lofthouse, R., *et al.* (1986). Gliosis in schizophrenia: a survey. *Biol Psychiatry* **21**: 1043–1050.

Roberts, G. W., Colter, N., Lofthouse, R., Johnstone, E. C., Crow, T. J. (1987). Is there gliosis in schizophrenia? Investigation of the temporal lobe. *Biol Psychiatry* **22**: 1459–1468.

Rund, B. R. (1998). A review of the longitudinal studies of cognitive decline in schizophrenia patients. *Schizophr Bull* **24**: 425–435.

Saykin, A. J., Shtasel, D. L., Gur, R. E., *et al.* (1994). Neuropsychological deficits in neuroleptic naive patients with first episode schizophrenia. *Arch Gen Psychiatry* **51**: 124–131.

Schlaepfer, T. E., Harris, G. J., Tien, A. Y., *et al.* (1994). Decreased regional cortical gray matter volume in schizophrenia. *Am J Psychiatry* **151**: 842–848.

Selemon, L. D., Rajkowska, G., Goldman-Rakic, P. S. (1995). Abnormally high neuronal density in the schizophrenic cortex: a morphometric analysis of prefrontal area 9 and occipital area 17. *Arch Gen Psychiatry* **52**: 805–818.

  (1998). Elevated neuronal density in prefrontal area 46 in brains from schizophrenic patients: application of a three-dimensional, stereologic counting method. *J Comp Neurol* **392**: 402–412.

Smith, A. (1964). Mental deterioration in chronic schizophrenia. *J Nerv Ment Dis* **139**: 479–487.

Stanley, J. A., Williamson, P. C., Drost, D. J., *et al.* (1995). An in vivo study of the prefrontal cortex of schizophrenic patients at different stages of illness via phosphorus magnetic resonance spectroscopy. *Arch Gen Psychiatry* **52**: 399–406.

Stevens, J. R. (1982). Neuropathology of schizophrenia. *Arch Gen Psychiatry* **39**: 1131–1139.

Thompson, P. M., Sower, A. C., Perrone-Bizzozero, N. I. (1998). Altered levels of the synaptosomal associated protein SNAP-25 in schizophrenia. *Biol Psychiatry* **43**: 239–243.

Weinberger, D. R. (1987). Implications of normal brain development for the pathogenesis of schizophrenia. *Arch Gen Psychiatry* **44**: 660–669.

Weinberger, D. R., McClure, R. K. (2002). Neurotoxicity, neuroplasticity, and magnetic resonance imaging morphometry: what is happening in the schizophrenic brain? *Arch Gen Psychiatry* **59**: 553–558.

Weinberger, D. R., Berman, K. F., Zec, R. F. (1986). Physiologic dysfunction of dorsolateral prefrontal cortex in schizophrenia. I. Regional cerebral blood flow evidence. *Arch Gen Psychiatry* **43**: 114–124.

Woods, B. T. (1998). Is schizophrenia a progressive neurodevelopmental disorder? Toward a unitary pathogenetic mechanism. *Am J Psychiatry* **155**: 1661–1670.

Wyatt, R. J. (1991). Neuroleptics and the natural course of schizophrenia. *Schizophr Bull* **17**: 325–351.

(1995). Early intervention for schizophrenia: can the course of the illness be altered? *Biol Psychiatry* **38**: 1–3.

Young, K. A., Manaye, K. F., Liang, C. H., Hicks, P. B., German, D. C. (2000). Reduced number of mediodorsal and anterior thalamic neurons in schizophrenia. *Biol Psychiatry* **47**: 944–953.

Zipursky, R. B., Lim, K. O., Sullivan, E. V., Brown, B. W., Pfefferbaum, A. (1992). Widespread cerebral gray matter volume deficits in schizophrenia. *Arch Gen Psychiatry* **49**: 195–205.

Zorrilla, L. T. E., Heaton, R. K, McAdams, L. A., *et al.* (2000). Cross-sectional study of older outpatients with schizophrenia and health comparison subjects: no differences in age-related decline. *Am J Psychiatry* **157**: 1324–1326.

21

Does disordered brain development occur across diagnostic boundaries?

Christian W. Kreipke[1], David R. Rosenberg[1], and Matcheri S. Keshavan[1,2]
[1]Wayne State University School of Medicine, Detroit, USA
[2]University of Pittsburgh School of Medicine, Pittsburgh, USA

The view that major psychiatric disorders such as schizophrenia and bipolar disorders (BPD) are distinct clinical entities is being increasingly challenged (Taylor, 1992). Several authors have proposed the concept of an expanded psychiatric continuum between affective disorders and schizophrenia and several lines of evidence support this notion. First, the cross-sectional and longitudinal co-occurrence of affective and schizophrenic symptoms is well known, leading to that diagnostic conundrum called schizoaffective disorder (Adler and Strakowski, 2003). Second, both affective disorder and schizophrenia demonstrate a high degree of genetic susceptibility; some recent gene mapping studies show common susceptibility genes for the two disorders (Berrettini, 2000). Third, BPD and schizophrenia also demonstrate some similarities in neurotransmitter and neurophysiological dysfunction (Moller, 2003). Finally, many newer atypical antipsychotic agents such as olanzapine and quetiapine, initially approved for the treatment of schizophrenia, are also being increasingly used in BPD, suggesting a therapeutic continuum (Moller, 2003).

Similar boundary issues exist between schizophrenia and other psychiatric disorders. Although obsessive–compulsive disorder (OCD) and schizophrenia are generally considered to be separate psychiatric disorders, comorbidities of the two illnesses are frequent, leading to the occasional diagnosis of schizo-obsessive disorder (Gross-Isseroff *et al.*, 2003). As will be reviewed below, neuroimaging studies show overlapping findings in these two illnesses, in particular abnormalities in the frontostriatal circuits. Attention-deficit hyperactivity disorder (ADHD) also frequently coexists with schizophrenia (Bellak *et al.*, 1987) and BPD (Kim and Miklowitz, 2002). Many children with ADHD have features of thought disorder similar to children with schizophrenia (Caplan *et al.*, 2002). Individuals at genetic risk for schizophrenia (Keshavan *et al.*, 2002a) and BPD (Chang *et al.*, 2000) also have an increased frequency of ADHD.

Neurodevelopment and Schizophrenia, ed. Matcheri S. Keshavan *et al.* Published by Cambridge University Press. © Cambridge University Press 2004.

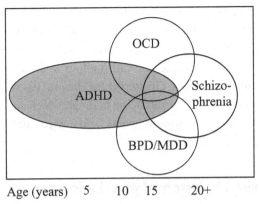

Fig. 21.1.   Developmental trajectories of diverse childhood/adolescent psychiatric disorders. OCD, obsessive–compulsive disorder; ADHD, attention-deficit hyperactivity disorder; BPD, bipolar disorder; MDD, major depressive disorder.

Not surprisingly, the pathophysiological characterization of the neurodevelopmental basis of these psychiatric disorders has been limited by comorbidity and symptom commonality. Distinct clinical phenotypes of illness expression have often been elusive. Nevertheless, technical advances in areas such as neuroimaging and genetics are capable of enhancing our understanding of the developmental neurobiological underpinnings across childhood/adolescent-onset neuropsychiatric disorders. The convergence of findings across major neuropsychiatric disorders in neurodiagnostic and treatment research presents a unique opportunity to deepen our understanding of the etiopathogenesis of childhood-onset neuropsychiatric disorders in the context of the clinically relevant question, "Which treatments for which child with which set of subgrouping characteristics?" Specifically, the combination of biological and behavioral/symptomatic predictor and outcome variables enables translational approaches to childhood-onset neuropsychiatric disorders and, in turn, may lead to new diagnostic and treatment modalities. Such an approach may also help to identify developmental biomarkers that are applicable across diagnostic boundaries as well as those that are specific to a particular condition, resulting in improved diagnosis and interventions in complex neurodevelopmental disorders.

In this chapter, we will focus on the neurodevelopmental basis of diagnostic overlap and symptom commonality by addressing similarities and differences in the neuroanatomical and functional neurochemical basis of three common childhood/adolescent-onset neuropsychiatric disorders: ADHD, OCD, and mood disorders, including major depressive disorder (MDD) and BPD. We chose these disorders because of the clinical commonalities with schizophrenia, as discussed above, and because of the known or presumed developmental origins of these disorders. Schizophrenia, BPD, and OCD have their onset in adolescence or early adulthood, and they may be preceded by symptoms similar to those in developmental disorders such as ADHD (Fig. 21.1). Each of the disorders is discussed in comparison with schizophrenia since the latter represents the main focus of this volume. We will only briefly describe the relevant findings in schizophrenia and will refer the reader to the appropriate chapter(s) for details. We will limit our pathophysiological discussion to the neuroimaging findings, which are the focus of our work, but will briefly consider common genetic and environmental etiologic factors that may cut across these disorders.

Neuroimaging and the pathological trajectory of psychiatric disorders

Recent advances in neuroimaging techniques have afforded clinicians and researchers the opportunity to study alterations in neurodevelopment as they relate to psychiatric disorders. Much of the intrinsic neural circuitry abnormalities underlying the pathological trajectory of psychiatric disorders may be elucidated. Further, this information may be used to explore the relationship between psychiatric disorders and commonalities that may exist. The following will outline current findings in structural abnormalities inherent to several psychiatric disorders as they relate to schizophrenia, in order to address the complexities of diagnostic overlap (see Table 21.1 for summary).

Attention-deficit hyperactivity disorder

ADHD is the most common childhood psychiatric disorder (Tannock, 1998). Consequently, it is not surprising that it has been studied with various brain imaging techniques to elucidate its developmental neurobiological mechanisms. A large literature has now accumulated and several brain structural alterations have been described.

Total cerebral volume

Zametkin et al. (1990) reported decreased cerebral metabolism throughout the brain in adult patients with ADHD. One of the most replicated findings in schizophrenia is that total brain volume is decreased (reviewed by Sowell et al., 2000); a study comparing 152 children and adolescents with ADHD (5–18 years of age) with 139 age- and sex-matched controls (Castellanos et al., 2002) demonstrated significantly smaller total cerebral volumes in children with ADHD persisting across the age range studied (Fig. 21.2). Total cerebral volume was comparably decreased in medicated and non-medicated patients with ADHD. Comparable reductions in total cerebral volume were observed in males and females. Decrease in cerebral volume was most marked in the white matter of unmedicated patients with ADHD. Specifically, significantly smaller total white matter volumes were observed

Table 21.1. Brief review of neuroanatomical abnormalities across several psychiatric disorders

	Schizophrenia	ADHD	OCD	MDD	BPD
Total brain	↓	↓	↔	↓	↔
Corpus callosum	↓	↓	↔	↑	↑
Prefrontal cortex	↓	↓		↓	
Hippocampus	↓		↓	↓	
Amygdala	↓		↑	↑	↑
Basal ganglia	↓	↓	↓	↓	↑
Thalamus	↓	↔	↑	↔	
Cingulate	↓		↑	↓	↓

ADHD, attention-deficit hyperactivity disorder; OCD, obsessive–computive disorder; MDD, major depressive disorder; BPD, bipolar disorder.

in unmedicated children with ADHD, compared with both medicated children with ADHD and controls. Medicated patients with ADHD did not differ from controls in total white matter volumes. This underscores the importance of controlling for potentially confounding factors such as medication status and age. Reductions in total brain volume is similar to that observed in schizophrenia (see Ch. 19).

Frontostriatal circuitry

As the executive, "decision-making" center of the brain, the prefrontal cortex and its striatal target fields have been considered key regions of interest in ADHD. Similar to reports of decreased prefrontal lobe activity (Andreasen *et al.*, 1992) and decreased striatal volumes (Keshavan *et al.*, 1998; Shihabuddin *et al.*, 1998) in schizophrenia, converging lines of evidence support reduced prefrontal and striatal volumes and hypoactivation of the prefrontal cortex and striatum in patients with ADHD (Aylward *et al.*, 1996; Bush *et al.*, 1999; Casey *et al.*, 1997; Castellanos *et al.*, 1994, 2001, 2002; Filipek *et al.*, 1997; Hynd *et al.*, 1990; Rubia *et al.*, 1999; Teicher *et al.*, 2000). Reversed asymmetry of the caudate nucleus has also been found in pediatric patients with ADHD (Hynd *et al.*, 1993). Reduced caudate volumes appear to be most pronounced in younger patients with ADHD, and

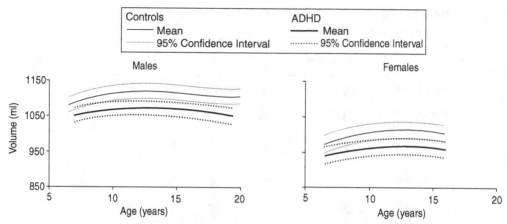

Fig. 21.2.   Predicted unadjusted longitudinal growth curves for total cerebral volumes for patients with attention-deficit hyperactivity disorder (ADHD) and controls. (Taken with permission from Castellanos, F. X., Lee, P. P., Sharp, W., *et al.*, 2002. Developmental trajectories of brain volume abnormalities in children and adolescents with attention-deficit/hyperactivity disorder. *JAMA* **288**: 1740–1748.)

the difference from controls disappears in adolescence as caudate volumes decrease with age (Castellanos *et al.*, 2002; Durston *et al.*, 2001; Fig. 21.3).

Proton magnetic resonance spectroscopy (MRS) investigations allow direct, in vivo, and non-invasive measurement of brain chemistry, including the putative neuronal marker *N*-acetyl aspartate (NAA). Consistent with volumetric reduction and hypoactivation in the striatum in patients with ADHD, decreased NAA levels and increased levels of choline, a critical membrane component believed to play a critical role in brain signal transduction, have been found in the left and right striatum in pediatric patients with ADHD (Birken and Oldendorf, 1989; Hesslinger *et al.*, 2001). This is consistent with reports of reductions in NAA and related gray matter volumes in frontal cortex and anterior cingulate cortex in childhood-onset schizophrenia and in unaffected offspring at increased risk for developing schizophrenia (Keshavan *et al.*, 1997; Sowell *et al.*, 2000). MacMaster *et al.* (2003) found increased frontostriatal glutamatergic levels in medication-free children with ADHD, aged 7–16 years, compared with case-matched controls. Reductions in NAA levels may result from excess glutamatergic excitotoxicity (Bartha *et al.*, 1998).

Vaidya *et al.* (1998) used functional magnetic resonance imaging (fMRI) to examine the effect of pharmacologic challenge with methylphenidate, a first-line treatment for ADHD (Rosenberg *et al.*, 2002a), in children with ADHD and healthy controls. Specifically, methylphenidate challenge resulted in distinct alterations in frontostriatal activity in the children with ADHD compared with the controls. Differences in methylphenidate-related activation were hypothesized to reflect

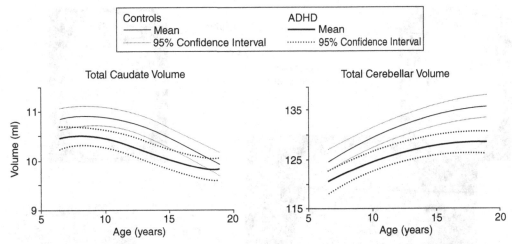

Fig. 21.3.   Predicted unadjusted longitudinal growth curves for total caudate and cerebellar volume for patients with attention-deficit hyperactivity disorder (ADHD) and controls. (Taken with permission from Castellanos, F. X., Lee, P. P., Sharp, W., *et al.*, 2002. Developmental trajectories of brain volume abnormalities in children and adolescents with attention-deficit/hyperactivity disorder. *JAMA* **288**: 1740–1748.)

alterations in frontostriatal dopamine systems in ADHD. A positron emission tomography investigation in children with ADHD that found high midbrain accumulation of [18F]-labeled dihydroxyphenylalanine, a putative marker of dopamine synthesis, provides additional support for dopamine dysfunction in ADHD (Ernst *et al.*, 1999). A shift in dopaminergic dysfunction in ADHD from the midbrain to frontal cortex during adolescence has been proposed (Ernst *et al.*, 1998, 1999; Schweitzer *et al.*, 2000).

Studies examining the corpus callosum have generally shown reductions in its size in ADHD (Castellanos, 1994; Hill *et al.*, 2003), similar to the corpus callosal reductions observed in schizophrenia (Shenton *et al.*, 2001). Increased attentional problems have been associated with greater reductions in corpus callosal size (Kayl *et al.*, 2000).

Obsessive–compulsive disorder

Neurobiological studies in various laboratories using diverse techniques have consistently found alterations in ventral prefrontostriatothalamic function in OCD associated with symptom severity and response to treatment (Rosenberg *et al.*, 2001; Fig. 21.4). Recent investigation in treatment-naive pediatric patients with OCD has suggested a neural network dysplasia, with reduced striatal volumes and increased anterior cingulate and thalamic volumes. Rosenberg and colleagues (2000a, 2001) have proposed that a reversible thalamocorticostriatal dysfunction in glutamatergic

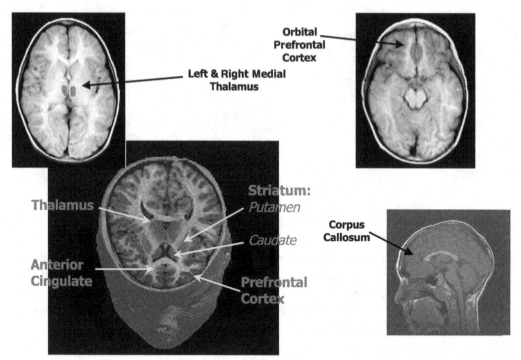

Fig. 21.4.   Brain regions implicated in the pathophysiology of obsessive–compulsive disorder. (Reprinted with permission from Rosenberg, D. R., MacMillan, S. N., Moore, G. J. Brain anatomy and chemistry may predict treatment response in paediatric obsessive–compulsive disorder. *Int J Neuropsychopharmacol* **4**: 179, 2001.) For a colour version of this figure, see www.cambridge.org/9780521126595.

neurotransmission may be critically involved in the pathogenesis and treatment response of pediatric patients with OCD (Fig. 21.5).

Total brain volume

In contrast to findings of reduced total cerebral volume in patients with ADHD and in those with schizophrenia, repeated investigation has revealed no significant differences in intracranial volume between treatment-naive pediatric patients with OCD and normal controls (Gilbert *et al.*, 2000; Rosenberg and Keshavan, 1998; Rosenberg *et al.*, 1997a). No significant changes in intracranial volume have been observed with treatment with a selective serotonin reuptake inhibitor or with cognitive behavioral therapy in pediatric patients with OCD (Gilbert *et al.*, 2000; Rosenberg *et al.*, 2000b).

Prefrontal cortex

Volumetric MRI investigation in treatment-naive pediatric patients with OCD compared with age- and sex-matched controls has demonstrated increased anterior

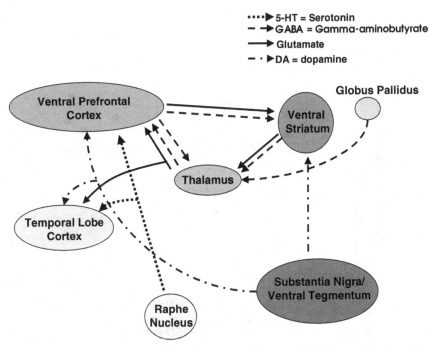

Fig. 21.5.   Schematic diagram showing selected aspects of corticostriatal connections in the neurodevelopment of obsessive–compulsive disorder. Arrows show the actions of different neurotransmitters. (Adapted by permission from D. R. Rosenberg and M. S. Keshavan. Toward
a neurodevelopmental model of obsessive–compulsive disorder. *Biol Psychiatry*, **43**: 623,
1998. Permission to reprint adaptation also from Farchione, T. R., MacMillan, S. N., Rosenberg, D. R. 2003. Obsessive–compulsive disorder as a fronto–striatal–thalamic dysfunction.
In *Mental and Behavioral Dysfunction in Movement Disorders*. Ed. Bedard, M. A., Agid, Y.,
Chouinard, S., *et al.* Totowa, NJ: Humana Press.)

cingulate volume in the former (Rosenberg and Keshavan, 1998; Fig. 21.6). These
observations contrast with cingulate volume reductions seen in schizophrenia
(Noga *et al.*, 1995; Takahashi *et al.*, 2003). The age-related increase in anterior
cingulate volume in healthy children appears to be absent in children with OCD.
Increased anterior cingulate volumes were positively correlated with increased OCD
symptom severity and inversely correlated with reduced striatal volumes. No significant differences were observed between children with OCD and controls in
dorsolateral prefrontal cortex, posterior cingulate, whole temporal lobe, amygdala,
hippocampus, or superior temporal gyrus volumes. By contrast, volumetric reductions have been seen in these structures in schizophrenia (reviewed by Shenton
et al., 2001). It should be noted that the increases in anterior cingulate volumes seen
in OCD have not been reported in pediatric patients with ADHD. Finally, reduced
NAA levels suggestive of neuronal dysfunction have been reported in the anterior

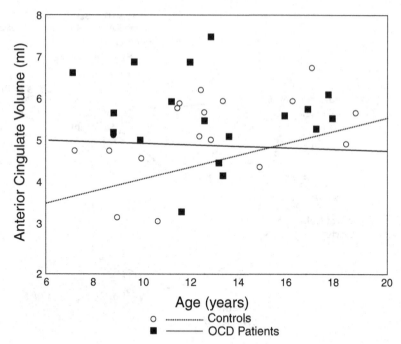

Fig. 21.6.   Anterior cingulate volume as a function of age for pediatric patients with obsessive–compulsive disorder and normal controls. Opposite neurodevelopmental trajectories in the patients compared with the healthy subjects may reflect an absence of early neuronal pruning in children with OCD. (Reprinted with permission from Rosenberg, D. R. Keshavan, M. S. Toward a neurodevelopmental model of obsessive–compulsive disorder. *Biol Psychiatry* **43**: 623, 1998.)

cingulate of pediatric patients with OCD (Ebert *et al.*, 1997). Reduced anterior cingulate glutamatergic concentrations have also been reported in pediatric patients with OCD, which increase to levels not significantly different from controls after effective treatment with the selective serotonin reuptake inhibitor paroxetine (Rosenberg *et al.*, 2002b). We have suggested that increased caudate glutamatergic concentrations coupled with reduced anterior cingulate glutamatergic concentrations in treatment-naive pediatric patients with OCD suggest a tonic–phasic dysregulation of the glutamatergic system involving the corticostriatal circuits in OCD (Rosenberg and Keshavan, 1998). Tonic cortical glutamatergic activity has an inhibitory influence on phasic stress-related glutamate release from the striatum, particularly the ventral striatum. Therefore, reduced tonic glutamatergic activity in the anterior cingulate might predispose to phasic glutamatergic overactivity in the striatum. The fact that caudate glutamatergic increase is reversible with paroxetine treatment further supports this idea.

Thalamus

The thalamus serves as the final subcortical relay station to various cortical structures, including the frontal cortex. There is evidence that thalamic volumes are reduced in first-episode neuroleptic drug-naive patients with schizophrenia (Gilbert *et al.*, 2001), whereas thalamic volumes are significantly increased in treatment-naive pediatric patients with OCD compared with controls. After 12 weeks of monodrug therapy with paroxetine, thalamic volumes decreased significantly to levels not significantly different from controls. Reduction in thalamic volumes in pediatric patients with OCD was positively correlated with reduction in OCD symptom severity, with higher pretreatment thalamic volumes predicting enhanced response to paroxetine. In contrast, thalamic volumes did not change significantly in treatment-naive pediatric patients with OCD treated for 12 weeks with cognitive behavioral therapy (Rosenberg *et al.*, 2000b). Consequently, reduction in thalamic volumes may be specific to treatment with a selective serotonin reuptake inhibitor rather than linked to a spontaneous resolution of symptoms or some more generalized treatment response.

Fitzgerald *et al.* (2000) used proton MRS to evaluate medial and lateral subregions of the thalamus since medial thalamic regions have been particularly implicated in OCD (Modell *et al.*, 1989). Reduced levels of NAA were found in medial, but not lateral, thalamus in pediatric patients with OCD. Increased thalamic volumes in pediatric patients with OCD were associated with lower levels of NAA, suggestive of neuronal dysfunction.

Basal ganglia

Similar to findings in patients with ADHD and schizophrenia, reduced striatal volumes have been observed in child and adolescent patients with OCD compared with controls, using both quantitative computed tomography (Luxenberg *et al.*, 1988) and volumetric MRI (Rosenberg *et al.*, 1997b). Reductions in striatal volumes were associated with increased OCD symptom severity, but not illness duration (Rosenberg *et al.*, 1997b). Consistent with reduced striatal volumes, increased ventricle to brain ratios and increased third ventricular volumes have been observed in children and adolescents with OCD compared with healthy controls (Behar *et al.*, 1984; Rosenberg *et al.*, 1997b).

Also, similar to reports in ADHD, reductions in NAA have been reported in the striatum in patients with OCD compared with controls (Bartha *et al.*, 1998; Ebert *et al.*, 1997). Bartha *et al.* (1998) proposed that this reduction in neuronal viability may be mediated by glutamatergic excitotoxicity. Therefore, Rosenberg *et al.* (2000a) measured caudate glutamatergic concentrations in treatment-naive pediatric patients with OCD before and after monodrug therapy with paroxetine and compared these with case-matched pediatric controls. The occipital cortex was also studied as a control region not implicated in the pathogenesis of OCD. Localized increased glutamatergic concentrations were observed in treatment-naive pediatric patients with OCD compared with controls in the caudate nucleus but not in the occipital cortex. Remarkably, after effective treatment with paroxetine, caudate glutamatergic concentrations decreased to levels not significantly different from those observed in controls. Reduction in caudate glutamatergic concentrations was positively correlated with reduction in OCD symptom severity, as measured by the Children's Yale Brown Obsessive Compulsive Scale. Increased caudate glutamatergic levels before treatment predicted better response to paroxetine, whereas decreased glutamatergic levels in the caudate pretreatment predicted a poorer response. There were no significant changes in occipital glutamatergic concentrations after paroxetine treatment. Reduction in caudate glutamatergic concentrations also appears to persist even after medication discontinuation if remission of OCD symptoms is maintained (Bolton *et al.*, 2001).

It should be noted that no significant changes in caudate glutamatergic concentrations were observed in 21 psychotropic drug-naive pediatric patients with OCD treated for 12 weeks with cognitive behavioral therapy (Benazon *et al.*, 2001). Therefore, the reduction in caudate glutamatergic concentrations may be specific to treatment with a selective serotonin reuptake inhibitor rather than reflecting a more generalized treatment response or spontaneous resolution of symptoms. It should be noted that increased striatal glutamate has been reported in medication-free pediatric patients with both OCD and ADHD (MacMaster *et al.*, 2003). This finding has to be viewed with caution, however, because the glutamine and glutamate resonances are not clearly resolved in the in vivo spectra.

The corpus callosum appears to be bigger in OCD than in normal controls (Rosenberg *et al.*, 1997a), which contrasts with the reductions in this structure seen in schizophrenia and ADHD. The mean signal intensity was also altered in patients with OCD, suggesting possibly an increase in myelination. However, not all studies show corpus callosum changes in OCD (Kellner *et al.*, 1991).

Major depressive disorder and bipolar disorder
Total brain volume

Steingard *et al.* (2002) observed smaller total brain volumes in adolescent patients with MDD compared with healthy adolescents. This is consistent with an MRI investigation that found reduced intracranial volumes in medication-free adult patients with MDD compared with controls (Brambilla *et al.*, 2001). No significant differences were observed in intracranial volume between patients with BPD and controls. Therefore, reduced total brain volumes appear to cut across diagnostic boundaries of ADHD and MDD but not OCD and BPD. A review of the literature by Soares and Mann (1997) suggested that left hemispheric lesions are more commonly associated with depression, whereas right-sided lesions appear to be more commonly associated with mania.

Frontal cortex

Reduced frontal lobe volumes have been consistently reported in adult and pediatric patients with MDD (Steingard *et al.*, 2002). These authors also noted reduced frontal white matter volumes and significantly larger frontal gray matter volumes in adolescent patients with MDD compared with healthy adolescents. It appears that patients with ADHD or MDD have reduced frontal white matter volumes compared with controls (Castellannos *et al.*, 2002), but the former also have reduced gray matter volumes. Striking left, but not right, volumetric reductions in the subgenual region of the prefrontal cortex, which are associated with reduced regional cerebral blood flow in this region, have been observed in adult patients with familial MDD or BPD (at least one first-degree relative with MDD or BPD) compared with that in patients with non-familial MDD or BPD (no evident family history) (Drevets, 2000). Botteron *et al.* (2002) also reported comparable left but not right volumetric reductions of the subgenual region of the prefrontal cortex in 30 young women aged 18–23 years with early-onset MDD and 18 women aged 24–52 years with recurrent MDD compared with matched controls. It should be noted that no significant differences from controls in left or right subgenual prefrontal cortex in patients with MDD or BPD were seen in other studies (Brambilla *et al.*, 2002; Bremner *et al.*, 2002). A recent investigation by Nolan *et al.* (2002) in 22 psychotropic drug-naive pediatric patients with MDD compared with 22 case-matched controls identified distinct neuroanatomic differences in left but not right prefrontal cortical volumes in familial but not non-familial MDD. Reduced left prefrontal cortical volume was correlated with increased depressive symptom severity and longer illness duration in familial but not non-familial MDD. Left-sided prefrontal cortical volume reduction in patients with familial MDD may represent a progressive rather than a static developmental effect and familial/genetic factors may be involved in pathogenesis given. However, since all investigations to date have been cross-sectional rather than longitudinal studies, definitive conclusions are premature.

Medial temporal cortex

MacMillan and colleagues (2003) have noted that volumetric abnormalities in the amygdala in pediatric patients with MDD may be more related to severity of anxiety than the severity of depression. Specifically, they observed increased bilateral amygdala hippocampal volumes in 23 treatment-naive pediatric patients with MDD compared with case-matched controls. Robust positive correlations were observed between increased amygdala–hippocampal volumes and increased severity of anxiety, but not with severity of depression or duration of illness. Amygdala volumes were larger in pediatric patients with MDD than in controls, while hippocampal volumes tended to be smaller in the MDD patients. Pine *et al.* (2001) has also found that excess fear in adolescence is a robust predictor for development of MDD in early adulthood. Moreover, in a recent fMRI study conducted by Thomas *et al.* (2001), measuring amygdala response to fearful faces in children with generalized anxiety disorder and panic disorder, children with MDD, and healthy controls, the magnitude of signal change in the amygdala was most associated with the severity of the child's anxiety in patients with MDD and generalized anxiety disorder.

When considering whether disordered brain development cuts across diagnostic boundaries, it is important to point out that increased amygdala volume is one of the more consistent findings observed in volumetric neuroimaging studies of adult patients with BPD (Altshuler *et al.*, 2000; Frodl *et al.*, 2002; Strakowski *et al.*, 1999). Increased amygdala activation in response to fearful facial affect has also been observed in fMRI studies conducted in patients with BPD (Thomas *et al.*, 2001). Pediatric MDD carries an increased risk for becoming BPD in adulthood (Geller *et al.*, 2001; Harrington *et al.*, 1990; Weissman *et al.*, 1999), and increased amygdala and reduced hippocampal volumes are seen in pediatric patients with MDD and in adults with first-episode MDD (Frodl *et al.*, 2002; MacMillan *et al.*, 2003). These findings contrast with those reporting decreased amygdala volumes in patients with schizophrenia (reviewed by Shenton *et al.*, 2001), and in those at risk for this disorder (Keshavan *et al.*, 2002b; Ch. 19). Longitudinal MRI studies are necessary to determine whether anatomic and functional alterations in the amygdala may serve as potential biomarkers of risk for development of BPD.

Only one available study has examined the corpus callosum in unipolar depression and this found an increase in size (Wu *et al.*, 1993). The corpus callosum also appears to be larger in BPD (Hauser *et al.*, 1989), and the striatum appears larger in first-episode BPD (Strakowski *et al.*, 2002). However, basal ganglia volumes appear to be reduced in depression (reviewed by Soares and Mann, 1997).

Other factors that may occur across psychiatric disorders

While advances in neuroimaging have afforded a new understanding of the developmental abnormalities associated with psychiatric disorders, genetics and other etiological factors, such as obstetric complications (OCs), contribute to our understanding of psychiatric disorders and further help to identify the inherent diagnostic overlap associated with psychiatric phenomena.

Genetic component

There is a substantial genetic component to both schizophrenia and ADHD. Early family, twin, and adoptee studies have shown a strong likelihood of genetic susceptibility in both ADHD and schizophrenia. Combined reports suggest that the mean concordance for schizophrenia within monozygotic twins is approximately 46% and within dizygotic pairs is approximately 14% (Gottesman, 1991; Moldin and Gottesman, 1997). The rate of ADHD in first-degree relatives of children diagnosed as having ADHD ranges from 16% to 25% (Biederman *et al.*, 1992, 1991).

Molecular genetic findings suggest that alterations in the dopaminergic system may underlie both ADHD and schizophrenia. Several groups have reported alterations in the gene encoding the dopamine D_4 receptor in children diagnosed with ADHD (Benjamin *et al.*, 1996; Ebstein *et al.*, 1996; LaHoste *et al.*, 1996). Cook *et al.* (1995) and Gill *et al.* (1997) have both reported an association between alterations in the gene encoding the dopamine transporter and ADHD. Alterations in the gene encoding catechol-*O*-methyltransferase (COMT), an enzyme that degrades dopamine, have been associated with schizophrenia (reviewed by Sawa and Snyder, 2002) and with BPD (Badner and Gershon, 2002). In animals with a targeted deletion of the COMT gene, decreased levels of dopamine are seen only in the prefrontal cortex (Gogos *et al.*, 1998). Therefore, changes affecting dopamine metabolism could lead to a decrease in prefrontal dopamine levels, and such deficits may underlie the executive function deficits seen in both schizophrenia and BPD.

A heritability component has been suggested in both OCD and BPD. However, by contrast with schizophrenia where replicable findings are beginning to emerge (O'Donovan *et al.*, 2003; Ch. 1), few replicated genetic susceptibility loci have been identified for OCD and BPD. One finding suggests linkage of BPD to a location on chromosome 18 (Berrettini *et al.*, 1994; Stine *et al.*, 1995). However, the large-scale National Institute of Mental Health Genetics Bipolar Group study (1997) did not find an association between BPD and chromosome 18.

Obstetric complications

While accumulating evidence points to the role of OCs in vulnerability for schizophrenia (Ch. 11), the diagnostic specificity and the etiological significance of this association remain unclear. Other severe psychiatric disorders, such as ADHD and psychotic affective disorder, have been linked with OCs; low birth weight, neonatal complications, and excessive bleeding have been associated with ADHD (Milberger *et al.*, 1997; Sprich-Buckminster *et al.*, 1993). OCs have been observed sporadically in BPD (reviewed by Buka and Fan, 1999) but could not be reliably replicated. Complications within these studies include small sample sizes and data obtained primarily in retrospect from maternal recall. A recent comprehensive study showed no excess in OCs in mania (Browne *et al.*, 2000).

Overall, OCs may increase the vulnerability for a range of severe mental disorders in a relatively non-specific way and may interact with genetic liability and later environmental risk factors (Verdoux and Sutter, 2002).

Conclusions

The studies described in this chapter indicate the impressive commonalities in neurodevelopmentally mediated pathophysiological alterations across several major psychiatric disorders. The similarities in pathophysiology are consistent with the observations of frequent comorbidity and diagnostic overlap. The similarity between ADHD and schizophrenia in abnormalities of the overall brain volume, corpus callosum size, and frontostriatal circuits is striking and is consistent with the increasing understanding of attentional impairment as a core feature of schizophrenia (Ch. 4). Additionally, observations of attentional problems are among the most robust premorbid predictors of later schizophrenia (Ch. 23). There is good evidence that ADHD also predicts the later emergence of BPD (Kim and Miklowitz, 2002). Interestingly, an association has also been proposed between ADHD and childhood OCD (Geller *et al.*, 2002). Therefore, attentional impairments in childhood may serve as the bridge connecting the commonalities between diverse psychiatric presentations in adulthood, such as OCD, BPD, and schizophrenia (Fig. 21.1). Considering the earlier onset of ADHD compared with the other disorders, it may even be suggested that attentional impairments, perhaps related to distributed cortical gray and white matter changes, especially in the prefrontal cortex, may represent a non-specific precursor for the later development psychiatric disorders, at least in some patients.

The comparisons between overlapping disorders also reveal some intriguing differences. For example, while schizophrenia and OCD share similar reductions in striatal volumes, OCD shows increased cingulate volumes while schizophrenia shows decreased volumes. Similarly, patients with BPD and possibly those with OCD show larger amygdala volumes, whereas smaller amygdala volumes are observed in schizophrenia. Patients with BPD may also show larger basal ganglia, unlike the schizophrenia patients. This suggests that different developmental trajectories may emerge during late childhood and adolescence from common neurodevelopmental precursors in childhood. These developmental trajectories may be related to differential pathoplastic responses of the subcortical brain structures, such as the cingulate and amygdala, and may mediate the emergence of distinct symptomatic presentations. It is useful to recall here that the amygdala and the cingulate are critically involved in affect regulation and conflict monitoring, respectively (Carter *et al.*, 1999; Ledoux, 2003). Consequently, the amygdala enlargements in BPD might represent a pathological hyperplasia in that region related to repeated activation in the context of highly valenced emotional states, such as the manic and depressive episodes. Likewise, the cingulate enlargement in OCD might reflect a hyperresponsive error-monitoring system. By comparison, failure of optimum functioning of the cingulate and amygdala may underlie the deficits in self-monitoring that lead to disorganized thinking and diminished affective responsivity, leading to blunted affect in schizophrenia.

These predictions can best be examined by an integrated approach to longitudinal follow-up studies of children at risk for a variety of major psychiatric disorders using the non-invasive neuroimaging techniques that are available. Such studies also allow us to clarify the common and distinct neurodevelopmental alterations across diverse disorders and help us to unravel the shared and distinct vulnerability factors of genetic or environmental origin. Additionally, mapping the developmental trajectories of adult psychiatric disorders can help in designing prevention strategies. Several longitudinal–epidemiological studies suggest that most adult psychiatric problems can be traced back to childhood disorders, either of the same type (i.e. homotypic continuity) or a different one (i.e. sequential comorbidity) (Kim-Cohen *et al.*, 2003). Improved knowledge of the common developmental basis of psychiatric disorders will clearly promote a life-course developmental approach to psychopathology and eventually improve treatment and prevention.

REFERENCES

Adler, C. M., Strakowski, S. M. (2003). Boundaries of schizophrenia. *Psychiatr Clin North Am* **26**: 1–23.

Altshuler, L. L., Bartzokis, G., Grieder, T., *et al.* (2000). An MRI study of temporal lobe structures in men with bipolar disorder or schizophrenia. *Biol Psychiatry* **48**: 147–162.

Andreasen, N. C., Rezai, K., Alliger, R., *et al.* (1992). Hypofrontality in neuroleptic-naive patients and in patients with chronic schizophrenia. Assessment with xenon 133 single-photon emission computed tomography and the Tower of London. *Arch Gen Psychiatry* **49**: 943–958.

Aylward, E. H., Reiss, A. L., Reader, M. J., *et al.* (1996). Basal ganglia volumes in children with attention-deficit hyperactivity disorder. *J Child Neurol* **11**: 112–115.

Badner, J. A., Gershon, E. S. (2002). Meta-analysis of whole-genome scans of bipolar disorder and schizophrenia. *Mol Psychiatry* **7**: 405–411.

Bartha, R., Stein, M. B., Williamson, P. C., *et al.* (1998). A short echo ^{1}H spectroscopy and volumetric MRI study of the corpus striatum in patients with obsessive–compulsive disorder and comparison subjects. *Am J Psychiatry* **155**: 1584–1591.

Behar, D., Rapoport, J. L., Berg, C. J., *et al.* (1984). Computerized tomography and neuropsychological test measures in adolescents with obsessive–compulsive disorder. *Am J Psychiatry* **141**: 363–369.

Bellak, L., Kay, S. R., Opler, L. A. (1987). Attention deficit disorder psychosis as a diagnostic category. *Psychiatr Dev* **5**: 239–263.

Benazon, N. R., Ager, J., Rosenberg, D. R. (2001). Cognitive behavior therapy in treatment-naive children and adolescents with obsessive–compulsive disorder: an open trial. *Behav Res Ther* **40**: 529–539.

Benjamin, J., Li, L., Patterson, C., *et al.* (1996). Population and familial association between the D4 dopamine receptor gene and measures of novelty seeking. *Nat Genet* **12**: 81–84.

Berrettini, W. (2000). Review of bipolar molecular linkage and association studies. *Curr Psychiatry Rep* **4**: 124–129.

Berrettini, W. H., Ferraro, T. N., Alexander, R. C., Buchberg, A. M., Vogel, W. H. (1994). Quantitative trait loci mapping of three loci controlling morphine preference using inbred mouse strains. *Nat Genet* **7**: 54–58.

Biederman, J., Faraone, S. V., Keenan, V., Tsuang, M. T. (1991). Evidence of familial association between attention deficit disorders and major affective disorder. *Arch Gen Psychiatry* **78**: 633–672.

Biederman, J., Faraone, S. V., Keenan, K., *et al.* (1992). Further evidence for familial-genetic risk factors in ADHD: patterns of comorbidity in probands and relatives in psychiatrically and pediatrically referred samples. *Arch Gen Psychiatry* **49**: 728–738.

Birken, D. L., Oldendorf, W. H. (1989). *N*-Acetyl-L-aspartic acid: a literature review of a compound prominent in ^{1}H-NMR spectroscopic studies of brain. *Neurosci Biobehav Rev* **13**: 23–31.

Bolton, J., Moore, G. J., MacMillan, S., Stewart, C. M., Rosenberg, D. R. (2001). Case study: caudate glutamatergic changes with paroxetine persist after medication discontinuation in pediatric OCD. *J Am Acad Child Adolesc Psychiatry* **40**: 903–906.

Botteron, K. N., Raichle, M. E., Drevets, W. C., Heath, A. C., Todd, R. D. (2002). Volumetric reduction in left subgenual prefrontal cortex in early onset depression. *Biol Psychiatry* **51**: 342–344.

Brambilla, P., Harenski, K., Nicoletti, M. A., *et al.* (2001). Anatomical MRI study of basal ganglia in bipolar disorder patients. *Psychiatry Res* **106**: 65–80.

Brambilla, P., Nicoletti, M. A., Harenski, K., *et al.* (2002). Anatomical MRI study of subgenual prefrontal cortex in bipolar and unipolar subjects. *Neuropsychopharmacology* **27**: 792–799.

Bremner, J. D., Vythilingam, M., Vermetten, E., *et al.* (2002). Reduced volume of orbitofrontal cortex in major depression. *Biol Psychiatry* **51**: 273–279.

Browne, R., Byrne, M., Mulryan, N., *et al.* (2000). Labor and delivery complications at birth and later mania. *Br J Psychiatry* **176**: 369–372.

Buka, S., Fan, A. (1999). Association of prenatal and perinatal complications with subsequent bipolar disorder and schizophrenia. *Schizophr Res* **39**: 113–119.

Bush, G., Frazier, J. A., Rauch, S. L., *et al.* (1999). Anterior cingulate cortex dysfunction in attention-deficit/hyperactivity disorder revealed by fMRI and the Counting Stroop. *Biol Psychiatry* **45**: 1542–1552.

Caplan, R., Guthrie, D., Tang, B., Nuechterlein, K. H., Asarnow, R. E. (2002). Thought disorder in attention-deficit hyperactivity disorder. *Int Rev Neurobiol* **49**: 269–284.

Carter, C. S., Botvinick, M. M., Cohen, J. D. (1999). The contribution of the anterior cingulate cortex to executive process in cognition. *Rev Neurosci* **10**: 49–57.

Casey, B. J., Castellanos, F. X., Giedd, J. N., *et al.* (1997). Implication of right frontostriatal circuitry in response inhibition and attention-deficit/hyperactivity disorder. *J Am Acad Child Adolesc Psychiatry* **36**: 374–383.

Castellanos, F. X., Giedd, J. N., Eckburg, P., *et al.* (1994). Quantitative morphology of the caudate nucleus in attention deficit hyperactivity disorder. *Am J Psychiatry* **151**: 1791–1796.

Castellanos, F. X., Giedd, J. N., Berquin, P. C., *et al.* (2001). Quantitative brain magnetic resonance imaging in girls with attention-deficit/hyperactivity disorder. *Arch Gen Psychiatry* **58**: 289–295.

Castellanos, F. X., Lee, P. P., Sharp, W., *et al.* (2002). Developmental trajectories of brain volume abnormalities in children and adolescents with attention-deficit/hyperactivity disorder. *J Am Mod Assoc* **288**: 1740–1748.

Chang, K. D., Steiner, H., Ketter, T. A. (2000). Psychiatric phenomenology of child and adolescent bipolar offspring. *J Am Acad Child Adolesc Psychiatry* **39**: 453–460.

Cook, E. H., Sterin, M. A., Krasowski, M. D., *et al.* (1995). Association of attention-deficit disorder and the dopamine transporter gene. *Am J Hum Genet* **56**: 993–998.

Drevets, W. C. (2000). Neuroimaging studies of mood disorders. *Biol Psychiatry* **48**: 813–829.

Durston, S., Hulshoff Pol, H. E., Casey, B. J., *et al.* (2001). Anatomical MRI of the developing human brain: what have we learned? *J Am Acad Child Adolesc Psychiatry* **40**: 1012–1020.

Ebert, D., Speck, O., Konig, A., *et al.* (1997). ^{1}H-magnetic resonance spectroscopy in obsessive–compulsive disorder: evidence for neuronal loss in the cingulate gyrus and the right striatum. *Psychiatry Res* **74**: 173–176.

Ebstein, R. P., Novick, O., Umansky, R., *et al.* (1996). Dopamine D4 receptor (D4DR) exon III polymorphism associated with the human personality trait of novelty seeking. *Nat Genet* **12**: 78–80.

Ernst, M., Zametkin, A. J., Matochik, J. A., Jons, P. J., Cohen, R. M. (1998). DOPA decarboxylase activity in attention deficit hyperactivity disorder adults. A [fluorine-18]fluorodopa positron emission tomographic study. *J Neurosci* **18**: 5901–5907.

Ernst, M., Zametkin, A. J., Matochik, J. A., *et al.* (1999). High midbrain [^{18}F]DOPA accumulation in children with attention deficit hyperactivity disorder. *Am J Psychiatry* **156**: 1209–1215.

Farchione, T. R., MacMillan, S. N., Rosenberg, D. R. (2003). Obsessive–compulsive disorder as a fronto–striatal–thalamic dysfunction. In *Mental and Behavioral Dysfunction in Movement Disorders*, ed. M. A. Bedord, Y. Agid, S. Chouinard, *et al.* Totowa, NJ: Humana Press, pp. 477–488.

Filipek, P. A., Semrud-Clikeman, M., Steingard, R. J., *et al.* (1997). Volumetric MRI analysis comparing attention-deficit hyperactivity disorder and normal controls. *Neurology* **48**: 589–601.

Fitzgerald, K. D., Moore, G. J., Paulson, L. D., Stewart, C. M., Rosenberg, D. R. (2000). Proton spectroscopic imaging of the thalamus in treatment-naive pediatric obsessive–compulsive disorder. *Biol Psychiatry* **48**: 55–72.

Frodl, T., Meisenzahl, E., Zetzsche, T., *et al.* (2002). Enlargement of the amygdala in patients with a first episode of major depression. *Biol Psychiatry* **51**: 708–714.

Geller, B., Zimerman, B., Williams, M., Bolhofner, K., Craney, J. L. (2001). Bipolar disorder at prospective follow-up of adults who had prepubertal major depressive disorder. *Am J Psychiatry* **158**: 125–127.

Geller, D. A., Biederman, J., Faraone, S. V., *et al.* (2002). Attention-deficit/hyperactivity disorder in children and adolescents with obsessive–compulsive disorder: fact or artifact? *J Am Acad Child Adolesc Psychiatry* **41**: 52–58.

Gilbert, A. R., Moore, G. J., Keshavan, M. S., *et al.* (2000). Decrease in thalamic volumes of pediatric patients with obsessive–compulsive disorder who are taking paroxetine. *Arch Gen Psychiatry* **57**: 449–456.

Gilbert, A. R., Rosenberg, D. R., Harenski, K., *et al.* (2001). Thalamic volumes in patients with first-episode schizophrenia. *Am J Psychiatry* **158**: 618–624.

Gill, M., Daly, G., Heron, S., Hawi, Z., Fitzgerald, M. (1997). Confirmation of association between attention deficit hyperactivity disorder and a dopamine transporter polymorphism. *Biol Psychiatry* **2**: 311–313.

Gogos, J. A., Morgan, M., Luine, V., *et al.* (1998). Catechol-*O*-methyltransferase-deficient mice exhibit sexually dimorphic changes in catecholamine levels and behavior. *Proc Natl Acad Sci USA* **95**: 9991–9996.

Gottesman, I. L. (1991). *Schizophrenia Genesis: The Origins of Madness.* New York: Freeman.

Gross-Isseroff, R., Hermesh, H., Zohar, J., Weizman, A. (2003). Neuroimaging communality between schizophrenia and obsessive–compulsive disorder: a putative basis for schizo-obsessive disorder? *World J Biol Psychiatry* **4**: 129–134.

Harrington, R., Fudge, H., Rutter, M., Pickles, A., Hill, J. (1990). Adult outcomes of childhood and adolescent depression: psychiatric status. *Arch Gen Psychiatry* **47**: 465–473.

Hauser, P., Dauphinais, I. D., Berrettini, W., *et al.* (1989). Corpus callosum dimensions measured by magnetic resonance imaging in bipolar affective disorder and schizophrenia. *Biol Psychiatry* **26**: 659–668.

Hesslinger, B., Thiel, T., Tebartz van Elst, L., Hennig, J., Ebert, D. (2001). Attention-deficit disorder in adults with or without hyperactivity: where is the difference? A study in humans using short echo ^{1}H-magnetic resonance spectroscopy. *Neurosci Lett* **304**: 117–119.

Hill, D. E., Yeo, R. A., *et al.* (2003). Magnetic resonance imaging correlates of attention-deficit/hyperactivity disorder in children. *Neuropsychology* **17**: 496–506.

Hynd, G. W., Semrud-Clikeman, M., Lorys, A. R., Novey, E. S., Eliopulos, D. (1990). Brain morphology in developmental dyslexia and attention deficit disorder/hyperactivity. *Arch Neurol* **47**: 919–926.

Hynd, G. W., Hern, K. L., Novey, E. S., *et al.* (1993). Attention deficit hyperactivity disorder and asymmetry of the caudate nucleus. *J Child Neurol* **8**: 339–347.

Kayl, A. E., Moore, III, B. D., Slopis, J. M., Jackson, E. F., Leeds, N. E. (2000). Quantitative morphology of the corpus callosum in children with neurofibromatosis and attention-deficit hyperactivity disorder. *J Child Neurol* **15**: 90–96.

Keshavan, M. S., Montrose, D. M., Pierri, J. N., *et al.* (1997). Magnetic resonance imaging and spectroscopy in offspring at risk for schizophrenia: preliminary studies. *Prog Neuropsychopharmacol Biol Psychiatry* **21**: 1285–1295.

Keshavan, M. S., Rosenberg, D., Sweeney, J. A., Pettegrew, J. W. (1998). Decreased caudate volume in neuroleptic-naive psychotic patients. *Am J Psychiatry* **155**: 774–778.

Keshavan, M. S., Sujata, M., Mehra, A., Montrose, D. M., Sweeney, J. A. (2002a). Psychosis proneness and ADHD in young relatives at risk for schizophrenia. *Schizophr Res* **59**: 85–92.

Keshavan, M. S., Dick, E., Mankowski, I., *et al.* (2002b). Decreased left amygdala and hippocampal volumes in young offspring at risk for schizophrenia. *Schizophr Res* **58**: 173–183.

Kellner, C. H., Jolley, R. R., Holgate, R. C., *et al.* (1991). Brain MRI in obsessive–compulsive disorder. *Psychiatry Res* **36**: 45–49.

Kim-Cohen, J., Caspi, A., Moffitt, T. E., *et al.* (2003). Prior juvenile diagnoses in adults with mental disorder: developmental follow-back of a prospective-longitudinal cohort. *Arch Gen Psychiatry* **60**: 709–717.

Kim, E. Y., Miklowitz, D. J. (2002). Childhood mania, attention deficit hyperactivity disorder and conduct disorder: a critical review of diagnostic dilemmas. *Bipolar Disord* **4**: 215–225.

LaHoste, G. J., Swanson, J. M., Wigal, S. B., *et al.* (1996). Dopamine D4 receptor gene polymorphism is associated with attention-deficit hyperactivity disorder. *Mol Psychiatry* **1**: 121–124.

Ledoux, J. (2003). The emotional brain, fear, and the amygdala. *Cell Mol Neurobiol* **23**: 727–738.

Luxenberg, J. S., Swedo, S. E., Flament, M. F., *et al.* (1988). Neuroanatomical abnormalities in obsessive–compulsive disorder detected with quantitative X-ray computed tomography. *Am J Psychiatry* **145**: 1089–1093.

MacMaster, F. P., Carrey, N., Sparkes, S., Khan, S., Kusumakar, V. (2003). Proton spectroscopy in medication free pediatric attention deficit hyperactivity disorder. *Biol Psychiatry* **53**: 184–187.

MacMillan, S. N., Szeszko, P. R., Moore, G. J., *et al.* (2003). Increased amygdala:hippocampal volumes associated with severity of anxiety in pediatric major depression. *J Child Adol Psychpharm* **13**: 65–73.

Milberger, S., Biederman, J., Faraone, S. X., Guite, J., Tsuang, M. T. (1997). Pregnancy, delivery, and infancy complications and attention deficit hyperactivity disorder: issues of gene–environment interaction. *Biol Psychiatry* **41**: 65–75.

Modell, J. G., Mountz, J. M., Curtis, G. C., Greden, J. F. (1989). Neurophysiologic dysfunction in basal ganglia/limbic striatal and thalamocortical circuits as a pathogenetic mechanism of obsessive–compulsive disorder. *J Neuropsychiatry Clin Neurosci* **1**: 27–36.

Moldin, S. O., Gottesman, I. I. (1997). At issue: genes, experiments and chance in schizophrenia-positioning for the 21st century. *Schizoph Bull* **23**: 547–561.

Moller, H. J. (2003). Bipolar disorder and schizophrenia: distinct illnesses or a continuum? *J Clin Psychiatry* **64**: 23–27.

National Institute of Mental Health Genetics Initiative Bipolar Group (1997). Genomic survey of bipolar illness in the NIMH Genetics Initiative pedigrees: a preliminary report. *Am J Med Gen Neuropsychiatr Genet* **74**: 227–237.

Noga, J. T., Aylward, E., Barta, P. E., Pearlson, G. D. (1995). Cingulate gyrus in schizophrenic patients and normal volunteers. *Psychiatry Res* **61**: 201–208.

Nolan, C. L., Moore, G. J., Madden, R., *et al.* (2002). Prefrontal cortical volume in childhood-onset major depression: preliminary findings. *Arch Gen Psychiatry* **59**: 173–179.

O'Donovan, M. C., Williams, N. M., Owen, M. J. (2003). Recent advances in the genetics of schizophrenia. *Hum Mol Genet* **12**(Suppl 2): R125–R133.

Pine, D. S., Cohen, P., Brook, J. (2001). Adolescent fears as predictors of depression. *Biol Psychiatry* **50**: 721–724.

Rosenberg, D. R., Keshavan, M. S., Dick, E. L., *et al.* (1997a). Corpus callosal morphology in treatment-naive pediatric obsessive–compulsive disorder. *Prog Neuropsychopharmacol Biol Psychiatry* **21**: 1269–1283.

Rosenberg, D. R., Keshavan, M. S., O'Hearn, K. M., *et al.* (1997b). Frontostriatal measurement in treatment-naive children with obsessive–compulsive disorder. *Arch Gen Psychiatry* **54**: 824–830.

Rosenberg, D. R., Keshavan, M. S. (1998). A. E. Bennett Research Award. Toward a neurodevelopmental model of obsessive–compulsive disorder. *Biol Psychiatry* **43**: 623–640.

Rosenberg, D. R., MacMaster, F. P., Keshavan, M. S., *et al.* (2000a). Decrease in caudate glutamatergic concentrations in pediatric obsessive–compulsive disorder patients taking paroxetine. *J Am Acad Child Adolesc Psychiatry* **39**: 1096–1103.

Rosenberg, D. R., Benazon, N. R., Gilbert, A., Sullivan, A., Moore, G. J. (2000b). Thalamic volume in pediatric obsessive–compulsive disorder patients before and after cognitive behavioral therapy. *Biol Psychiatry* **48**: 294–300.

Rosenberg, D. R., MacMillan, S. N., Moore, G. J. (2001). Brain anatomy and chemistry may predict treatment response in pediatric obsessive–compulsive disorder. *Int J Neuropsychopharmacol* **4**: 179–190.

Rosenberg, D. R., Davanzo, P. A., Gershon, S. (2002a). *Pharmacotherapy for Child and Adolescent Psychiatric Disorders*, 2nd edn (revised and expanded). New York: Marcel Dekker.

Rosenberg, D. R., Madden, R., Tang, J., *et al.* (2002b). Anterior cingulate glutamate and treatment response in pediatric OCD. In *Scientific Proceedings of the 49th Annual Meeting of the American Academy of Child and Adolescent Psychiatry*. Washington DC: American Academy of Child and Adolescent Psychiatry, Vol. D18, p. 118.

Rubia, K., Overmeyer, S., Taylor, E., *et al.* (1999). Hypofrontality in attention deficit hyperactivity disorder during higher-order motor control: a study with functional MRI. *Am J Psychiatry* **156**: 891–896.

Sawa, A., Snyder, S. (2002). Schizophrenia: diverse approaches to a complex disease. *Science* **296**: 692–695.

Schweitzer, J. B., Anderson, C., Ernst, M. (2000). Attention-deficit hyperactivity disorder: neuroimaging and behavioral/cognitive probes. In *Functional Neuroimaging in Child Psychiatry*, ed. M. Ernst, J. Rumsey. Cambridge, UK: Cambridge University Press, pp. 278–297.

Shenton, M. E., Dickey, C. C., Frumin, M., McCarley, R. W. (2001). A review of MRI findings in schizophrenia. *Schizophr Res* **49**: 1–52.

Shihabuddin, L., Buchsbaum, M. S., Hazlett, E. A., *et al.* (1998). Dorsal striatal size, shape, and metabolic rate in never-medicated and previously medicated schizophrenics performing a verbal learning task. *Arch Gen Psychiatry* **55**: 235–243.

Soares, J. C., Mann, J. J. (1997). The anatomy of mood disorders: review of structural neuroimaging studies. *Biol Psychiatry* **41**: 86–106.

Sowell, E. R., Toga, A. W., Asarnow, R. (2000). Brain abnormalities observed in childhood-onset schizophrenia: a review of the structural magnetic resonance imaging literature. *Ment Retard Dev Disabil Res Rev* **6**: 180–185.

Sprich-Buckminster, S., Biederman, J., Milberger, S., Faraone, S. W., Lehman, B. K. (1993). Are perinatal complications relevant to the manifestation of ADD? Issues of comorbidity and familiality. *J Am Acad Child Adolesc Psychiatry* **32**: 1032–1037.

Steingard, R. J., Renshaw, P. F., Hennen, J., *et al.* (2002). Smaller frontal lobe white matter volumes in depressed adolescents. *Biol Psychiatry* **52**: 413–417.

Stine, O. C., Xu, J., Koskela, R., *et al.* (1995). Evidence for linkage of bipolar disorder to chromosome 18 with a parent-of-origin effect. *Am J Hum Genet* **57**: 1384–1394.

Strakowski, S. M., DelBello, M. P., Sax, K. W., *et al.* (1999). Brain magnetic resonance imaging of structural abnormalities in bipolar disorder. *Arch Gen Psychiatry* **56**: 254–260.

Strakowski, S. M., DelBello, M. P., Zimmerman, M. E., *et al.* (2002). Ventricular and periventricular structural volumes in first- versus multiple-episode bipolar disorder. *Am J Psychiatry* **159**: 1841–1847.

Takahashi, T., Suzuki, M., Kawasaki, Y., *et al.* (2003). Perigenual cingulate gyrus volume in patients with schizophrenia: a magnetic resonance imaging study. *Biol Psychiatry* **53**: 593–600.

Tannock, R. (1998). Attention deficit hyperactivity disorder: advances in cognitive, neurobiological, and genetic research. *J Child Psychol Psychiatry* **39**: 65–99.

Taylor, M. A. (1992). Are schizophrenia and affective disorder related? A selective literature review. *Am J Psychiatry* **149**: 22–32.

Teicher, M. H., Anderson, C. M., Polcari, A., *et al.* (2000). Functional deficits in basal ganglia of children with attention-deficit/hyperactivity disorder shown with functional magnetic resonance imaging relaxometry. *Nat Med* **6**: 470–473.

Thomas, K. M., Drevets, W. C., Dahl, R. E., *et al.* (2001). Amygdala response to fearful faces in anxious and depressed children. *Arch Gen Psychiatry* **58**: 1057–1063.

Vaidya, C. J., Austin, G., Kirkorian, G., *et al.* (1998). Selective effects of methylphenidate in attention deficit hyperactivity disorder: a functional magnetic resonance study. *Proc Natl Acad Sci USA* **95**: 14494–14499.

Verdoux, H., Sutter, A. L. (2002). Perinatal risk factors for schizophrenia: diagnostic specificity and relationships with maternal psychopathology. *Am J Med Genet* **114**: 898–905.

Weissman, M. M., Wolk, S., Wickramaratne, P., *et al.* (1999). Children with prepubertal-onset major depressive disorder and anxiety grown up. *Arch Gen Psychiatry* **56**: 794–801.

Wu, J. C., Buchsbaum, M. S., Johnson, J. C., *et al.* (1993). Magnetic resonance and positron emission tomography imaging of the corpus callosum: size, shape and metabolic rate in unipolar depression. *J Affect Disord* **28**: 15–25.

Zametkin, A. J., Nordahl, T. E., Gross, M., *et al.* (1990). Cerebral glucose metabolism in adults with hyperactivity of childhood onset. *N Engl J Med* **323**: 1361–1366.

Part IV

Clinical implications

22

Can one identify preschizophrenia children?

Eugenia Kravariti, Paola Dazzan, Paul Fearon, and Robin M. Murray

Institute of Psychiatry, King's College, London, UK

The 1980s and 1990s saw a surge of neurodevelopmental theories of schizophrenia, which challenged the traditional notion of the disorder as an early form of dementia or other degenerative condition (Kraepelin, 1919). Some early versions of the neurodevelopmental hypothesis – sometimes unkindly termed "doomed from the womb" theories – saw schizophrenia as the inevitable consequence of an early brain lesion (Murray and Lewis, 1987; Weinberger, 1987). More recently, however, it has become increasingly accepted that the likelihood of schizophrenia developing is probabilistic rather than deterministic (Fearon *et al.*, 2001).

The postulated aberration in neurodevelopment was initially thought to be silent until late adolescence or early adulthood. It is now hypothesised to give rise to subtle brain abnormalities, which determine the underlying susceptibility to schizophrenia, and translate into subtle neuro-behavioral deficits that are evident throughout development (Murray, 1994). Therefore, identifying and characterizing the early-emerging markers of the schizophrenia diathesis offers the theoretical possibility of predicting the disorder. However, childhood antecedents of schizophrenia may variably reflect (i) integral components of the schizophrenia diathesis, (ii) non-specific factors that potentiate this predisposition, or (iii) early manifestations of the disorder itself (Dworkin and Cornblatt, 1995). While all three types of antecedent are relevant to estimating *schizophrenia risk*, only the third one is directly relevant to establishing *preschizophrenic status*, and, hence, to predicting with certainty which individuals will express the disorder.

In this chapter, we will explore the nature of the childhood antecedents of schizophrenia, addressing the following questions. Are children who develop schizophrenia in adulthood distinguishable from control children? How strong is the association between the distinguishing features of preschizophrenia children as a group and the later development of the disorder? How accurately can we identify

Neurodevelopment and Schizophrenia, ed. Matcheri S. Keshavan *et al.* Published by Cambridge University Press. © Cambridge University Press 2004.

Table 22.1. Predicting schizophrenia: neurointegrative risk factors in population-based, high-risk and archival–observational studies

Risk factor	OR/(RR)	SEN (%)	SPE (%)	PPV (%)	NPV (%)
Population-based studies					
Delayed developmental milestones at 2 yrs (Jones et al., 1994)[a]	4.8	7	98	3	99
Learned to stand at or after 12 months (Isohanni et al., 2001)[b]	(1.4)	–	–	–	–
Excess of neurological signs at 3 yrs (Cannon et al., 2002)[c]	4.6	–	–	–	–
Unusual movements at 7 yrs (Rosso et al., 2000)[d]	4.4	15	96	3	99
Motor coordination dysfunction at 7 yrs (Rosso et al., 2000)[d]	2.4	11	96	2	99
High-risk studies					
Deviance on a composite index of attentional, perceptual and motor dysfunctioning at 8–15 yrs (Marcus et al., 1987)[e]	–	89	64	22	98
Gross motor skills at 7–12 yrs (Erlenmeyer-Kimling et al., 2000)[f]	–	75	73	33	94
Archival-observational studies					
Postural hand abnormalities in the first 2 yrs of life (Walker et al., 1994)[g]	7.9[g]	63	82	–	–
Choreoathetoid movements in the first 2 yrs of life (Walker et al., 1994)[g]	8.2[g]	23	96	–	–

OR, odds ratio; RR, risk ratio (the ratio between the observed and the expected cases); SEN, sensitivity; SPE, specificity; PPV, positive predictive value; NPV, negative predictive value.

[a]The British MRC National Survey of Health and Development of 1946 followed prospectively a stratified random sample (4746 alive at 16 years) of 13 687 births in Britain during the week 3–9 March 1946. Thirty subjects developed schizophrenia at ages 16–43 and were compared with the remaining 4716 subjects.

[b]The Northern Finland Birth Cohort Study (Isohanni et al., 1998, 1999, 2001) followed prospectively 96% of all births in Northern Finland in 1966 (12 058 liveborn children). Psychiatric outcome was established at 16–28 years (58 subjects had developed schizophrenia), and the comparison group included individuals with no hospital-treated psychiatric outcome (Isohanni et al., 1998, 1999).

[c]The Dunedin Birth Cohort Study followed prospectively 91% (1037) of all children born between April 1972 and March 1973 in Dunedin (New Zealand). At age 26, 36 had developed schizophreniform disorder, 20 mania, and 278 anxiety/depression. These diagnostic groups were each compared with the remainder of the cohort (healthy control group).

[d]The Philadelphia birth cohort study (Bearden et al., 2000; Rosso et al., 2000) followed prospectively over 90% (9236) of all deliveries at two inner city hospital obstetric wards in Philadelphia between 1959 and 1966. The cohort included 72 subjects who developed schizophrenia/schizoaffective disorder at ages 19–36, 63 healthy siblings, and 7941 non-psychiatric controls.

[e]The National Institute of Mental Health (NIMH) Israeli Kibbutz–City High-Risk Study followed prospectively 50 offspring of schizophrenia parents and 50 offspring of psychiatrically normal parents. Diagnostic outcome

preschizophrenia children on the basis of these characteristics? Are there early risk factors that, in isolation or in combination, flag the preschizophrenia status? These questions, including the putative neurobiological predictions of the schizophrenia illness (Ch. 23), are also addressed elsewhere in this volume.

Where they are available from the primary sources or computable through information derived from the text, the following association indexes and predictive parameters will be reported: the *odds ratio* (OR) is the likelihood of developing schizophrenia in the children who test positive for the predictor relative to those who do not. *Sensitivity* is the percentage of children with adult schizophrenia outcomes who test positive for the predictor. *Specificity* is the percentage of children with normal adult outcomes who test negative for the predictor. *Positive predictive value* is the probability of developing adult schizophrenia given the presence of the predictor in childhood. *Negative predictive value* is the probability of escaping adult schizophrenia given the absence of the predictor in childhood.

We will place particular emphasis on prospective population-based, high-risk, and follow-back studies. All three types of study provide relatively unbiased information, as both researchers and informants do not know which subjects will develop schizophrenia, and the data collected are contemporaneous rather than retrospective. In addition, general population cohorts are less confounded by the selection and information biases usually associated with case–control studies.

Neurointegrative predictors

Population-based studies

Unusual movements and coordination problems in mid-childhood were significantly associated with adult schizophrenia in the Philadelphia 1959–1966 Birth

---

was established at 26–32 years (nine high-risk subjects had developed schizophrenia-spectrum disorders). The predictive validity of neurobehavioral deviance was estimated in a subgroup of 46 high-risk and 44 control offspring.

f The New York High-Risk Project (Cornblatt *et al.*, 1999; Erlenmeyer-Kimling and Cornblatt 1992; Erlenmeyer-Kimling *et al.*, 2000; Ott *et al.*, 1998) recruited offspring of schizophrenia, affectively ill, and psychiatrically normal parents in 1971–2 (sample A: 206, mean age 9.5 years) and 1977–9 (sample B: 150, mean age 9.0 years) and followed them prospectively. Erlenmeyer-Kimling *et al.* (2000) assessed the predictive validity of gross motor skills in a sample of 79 offspring of schizophrenia parents. Diagnostic outcome was established at a mean age of 30.7 years (12 offspring had developed schizophrenia-related psychoses).

g Walker *et al.* (1994) observed childhood home videos of 30 schizophrenia patients and their 28 healthy siblings, 19 affective disorder patients and their 14 siblings, and 21 subjects from families with no mental illness. The OR, sensitivity, specificity, positive and negative predictive values reported here refer to the comparison of the preschizophrenia subjects with their healthy siblings.

Cohort Study (Rosso *et al.*, 2000). The positive predictive value of these indices remained low, however (Table 22.1). An excess of motor coordination dysfunction was also observed in the unaffected siblings of subjects with adult schizophrenia, suggesting that coordination problems might be related to a genetic vulnerability to develop the disorder.

Individuals who developed schizophrenia in the 1946 British birth cohort study (MRC National Survey of Health and Development; Jones *et al.*, 1994) were 4.8 times more likely to have delayed milestones (sitting, standing, walking, and talking) at age 2 (Table 22.1). However, the probability of developing schizophrenia was only 3% (Table 22.1). The authors indicated that ". . . no child destined to develop schizophrenia could be singled out as a late walker." Subjects with a diagnosis of childhood affective disorder (but not those with an adult-onset affective disorder) according to an anxiety–depression rating also attained later motor milestones and had an excess of grimaces and twitches at age 15 (van Os *et al.*, 1997). Therefore, although there were some similarities between the antecedents of schizophrenia and those of affective disorders, the effect on the latter was smaller and more evident in those with an early onset. Age at learning to stand, walk, or become potty-trained in the Northern Finland 1966 Birth Cohort Study (Isohanni *et al.*, 2001) showed a linear association not only with schizophrenia (Table 22.1) but also with other psychoses. By contrast, motor problems (more than 0.3 standard deviation [SD]) and an excess of neurological signs (OR, 4.6) in the Dunedin study (Cannon *et al.*, 2002) were present in children who developed adult schizophreniform, but not manic or anxiety/depression, outcomes. Similarly, children who developed adult schizophrenia in the 1946 British cohort and in the 1958 cohort (National Child Development Study of 1958; Done *et al.*, 1994) studies showed more "hand control and speech problems" than either children who remained well or those who developed affective psychosis (Crow *et al.*, 1995; Done *et al.*, 1994; Leask *et al.*, 2002).

High-risk studies

Fish (Fish, 1977; Fish *et al.*, 1992) created the term "pandevelopmental retardation" to refer to abnormalities in physical growth, gross motor development and visual–motor development that are frequently observed in subjects who develop schizophrenia (Fish, 1987). Hyperkinesis, poor coordination, motor dysfunction, and perceptual signs were present in eight of the nine children who later developed schizophrenia or schizoid personality disorder in the Israeli High Risk Study (Marcus *et al.*, 1987). Similarly, impairment in gross motor skills in the New York High Risk Study was predictive of a future diagnosis of schizophrenia with a reasonably high sensitivity and specificity (Erlenmeyer-Kimling *et al.*, 2000). However, even children with grossly abnormal motor skills only had a 33% probability of developing schizophrenia (Table 22.1).

Archival–observational studies

In a study of sibships filmed from infancy through at least the first 5 years of life, each including one offspring who later developed schizophrenia and normal offspring, viewers blind to the subjects' diagnosis were able to identify the preschizophrenia siblings on the basis of neuromotor abnormalities (Walker *et al.*, 1994). Those who would develop schizophrenia were 7.9 times more likely to show postural hand abnormalities, and 8.2 times more likely to show choreo-athetoid movements than their control siblings. These group differences were only significant until 2 years of age, after which they tended to disappear. It is possible that preschizophrenia children have an impaired cortical modulation on subcortical structures, as supported by evidence of disrupted connectivity in patients with schizophrenia (Rosso *et al.*, 2000).

Such neurodevelopmental deficits could be the consequence of pregnancy and delivery complications (for example, fetal hypoxia), which have been associated with both schizophrenia (Geddes and Lawrie, 1995; McGrath and Murray, 1995; McNeil, 1995) and unusual movements (Rosso *et al.*, 2000). Alternatively, obstetric complications may just play a non-specific, precipitating, or facilitating role in subjects with a genetic liability to schizophrenia (Cannon *et al.*, 2000a).

Neuropsychological predictors

Population-based studies

Prospective investigations of population-based samples have reported persistent intellectual deficits, language pathology, and educational failures in preschizophrenia children and adolescents (Bearden *et al.*, 2000; Cannon *et al.*, 1999, 2000b; Isohanni *et al.*, 1998, 1999; Jones and Done, 1997; Jones *et al.*, 1994), with the respective functional abnormalities being relatively stable across developmental periods (Cannon *et al.*, 2000b; Jones and Done, 1997).

Individuals destined to develop schizophrenia in the Philadelphia Birth Cohort Study showed intellectual abnormalities as early as 4 and 7 years of age (Cannon *et al.*, 2000b); intelligence quotient (IQ) category at either age emerged as a significant predictor of adult schizophrenia (Cannon *et al.*, 2000b). These findings were supplemented by the 1946 and 1958 British birth cohort studies (Jones and Done, 1997), which reported deficits in intellectual capacity, verbal and non-verbal reasoning, reading comprehension, and mathematics at various age points between 7 and 16 years of age in preschizophrenia individuals. Repeating a school grade or receiving special education at age 14 (mainly owing to low IQ) also predicted future schizophrenia in the Northern Finland Birth Cohort Study (Isohanni *et al.*, 1998). Similarly, poor intellectual functioning in a national sample of 18-year-old male conscripts to the Swedish army emerged as a strong predictor of future schizophrenia (David *et al.*, 1997), a finding replicated in the national Israeli cohort of males aged 16–17 years (Davidson *et al.*, 1999).

A common finding in nearly all of the above studies is a linear association between intellectual functioning and the risk for schizophrenia: the latter appears to be a function of performance over the entire range of population scores, increasing progressively as ability declines (Cannon *et al.*, 1999, 2000b; David *et al.*, 1997; Davidson *et al.*, 1999; Jones and Done, 1997; Jones *et al.*, 1994). The Philadelphia Birth Cohort Study, for example, reported a 30–60% increase in schizophrenia risk per unit decrease in ability category (divided into five performance levels), such that individuals scoring in the deficient range were five to six times more likely to become schizophrenia than those scoring in the high-average to superior range (Cannon *et al.*, 1999). Similarly, David *et al.* (1997) reported a nine-fold increase in schizophrenia risk among conscripts scoring in the lowest IQ band compared with those falling within the highest one.

Despite the significant increase in schizophrenia risk in the lower end of the IQ distribution, in no study did the disorder arise solely from a population subgroup with low IQ, nor was there evidence of a subgroup with very low scores (Cannon *et al.*, 1999, 2000b; David *et al.*, 1997; Davidson *et al.*, 1999; Jones and Done, 1997; Jones *et al.*, 1994). Rather, the IQ distribution of the schizophrenia population as a whole is shifted downward in a systematic fashion, most likely reflecting an effect on each individual. This effect is rather subtle: IQ data at age 11 examined together for the 1946 and 1958 birth cohorts revealed a shift of the schizophrenia population mean by < 0.5 SD (Jones and Done, 1997). No single child destined to develop schizophrenia in the former cohort could be singled out as having learning difficulties (Jones *et al.*, 1994).

Contrary to the prevailing view that schizophrenia risk increases linearly with decreasing intellectual capacity, the Northern Finland Birth Cohort Study (Isohanni *et al.*, 1999) failed to confirm linearity in the association between educational attainment and schizophrenia outcome, raising the possibility that it is distance from the cognitive norm – in either direction – that increases the odds for the disorder. Excellent school performance among 16-year-old males in the latter cohort was associated with nearly a four-fold increase in schizophrenia risk, with 11% of the preschizophrenia boys compared with only 3% of the comparison group (with no hospital-treated psychiatric outcome) obtaining excellent school marks. In accord with this finding, the proportion of preschizophrenia cases falling within the highest IQ category among the Israeli males aged 16–17 years was six times higher than that of the comparison subjects (with no hospital-treated psychiatric outcome) (Davidson *et al.*, 1999). It remains to be seen whether these surprising findings will be confirmed in other populations.

Premorbid language dysfunction is one of the most potent predictors of future schizophrenia. Abnormal summary ratings of speech intelligibility at age 7 were associated with a greater than 12-fold increase in risk for adult schizophrenia in the Philadelphia cohort (Bearden *et al.*, 2000). Similarly, the evidence for abnormal speech development prior to schizophrenia is strong in the two British birth cohorts (Jones and Done, 1997). In the 1958 birth cohort, the relevant abnormalities are more than reflections of developmental timing: oral ability and quality of speech at 7 and 11 years were more frequently rated as qualitatively abnormal in the preschizophrenia children; speech defects (not caused by structural problems) persisted throughout childhood and adolescence in the 1946 cohort, being associated with a three-fold increase in schizophrenia risk.

Although the large sample sizes (ranging from approximately 5000 to 50 000 individuals) in these epidemiological studies provide sufficient statistical evidence for the predictive potential of neuropsychological abnormalities, it would be misleading to conclude that the latter can be used as effective population screens for the identification of individuals at true risk for schizophrenia. A particular limitation is the extent to which premorbid neuropsychological deficits can distinguish between schizophrenia and other psychiatric disorders. Impairments in general ability have also been recorded in the early biographies of individuals with other psychoses and anxiety or depressive disorders, with any distinction between the respective groups simply being one of magnitude: preschizophrenia individuals usually perform worse than the other patient groups, which also perform below the norm (David *et al.*, 1997; Davidson *et al.*, 1999; Jones and Done, 1997). Indeed, the association between receiving special education or repeating a school grade and the diagnostic category of "other psychoses" in the Finnish cohort was even stronger than that with schizophrenia (Isohanni *et al.*, 1998). A possible exception to this rather undifferentiated pattern of associations is the one between speech difficulties and future schizophrenia. The only school-based assessment that distinguished the preschizophrenia children from the other patient groups in the British 1958 cohort was the qualitative evaluation of "speech difficulties" at both 7 and 11 years (Jones and Done, 1997).

A second problem is the significant impact on a population level of the false-negative properties carried by even highly sensitive and specific screens, when used for low-prevalence disorders such as schizophrenia (O'Toole, 2000). Table 22.2 presents the predictive profiles of the neuropsychological and educational risk factors examined in the various studies. Although the specificity of the various predictors is moderate to high (53–99%), their sensitivity is less satisfactory (11–55%), and only a small proportion (1–17%) of individuals falling within the "impaired" range on the different measures eventually go on to develop schizophrenia. For

Table 22.2. Predicting schizophrenia: neuropsychological and educational risk factors in population-based studies

Risk factor	OR	SEN (%)	SPE (%)	PPV (%)	NPV (%)
IQ at 4 yrs (Cannon et al., 1999)[a]	1.3[b]	30	85	2	99
IQ at 7 yrs (Cannon et al., 1999)[a]	1.6[b]	33	83	2	99
IQ at 11 and 15 yrs (Jones et al., 1994)[c]	0.6 and 0.5[b]	–	–	–	–
IQ at 16–17 yrs (Davidson et al., 1999)[d]	1.6	54	53	–	–
IQ < 96 at 18 yrs (David et al., 1997)[e]	3.5–8.6	55	67	1	100
Class below age level or special education at 14 yrs (Isohanni et al., 1998)[f]	2.8	17	93	3	99
Excellent school marks at 16 yrs (Isohanni et al., 1999)[f]	3.8	11	97	4	99
Abnormal speech at 7 yrs (Bearden et al., 2000)[a]	12.7	14	99	17	99
Abnormal speech at 2–15 yrs (Jones et al., 1994)[c]	2.8	–	–	–	–
Expressive language at 7 yrs (Bearden et al., 2000)[a]	0.7	–	–	–	–

OR, odds ratio; SEN, sensitivity; SPE, specificity; PPV, positive predictive value; NPV, negative predictive value; IQ, intelligence quotient.

[a]See footnote d in Table 22.1.

[b]Odds ratio for linear trend, i.e., that associated with moving a category (e.g. tertile or quintile) of score distribution.

[c]See footnote a in Table 22.1.

[d]The National Israeli sample of 16–17-year-old males included 509 subjects who developed schizophrenia by the age of 26, and 9215 controls who did not appear in the national psychiatric registry by the same age (Davidson et al., 1999).

[e]A national sample of 49 968 male conscripts to the Swedish army (David et al., 1997): 195 subjects developed schizophrenia by the age of 33–34 and were compared with 49 773 individuals with no or other psychotic outcomes. OR values (unadjusted for confounders) were estimated separately for each IQ band (< 74, 74–81, 82–89, 90–95) by David et al. (1997); SEN, SPE, PPV, and NPV were estimated for all the IQ (< 96) bands together by the present authors.

[f]See footnote b, in Table 22.1.

example, receiving special education or repeating a school grade (mainly owing to low IQ) at 14 years of age in the Northern Finland Birth Cohort Study (Isohanni et al., 1998) correctly predicted 10 of the 58 cases of schizophrenia (sensitivity, 17%) and 4986 of the 5351 non-cases (specificity, 93%). However, of the 375 individuals repeating a class or receiving special education at age 14, only 10 went on to develop schizophrenia (positive predictive value, 3%). It is, therefore, unrealistic to target early identification and prevention programs for schizophrenia on individuals with deviant cognitive functioning or poor educational achievement. This observation applies to all the remaining risk factors identified in the population-based studies reviewed in this section (Table 22.2).

High-risk studies

The "high-risk" strategy reduces the chances of false positives in the face of low prevalence disorders by studying individuals whose risk for developing schizophrenia is high, thus increasing the observed prevalence of the disorder in the sample studied: children of one schizophrenia parent can be up to 15 times more likely to develop the disorder than members of the general population. In addition, unlike population-based studies, which usually study general aspects of development, research in high-risk groups is a longitudinal quest for variables that predict the disorder (Erlenmeyer-Kimling et al., 2000). As such, the high-risk paradigm usually includes measurements of particular relevance to schizophrenia.

Impaired attention is the most extensively investigated and validated neuropsychological predictor in the high-risk literature. For example, the preschizophrenia offspring of affected parents in the Copenhagen High Risk Study displayed poor concentration from infancy (Parnas et al., 1982). Similarly, childhood attentional deficits in the Israeli high-risk sample successfully predicted the development of schizophrenia-spectrum disorders (Mirsky et al., 1995). In addition, in the New York High Risk Project, attentional deficits predicted schizophrenia-related psychoses as opposed to other psychiatric outcomes (Erlenmeyer-Kimling et al., 2000), were more prevalent among children of schizophrenia parents than offspring of affectively ill patients (Cornblatt and Erlenmeyer-Kimling, 1985; Cornblatt et al., 1992; Erlenmeyer-Kimling et al., 2000; Freedman et al., 1998), and displayed the greatest predictive power within the group at genetic risk for schizophrenia (Cornblatt and Erlenmeyer-Kimling, 1985; Cornblatt et al., 1992). These findings attest both to the predictive validity and the diagnostic specificity of attentional dysfunction in high-risk studies (Table 22.3).

Although other cognitive functions have been less extensively investigated, memory dysfunction, IQ change, and subtest scatter in standard intelligence tests may provide sensitive indicators of the preschizophrenia state (Erlenmeyer-Kimling et al., 2000; Ott et al., 1998). The use of intelligence scores from the Revised Wechsler Intelligence Scale for Children (WISC-R) or the Revised Adult Scale (WAIS-R) in the New York High Risk Project achieved one of the best predictive profiles reported in the high-risk literature to date, with a false-positive rate (equal to 1 minus specificity) of just 2–5% (Ott et al., 1998) (Table 22.3).

However, the focus on single neuropsychological constructs is less promising than using clusters of cognitive and neurobehavioral variables. Combining an attentional screen with behavioral ratings in the New York High Risk Project enhanced

Table 22.3. Predicting schizophrenia: neuropsychological risk factors in high-risk studies[a]

Risk factor	SEN (%)	SPE (%)	PPV (%)	NPV (%)
Attention deficits at 12 yrs (Cornblatt *et al.*, 1999)[b]	67	79	19	97
Attention deficits at 12 yrs and behavior ratings at 12–17 yrs (Cornblatt *et al.*, 1999)[b]	83	90	38.5	99
Attention deviance at 7–12 yrs (Erlenmeyer-Kimling *et al.*, 2000)[c]	58	82	37	92
Memory deficits at 7–12 yrs (Erlenmeyer-Kimling *et al.*, 2000)[c]	83	72	34.5	96
Attention deviance, memory and gross motor skills at 7–12 yrs (Erlenmeyer-Kimling *et al.*, 2000)[c]	50	90	46	91
WISC(-R) or WAIS(-R) subtest scatter at 15 yrs, change in Full Scale IQ and Vocabulary between 9 and 15 yrs, Picture Arrangement minus Vocabulary score at 9 yrs and parental risk (Ott *et al.*, 1998)[d]	54–85	95–98	61–70	96–99
WISC(-R) or WAIS(-R) subtest scatter at 15 yrs and Picture Arrangement minus Vocabulary score at 9 yrs (Ott *et al.*, 1998)[e]	56	90	62.5	87

SEN, sensitivity; SPE, specificity; PPV, positive predictive value; NPV, negative predictive value.

[a]Data from the New York High Risk Project (see footnote *f*, Table 22.1).

[b]The predictive validity of sustained attention – alone or in conjunction with behavioral ratings – was assessed in a mixed sample of 21 offspring of schizophrenia parents, 26 children of affectively ill parents, and 40 offspring of psychiatrically normal parents (total, 87). Diagnostic outcome was last updated when the subjects were in their early thirties.

[c]The predictive validity of attention, memory, and motor skills (each alone or in conjunction with the other predictors) was assessed in a sample of 79 offspring of schizophrenia parents. Diagnostic outcome was established at a mean age of 30.7 years (12 offspring had developed schizophrenia-related psychoses).

[d]The accuracy of a logistic regression model (including variables from Wechsler Intelligence Scales for Children and Adults) was examined for prediction of schizophrenia-related psychoses (versus no diagnosis) in a mixed sample of 157 high- and low-risk children (offspring of schizophrenia, affectively ill, and psychiatrically normal parents). The diagnostic outcome was established at the mean ages of 30.17 years (sample A) and 22.09 years (sample B). The ranges of SEN, SPE, PPV and NPV resulted from varying the predicted cut-off probability.

[e]The predictive accuracy of WISC(-R)/WAIS(-R)-derived variables was examined in a sample of 39 offspring of schizophrenia parents derived from the sample described in footnote *d* of this table.

measurably the overall accuracy of the attentional model, reducing false positives by half (Cornblatt *et al.*, 1999). Similarly, combining deficits in attention, verbal memory, and gross motor skills in the above study achieved higher precision than any of the contributing variables alone (Erlenmeyer-Kimling *et al.*, 2000).

Table 22.3 presents the predictive profiles of selected neuropsychological predictors used in high-risk studies. As expected from measures specifically selected for their relevance to schizophrenia, and from the increased prevalence of the disorder in the relatively small samples screened, the examined predictors show moderate-to-high sensitivity, with 50–85% of future spectrum cases being correctly identified. Of all subjects predicted to develop schizophrenia-related psychoses, 19–70% went on to develop the outcome of interest, and, almost invariably, over 90% of "non-deviant" performers did not develop schizophrenia or related psychoses. However, the false-positive rates can sometimes be substantial. Although in some models (Erlenmeyer-Kimling *et al.*, 2000; Ott *et al.*, 1998), only 2–10% of non-cases are falsely predicted to develop spectrum disorders, about a third of non-cases are false positives in others (Erlenmeyer-Kimling *et al.*, 2000) (Table 22.3). In addition, the predictive performance of the reviewed models cannot be extrapolated to the general population, since only about 10–15% of future schizophrenia patients have an ill parent, and the normal control samples in the existing high-risk studies are relatively small (Erlenmeyer-Kimling *et al.*, 2000).

Behavioral predictors

Population-based studies

Teacher-rated behavioral deviance emerged as a potent predictor of adult schizophrenia in the 1946 and 1958 British birth cohort studies. In the 1946 study, social anxiety at age 15 showed a significant linear association with schizophrenia, such that individuals scoring within the highest tertile were six times more likely to develop the disorder relative to those scoring in the lowest tertile (Jones *et al.*, 1994). Teacher-rated anxiety was also a prominent characteristic of the preschizophrenia 7-year-old males of the 1958 study (Crow *et al.*, 1995), as were hostility and inconsequential behavior: 50% of the preschizophrenia males compared with only 10% of normal controls received abnormal global ratings of over-reactive behavior. A clear gender effect was noted in the 1958 study: the 7-year-old girls who later developed schizophrenia were hardly distinguishable from normal controls. Even though they were finally rated as more withdrawn, depressed, and likely to dismiss adult values in later childhood (age 11), they showed no evidence of over-reactive behavior at any time point, with the exception of a trend towards adult-directed hostility at age 11. By then, depression and a trend for dismissal of adult values were also added to the behavioral profile of the preschizophrenia males. In contrast to the preschizophrenia children, the preaffective children were unremarkable in their profiles, with the exception of hostility at age 7 (boys) and restlessness at either 7 (boys) or 11 (girls) years of age. The behavioral abnormalities of the preneurotic individuals were similar to those of the preschizophrenia group, although they emerged at a slightly later stage of development and were present in the females rather than the males (Crow *et al.*, 1995).

Table 22.4. Predicting schizophrenia: behavioral risk factors in population-based and high-risk studies

Risk factor	OR	SEN (%)	SPE (%)	PPV (%)	NPV (%)
Population-based studies					
Global social maladjustment at 7 yrs (Bearden *et al.*, 2000)[a]	2.54	29	86	2	99
Focal behavioral deviance at 4 yrs (Bearden *et al.*, 2000)[a]	1.68	33	81	1	99
Focal behavioral deviance at 7 yrs (Bearden *et al.*, 2000)[a]	1.65	31	81	2	99
Poor social functioning at 16–17 yrs (males) (Davidson *et al.*, 1999)[b]	4.37	48	88		
Poor organizational ability at 16–17 yrs (males) (Davidson *et al.*, 1999)[b]	2.03	30	88		
High-risk studies					
Behavior problems at 15 yrs (males) (Olin and Mednick, 1996)[c]					
a. Disciplinary problems		39	96	88	71
b. Teacher-predicted future emotional or psychotic problems		43	88	67	73
c. Repeated a grade		29	96	80	73
d. Disturbs class with inappropriate behavior		50	82	64	72
e. Emotional reaction persists; high-strung		40	85	60	72
f. Lonely and rejected by peers		44	82	58	71
g. Treated by psychologist for problem		36	86	57	73
h. Easily excited or irritated		41	82	58	69
Behavior problems at 15 yrs (females) (Olin and Mednick, 1996)[c]					
a. Teacher-predicted future emotional or psychotic problems		30	97	75	82
b. Nervousness		46	82	45	82

OR, odds ratio; SEN, sensitivity; SPE, specificity; PPV, positive predictive value; NPV, negative predictive value.

[a]See footnote *d* in Table 22.1.

[b]See footnote *d* in Table 22.2.

[c]The Copenhagen High Risk Project (Olin and Mednick, 1996) recruited 207 offspring of mothers with severe schizophrenia and 104 matched control offspring of parents and grandparents with no history of psychiatric hospitalization (mean age 15.1 yrs). At a mean age of 42 years, 33 subjects had developed schizophrenia, 10 schizophrenia-associated psychosis, and 46 schizotypal or paranoid personality disorder. The predictive parameters refer to the comparison of the preschizophrenia group with those with non-psychiatric outcomes.

Global social maladjustment at 7 years of age was a potent predictor of later schizophrenia in the Philadelphia Birth Cohort Study (Cannon *et al.*, 1999) (Table 22.4). In addition, signs of behavioral deviance such as meaningless laughter, excessive crying, echolalia, thumb-sucking, and nail biting (focal deviance) at ages 4 and 7 were predictive of both schizophrenia (Table 22.4) and unaffected sibling status (Bearden *et al.*, 2000). The authors commented that focal behavioral deviance may reflect the underlying genetic susceptibility to schizophrenia, whereas global social maladjustment is likely to predate the onset of the clinical phenotype (Bearden *et al.*, 2000).

Behavioral assessments of males aged 16–17 years in the national Israeli cohort indicated significant differences in measures of social functioning, individual autonomy, and organizational ability between subjects who later developed schizophrenia and healthy controls (Davidson *et al.*, 1999) (Table 22.4). Using the social functioning scale alone with a cut-off point of the lowest two quintiles accurately predicted group membership in 43% of future cases and 93% of controls.

High-risk studies

In the seminal study of Barbara Fish (1987), half of the preschizophrenia children with chronic disturbance from childhood had been abnormally quiet infants with flat affect, who developed withdrawn or explosive and non-compliant behavior by the age of 3 years.

Eight of the nine adults who received schizophrenia-spectrum diagnoses in the National Institute of Mental Health (NIMH) Israeli Kibbutz–City High Risk Study had shown antisocial and/or withdrawn behavior in childhood (Marcus *et al.*, 1987). These abnormalities were mainly evident in the males. According to teachers and parents, females had shown adequate interpersonal adjustment and less overt dysfunctioning, even though the girls themselves had reported acute feelings of rejection and not belonging.

Teacher ratings of social dysfunction and behavioral deviance among 15-year-old males were among the best predictors of future schizophrenia in the Copenhagen High Risk Study (Olin and Mednick, 1996) (Table 22.4). Compared with normal controls, preschizophrenia males were more likely to pose discipline problems and disturb the class, to be emotionally reactive and easily excited, to have been treated by a school psychologist or repeated a grade, and to be lonely and rejected by their peers. While both males and females with a schizophrenia outcome were significantly more likely than normal controls to receive a prediction of future psychosis by their teachers, the only other item to have predictive value for females was nervousness. These behavioral indices predicted future schizophrenia with low to moderate sensitivity, high specificity, and moderate to high positive and negative predictive values (Table 22.4). Compared with males with other diagnostic outcomes, preschizophrenia boys showed more externalized signs of abnormality, educational failures, and interpersonal difficulties, and received more predictions of future psychosis. Preschizophrenia girls were clearly distinguishable only from those with non-psychotic psychiatric outcomes, showing more internalized signs of abnormality and being more prone to psychotic and emotional problems (Olin and Mednick, 1996).

Archival–observational studies

In a preliminary study of sibships filmed from infancy through at least the first 5 years of life, each including a preschizophrenia child (Walker and Lewine, 1990), viewers blind to the subjects' adult psychiatric outcome were able to identify the future cases at levels well above chance: 25 of their 32 judgements were correct ($P < 0.05$). Furthermore, the distinguishing behavioral features of the target children compared with their control sibling(s) (i.e. less responsiveness, eye contact, and positive affect) were apparent at a gross level of analysis, as the viewers were not instructed to use specific criteria. Similarly, on extending the above study to a larger sample, Walker *et al.* (1993) observed lower rates of joy expressions and increased negative affect in the future cases compared with same-gender siblings.

The emotional blunting of infants, children, and adolescents destined to develop schizophrenia (Fish, 1987; Walker *et al.*, 1993) is consistent with the lack of hedonic capacity observed in affected adults, suggesting continuity between some schizophrenia antecedents and the clinical syndrome. Other evidence in support of this notion comes from a retrospective study. Baum and Walker (1995) found positive correlations between withdrawal in childhood and adolescence and psychomotor poverty in adult schizophrenia. Taken together, these findings suggest that certain primary negative or deficit symptoms may be enduring traits, manifested across the lifespan of schizophrenia patients.

Conclusions

Using a statistical analogy, the null hypothesis that preschizophrenia children *as a group* cannot be identified on the basis of early developmental, cognitive, social, and behavioral characteristics can be rejected. Subtle, yet detectable, abnormalities in all these functional domains have been reliably reported in preschizophrenia children, achieving a statistically significant predictive status in epidemiological, high-risk and archival–observational studies. However, the predictive profile of these characteristics on a population level advises against their use as schizophrenia screens in unselected populations. To date, no single predictor or composite model has shown sufficient sensitivity, specificity, and positive/negative predictive values. In the various studies reviewed, 11–93% of individuals with adult-onset schizophrenia were missed on the basis of their childhood characteristics; 1–47% were falsely predicted to develop the disorder; as few as 12% or as many as 99% of youths with a given deviant characteristic *did not* develop schizophrenia as adults; and as many as 31% of children with no detectable deviance did so. On a population level, the misclassification rate can be substantial. Despite the promise of the various predictors as tools for estimating *schizophrenia risk*, no single or composite marker of the *preschizophrenia status* has been detected so far. The lack of complete specificity to schizophrenia and the overlapping distributions of the predictors in normal and preschizophrenia populations suggest that predicting the disorder on an *individual basis* is still not feasible.

However, it is becoming increasingly clear that combining risk indicators from different functional domains can impressively enhance the accuracy of predictive models. In addition, the measures investigated by the high-risk paradigm can aid in the identification of truly vulnerable individuals within the high-risk population. Although the misclassification rates are still sufficiently high to prevent the implementation of invasive protocols for preventive intervention, this subgroup may potentially form a target for cognitive intervention treatments.

REFERENCES

Baum, K. M., Walker, E. F. (1995). Childhood behavioral precursors of adult symptom dimensions in schizophrenia. *Schizophr Res* **16**: 111–120.

Bearden, C. E., Rosso, I. M., Hollister, J. M., *et al.* (2000). A prospective cohort study of childhood behavioral deviance and language abnormalities as predictors of adult schizophrenia. *Schizophr Bull* **26**: 395–410.

Cannon, T. D., Rosso, I. M., Bearden, C. E., Sanchez, L. E., Hadley, T. (1999). A prospective cohort study of neurodevelopmental processes in the genesis and epigenesis of schizophrenia. *Dev Psychopathol* **11**: 467–485.

Cannon, T. D., Rosso, I. M., Hollister, J. M., *et al.* (2000a). A prospective cohort study of genetic and perinatal influences in the etiology of schizophrenia. *Schizophr Bull* **26**: 351–366.

Cannon, T. D., Bearden, C. E., Hollister, J. M., *et al.* (2000b). Childhood cognitive functioning in schizophrenia patients and their unaffected siblings: a prospective cohort study. *Schizophr Bull* **26**: 379–393.

Cannon, M., Caspi, A., Moffitt, T. E., *et al.* (2002). Evidence for early-childhood, pandevelopmental impairment specific to schizophreniform disorder: results from a longitudinal birth cohort. *Arch Gen Psychiatry* **59**: 449–456.

Cornblatt, B. A., Erlenmeyer-Kimling, L. (1985). Global attentional deviance as a marker of risk for schizophrenia: specificity and predictive validity. *J Abnorm Psychol* **94**: 470–486.

Cornblatt, B. A., Lenzenweger, M. F., Dworkin, R. H., Erlenmeyer-Kimling, L. (1992). Childhood attentional dysfunctions predict social deficits in unaffected adults at risk for schizophrenia. *Br J Psychiatry* **18**(Suppl.): 59–64.

Cornblatt, B. A., Obuchowski, M., Roberts, S., Pollack, S., Erlenmeyer-Kimling, L. (1999). Cognitive and behavioral precursors of schizophrenia. *Dev Psychopathol* **11**: 487–508.

Crow, T. J., Done, D. J., Sacker, A. (1995). Childhood precursors of psychosis as clues to its evolutionary origins. *Eur Arch Psychiatry Clin Neurosci* **245**: 61–69.

David, A. S., Malmberg, A., Brandt, L., Allebeck, P., Lewis, G. (1997). I. Q. and risk for schizophrenia: a population-based cohort study. *Psychol Med* **27**: 1311–1323.

Davidson, M., Reichenberg, A., Rabinowitz, J., *et al.* (1999). Behavioral and intellectual markers for schizophrenia in apparently healthy male adolescents. *Am J Psychiatry* **156**: 1328–1335.

Done, D. J., Crow, T. J., Johnstone, E. C., Sacker, A. (1994). Childhood antecedents of schizophrenia and affective illness: social adjustment at ages 7 and 11. *Br Med J* **309**: 699–703.

Dworkin, R. H., Cornblatt, B. A. (1995). Predicting schizophrenia. *Lancet* **345**: 139–140.

Erlenmeyer-Kimling, L., Cornblatt, B. A. (1992). A summary of attentional findings in the New York High-Risk Project. *J Psychiatr Res* **26**: 405–426.

Erlenmeyer-Kimling, L., Rock, D., Roberts, S. A., *et al.* (2000). Attention, memory, and motor skills as childhood predictors of schizophrenia-related psychoses: the New York High-Risk Project. *Am J Psychiatry* **157**: 1416–1422.

Fearon, P., Cannon, M., Murray, R. M. (2001). A critique of the idea and science of risk-factor research in schizophrenia. *Int J Ment Health* **30**: 82–90.

Fish, B. (1977). Neurobiologic antecedents of schizophrenia in children. Evidence for an inherited, congenital neurointegrative defect. *Arch Gen Psychiatry* **34**: 1297–1313.

   (1987). Infant predictors of the longitudinal course of schizophrenia development. *Schizophr Bull* **13**: 395–409.

Fish, B., Marcus, J., Hans, S. L., Auerbach, J. G., Perdue, S. (1992). Infants at risk for schizophrenia: sequelae of a genetic neurointegrative defect. A review and replication analysis of pandysmaturation in the Jerusalem infant development study. *Arch Gen Psychiatry* **49**: 221–235.

Freedman, L. R., Rock, D., Roberts, S. A., Cornblatt, B. A., Erlenmeyer-Kimling, L. (1998). The New York High-Risk Project: attention, anhedonia and social outcome. *Schizophr Res* **30**: 1–9.

Geddes, J. R., Lawrie, S. M. (1995). Obstetric complications and schizophrenia: a meta-analysis. *Br J Psychiatry* **167**: 786–793.

Isohanni, I., Jarvelin, M.-R., Nieminen, P., *et al.* (1998). School performance as a predictor of psychiatric hospitalization in adult life. A 28-year follow-up in the northern finland 1966 birth cohort. *Psychol Med* **28**: 967–974.

Isohanni, I., Jarvelin, M. R., Jones, P., Jokelainen, J., Isohanni, M. (1999). Can excellent school performance be a precursor of schizophrenia? A 28-year follow-up in the Northern Finland 1966 birth cohort. *Acta Psychiatr Scand* **100**: 17–26.

Isohanni, M., Jones, P. B., Moilanen, K., *et al.* (2001). Early developmental milestones in adult schizophrenia and other psychoses. A 31-year follow-up of the Northern Finland 1966 Birth Cohort. *Schizophr Res* **52**: 1–19.

Jones, P., Done, D. J. (1997). From birth to onset: a developmental perspective of schizophrenia in two national birth cohorts. In *Neurodevelopment and Adult Psychopathology*, ed. M. S. Keshavan, R. M. Murray. Cambridge, UK: Cambridge University Press, pp. 119–136.

Jones, P., Rodgers, B., Murray, R., Marmot, M. (1994). Child developmental risk factors for adult schizophrenia in the British 1946 birth cohort. *Lancet* **344**: 1398–1402.

Kraepelin, E. (1919). *Dementia Praecox and Paraphrenia*. Edinburgh: Livingston.

Leask, S. J., Done, D. J., Crow, T. J. (2002). Adult psychosis, common childhood infections and neurological soft signs in a national birth cohort. *Br J Psychiatry* **181**: 387–392.

Marcus, J., Hans, S. L., Nagler, S., *et al.* (1987). Review of the NIMH Israeli Kibbutz-City Study and the Jerusalem Infant Development Study. *Schizophr Bull* **13**: 425–438.

McGrath, J., Murray, R. M. (1995). Risk factors for schizophrenia: from conception to birth. In *Schizophrenia*, ed. S. Hirsh, D. Weinberger. Oxford: Blackwell, pp. 187–205.

McNeil, T. F. (1995). Perinatal risk factors and schizophrenia: selective review and methodological concerns. *Epidemiol Rev* **17**: 107–112.

Mirsky, A. F., Ingraham, L. J., Kugelmass, S. (1995). Neuropsychological assessment of attention and its pathology in the Israeli cohort. *Schizophr Bull* **21**: 193–204.

Murray, R. M. (1994). Neurodevelopmental schizophrenia: the rediscovery of dementia praecox. *Br J Psychiatry* **165**: 6–12.

Murray, R. M., Lewis, S. W. (1987). Is schizophrenia a neurodevelopmental disorder? *Br Med J (Clin Res Ed)* **295**: 681–682.

Olin, S. C., Mednick, S. A. (1996). Risk factors of psychosis: identifying vulnerable populations premorbidly. *Schizophr Bull* **22**: 223–240.

O'Toole, B. I. (2000). Screening for low prevalence disorders. *Aust N Z J Psychiatry* **34**(Suppl): S39–S46.

Ott, S. L., Spinelli, S., Rock, D., *et al.* (1998). The New York High-Risk Project: social and general intelligence in children at risk for schizophrenia. *Schizophr Res* **31**: 1–11.

Parnas, J., Schulsinger, F., Schulsinger, H., Mednick, S. A., Teasdale, T. W. (1982). Behavioral precursors of schizophrenia spectrum. A prospective study. *Arch Gen Psychiatry* **39**: 658–664.

Rosso, I. M., Bearden, C. E., Hollister, J. M., *et al.* (2000). Childhood neuromotor dysfunction in schizophrenia patients and their unaffected siblings: a prospective cohort study. *Schizophr Bull* **26**: 367–378.

van Os, J., Jones, P. B., Lewis, S., Wadsworth, M., Murray, R. M. (1997). Developmental precursors of affective illness in a general population birth cohort. *Arch Gen Psychiatry* **54**: 625–631.

Walker, E., Lewine, R. J. (1990). Prediction of adult-onset schizophrenia from childhood home movies of the patients. *Am J Psychiatry* **147**: 1052–1056.

Walker, E. F., Grimes, K. E., Davis, D. M., Smith, A. J. (1993). Childhood precursors of schizophrenia: facial expressions of emotion. *Am J Psychiatry* **150**: 1654–1660.

Walker, E. F., Savoie, T., Davis, D. (1994). Neuromotor precursors of schizophrenia. *Schizophr Bull* **20**: 441–451.

Weinberger, D. R. (1987). Implications of normal brain development for the pathogenesis of schizophrenia. *Arch Gen Psychiatry* **44**: 660–669.

23

High-risk studies, brain development, and schizophrenia

Matcheri S. Keshavan

University of Pittsburgh School of Medicine, Pittsburgh and
Wayne State University School of Medicine, Detroit, USA

Research on schizophrenia since the 1970s is conspicuous for its "shift to the left," emphasizing earlier phases of schizophrenia. This shift toward *first-episode studies* replaced earlier cross-sectionally designed neurobiological studies of mostly those with chronic schizophrenia, thus minimizing the confounds of chronicity and treatment effects (Keshavan and Schooler, 1992). During the 1990s, attention shifted further left, underscoring the importance of studying the *prodromal phase* of schizophrenia with a glimmer of hope for secondary, and possibly primary prevention (McGorry, 1998). Neurodevelopmental models of schizophrenia (Murray and Lewis, 1987; Weinberger, 1987) have spurred the characterization of the *premorbid phase* of schizophrenia. Studies of the premorbid phase help us to identify neurodevelopmentally mediated vulnerability factors, examine the evolution of the early phase of schizophrenia, unravel the premorbid pathophysiology without the potential confounds of illness or treatment effects, and facilitate early diagnosis and preventive intervention (Cornblatt and Obuchowski, 1997; Ch. 24).

This chapter will review the several approaches to investigate premorbid risk for schizophrenia. What follows will be a critical appraisal of the existing studies focusing on the populations at risk for schizophrenia, the issues surrounding study design, predictive and outcome factors identified so far, and the timing of the studies. Conceptual and methodological issues and future directions will also be discussed. Specifically, we will address the following questions. *Who* are the most likely individuals that, when studied, will reveal useful insight about the nature of vulnerability to schizophrenia? *How* should such studies be designed, and what are the methodological issues that need to be addressed in these studies? *What* neurodevelopmental predictors, and/outcome measures, if studied, are likely to yield the best insights? *When* (i.e. during which critical periods of development) is it most fruitful to assess the risk factors? Focused, hypothesis-driven studies

Neurodevelopment and Schizophrenia, ed. Matcheri S. Keshavan *et al.* Published by Cambridge University Press. © Cambridge University Press 2004.

mindful of the above questions and deploying state of the art neurobiological tools of assessment are likely to provide fresh impetus to this important, rather neglected field of research. They are reviewed here.

At-risk populations

Studies of premorbid risk refer to the investigation of individuals who are considered more vulnerable to develop schizophrenia than are individuals in the general population. Studies of risk for schizophrenia can be retrospective or "follow-back" investigations (Walker *et al.*, 1993) or prospective. Prospective studies could involve longitudinal investigation of large cohorts of unselected general populations (such as birth cohorts) or individuals selected for one or other index of high-risk (HR). These studies have utilized genetic propensity, neurobehavioral markers, or psychopathology to identify the risk status. In this section, we will outline the potential merits and disadvantages of these strategies, review the lessons learned from the early first HR studies and present a rationale for more focused next-generation studies to examine premorbid risk.

General population cohort studies

Longitudinal studies of general population samples have been used to investigate developmental antecedents of schizophrenia. Two British birth cohorts, the MRC National Survey of Health and Development of 1946 (Jones *et al.*, 1994) and the National Child Development Study of 1958 (Done *et al.*, 1994), in which the participants have lived through most of the age of risk, showed that children destined to develop schizophrenia could be differentiated based on motor and cognitive dysfunction throughout childhood. David *et al.* (1997) showed a significant association between low intelligence quotient (IQ) score and later schizophrenia in a cohort study of male Swedish conscripts. Population-based cohort studies have also revealed valuable information about potential etiological variables; the North Finland Birth Cohort (Rantakallio *et al.*, 1997) and the UK National Child Development Study (Leask *et al.*, 2002) revealed associations between childhood infections and later schizophrenia. Risk for schizophrenia has been associated in birth cohort studies with urban place of birth (Harrison and Owen, 2003), migration (Cantor-Graae *et al.*, 2003), paternal age (Brown *et al.*, 2002), birth order (Kemppainen *et al.*, 2001), exposure to prenatal rubella (Brown *et al.*, 2001), and low maternal and birth weights (Wahlbeck *et al.*, 2001).

The main advantage with general population cohort studies is that they are an unbiased estimate of the at-risk population; hence the findings, however limited, are generalizable and can be specifically applied to this illness. However, there are limitations. First, large population samples are needed to yield a sufficient number of cases, and the number of predictive variables is often inadequate to address the specific questions. Second, birth cohort studies involve prolonged follow-up periods and are very expensive, leading to a delay of several decades before gaining predictive knowledge. However, prospective studies of young adult and adolescent cohorts (e.g. Davidson *et al.*, 1999) may have an advantage of requiring a shorter follow-up. Third, birth cohort studies are limited by "cohort effects," which refer to variation in illness characteristics (such as age of onset) over time among individuals defined by shared temporal features such as year of birth. This could lead to variable findings between studies, and bias in interpretation of data (Di Maggio *et al.*, 2001). Finally, since large populations are involved, and most cohort studies were not begun with schizophrenia-related research questions in mind, the data collected at the outset are not fine-grained enough to ascertain neurodevelopmental antecedents of schizophrenia with any degree of specificity (Jones and Tarrant, 1999).

Follow-back and retrospective studies

Follow-back studies examine precursors of adult-onset psychopathology by examining medical or scholastic archives of individuals with known outcome in adulthood. Using this approach (archival–observational approach), Walker and colleagues (Walker and Lewine, 1990; Walker *et al.*, 1993) collected old home movies from families of schizophrenia patients. Children who later developed schizophrenia were characterized by subtle but significant neuromotor abnormalities compared with their unaffected siblings. These provocative findings support the view that dysmaturation of motor systems may occur in the future schizophrenia patient even in early childhood. This approach is relatively free from recall bias (because of the archival source of information), and a representative sample of the schizophrenia population is obtained; hence the findings are fairly generalizable to both genetic and non-genetic forms of schizophrenia, unlike the genetic HR studies. However, the information available for such studies is severely limited and may or may not be related to pathophysiological questions of the premorbid diathesis.

One needs to make a distinction between "follow-back" and retrospective studies; the former utilize archival sources of information that are relatively unbiased whereas the latter are limited by the problems of recall bias. Retrospective studies rely on chart-review data and other historical sources of information. The high prevalence of behavioral and cognitive difficulties in the general population can make them likely to be selectively attributed to the illness. Further, the information obtained in any retrospective analysis is likely to be biased; can be variable, depending on the doctor's record-keeping practices; and often is too sketchy to allow examination of specific neurodevelopmental hypotheses.

Genetic high-risk studies

Genetic factors are among the best-established etiological factors in schizophrenia. Prospectively studying relatives of schizophrenia patients with enhanced genetic risk should, therefore, be instructive in our search of markers that may predict the onset of the illness. Pearson and Kley (1957) first recognized the benefits of this HR approach. The risk of schizophrenia increases relative to the general population in proportion to the proximity of the relationship and the number of affected relatives. Offspring of parents with schizophrenia represent an attractive HR population for study since having one schizophrenia parent entails about 13% risk of developing the illness, and having two schizophrenia parents increases the risk to about 40% (Gottesman and Shields, 1982). In terms of the risk, having a first-degree relative with schizophrenia increases the risk by five times in parents, eight times in siblings, 13 times in children with one schizophrenia parent and 40 times in children of two schizophrenia parents compared with the general population (where it is about 1%). Heritability of schizophrenia, calculated from correlations of liability in monozygotic and dizygotic twins and presuming that schizophrenia is multifactorial–polygenic in inheritance, is estimated to be 60–90% (Gottesman, 1991; Kendler, 2002; McGuffin et al., 1984).

Mednick and several other investigators initiated HR studies in the early 1960s and 1970s and some of these "first-generation" studies have continued to date (Table 23.1). These studies typically involved follow-up of offspring of schizophrenia parents, though younger siblings (Maier et al., 1992; Saitoh et al., 1984; Weinberger et al., 1981) and discordant monozygotic twins have also been studied as at-risk populations (Reveley et al., 1982; Suddath et al., 1990). An advantage of the twin approach is that this is an elegant way to tease apart genetic from non-genetic developmental risk factors in the vulnerability to schizophrenia. However, twin studies are limited by difficulties in generalizability of twin data to the non-twin population, increased frequency of obstetric complications associated with twin births, and problems in determining zygosity.

Three HR studies, the New York Infant Study (Fish et al., 1992), the Swedish High Risk Study (McNeil et al., 1993), and the Israeli Infant Study (Marcus et al., 1993) followed the offspring from birth onwards. The New York High Risk Project (NYHRP) (Erlenmeyer-Kimling et al., 1995) and the Israeli Kibbutz High Risk Study (Mirsky et al., 1995) involved offspring from elementary school ages; the Copenhagen High Risk Project (CHRP) (Mednick et al., 1987) and the Edinburgh High Risk Study (Johnstone et al., 2003) followed the subjects from adolescence onwards. Some, but not all of these studies have followed subjects through the risk period and have provided data on risk for schizophrenia and related disorders. Rates of axis I schizophrenia and related psychotic disorders among the offspring

Table 23.1. High-risk studies in schizophrenia[a]

Study	Sample	Beginning year/duration of follow-up	Main predictors	Outcome
New York Infant High Risk Study (Fish et al., 1992)	12 HR offspring; 12 controls	1952/> 30 years follow-up from infancy	Pandysmaturation, predicted outcome	Scz, 8%; spectrum PD, 50%
Boston Providence High Risk Study (Goldstein et al., 2000)	118 HR Scz; 126 HR Aff	1959/7 years	Low IQ at age 7 associated with risk for Scz	
Copenhagen High Risk Project (Parnas et al., 1993)	207 HR offspring; 104 controls; mean age 15 years	1962/30+ years	Poor affective control; psychoticism on MMPI; institutional care; unstable early rearing	Psychosis, 20.8%; spectrum PD, 21.9%
Israel High Risk Study (Mirsky et al., 1995)	25 HR; 25 controls; all raised in kibbutz; age 8–14 years	1964/27 years	Poor neurobehavioral functioning; anxiety; undesirable behavior	Scz, 8%; Aff, 24%
Rochester High Risk Study (Wynne et al., 1987)	HR Scz 20; HR Aff 38	1972/10+ years follow-up from infancy	Parental psychopathology and family variables predict school functioning in the offspring	52% of offspring with psychopathology
Jerusalem Infant Study (Marcus et al., 1987)	HR Scz 29; other 30; controls 27	1973/20+ years	Poor neurobehavioral functioning	4.1% Scz among HR Scz; 0% in controls
New York High Risk Project (Erlenmeyer-Kimling et al., 1995)	63 HR offspring; 100 controls; 43 psychiatric controls	1971/20+ years	Attentional impairment; poor verbal memory; motor abnormalities; behavioral problems; psychoticism on MMPI	Psychosis, 18.6%; spectrum PD, 18.1%
Finnish Adoptive Family Study (Tienari et al., 1994)	180 offspring of Scz mothers adopted away; 200 offspring of mentally well mothers	1974/20+ years	Communication deviance in parents associated with schizophrenia risk	Scz, 5.2%; psychosis, 7.8%
Edinburgh High Risk Study (Johnstone et al., 2003)	162 HR Scz; 36 controls	1994/5+ years followed up from adolescence/early adulthood	Childhood behavioral abnormalities; self and interviewer rated schizotypy; drug abuse; major life events; temporal lobe volume reductions	18 of 162 (11%) developed Scz

HR, high risk; Scz, schizophrenia; PD, personality disorder; Aff, affective disorder; MMPI, Minnesota Multiphasic Personality Inventory.
[a]Includes only studies with published data pertaining to psychopathological outcome at follow-up.

Table 23.2. Relative advantages and limitations of prospective research designs to assess developmental premorbid risk

	General population cohort studies	Genetic HR studies	Neurobehavioral HR studies	Clinical HR studies	"Enhanced" Clinical/genetic HR studies
Statistical power/cost	−	±	±	+	+
Feasible number of predictors	±	±	±	+	+
Generalizability to schizophrenia	+	−	−	±	±
Specificity to schizophrenia	+	+	±	−	+

HR, high risk; −, weakness; ±, questionable; +, strength.

of schizophrenia patients have ranged from 8% (NYHRP studies) to 21% (CHRP study), and these risks have been substantially higher than in control offspring. Offspring of schizophrenia parents also have significantly elevated risk for cluster A personality disorders (Erlenmeyer-Kimling *et al.*, 1995).

The prospective HR approaches are free from recall bias. Since subjects with a genetic propensity for a known disorder are studied, it is feasible to examine putative, disease-specific predictors. The main disadvantage of the earlier HR studies, however, is the lack of statistical power, and the relatively modest cost effectiveness of the studies. Large samples of subjects will need to be studied, potentially limiting the number of feasible predictive variables. Another disadvantage is that the findings may be generalizable to only patients with familial schizophrenia. Finally, the low reproductive rates of schizophrenia patients make it hard to recruit adequate numbers of offspring. Despite these shortcomings, studies of HR offspring have indicated that some individuals with genetic risk show evidence of increased liability to schizophrenia. However, the findings are highly variable across studies and often lack specificity (Gooding and Iacono, 1995; Niemi *et al.*, 2003; Sarfati and Hardy-Bayle, 2002; reviewed by Cornblatt and Obuchowski, 1997; Erlenmeyer-Kimling, 2000) (Table 23.2).

"Neurobehavioral" high-risk strategies

The genetic HR strategy is likely to overlook the majority of schizophrenia patients who do not have an affected relative. Nearly 63% of persons with schizophrenia have neither a first- nor a second-degree relative with this illness (Gottesman and Erlenmeyer-Kimling, 2001). Because of this, an alternative strategy has been utilized: using one or other neurobehavioral characteristics to define risk. For this purpose, the putative neurobehavioral marker(s) has to be a valid and relatively specific characteristic of the schizophrenia diathesis. Both population-based and clinic-based samples have been used. Some studies have used psychometric indices of deviation (e.g. high scores on the Minnesota Multiphasic Personality Inventory [MMPI]; Carter *et al.*, 1999) or schizotypal personality features (Lenzenweger, 1994; Siever, 1994). Performance on questionnaires such as the Magical Ideation Scale and the Perceptual Aberration Scale (Chapman *et al.*, 1976, 1978) have also been used to identify schizotypal subjects for this purpose. Using MMPI scores obtained during the ninth grade in 15 000 adolescents, Hanson *et al.* (1990) observed that those who later developed schizophrenia were characterized by elevations in the schizophrenia and the psychopathic deviate scales.

Other studies have used psychophysiological measures. Venables *et al.* (1978) observed that electrodermal hyper-responsiveness in early childhood was predictive of deviant smooth pursuit eye movements (SPEM) later, though it was not predictive of a schizophrenia outcome. Josiassen *et al.* (1985) have shown reduced amplitudes on late positive evoked response potentials in college students with extreme scores on Chapman's psychosis proneness scales. Lencz *et al.* (1993) have observed an association between deviant SPEM and schizotypal personality traits. Collectively, these observations suggest that certain personality characteristics such as schizotypy may be related to physiological indices such as SPEM, evoked response potentials, and electrodermal responsiveness. However, none of these measures have been shown in prospective studies to predict schizophrenia outcome reliably at follow-up (Cornblatt and Obuchowski, 1997).

Like the genetic HR strategies, the neurobehavioral HR strategy is free from recall bias. However, its utility will depend on the choice of the markers used; in a longitudinal study, the initial choice of predictive measures will be guided by the state of understanding of the illness at that time, which is a "moving target" that surely changes over time. The longer the duration of follow-up, the more likely it is that advances in the field would have made prior predictive markers increasingly out of date. Further, normative data for developmental changes are often lacking; thus, it is difficult to be certain by what age these measures have "stabilized." For this reason, it is unwise to conduct long-term follow-up studies using this strategy. The biobehavioral measures often lack specificity for schizophrenia; the significance of these markers for the pathophysiology of schizophrenia is also often unclear (i.e. construct validity). Finally, this strategy also suffers from a lack of statistical power, and is ineffective in cost terms (Table 23.2).

Clinical high-risk strategies

The onset of schizophrenia in adolescence or early adulthood is preceded by a period of non-specific, subthreshold psychotic-like and negative symptoms for weeks to years. This prodromal phase is essentially a retrospective concept. However, in recent years, there has been an increasing interest in prospectively characterizing the prodromal signs and symptoms of schizophrenia, with the hope of potentially diagnosing, and even intervening, early in the illness (McGlashan, 1998). The goal in these studies is to identify potential clinical predictors of "conversion" to psychosis and schizophrenia during follow-up. This approach seeks to identify individuals at risk for psychosis in a clinically defined sample, hence the term clinical HR strategy (Lencz *et al.*, 2001). To pursue this goal, an attempt has been made to operationalize criteria for prospective characterization of the prodrome (Yung *et al.*, 1998). Recent data suggest that early pharmacotherapeutic intervention in the prodromal phase may potentially reduce the rate of "conversion" to psychotic disorders (McGorry *et al.*, 2002). However, the difficulty with this approach is that many persons who may not have converted to schizophrenia could receive unnecessary treatment. The definition of the prodrome, therefore, needs to be stringent and to include trait-related (family history, personality traits) and state-related psychopathological criteria (subthreshold positive and negative symptoms) and functional impairment (Yung *et al.*, 1998).

Using a clinical HR strategy, the frequency of conversion to psychosis in prospectively characterized prodromal samples has been reported to be approximately 41% over 12 months in the Melbourne PACE clinic study (Yung *et al.*, 2003). In the Melbourne study, highly significant predictors of psychosis included prolonged prodromal symptoms, poor functioning at intake, low-grade psychotic symptoms, depression, and disorganization. Combining some predictive measures yielded good sensitivity (86%), specificity (91%), positive predictive value (80%), and negative predictive value (94%) for the emergence of psychosis within 6 months. One of the advantages of the clinical HR strategy is its generalizability to schizophrenia but a relative lack of specificity. Another advantage is that given the temporal proximity of prodromal symptoms to schizophrenia, the follow-up durations needed are shorter.

"Enhanced" high-risk strategies

One way to enhance the power of HR studies is to combine the genetic and psychobiological and/or clinical HR strategies, rather than use any one approach alone. In this way, subjects could be selected initially for the presence of an affected relative, and then only those that also showed one or other psychobiological markers (such as a personality deviation, SPEM impairment, attentional deviation, or evoked response potential abnormality) or those with prodromal symptomatology (using one or other operational definitions) would be finally included (Yung *et al.*, 1998). Such an approach is supported by the observation that, among offspring of schizophrenia parents, those with a deviant MMPI score had a higher risk of manifesting a schizophrenia outcome (Moldin *et al.*, 1991) and that global attentional deviance was predictive of the subsequent emergence of schizophrenia among the HR offspring (Cornblatt and Erlenmeyer-Kimling, 1989). Such an "enhanced HR strategy" suffers from the difficulty that findings from this design cannot be generalized to all of schizophrenia because a narrowly defined population is studied. However, this approach is likely to have more statistical power to detect differences from controls and can, therefore, be used to conduct the newer "second-generation" HR studies involving more expensive neurobiological studies (Table 23.2).

Methodological issues

As discussed above, all the strategies described seeking to elucidate premorbid neurodevelopmental risk factors have methodological limitations. Lack of statistical power, increased cost owing to prolonged follow-up and the use of ill-established and "dated" predictive measures characterize the HR and birth cohort studies; the problems of recall bias and the inadequacy of retrospective information are limitations of retrospective studies. Studies of genetic "ultra-HR" populations such as discordant monozygotic twins and children of two parents with schizophrenia are limited by the fact that these are rare populations to find. Other methodological issues that have plagued the previous HR studies are worth considering.

Reliability of parental diagnoses

Early HR studies were initiated at a time when explicit diagnostic criteria for psychiatric disorders had not yet been developed, and structured psychiatric diagnostic interviews were not used for obtaining reliable information for the diagnosis. Therefore, many patients diagnosed as schizophrenic in these studies may not fulfill the current DSM-IV (American Psychiatric Association, 1994) criteria for this illness. Diagnostic criteria are bound to change over time, but availability of comprehensive clinical information at baseline is critical to enable the researcher to apply future diagnostic schema to such information.

Specificity to schizophrenia

Several of the early HR studies lacked psychiatric control groups (i.e. offspring of parents with non-schizophrenic disorders) and so failed to examine the issue of specificity. It is known that individuals at genetic risk for schizophrenia are at an increased risk for non-schizophrenic psychiatric disorders (Amminger *et al.*, 1999). It remains unclear whether this is from a transmitted risk for a broad range of psychopathology or whether non-schizophrenic psychopathology is a precursor, or a milder manifestation, of schizophrenia. Follow-back studies and prospective birth cohort studies have shown that individuals with schizophrenia in adult life frequently have prior histories of childhood internalizing and externalizing disorders (Kim-Cohen *et al.*, 2003). These disorders may also precede other psychiatric disorders. The issue of diagnostic specificity can best be addressed in HR studies by having appropriate psychiatric control groups.

Generalizability to schizophrenia

The HR studies have often suffered from difficulties in generalizability to schizophrenia. Children of schizophrenia patients are fewer and paternity may often be uncertain. For these reasons, only children of female schizophrenia patients were included in many studies (Fish *et al.*, 1992; Parnas *et al.*, 1993; Tienari *et al.*, 1994). The etiological factors among offspring of schizophrenia mothers may involve a higher risk of non-genetic factors (such as alcohol/drug use during pregnancy and increased perinatal complications) interacting with the genetic factors; therefore, the causative risk factors may differ depending on which parent had the illness (Verdoux and Sutter, 2002). Some studies excluded offspring because of lack of intact families (e.g. Erlenmeyer-Kimling *et al.*, 1995). There are practical difficulties in conducting longitudinal studies of offspring from non-intact families. Recruiting non-representative samples of HR subjects could lead to loss of critical information on risk factors, leading to the problem of throwing the "baby out with the bathwater."

Predictive and outcome measures

The emerging neurodevelopmental models of schizophrenia have led to a search for the possible developmentally mediated and trait-related alterations that may precede schizophrenia. A trait marker, to be useful in studies of familial vulnerability to schizophrenia, should (i) robustly distinguish the individuals with the illness from control populations; (ii) be stable over time; (iii) have greater prevalence in family members of patients identified schizophrenia patients than in the general population and be associated with psychotic spectrum disorder in family members; (iv) be correlated with subsequent development of psychotic spectrum illness in HR children and precede the development of clinical manifestations of psychotic spectrum disease; and (v) be relatively non-invasive and reliable (Garver, 1987; Sarfati and Hardy-Bayle, 2002). While none of the biobehavioral markers so far studied in HR studies fulfills all of these criteria (Table 23.3), some are relatively more promising. Nevertheless, biological and neurobehavioral variables that may not strictly meet the above criteria may still be of considerable interest for prediction and prevention purposes. Nuechterlein *et al.* (1992) have described mediating vulnerability factors that may be intervening variables between risk factors

Table 23.3. Relative advantages and disadvantages of putative neurobehavioral and biological markers for use in prospective high-risk studies

	Sensitivity	Specificity	Heritability	Stability	Predictive power
Cognitive					
Attentional impairment	+	±	+	+	+
Psychophysiological					
Smooth pursuit eye movements	+	±	+	?	?
P300[a]	−	−	±	±	?
P50[a]	+	±	?	?	?
Neurobiological					
MRI	+	±	±	+	±
¹H MRS (NAA)	+	±	+	±	?
³¹P MRS (PME)	+	±	?	?	?

MRI, magnetic resonance imaging; MRS, magnetic resonance spectroscopy; NAA, *N*-acetyl aspartate; PME, phosphomonoesters; +, good; ±, inconsistent; −, unsatisfactory; ?, data unavailable.
[a]Components of cognitive evoked response potentials.

and symptoms. An example is social cognitive deficits, which may mediate the relation between cognitive impairment and psychopathology in predisposition to schizophrenia (Keshavan and Hogarty, 1999). In this review, we confine ourselves to a discussion of risk markers in the conventional sense. Further details are also provided on this issue in Ch. 22.

Predictive measures
Cognitive deficits

The strongest evidence of impairment in relatives of schizophrenia patients appears to be in sustained attention, abstract thinking, and perceptual motor speed (Kremen *et al.*, 1994). Among the various neuropsychological measures, the continuous performance test appears to be consistently associated with liability to schizophrenia (Cornblatt and Keilp, 1994). In the NYHRP, attentional impairment in childhood predicted 58% of the HR subjects who developed schizophrenia spectrum disorders in adulthood (Erlenmeyer-Kimling, 2000). Attentional impairment is trait related, stable over time, and related to genetic vulnerability (Michie *et al.*, 2000). Gross motor skills were also abnormal in 75% of offspring, while false-positive rates were 27%. Short-term verbal memory was impaired in 83% of offspring who later developed schizophrenia (Erlenmeyer-Kimling, 2000), showing a high sensitivity but with relatively high false-positive rates (28%). By contrast, attentional impairments had lower sensitivity (58%) and also lower false-positive rates (18%).

In summary, therefore, attentional impairments may be among the most useful neurobehavioral measures for prediction of outcome in HR offspring at risk for schizophrenia.

Neuromotor and minor physical anomalies

Fish (1984) originally observed neuromotor deviations in about a half of the off-spring subjects in her infant and children study, a pattern she termed "pandysmaturation." Similar neuromotor dysfunctions have been observed in other studies, including the NYHRP (Erlenmeyer-Kimling, 2000), and may predict affective flattening in adolescence (Dworkin *et al.*, 1993).

Minor physical anomalies such as malformations of the ear or palate and facial dysmorphology may provide important clues to understanding schizophrenia spectrum disorders from a neurodevelopmental perspective. Offspring of schizophrenia parents with a high number of minor physical anomalies have been found to develop schizophrenia spectrum disorders more often than other psychopathology (Dworkin *et al.*, 1993). In the Edinburgh High Risk Study (EHRS), minor physical anomalies were elevated in the HR subjects compared with controls but did not predict psychotic symptoms (Lawrie *et al.*, 2001).

Electrophysiological measures

A physiological measure that has received attention in HR studies is eye tracking abnormality (Levy *et al.*, 1994), seen in approximately 50% of adult relatives; studies of SPEMs in adolescent HR subjects have shown significant dysfunction compared with healthy comparison subjects (Ross, 2003). However, this measure has not been investigated as a predictor of schizophrenia risk in prospective studies. Cognitive evoked response potentials have also been proposed as measures of liability; prolonged latency and reduced amplitude of N100, P300, and P50 components have been observed among relatives (Friedman and Squires-Wheeler, 1994). Abnormal auditory event potentials (Schreiber *et al.*, 1989) and electrodermal hypo- or hyper-responsiveness (Dykes *et al.*, 1992; Hollister *et al.*, 1994) have also been demonstrated, albeit less consistently.

Neurobiological measures

The advent of in vivo structural and physiological neuroimaging studies since the early 1980s has raised the possibility that altered brain structure and function could be detected in the premorbid phase of schizophrenia. New in vivo approaches to examine the brain biology of abnormal neurodevelopment are being developed. Several studies, including our own (Keshavan *et al.*, 2002a; Lawrie *et al.*, 1999; Schreiber *et al.*, 1999; Seidman *et al.*, 2002), have shown evidence of structural brain abnormalities in young relatives of schizophrenia parents. In recent years, two prospective HR follow-up studies have been initiated, the EHRS and the Pittsburgh Risk Evaluation Program (PREP). The EHRS has made important observations regarding the neurobehavioral and neurobiological predictors of the emergence of psychosis among young HR relatives: these include self- and observer-rated schizotypy, school behavior abnormalities, and medial temporal volume reductions (reviewed by Johnstone et al., 2003; Miller et al., 2002). Cross-sectional data from the PREP have provided preliminary magnetic resonance spectroscopy (MRS) data suggesting that reductions in N-acetylaspartate (an in vivo marker of neuronal integrity) can be detected in offspring at risk for schizophrenia (Keshavan et al., 1997). Similar reductions have been observed in adult relatives of schizophrenia patients (Callicott et al., 1998). Blood oxygenation level-dependent and contrast functional magnetic resonance imaging enables abnormal regional brain activation to be studied in adolescent HR subjects. In a preliminary study, reduced activation in prefrontal brain regions was seen in HR adolescents during a spatial working memory task (Keshavan et al., 2002b). In vivo phosphorus MRS studies in HR subjects have shown alterations in membrane phospholipid metabolism (decreased phosphomonoesters, which are precursors of membrane phospholipids) similar to those seen in first-episode schizophrenia (Keshavan et al., 2003); similar results have been observed by Klemm et al. (2001). Overall, data regarding the predictive value of neuroimaging measures for the development of psychotic symptoms are still sparse, since HR studies incorporating such measures have started only recently, and only limited follow-up data are available (Johnstone et al., 2003).

Outcome measures

The choice of outcome measures is also critical in designing HR studies. Developmental pathways can vary widely between individuals; one specific etiological factor can lead to diverse psychopathological outcomes (multi-finality), and several etiological variables and several developmental pathways can lead to a common clinical outcome (equi-finality) (Von Bertalanffy, 1968). The failure to identify reliable predictors of future illness in previous HR studies may have been related to the use of narrowly defined schizophrenia as the gold standard in assessing outcome. The likelihood of the adolescent relatives at risk for developing schizophrenia actually being diagnosed with schizophrenia during the span of follow-up in these studies was relatively small; in HR follow-up studies, the schizophrenia-related psychotic disorders (schizophrenia, schizoaffective disorders, and schizophreniform disorders) occurred in 16–18% of offspring of subjects followed up into adulthood (Erlenmeyer-Kimling et al., 1995). However, retrospective analyses as well as follow-up studies of young at-risk individuals suggest that many individuals develop behavioral and emotional disturbances that may represent features of a "broad" schizophrenia spectrum of psychopathology. These features form three groups.

The non-schizophrenia psychiatric disorders (non-schizophrenia psychotic disorders, mood and anxiety disorders)　Prospective studies have shown that adolescents with non-psychotic psychiatric diagnoses have a significantly increased frequency of subsequent emergence of schizophrenia (Amminger *et al.*, 1999; Hafner, 1990; Weiser *et al.*, 2001).

Schizotypy　This represents a set of personality dimensions that may underlie the predisposition to schizophrenia. Approximately 16–20% of high risk offspring develop cluster A personality disorders (Erlenmeyer-Kimling *et al.*, 1995); adolescents with schizotypal personality traits appear to be at a particularly higher risk for future psychosis (Chapman *et al.*, 1994; Kwapil, 1998; Kwapil *et al.*, 1997).

Attenuated psychotic and negative symptoms　Several studies have shown that the emergence of subthreshold or attenuated psychotic symptoms during childhood or adolescence, and brief intermittent psychotic symptoms, have a high predictive value for the future development of schizophrenia (Klosterkotter *et al.*, 2001; Poulton *et al.*, 2000) or of full-blown psychotic episodes (Yung *et al.*, 2003).

Each of these categories of broad-spectrum psychopathology can be operationally defined; taken together, one or other of these manifestations may be seen in at least one third of adolescent relatives at familial risk for schizophrenia. The schizophrenia spectrum of psychopathology can, therefore, provide us with a point of entry for identifying individuals at risk for schizophrenia; characterization of the biobehavioral predictors of such broad-spectrum psychopathology is likely to help us eventually to predict the emergence of schizophrenia by a "close-in" strategy. This approach may be of advantage from a public health point of view, since such data may allow more than one outcome to be identified, as well as prevented (Jones and Tarrant, 1999).

Critical periods of development

Certain periods during development may be particularly sensitive for the impact of adverse biological or environmental influences. Such "sensitive" periods include the fetal, neonatal, and early childhood periods, as well as adolescence. Studies of adolescent individuals at risk for schizophrenia are advantageous in studies of premorbid risk for schizophrenia for several reasons. First, adolescence is characterized by continuing experience-dependent reorganization of neural structures. Neurobiological phenomena that undergo major changes during such critical periods (e.g. delta sleep, neuronal membrane synthesis, and cortical gray matter structure) are also abnormal in schizophrenia, suggesting that an abnormality in the peri-adolescent brain maturational processes may underlie pathogenesis of schizophrenia (Feinberg, 1982; Keshavan and Hogarty, 1999). Second, adolescence represents a developmental period most proximal to the illness onset; follow-up of adolescent HR subjects may, therefore, be cost effective since a shorter duration of follow-up may be needed to determine outcome. Third, genetic HR studies (reviewed by Gooding and Iacono, 1995) suggest that at least a subgroup of HR subjects may become increasingly deviant with age during childhood and adolescence. Finally, recent data support the predictive ability of neurobehavioral indices in adolescence for schizophrenia-related outcome. General population cohort studies (Gunnell et al., 2002) and "historical" prospective (or follow-back) studies (Davidson et al., 1999) have shown that schizophrenia could be predicted by deficits in social and intellectual functioning that were evident during adolescence. Neurobehavioral and neurobiological characterization of adolescent HR subjects is, therefore, likely to be fruitful; however, it is important to ensure that the variables being examined have temporally stabilized, because of the enormous influence of age on several biological parameters of interest.

Conclusions

Studies of HR subjects have revealed impaired attentional and neurobehavioral abnormalities in individuals at genetic risk for schizophrenia. These observations are consistent with the neurodevelopmental basis of schizophrenia and may have some predictive value. Further, these findings provide a good foundation for future studies; the goal of future HR studies is to elucidate the premorbid neurobiological risk for schizophrenia and utilize such knowledge for early identification and intervention in this illness. The following caveats are worth keeping in mind while designing such studies.

First, previous HR studies were limited by their expense, as they involved prolonged follow-up periods with the likelihood of only a small proportion of the individuals developing the illness. Table 23.2 outlines the merits and disadvantages of the various approaches to studying premorbid developmental risk. It is proposed in this review that an "enhanced" HR strategy that involves a genetically at-risk population and the use of putative neurobehavioral/psychopathological markers of risk for further selection of participants may increase the likelihood of identifying premorbid risk indicators in schizophrenia. Using a narrow approach of identifying only individuals with a genetic predisposition to schizophrenia is likely to limit generalizability of HR studies to schizophrenia; an alternative is to define risk broadly, using both vulnerability indicators (family history, biological markers) as well as prodromal psychopathological indicators (e.g. "subthreshold" psychotic and negative symptoms) (Yung et al., 1998). Such individuals are difficult to identify and characterize reliably, however. Carefully coordinated, multicenter studies of broadly defined HR subjects are a valuable approach toward enhancing statistical power.

Second, the first-generation HR studies have often been explorative, at least in part, because of the lack of adequate theoretical models. Since the 1980s, newer conceptualizations such as the neurodevelopmental models of schizophrenia have generated many testable predictions; the advent of non-invasive methodologies such as structural and functional neuroimaging allow testing of such predictions. Future HR studies are, therefore, likely to be more hypothesis driven. The choice of predictive measures in future HR studies should be driven by the emerging neurobiological hypotheses of schizophrenia. Among the promising predictive markers are neurobehavioral indices such as attentional impairment and neuroimaging measures reflecting the integrity of frontotemporal and subcortical brain structures. The follow-up studies should also include a broad range of outcome measures since previous studies have suggested that risk is increased not only for schizophrenia but also for a broader spectrum of schizophrenia-related psychopathology. Issues of sensitivity, specificity, and generalizability should also be carefully considered.

Third, the question of when might it be most fruitful to study premorbid risk for schizophrenia should also draw upon ongoing newer scientific research in schizophrenia. Adolescence is increasingly viewed as a critical period of development during which the schizophrenia diathesis might unfold. Studies of adolescent HR subjects also offer the advantage of proximity to the onset of schizophrenic illness and are, therefore, likely to be cost efficient.

Fourth, schizophrenia is a complex multifactorial and polygenic disorder considered to result from an interaction between genetic and environmental factors. Genetic linkage and candidate gene association studies have implicated various loci and genes in predisposition to schizophrenia. These include polymorphisms in the genes encoding catechol-O-methyltransferase, regulatory G-protein signaling (RGS4), neuregulin, and dysbindin, among others (Harrison and Owen, 2003). Large-scale association studies that examine many gene polymorphisms simultaneously are required to predict genetic risk for schizophrenia. The known ethnic divergence of gene polymorphisms makes it important to construct a database of polymorphisms related to schizophrenia in each ethnic group. Few studies so far have examined the value of specific genetic polymorphisms in combination with environmental risk factors for predicting the risk for psychoses among HR subjects.

Finally, while this review has focused on premorbid neurodevelopmental antecedents of schizophrenia, the approaches discussed herein are applicable to other neuropsychiatrisc developmental disorders as well. Bipolar disorder, which has been considered to have neurodevelopmental origins (Nasrallah and Tolbert,

1997), also has an onset in late adolescence or early adulthood; obsessive compulsive disorder has also been recently viewed as a neurodevelopmental disorder (Ch. 21).

Recent advances in developmental neurobiology and neuroscience make it reasonable to expect a paradigm shift in research on schizophrenia. Studies of vulnerability as well as protective factors and studies of nature as well as nurture are needed. It is critical that such research is linked meaningfully to our efforts for early detection and intervention of this debilitating disorder. It is hoped that the third millennium will usher in a new generation of research studies on HR populations and move us closer to piecing together the puzzle of schizophrenia.

Acknowledgements

This work was supported in part by NIMH grants MH 01180, MH 64023, and MH 45156, and by a NARSAD grant.

REFERENCES

American Psychiatric Association (1994). Diagnostic and Statistical Manual of Mental Disorders, 4th edn. Washington, DC: American Psychiatric Press.

Amminger, G. P., Pape, S., Rock, D., et al. (1999). Relationship between childhood behavioral disturbance and later schizophrenia in the New York High-risk Project. Am J Psychiatry 156: 525–530.

Brown, A. S., Schaefer, C. A., Wyatt, R. J., et al. (2002). Paternal age and risk of schizophrenia in adult offspring. Am J Psychiatry 159: 1528–1533.

Brown, R. T., Freeman, W. S., Perrin, J. M., et al. (2001). Prevalence and assessment of attention-deficit/hyperactivity disorder in primary care settings. Pediatrics 107: E43.

Callicott, J. H., Egan, M. F., Bertolino, A., et al. (1998). Hippocampal N-acetyl aspartate in unaffected siblings of patients with schizophrenia: a possible intermediate neurobiological phenotype. Biol Psychiatry 44: 941–950. [Erratum in Biol Psychiatry (1999). 45: 244.]

Cantor-Graae, E., Pedersen, C. B., McNeil, T. F., Mortensen, P. B. (2003). Migration as a risk factor for schizophrenia: a Danish population-based cohort study. Br J Psychiatry 182: 117–122.

Carter, J. W., Parnas, J., Cannon, T. D., Schulsinger, F., Mednick, S. A. (1999). MMPI variables predictive of schizophrenia in the Copenhagen High-risk Project: a 25-year follow-up. Acta Psychiatr Scand 99: 432–440.

Chapman, L. J., Chapman, J. P., Raulin, M. L. (1976). Scales for physical and social anhedonia. J Abnorm Psychol 85: 374–382.

(1978). Body-image aberration in schizophrenia. J Abnorm Psychol 87: 399–407.

Chapman, L. J., Chapman, J. P., Kwapil, T. R., Eckblad, M., Zinser, M. C. (1994). Putatively psychosis-prone subjects 10 years later. J Abnorm Psychol 103: 171–183.

Cornblatt, B., Erlenmeyer-Kimling, L. (1989). Attention and schizophrenia. Schizophr Res 2: 58.

Cornblatt, B. A., Keilp, J. G. (1994). Impaired attention, genetics, and the pathophysiology of schizophrenia. *Schizophr Bull* **20**: 31–46.

Cornblatt, B., Obuchowski, M. (1997). Update of high risk research: 1987–1997. *Int Rev Psychiatry* **9**: 437–447.

David, A. S., Malmberg, A., Brandt, L., Allebeck, P., Lewis, G. (1997). IQ and risk for schizophrenia: a population-based cohort study. *Psychol Med* **27**: 1311–1323.

Davidson, M., Reichenberg, A., Rabinowitz, J., *et al.* (1999). Behavioral and intellectual markers for schizophrenia in apparently healthy male adolescents. *Am J Psychiatry* **156**: 1328–1335.

Di Maggio, C., Martinez, M., Menard, J. F., Petit, M., Thibaut, F. (2001). Evidence of a cohort effect for age at onset of schizophrenia. *Am J Psychiatry* **158**: 489–492.

Done, D. J., Crow, T. J., Johnstone, E. C., Sacker, A. (1994). Childhood antecedents of schizophrenia and affective illness: social adjustments at ages 7 and 11. *Br Med J* **309**: 699–703.

Dworkin, R. H., Cornblatt, B. A., Friedmann, R., *et al.* (1993). Childhood precursors of affective vs. social deficits in adolescents at risk for schizophrenia. *Schizophr Bull* **19**: 563–577.

Dykes, K. L., Mednick, S. A., Machon, R. A., Praestholm, J., Parnas, J. (1992). Adult third ventricle width and infant behavioral arousal in groups at high and low risk for schizophrenia. *Schizophr Res* **7**: 13–18.

Erlenmeyer-Kimling, L. (2000). Neurobehavioral deficits in offspring of schizophrenic parents: liability indicators and predictors of illness. *Am J Med Genet* **97**: 65–71.

Erlenmeyer-Kimling, L., Squires-Wheeler, E., Hilldoff-Adamo, U. H., *et al.* (1995). The New York High-risk Project. Psychoses and cluster A personality disorders in offspring of schizophrenic parents at 23 years of follow-up. *Arch Gen Psychiatry* **52**: 857–865.

Feinberg, I. (1982). Schizophrenia and late maturational brain changes in man. *Psychopharmacol Bull* **18**: 29–31.

Fish, B. (1984). Characteristics and sequelae of the neurointegrative disorder in infants at risk for schizophrenia: 1952–1982. In *Children at Risk for Schizophrenia: A Longitudinal Perspective*, ed. N. F. Watt, E. J. Anthony, L. C. Wynne, J. E. Rolf. New York: Cambridge University Press, pp. 423–439.

Fish, B., Marcus, J., Hans, S. L., Auerbach, J. G., Perdue, S. (1992). Infants at risk for schizophrenia: sequelae of a genetic neurointegrative defect. A review and replication analysis of pandysmaturation in the Jerusalem infant development study. *Arch Gen Psychiatry* **49**: 221–235.

Friedman, D., Squires-Wheeler, E. (1994). Event-related potentials (ERPs) as indicators for risk for schizophrenia. *Schizophr Bull* **20**: 63–74.

Garver, D. L. (1987). Methodological issues facing the interpretation of high-risk studies: biological heterogeneity. *Schizophr Bull* **13**: 525–529.

Goldstein, J. M., Seidman, L. J., Buka, S. L., *et al.* (2000). Impact of genetic vulnerability and hypoxia on overall intelligence by age 7 in offspring at high risk for schizophrenia compared with affective psychoses. *Schizophr Bull* **26**: 323–334.

Gooding, D. C., Iacono, W. G. (1995). Schizophrenia through the lens of a developmental psychopathology perspective. In *Developmental Psychopathology: Risk, Disorder, and Adaptation*, Vol. 2, ed. D. Cicchetti, D. J. Cohen. New York: Wiley, pp. 535–580.

Gottesman, I. I. (1991). *Schizophrenia Genesis: The Origins of Madness*. New York: W. H. Freeman.

Gottesman, I. I., Erlenmeyer-Kimling, L. (2001). Family and twin strategies as a head start in defining prodromes and endophenotypes for hypothetical early-interventions in schizophrenia. *Schizophr Res* **51**: 93–102.

Gottesman, I. I., Shields, J. (1982). *Schizophrenia: The Epigenetic Puzzle.* New York: Cambridge University Press.

Gunnell, D., Harrison, G., Rasmussen, F., Fouskakis, D., Tynelius, P. (2002). Associations between premorbid intellectual performance, early-life exposures and early-onset schizophrenia. Cohort study. *Br J Psychiatry* **181**: 298–305.

Hafner, H. (1990). New perspectives in the epidemiology of schizophrenia. In *Search for the Causes of Schizophrenia*, Vol. II, ed. H. Hafner, W. F. Gattaz. Berlin: Springer-Verlag, pp. 408–431.

Hanson, D. R., Gottesman, I. I., Heston, L. L. (1990). Long-range schizophrenia forecasting: many a slip twixt cup and lip. In *Risk and Protective Factors in the Development of Psychopathology*, ed. J. Rolf, A. Masten, D. Cicchetti, K. Nuechterlein, S. Weintraub. New York: Cambridge University Press.

Harrison, P. J., Owen, M. J. (2003). Genes for schizophrenia? Recent findings and their pathophysiological implications. *Lancet* **361**: 417–419.

Hollister, J. M., Mednick, S. A., Brennan, P., Cannon, T. D. (1994). Impaired autonomic nervous system-habituation in those at genetic risk for schizophrenia. *Arch Gen Psychiatry* **51**: 552–558.

Johnstone, E. C., Russell, K. D., Harrison, L. K., Lawrie, S. M. J. (2003). The Edinburgh High Risk Study: current status and future prospects. *World Psychiatry* **2**: 45–49.

Jones, P. B., Tarrant, C. J. (1999). Specificity of developmental precursors to schizophrenia and affective disorders. *Schizophr Res* **39**: 121–125.

Jones, P., Rodgers, B., Murray, R., Marmot, M. (1994). Child developmental risk factors for adult schizophrenia in the British 1946 birth cohort. *Lancet* **344**: 1398–1402.

Josiassen, R. C., Shagass, C., Roemer, R. A., Straumanis, J. J. (1985). Attention-related effects on somatosensory evoked potentials in college students at high risk for psychopathology. *J Abnorm Psychiatry* **94**: 507–518.

Kemppainen, L., Veijola, J., Jokelainen, J., *et al.* (2001). Birth order and risk for schizophrenia: a 31-year follow-up of the Northern Finland 1966 Birth Cohort. *Acta Psychiatr Scand* **104**: 148–152.

Kendler, K. S. (2002). Hierarchy and heritability: the role of diagnosis and modeling in psychiatric genetics. *Am J Psychiatry* **159**: 515–518.

Keshavan, M. S., Hogarty, G. E. (1999). Brain maturational processes and delayed onset in schizophrenia. *Dev Psychopathol* **11**: 525–543.

Keshavan, M. S., Schooler, N. R. (1992). First-episode studies of schizophrenia: criteria and characterization. *Schizophr Bull* **18**: 491–513.

Keshavan, M. S., Montrose, D. M., Pierri, J. N., *et al.* (1997). Magnetic resonance imaging and spectroscopy in offspring at risk for schizophrenia: preliminary studies. *Prog Neuropsychopharmacol Biol Psychiatry* **21**: 1285–1295.

Keshavan, M. S., Dick, E., Mankowski, I., *et al.* (2002a). Decreased left amygdala and hippocampal volumes in young offspring at risk for schizophrenia. *Schizophr Res* **58**: 173–183.

Keshavan, M. S., Diwadkar, V. A., Spencer, S. M., *et al.* (2002b). A preliminary functional magnetic resonance imaging study in offspring of schizophrenic parents. *Prog Neuropsychopharmacol Biol Psychiatry* **26**: 1143–1149.

Keshavan, M. S., Stanley, J. A., Montrose, D. M., Minshew, N. J., Pettegrew, J. W. (2003). Prefrontal membrane phospholipid metabolism of child and adolescent offspring at risk for schizophrenia or schizoaffective disorder: an in vivo (31)P MRS study. *Mol Psychiatry* **8**: 316–323.

Kim-Cohen, J., Caspi, A., Moffitt, T. E., *et al.* (2003). Prior juvenile diagnoses in adults with mental disorder: developmental follow-back of a prospective-longitudinal cohort. *Arch Gen Psychiatry* **60**: 709–717.

Klemm, S., Rzanny, R., Riehemann, S., *et al.* (2001). Cerebral phosphate metabolism in first-degree relatives of patients with schizophrenia. *Am J Psychiatry* **158**: 958–960.

Klosterkotter, J., Hellmich, M., Steinmeyer, E. M., Schultze-Lutter, F. (2001). Diagnosing schizophrenia in the initial prodromal phase. *Arch Gen Psychiatry* **58**: 158–164.

Kremen, W. S., Seidman, L. J., Pepple, J. R., *et al.* (1994). Neuropsychological risk indicators for schizophrenia: a review of family studies. *Schizophr Bull* **20**: 103–119.

Kwapil, T. R. (1998). Social anhedonia as a predictor of the development of schizophrenia-spectrum disorders. *J Abnorm Psychol* **107**: 558–565.

Kwapil, T. R., Miller, M. B., Zinser, M. C., Chapman, J., Chapman, L. J. (1997). Magical ideation and social anhedonia as predictors of psychosis proneness: a partial replication. *J Abnorm Psychol* **106**: 491–495.

Lawrie, S. M., Whalley, H., Kestelman, J. N., *et al.* (1999). Magnetic resonance imaging of brain in people at high risk of developing schizophrenia. [See comments] *Lancet* **353**: 30–33.

Lawrie, S. M., Byrne, M., Miller, P., *et al.* (2001). Neurodevelopmental indices and the development of psychotic symptoms in subjects at high risk of schizophrenia. *Br J Psychiatry* **178**: 524–530.

Leask, S. J., Done, D. J., Crow, T. J. (2002). Adult psychosis, common childhood infections and neurological soft signs in a national birth cohort. *Br J Psychiatry* **181**: 387–392.

Lencz, T., Raine, A., Scerbo, A., *et al.* (1993). Impaired eye tracking in undergraduates with schizotypal personality disorder. *Am J Psychiatry* **150**: 152–154.

Lencz, T., Cornblatt, B., Bilder, R. M. (2001). Neurodevelopmental models of schizophrenia: pathophysiologic synthesis and directions for intervention research. *Psychopharmacol Bull* **35**: 95–125.

Lenzenweger, M. F. (1994). Psychometric high-risk paradigm, perceptual aberrations, and schizotypy: an update. *Schizophr Bull* **20**: 121–135.

Levy, D. L., Holzman, P. S., Matthysse, S., Mendell, N. R. (1994). Eye tracking and schizophrenia: a selective review. *Schizophr Bull* **20**: 47–62.

Maier, W., Franke, P., Hain, C., Kipp, B., Rist, F. (1992). Neuropsychological indicators of the vulnerability to schizophrenia. *Prog Neuropsychopharmacol Biol Psychiatry* **16**: 703–715.

Marcus, J., Hans, S. L., Nagler, S., *et al.* (1987). Review of the NIMH Israeli Kibbutz-City Study and the Jerusalem Infant Development Study. *Schizophr Bull* **13**: 425–438.

Marcus, J., Hans, S. L., Auerbach, J. G., Auerbach, A. G. (1993). Children at risk for schizophrenia: the Jerusalem Infant Development Study. II. Neurobehavioral deficits at school age. *Arch Gen Psychiatry* **50**: 797–809.

McGlashan, T. H. (1998). Early detection and intervention of schizophrenia: rationale and research. *Br J Psychiatry* **172**: 3–6.

McGorry, P. D. (1998). "A stitch in time" . . . the scope for preventive strategies in early psychosis. *Eur Arch Psychiatry Clin Neurosci* **248**: 22–31.

McGorry, P. D., Yung, A. R., Phillips, L. J., *et al.* (2002). Randomized controlled trial of interventions designed to reduce the risk of progression to first-episode psychosis in a clinical sample with subthreshold symptoms. *Arch Gen Psychiatry* **59**: 921–928.

McGuffin, P., Farmer, A. E., Gottesman, I. I., Murray, R. M., Reveley, A. M. (1984). Twin concordance for operationally defined schizophrenia. Confirmation of familiality and heritability. *Arch Gen Psychiatry* **41**: 541–545.

McNeil, T. F., Harty, B., Blennow, G., Cantor-Graae, E. (1993). Neuromotor deviation in offspring of psychotic mothers: a selective developmental deficiency in two groups of children at heightened psychiatric risk? *J Psychiatr Res* **27**: 39–54.

Mednick, S. A., Parnas, J., Schulsinger, F. (1987). The Copenhagen High-risk Project, 1962–1986. *Schizophr Bull* **13**: 485–495.

Michie, P. T., Kent, A., Stienstra, R., *et al.* (2000). Phenotypic markers as risk factors in schizophrenia: neurocognitive functions. *Aust NZ J Psychiatry* **34**(Suppl): S74–S85.

Miller, P., Byrne, M., Hodges, A., *et al.* (2002). Schizotypal components in people at high risk of developing schizophrenia: early findings from the Edinburgh High Risk Study. *Br J Psychiatry* **180**: 179–184.

Mirsky, A. F., Kugelmass, S., Ingraham, L. J., Frenkel, E., Nathan, M. (1995). Overview and summary: twenty-five year follow-up of high-risk children. *Schizophr Bull* **21**: 227–239.

Moldin, S. O., Gottesman, I. I., Rice, J., Erlenmeyer-Kimling, L. (1991). Replicated psychometric correlates of schizophrenia. *Am J Psychiatry* **148**: 762–767.

Murray, R. M., Lewis, S. W. (1987). Is schizophrenia a neurodevelopmental disorder? [Editorial] *Br Med J (Clin Res Ed)* **295**: 681–682.

Nasrallah, H. A., Tolbert, H. A. (1997). Neurobiology and neuroplasticity in schizophrenia. Continuity across the life cycle. [Comment] *Arch Gen Psychiatry* **54**: 913–914.

Niemi, L. T., Suvisaari, J. M., Tuulio-Henriksson, A., Lonnqvist, J. K. (2003). Childhood developmental abnormalities in schizophrenia: evidence from high-risk studies. *Schizophr Res* **60**: 239–258.

Nuechterlein, K. H., Dawson, M. E., Gitlin, M., *et al.* (1992). Developmental processes in schizophrenic disorders: longitudinal studies of vulnerability and stress. *Schizophr Bull* **18**: 387–425.

Parnas, J., Cannon, T. D., Jacobsen, B., *et al.* (1993). Lifetime DSM-III-R diagnostic outcomes in the offspring of schizophrenic mothers. Results from the Copenhagen High-risk Study. *Arch Gen Psychiatry* **50**: 707–714.

Pearson, J. S., Kley, I. B. (1957). On the application of genetic expectancies as age specific base rates in the study of human behavior disorders. *Psychol Bull* **54**: 406–420.

Poulton, R. A. C., Moffitt, T. E., Cannon, M., Murray, R., Harrington, H. (2000). Children's self-reported psychotic symptoms and adult schizophreniform disorder: a 15-year longitudinal study. *Arch Gen Psychiatry* **57**: 1053–1058.

Rantakallio, P., Jones, P. B., Moring, J., von Wendt, L. (1997). Association between central nervous system infections during childhood and adult onset schizophrenia and other psychoses: a 28-year follow-up. *Int J Epidemiol* **26**: 837–843.

Reveley, A. M., Reveley, M. A., Clifford, C. A., Murray, R. M. (1982). Cerebral ventricular size in twins discordant for schizophrenia. *Lancet* **i**: 540–541.

Ross, R. G. (2003). Early expression of a pathophysiological feature of schizophrenia: saccadic intrusions into smooth-pursuit eye movements in school-age children vulnerable to schizophrenia. *J Am Acad Child Adolesc Psychiatry* **42**: 468–476.

Saitoh, O., Niwa, S., Hiramatsu, K., *et al.* (1984). Abnormalities in late positive components of event-related potentials may reflect genetic predisposition to schizophrenia. *Biol Psychiatry* **19**: 293–303.

Sarfati, Y., Hardy-Bayle, M. C. (2002). Could cognitive vulnerability identify high-risk subjects for schizophrenia? *Am J Med Genet* **114**: 893–897.

Schreiber, H., Stolz, G., Rothmeier, J., Kornhuber, H. H., Born, J. (1989). Prolonged latencies of the N2 and P3 of the auditory event-related potential in children at risk for schizophrenia. A preliminary report. *Eur Arch Psychiatry Neurol Sci* **238**: 185–188.

Schreiber, H., Baur-Seack, K., Kornhuber, H. H., *et al.* (1999). Brain morphology in adolescents at genetic risk for schizophrenia assessed by qualitative and quantitative magnetic resonance imaging. *Schizophr Res* **40**: 81–84.

Seidman, L. J., Faraone, S. V., Goldstein, J. M., *et al.* (2002). Left hippocampal volume as a vulnerability indicator for schizophrenia: a magnetic resonance imaging morphometric study of nonpsychotic first-degree relatives. *Arch Gen Psychiatry* **59**: 839–849.

Siever, L. J. (1994). Biologic factors in schizotypal personal disorders. *Acta Psychiatr Scand* **384**: 45–50.

Suddath, R. L., Christison, G. W., Torrey, E. F., Casanova, M. F., Weinberger, D. R. (1990). Anatomical abnormalities in the brains of monozygotic twins discordant for schizophrenia. *N Engl J Med* **322**: 789–794.

Tienari, P., Wynne, L. C., Moring, J., *et al.* (1994). The Finnish adoptive family study of schizophrenia: implications for family research. *Br J Psychiatry* **164**: 20–26.

Venables, P. H., Mednick, S. A., Schulsinger, S. F., *et al.* (1978). Screening for risk in mental illness. In *Cognitive Defects in the Development of Mental Illness*, ed. G. M. Serban. New York: Brunner/Mazel, pp. 273–303.

Verdoux, H., Sutter, A. L. (2002). Perinatal risk factors for schizophrenia: diagnostic specificity and relationships with maternal psychopathology. *Am J Med Genet* **114**: 898–905.

Von Bertalanffy, K. (1968). *General Systems Theory*. New York: Brazilier.

Wahlbeck, K., Forsen, T., Osmond, C., Barker, D. J., Eriksson, J. G. (2001). Association of schizophrenia with low maternal body mass index, small size at birth, and thinness during childhood. *Arch Gen Psychiatry* **58**: 48–52.

Walker, E., Lewine, R. (1990). Prediction of adult onset schizophrenia from childhood movies of patients. *Am J Psychiatry* **147**: 1052–1056.

Walker, E., Grimes, K., Davis, D., Smith, A. (1993). Childhood precursors of schizophrenia: facial expressions of emotion. *Am J Psychiatry* **150**: 1654–1660.

Weinberger, D. R. (1987). Implications of normal brain development for the pathogenesis of schizophrenia. *Arch Gen Psychiatry* **44**: 660–669.

Weinberger, D. R., DeLisi, L. E., Neophytides, A. N., Wyatt, R. J. (1981). Familial aspects of CT scan abnormalities in chronic schizophrenic patients. *Psychiatry Res* **4**: 65–71.

Weiser, M., Reichenberg, A., Rabinowitz, J., *et al.* (2001). Association between nonpsychotic psychiatric diagnoses in adolescent males and subsequent onset of schizophrenia. *Arch Gen Psychiatry* **58**: 959–964.

Wynne, L. C., Cole, R. E., Perkins, P. (1987). University of Rochester child and family study: risk research in progress. *Schizophr Bull* **13**: 463–476.

Yung, A. R., Phillips, L. J., McGorry, P. D., *et al.* (1998). Prediction of psychosis. A step towards indicated prevention of schizophrenia. *Br J Psychiatry Suppl* **172**: 14–20.

Yung, A. R., Phillips, L. J., Yuen, H. P., *et al.* (2003). Psychosis prediction: 12-month follow up of a high-risk ("prodromal") group. *Schizophr Res* **60**: 21–32.

24

Developmental models and hypothesis-driven early interventions in schizophrenia

Matcheri S. Keshavan[1] and Barbara A. Cornblatt[2]

[1] University of Pittsburgh School of Medicine, Pittsburgh and
Wayne State University School of Medicine, Detroit, USA
[2] Recognition and Prevention Program, Lake Success, New York, USA

As evident by several chapters in this volume, schizophrenia research in recent decades has been dominated by neurodevelopmental theories. During recent years, at least three types of pathophysiological models have been proposed, those that posit altered pre- or perinatal brain development (Murray and Lewis, 1987; Weinberger, 1987), those proposing peri-adolescent developmental abnormalities (Feinberg, 1982–83; Keshavan *et al.*, 1994; McGlashan and Hoffman, 2000), and those that argue for neuronal degenerative processes after illness onset (Lieberman *et al.*, 1997; Ch. 20). There is clearly a need for a unifying hypothesis. In this chapter, the lines of evidence from both clinical observations and neurobiological research leading to the three seemingly conflicting models are reviewed, and an alternative model that potentially integrates all three is outlined. We will also discuss the possible remediative and preventive treatment options suggested by the three current pathophysiological models, and review the data that have emerged so far from the prevention programs generated by these models (Table 24.1). We end by describing the way in which the unifying model newly proposed here provides an integrated theoretical foundation for prevention and early intervention in schizophrenia.

Clinical "facts" about the early course of schizophrenia

From the clinical perspective, consistent observations about the developmental course of schizophrenia can be viewed to support, at least in part, each of three currently competing pathophysiological models.

The premorbid phase is characterized by cognitive impairments

Clinical, genetic high-risk, and epidemiological studies report premorbid cognitive, academic, and social deficits that are typically quite subtle, yet, in many cases,

Neurodevelopment and Schizophrenia, ed. Matcheri S. Keshavan *et al.* Published by Cambridge University Press. © Cambridge University Press 2004.

Table 24.1. Phases of early schizophrenia outlining the clinical features, pathophysiology, etiology, and hypothesis-based preventive interventions

Phase of illness	Premorbid phase	Prodromal phase	Post-illness onset deterioration
Characteristic clinical features	Impairments in cognitive and neuromotor functions and social skills	Gradual progression of cognitive, affective, social, and educational difficulties, and subthreshold psychotic-like symptoms	Further functional decline and possible progression in cognitive impairments and negative symptoms
Proposed pathophysiology	Neuronal proliferation or migration? Glutamatergic hypofunction	Neuronal pruning/ myelination processes; tonic glutamate/ dopamine hypofunction (early prodrome) and phasic excess (late prodrome)	Excitoxicity (possibly glutamatergically mediated) and oxidative stress
Likely etiologic factors	Genetic factors; early brain adversity (pre/perinatal complications, viruses, malnutrition, maternal drug use), abuse/ neglect, parental age	Psychosocial stress; hormonal changes; drug use and misuse	Relapses; psychosocial stress; substance misuse
Strategies for preventive intervention	*Primary (universal or selective) prevention:* early detection, counseling re risk factors for high-risk parents; improved pre/prenatal care	*Secondary (indicated) prevention:* cognitive remediation, Omega-3 fatty acids (early prodrome); CBT, low-dose antipsychotics, antianxiety, antidepressant, mood stabilizer of antipsychotic medications; glutamate agonists (late prodrome)	*Tertiary prevention:* relapse prevention; adherence promotion; cognitive remediation; Omega-3 fatty acid supplementation; glutamatergic modulators, (ampakenes, glycine, memantine)

CBT, cognitive behavioral therapy.

date back to early development (Done *et al.*, 1994; Jones and Cannon, 1998). In particular, impaired cognition in areas such as attention and working memory appear to be early enduring core characteristics of schizophrenia, which support the involvement of pre- or perinatal brain abnormalities (Cornblatt and Malhotra, 2001; Elvevag and Goldberg, 2000; Erlenmeyer-Kimling *et al.*, 1995). These early deficits have been increasingly viewed as signs of an underlying vulnerability to illness that is dormant clinically (in terms of psychosis) but, nevertheless, suggests a fulminating process that will eventually lead to schizophrenia. This is one of the primary justifications for early intervention, since it is currently believed that preemptive treatment may stop, or at least reduce, the emergence of psychosis.

The prodromal phase is characterized by emergence of subthreshold symptoms

When they do begin to emerge in schizophrenia, psychotic symptoms have a characteristic onset in late adolescence or early adulthood (Hafner *et al.*, 1993). However, recent research has demonstrated that, for many patients, there is a developmental period between the premorbid and psychotic phases, currently widely referred to as schizophrenia "prodrome." During this phase, which can last from months to years, some premorbid deficits appear to progress (e.g. school and social difficulties) while, at the same time, new clinical symptoms begin to emerge, most notably subthreshold (or "attenuated") positive symptoms. This pattern of evolving difficulties is consistent with a peri-adolescent pathogenesis. At present, premorbid deficits cannot be identified with sufficient accuracy to attempt preventive intervention. However, based on the early intervention findings reported since the mid-1990s, it is now widely believed that prodromal signs and symptoms can be reliably identified and treated effectively, with the expectation that this will prevent, or at minimum contain, the progression into florid schizophrenia.

Early psychosis may be associated with further functional decline

There appears to be some deterioration during the early course of schizophrenia, at least in a subgroup of patients (McGlashan and Fenton, 1993). While the positive symptoms appear to stabilize after the first year of illness (Eaton *et al.*, 1995), primary negative symptoms appear to progress during the first 5 years of the illness (Fenton and McGlashan, 1994). Overall functional ability also appears to worsen during the first few years of the illness (Ch. 20).

Clinical observations can inform us about pathophysiology

The "early" developmental model and premorbid alterations

The well-known premorbid abnormalities in schizophrenia (reviewed by Haas and Sweeney, 1992) have suggested that this illness may have its roots early in development. The observed brain abnormalities in schizophrenia have been thought to stem primarily from one or other causal factors intra- or perinatally, perhaps during the second half of gestation. In these early neurodevelopmental models (Murray and Lewis, 1987; Weinberger, 1987), a fixed lesion from early life interacts with normal brain maturation occurring later. Consistent with this view, neuropathological observations suggest altered cytoarchitecture indicative of possible early developmental errors in neural genesis or migration (Akbarian *et al.*, 1993; Kovelman and Scheibel, 1984; Weinberger, 1995). High-risk studies have shown neurointegrative and cognitive deficits in preschizophrenia children dating back to early childhood (Erlenmeyer-Kimling and Cornblatt, 1992; Fish, 1987). Additionally, birth cohort studies have found that children and adolescents who developed schizophrenia at a later date had several characteristic abnormalities such as poorer intellectual and social functioning and language deficits while young. Regional brain structural (Ch. 19) and metabolic abnormalities as shown by magnetic resonance spectroscopy (MRS) studies (Keshavan *et al.*, 2003) have also been seen in young relatives of schizophrenia patients.

The "late" developmental model and the peri-adolescent beginning of illness

Based on the typical adolescent onset of schizophrenic illness, an alternative view has been proposed that the pathophysiology of this disorder has its onset in postnatal life. Based on data that indicate substantial changes in brain biology during adolescence, Feinberg (1982–83, 1990) initially proposed that schizophrenia may result from an abnormality in peri-adolescent synaptic pruning, though this model did not clarify whether too much, too little, or the wrong synapses were being pruned.

Adolescence is characterized by substantive changes in several in vivo neurobiological measures that may indirectly reflect changes in synapse density. Delta sleep, which represents the summed postsynaptic potentials in large assemblies of cortical and subcortical axons and dendrites, dramatically decreases during adolescence (Feinberg, 1982–83). Peri-adolescent reductions are also seen in synthesis of membrane phospholipids, as measured by phosphorus-3 magnetic resonance MRS studies (Pettegrew *et al.*, 1991), cortical gray matter volume (Jernigan and Tallal, 1990), and regional prefrontal metabolism (Chugani *et al.*, 1987). In schizophrenia, similar, but more pronounced decrements are seen, relative to healthy controls, in delta sleep (Keshavan *et al.*, 1998a), membrane synthesis (Pettegrew *et al.*, 1991), gray matter volume (Zipursky, 1992), and prefrontal metabolism (Andreasen *et al.*, 1992). These observations indirectly suggest the possibility in schizophrenia of an exaggeration of the normative process of synaptic pruning in certain brain regions such as prefrontal cortex (Pettegrew *et al.*, 1997; Keshavan *et al.*, 1994).

Neural network modeling studies also support the view that schizophrenia may be associated with synaptic or axonal pruning, but not neuronal cell death (Hoffman and McGlashan, 1997; McGlashan and Hoffman, 2000). Neuropathological studies show reduction in the synapse-rich neuropil and a consequent increase in cortical neuron density (Selemon *et al.*, 1995). Reductions have also been reported in the expression of synaptophysin, a synaptic marker (Eastwood and Harrison, 1995; Glantz and Lewis, 1997), and in the density of dendritic spines (Garey *et al.*, 1998; Ch. 17). These observations suggest an overall reduction of cortical synapse-rich neuropil in schizophrenia. This may lead to reduced neuronal plasticity. The net effect of reduced neuropil may, therefore, be a compromised neuronal capacity to modulate the normal academic, familial, and interpersonal demands of adolescence. When a critical threshold of such neuropil loss is exceeded, symptoms and signs of schizophrenia may appear.

The neurodegenerative model and deterioration after the onset of illness

Kraepelin (1919) suggested that schizophrenia may be associated with acquired neurodegenerative changes beginning in early adulthood, a view that led to the term dementia praecox. This view continues to receive support from several lines of clinical evidence (see also Ch. 20). First, some, though not all, schizophrenia patients may have a deteriorating rather than static course, at least during the first few years of their illness (Loebel *et al.*, 1992; McGlashan and Fenton, 1993). Moreover, patients typically appear to take longer to recover and show less-complete recovery after each successive episode of illness (Lieberman *et al.*, 1996). Second, early treatment with antipsychotic drugs may arrest disease progression in some schizophrenia patients (Wyatt, 1991). Third, prolonged untreated illness predicts a poorer outcome, suggesting a possible "neurotoxic" effect of psychosis (Lieberman, 1993). Fourth, progressive structural alterations may be seen in the brains of some schizophrenia patients in some studies (DeLisi, 1995; Thompson *et al.*, 2001), though others show no change (Jaskiw *et al.*, 1994) and still others show increases in temporal lobe structures (Keshavan *et al.*, 1998b; Lieberman *et al.*, 2001). Alterations in neurophysiological (P300 component of the cognitive evoked response potentials) indices are also consistent with ongoing cerebral degeneration in a significant subgroup of schizophrenia patients (Mathalon *et al.*, 2000).

Pathophysiology may be explained by an integrative neurochemical model

The three models discussed above may seem to conflict on the surface but can be reconciled. Studies of neurochemical and molecular mechanisms that regulate early brain development, postnatal brain plasticity, and brain degeneration can potentially help to understand the many complexities of schizophrenia. The glutamatergic system, which involves excitatory amino acid neurotransmitters, has recently attracted considerable interest as a candidate mechanism that unifies the multiple underlying pathophysiological processes. The glutamatergic hypothesis is supported by several lines of converging evidence, including (i) observations of similarities between the clinical manifestations of schizophrenia and psychosis caused by phencyclidine, a N-methyl-D-aspartate (NMDA) receptor antagonist (Coyle, 1996; Javitt and Zukin, 1991; Tamminga, 1998); (ii) reductions in cerebrospinal fluid glutamate levels in schizophrenia (Kim *et al.*, 1980); (iii) altered glutamate metabolism in schizophrenia (Tsai *et al.*, 1995); and (iv) altered gene expression for NMDA receptor subunits in affected individuals (Akbarian *et al.*, 1996). This hypothesis can be formulated in a "three-hit" model that incorporates all three phases discussed above: the early, late developmental, and neurodegenerative processes of illness. Furthermore, glutamatergic dysfunction ties together several known "facts" about schizophrenia: the premorbid deficits seen in many patients, the onset during adolescence, the relatively enduring cognitive impairments and negative symptoms, the "phasic" features of the illness such as psychoses, the role of dopamine, and the deterioration in the early course of illness seen in some patients (Keshavan, 1999). We discuss these aspects of the model below.

Glutamate is the predominant excitatory neurotransmitter in the mammalian brain. Glutamate is now known to be critical for neuronal migration and neuronal survival during early development, for neuronal plasticity during adolescence, and for neuronal excitability and viability throughout life. Therefore, acting via NMDA receptors, glutamate is likely to be essential for normal neuronal migration in early development (Behar *et al.*, 1999). The immature brain may be selectively vulnerable to NMDA-mediated excitotoxicity occurring during hypoxia–ischemia and other insults. Such insults during a critical developmental period (such as the second or the third trimester of pregnancy) can lead to glutamatergic neuronal loss or receptor hypofunction (Olney and Farber, 1995); this may generate dysplastic neural networks manifesting as *premorbid brain abnormalities*. In addition, sustained activity of NMDA receptors is needed for synaptic survival. Absence of activity-dependent synaptic change as a result of persistent hypofunction of NMDA receptors may lead to excessive peri-adolescent synaptic pruning, hypothesized to underlie the *adolescent onset* of schizophrenia (Keshavan, 1999).

Glutamate, especially the NMDA receptors, may also be critical for cognition and working memory mechanisms (Goff and Coyle, 2001). Therefore, persistent or "tonic" glutamatergic hypofunction may lead to the *enduring cognitive deficits characterizing the schizophrenic* illness. Corticostriatal glutamatergic neurons exert excitatory control over dopaminergic inputs to the prefrontal cortex and tonically inhibit mesolimbic dopamine neurons. Glutamatergic hypotransmission could, therefore, decrease tonic prefrontal dopamine release, and increase phasic stress-induced mesolimbic dopamine release (Moghaddam, 2002). A dysregulation of the tonic–phasic dopamine system may account for the *positive* and *negative symptoms* of schizophrenia (Grace, 1993).

Excess phasic release of glutamate during recurrent psychotic exacerbations can cause excitotoxic cell or dendrite loss via NMDA receptor-mediated calcium influx into cells, or oxidative stress (Goff and Coyle, 2001). This may explain the *neurodeteriorative changes* that may occur in some patients with untreated schizophrenic illness.

It may be seen from the above discussion that glutamate may play a role in each of the characteristic components of schizophrenic illness: premorbid cognitive deficits, adolescent onset of the illness, and early deterioration. Glutamatergic dysfunction may serve as a unitary explanation that links these observations together. The schizophrenia syndrome may result from the cumulative effect of a possibly genetically mediated hypoplasia in early and late maturational processes of brain development interacting with adverse psychosocial factors during adolescence and early adulthood and possible neurotoxic effects of untreated psychosis early in the schizophrenic illness. The premorbid vulnerability to schizophrenia may be caused by multiple genetic and environmental factors interacting to affect early brain development. The adolescent onset of the disorder may be determined by late brain maturational processes, as well as the stresses unique to adolescence. It is likely that early brain developmental defects (e.g. neuromigrational errors or defective neuronal proliferation) may predispose to excessive postnatal synaptic pruning and/or neuronal apoptosis, leading to the schizophrenic endophenotype. The development of a deficit state and of persistent psychopathology after illness onset may be determined by the possible neurotoxic effect of continuing psychotic illness.

Excitotoxic neuronal loss, interacting with genetic factors, may result from early brain adversity (viruses, malnutrition, or perinatal trauma) and lead to selective loss of NMDA receptor-bearing glutamatergic neurons in cortical and subcortical structures. This would account for the premorbid neurocognitive abnormalities seen among children and adolescents at risk for schizophrenia. The normative synaptic pruning process that sets in around late childhood and adolescence may interact with the state of reduced tonic glutamatergic neurotransmission, perhaps acting via NMDA receptors, to result in a net excess of synapse elimination in the cortical and subcortical structures. Reduced activity in the corticostriatal glutamatergic neurons would lead to diminished tonic cortical dopamine release because of reduced mesocortical dopamine release, which comes "on line" during adolescence. Recent data (Scott *et al.*, 2002) have suggested that NMDA agonists may shift the balance of dopamine signaling toward the D_1 receptor and away from the D_2 receptors, by recruiting D_1 receptors to the plasma membrane; this may account for the therapeutic effects of glutamatergic agonists such as glycine and d-cycloserine in improving negative symptoms and cognitive deficits in schizophrenia. The interpersonal and cognitive deficits could lead to an inability to handle the psychosocial stresses unique to adolescence and early adulthood (Keshavan and Hogarty, 1999). Such stresses, in turn, may lead to an upregulation of the subcortical dopaminergic neurons; the behavioral response to stress-induced phasic glutamate and dopamine release is, therefore, likely to be exaggerated, leading to positive psychotic symptoms. If untreated, persistent dopaminergic, and consequent phasic glutamatergic, excess could lead to further excitotoxic brain damage, perhaps by increasing oxidative stress.

Other similar, integrative models view schizophrenia as a lifetime disorder of brain development, plasticity, and aging (DeLisi, 1997; Lieberman *et al.*, 1997; Olney and Farber, 1995). In this chapter, we attempt to extend these models by proposing that the successive premorbid, morbid, and post-onset pathology of schizophrenia results from a glutamatergic dysfunction at critical windows of vulnerability during early and late developmental phases, and the early course of this illness. Each of the steps of dysfunction in glutamatergic functioning in this model could increase the risk for the subsequent step, leading to a pathophysiological cascade.

Toward an understanding of etiological factors

Both biological and psychosocial factors might be involved in the causation of the proposed developmental brain abnormalities. In regard to early premorbid alterations, epidemiological data suggest associations between intrauterine or perinatal brain insult (Ch. 11), exposure to viral infection (Mednick *et al.*, 1988), early malnutrition (Susser and Lin, 1992; see Ch. 9, this volume), and subsequent emergence of schizophrenia. The etiologic factors underlying peri-adolescent brain developmental deviations are less clear. Genetic factors may clearly be involved, perhaps involving genes regulating such maturational processes as myelination (Ch. 1 and the discussion of synaptic/neuronal pruning earlier in this chapter). In addition to glutamate, other neurotransmitters such as gamma-aminobutyric acid (GABA) or neurotrophic factors such as brain-derived neurotrophic factor may be involved in disordered pruning processes. Pathology involving one or more of such genes might lead to excessive or disordered pruning, or a premature loss of neuronal plasticity. The psychosocial challenges initiated by the interpersonal and academic demands of adolescence and young adulthood might interact with cognitive limitations (especially social cognition) leading to the emergence of psychopathology (Keshavan and Hogarty, 1999). The hormonal changes that characterize adolescence also take their toll. Finally, adolescence is the period when substance use becomes increasingly prevalent and this may interact with pre-existing risk to lead to psychopathology.

At least a subgroup of schizophrenia patients may have progressive brain deteriorative processes following illness onset. Proposed mechanisms for such neurodegeneration include oxidative stress (Coyle, 1996) or neurochemical sensitization from repeated exposure to neurochemical stressors (Lieberman *et al.*, 1997). However, one needs also to entertain the possibility that the observed neurobiological changes during the course of the illness may be plastic adaptations of the nervous system to being psychotic or cognitively impoverished (Weinberger and McClure, 2002).

Strategies for preventive intervention suggested by current pathophysiological models

Therapeutic interventions in schizophrenia, which have historically been derived from serendipitous observations, are being increasingly guided by recent pathophysiological models such as those proposed here. Several specific predictions, as outlined below, can be generated from these models and have already begun to yield promising findings in the literature. We will organize preventive interventions into the classic domains of primary, secondary, and tertiary preventions. We will also consider preventive strategies under the three categories proposed by the widely cited Institute of Medicine report: universal (targeting the general population), selective (targeting subject groups selected by the presence of one or more risk factors) and indicated (preventing the illness in at-risk persons with symptoms but not yet meeting diagnostic criteria) (Mrazek and Haggarty, 1994).

Premorbid phase: primary (universal or selective) prevention efforts

It is clear from the above discussion that, while schizophrenia begins in late adolescence or early adulthood, the seeds of schizophrenia are planted early in a long-term neurodevelopmental process eventually leading to deviant brain functioning. It is also evident that multiple and sequential etiological factors may interactively and additively contribute to the emergence of the illness. This view suggests that preventive treatments may be tailored to the stage of evolution of the disease processes in individuals predisposed to the disorder. However, prevention studies must first define their target population. The identification of risk factors is critical for accurately selecting the at-risk individuals most appropriate for preventive treatment. Considerable ongoing research is currently devoted to the identification and validation of such risk factors (Chs. 9–11).

The role of *universal* (population-based) interventions designed to prevent schizophrenia remains speculative. As reviewed elsewhere in this volume (Chs. 9–11), the widely reported risk factors for schizophrenia include genetic factors, season and place of birth, pregnancy and birth complications, antenatal exposure to viruses, and nutritional anomalies. Vaccinations and interventions related to improving prenatal nutrition and antenatal care appear to be plausible options for universal prevention. However, such interventions are not cost effective (Cuijpers, 2003; McGrath, 2000).

Selected preventive intervention targets a population or population subgroup identified to be at risk for illness based on biological, psychological, or social difficulties. At present, primary prevention initiated during the premorbid stage most feasibly will target individuals at genetic risk for schizophrenia. This is because the identification of such at-risk individuals is initially based on family history, so can begin at any developmental stage and can precede the emergence of clinical symptoms. Interventions for the families of genetically at-risk individuals are possible at present and include genetic counseling, family planning, and prenatal care for schizophrenia mothers. In the future, however, it will hopefully be possible to design interventions that are specific to those genetically at-risk individuals who display neurobehavioral and neurobiological precursors found to be accurate predictors of later illness by ongoing studies (e.g. Johnstone *et al.*, 2003; Keshavan *et al.*, 2003). For example, a program for an adolescent at genetic risk for schizophrenia who also displays cognitive and social deficits might include improvement of the home environment, prevention of abuse and neglect, a structured school environment combined with cognitive remediation, and possibly social skills training (Keshavan and Hogarty, 1999). While we do not have concrete evidence about the effectiveness of these interventions to actually prevent schizophrenia, most have been established to reduce suffering at an individual level (Christodolou, 1991) and, therefore, have an intrinsic therapeutic value. Cuijpers (2003) has suggested strategies that can potentially increase statistical power in such prevention studies: (i) placing increased emphasis on high-incidence groups, those with multiple risk factors, and those with multiple disorders; (ii) strengthening the effects of prevention programs; and (iii) increased use of cumulative meta-analyses to improve utilization of data from a large number of trials.

Prodromal phase: secondary (indicated) prevention strategies

Because the presence of attenuated positive symptoms is a primary criterion for identifying the prodromal phase of schizophrenia, it is assumed that the process leading to psychosis has already begun and secondary prevention will be the desirable approach. In the Mrazek and Haggarty (1994) classification, such approaches would be considered to represent an indicated prevention, since already evident but not yet diagnosable symptoms are being addressed.

Low-dose atypical antipsychotic drugs

The view that the attenuated psychotic-like symptoms characterizing the prodrome might be mediated by phasic dopaminergic excess has encouraged early treatment with low doses of dopamine-blocking drugs. In a single blind design study in Melbourne, Australia, McGorry *et al.* (2002) compared low-dose risperidone plus cognitive behavioral therapy with a needs-based intervention (i.e. counseling and case management) for 6 months. This was followed by a 6-month observation period of all patients on needs-based therapy only. The combined specific intervention led to a significant preventive treatment effect in a modest sized population of 60 subjects. However, it was difficult to determine the relative contribution of the pharmacological and non-pharmacological interventions for the prevention of progression into frank psychosis. The differential effect of risperidone and cognitive behavioral therapy for psychosis prevention is currently being investigated by the Melbourne group in a controlled three-cell trial comparing risperidone, cognitive behavioral therapy, and needs-based treatment.

There have been other, smaller trials that are beginning to yield data supportive of early interventions with low-dose antipsychotic drugs. Using a double-blind, multicenter approach McGlashan *et al.* (2003a) compared the efficacy of olanzapine plus supportive and family therapy versus supportive and family therapy alone. The study involved 1 year of active treatment (McGlashan, 2003b) followed by another 12 months of observation. Focus was on change in prodromal and other psychopathology ratings and rates of conversion to psychosis. Preliminary results (Woods *et al.*, 2003) suggest a modest improvement in symptoms associated with olanzapine treatment, although final results have not yet been reported and the potential for the prevention of psychosis remains unknown.

The German Schizophrenia Network has similarly used a 12 month active treatment and 12 month observation phase. Using a randomized, open-label design, amisulpiride was compared with psychological management for "late" prodromal symptoms suggested by attenuated psychotic symptoms (Ruhrmann *et al.*, 2002). Cannon *et al.* (2002) used low-dose risperidone in a small open-label trial for 3 months with four prodromal patients, and six with first-episode schizophrenia and have reported some preliminary positive results.

Naturalistic treatment studies

A different intervention strategy has been adopted by the Zucker Hillside Recognition and Prevention program, which has been ongoing in New York since 1998. In this program, adolescents and young adults between the ages of 12 and 22 who are considered to be in the prodromal stage of schizophrenia participate in both treatment and research studies (Cornblatt *et al.*, 2002). Treatment is provided within a naturalistic framework, in that clinicians (who are independent of the research team) prescribe medication according to best-care standards. This has provided essential observational data about the types and efficacy of medication currently prescribed to treat prodromal symptoms, data that have otherwise not been available. Preliminary findings generated by this initial research strategy are consistent with other prodromal studies in indicating that antipsychotic drugs, used either alone or in conjunction with other psychotropic medications, are most effective for late prodromal symptoms. However, unlike other studies, the data also indicate that antidepressants may be an effective alternative to antipsychotic drugs for individuals in the earlier prodromal stages, when attenuated positive symptoms are more moderate. The non-randomized naturalistic design of the Recognition and Prevention longitudinal study introduces many confounds. However, the results of such observations suggest the need for more rigorous controlled studies. A formal clinical trial is currently underway in this program to determine whether antidepressants do have a protective effect if initiated sufficiently early in the illness process (Cornblatt *et al.*, 2003).

Non-antipsychotic medications

Neurodevelopmental models, discussed above, have also suggested therapeutic trials of drugs with alternative putative (non-dopamine-related) mechanisms of action. Berger *et al.* (2004) have been conducting a 1 year trial with low-dose lithium, the definitive results of which are expected soon. Using predictions derived from the glutamatergic and membrane models of schizophrenia, respectively, Woods *et al.* (2002) have conducted a 2 month trial of glycine and a 3 month study with ethyl eicosopentaenoic acid, an omega-3 fatty acid. Outcome measures have included psychopathology ratings and rates of conversion into psychosis, cognitive assessments, neuroimaging, and in vitro measures of structural cortical and cell membrane integrity. The results are awaited.

Psychotherapeutic treatments

It has been suggested (Ch. 20) that cognitive decline has largely occurred in schizophrenia by the time of the first psychotic presentation. Therefore, a window of opportunity exists during the early prodromal period, which is characterized by non-specific behavioral signs and precedes the more schizophrenia-like features of the late prodromal phase. The German Schizophrenia Network has been conducting a 12 month non-pharmacological intervention of up to 26 sessions of cognitive behavioral therapy over 6 months plus monitoring compared with monitoring alone in a group of prodromal patients (Morrison *et al.*, 2002). Bechdolf and

Wagner (2003) compared a multimodal psychotherapeutic intervention with clinical management for symptoms suggestive of an "early" prodrome (genetic/obstetric risk in combination plus functional decline as evidenced by a Global Assessment of Functioning assessment fall of > 30 points) or "basic symptoms" deemed to be below the level of attenuated positive symptomatology. Results of these trials are awaited.

Strategies after onset of schizophrenia: toward tertiary prevention

As discussed above, treatments that modulate glutamatergic neurotransmission may have a protective effect on the progression of the schizophrenia illness. Recent studies have suggested the potential benefit of drugs reducing glutamate release, such as lamotrigene; NMDA receptor antagonists such as memantine; and agents that reduce the glutamate α-amino-3-hydroxy-5-methyl-4-isoxazole propionate (AMPA) receptor activity, such as topiramate. Such potential treatments are worth further exploration (Deutsch *et al.*, 2001). The beneficial effects of atypical antipsychotic drugs such as clozapine have been linked to their ability to modulate glutamatergic neurotransmission (Arnt and Skarsfeldt, 1998; Meltzer, 1994). Treatments that seek to enhance glutamatergic neurotransmission, such as glycine, L-serine, and D-cycloserine have also been found to be promising in the treatment of negative and cognitive symptoms of schizophrenia (Heresco-Levy and Javitt, 1998).

Another unanswered question is whether early introduction of antioxidant treatments can potentially mitigate the neurotoxic effects of oxidative stress in early schizophrenia. Cognitive remediation studies have begun to provide encouraging results in regard to improvements in functional outcome when introduced early in the course of schizophrenia (Hogarty *et al.*, unpublished data). Well-designed and carefully thought out clinical trials are needed to investigate these questions further.

In summary, the rationale for preventive interventions in schizophrenia goes beyond face validity alone and is rapidly gaining acceptance in the field. However, as our knowledge matures, it will be necessary to replicate the findings of the handful of early prevention studies more extensively, validate the criteria currently defining the prodrome more conclusively, extend the range of potential interventions further to include treatments other than antipsychotic drugs, and target specific prodromal and possibly premorbid phases of illness. Evidence-based demonstration of cost effectiveness of such interventions are critically needed if this field of research is to sustain and solidify this paradigm shift.

Acknowledgements

This work was supported in part by NIMH grants MH 45156 and MH 64023.

REFERENCES

Akbarian, S., Bunney, W. E., Potkin, S. G., *et al.* (1993). Altered distribution of nicotamine-adenine dinucleotide phosphate-diaphorase cells in frontal lobe of schizophrenics implies disturbances of cortical development. *Arch Gen Psychiatry* **50**: 169–177.

Akbarian, S., Sucher, N., Bradley, D., *et al.* (1996). Selective alterations in gene expression for NMDA receptor subunits in prefrontal cortex of schizophrenics. *J Neurosci* **16**: 19–30.

Andreasen, N., Rezai, K., Alliger, R., *et al.* (1992). Hypofrontality in neuroleptic-naive patients with chronic schizophrenia. Assessment with xenon 133 single-photon emission computed tomography and the Tower of London. *Arch Gen Psychiatry* **49**: 943–958.

Arnt, J., Skarsfeldt, T. (1998). Do novel antipsychotics have similar pharmacological characteristics? A review of the evidence. *Neuropsychopharmacology* **18**: 63–101.

Bechdolf, A., Wagner, M. (2003). Cognitive behavioral therapy in the prepsychotic phase: an exploratory study. *Schizophr Res* **60**(Suppl.): 319.

Behar, T. N., Scott, C. A., Greene, C. L., *et al.* (1999). Glutamate acting at NMDA receptors stimulates embryonic cortical neuronal migration. *J Neurosci* **19**: 4449–4461.

Berger, G. E., Profitt, T. M., McConchie, M. A., *et al.* (2004). Ethyl-eicosapentaenoic acid (E-EPA) supplementation in early psychosis, *Schizophr Res* **67**: 7.

Cannon, T. D., Huttunen, M. O., Dahlstrom, M., *et al.* (2002). Antipsychotic drug treatment in the prodromal phase of schizophrenia. *Am J Psychiatry* **159**: 1230–1232.

Christodolou, G. N. (1991). Prevention of psychopathology with early interventions. *Psychother Psychosom* **55**: 201–207.

Chugani, H. T., Phelps, M. E., Mazziotta, J. C. (1987). Positron-emission tomography study of human brain functional development. *Ann Neurol* **22**: 487–497.

Cornblatt, B. A., Malhotra, A. K. (2001). Impaired attention as an endophenotype for molecular genetic studies of schizophrenia. *Am J Med Genet* **105**: 11–15.

Cornblatt, B., Lencz, T., Correll, C., Author, A., Smith, C. (2002). Treating the prodrome naturalistic findings from the RAP Program. *Acta Psychiatr Scand* **106**(S413): 44.

Cornblatt, B. A., Lencz, T., Smith, C. W., *et al.* (2003). The schizophrenia program revisited: a neurodevelopmental perspective. *Schizophr Bull* **29**: 633–651.

Coyle, J. T. (1996). The glutamatergic dysfunction hypothesis for schizophrenia. *Harvard Rev Psychiatry* **3**: 241–253.

Cuijpers, P. (2003). Examining the effects of prevention programs on the incidence of new cases of mental disorders: the lack of statistical power. *Am J Psychiatry* **160**: 1385–1391.

DeLisi, L. E. (1995). A prospective follow-up study of brain morphology and cognition in first-episode schizophrenic patients: preliminary findings. *Biol Psychiatry* **38**: 349–360.

(1997). Is schizophrenia a lifetime disorder of brain plasticity, growth, and aging? *Schizophr Res* **23**: 119–129.

Deutsch, S. I., Rosse, R. B., Schwartz, B. L., Mastropaolo, J. (2001). A revised excitotoxic hypothesis of schizophrenia: therapeutic implications. *Clin Neuropharmacol* **24**: 43–49.

Done, D. J., Crow, T. J., Johnstone, E. C., Sacker, A. (1994). Childhood antecedents of schizophrenia and affective illness: social adjustment at ages 7 and 11. *Br Med J* **309**: 699–703.

Eastwood, S. L., Harrison, P. J. (1995). Decreased synaptophysin in the medical temporal lobe in schizophrenia demonstrated using immunoautoradiography. *Neuroscience* **69**: 339–343.

Eaton, W. W., Thara, R., Federman, B., Melton, B., Liang, K. Y. (1995). Structure and course of positive and negative symptoms in schizophrenia. *Arch Gen Psychiatry* **52**: 127–134.

Elvevag, B., Goldberg, T. E. (2000). Cognitive impairment in schizophrenia is the core of the disorder. *Crit Rev Neurobiol* **14**: 1–21.

Erlenmeyer-Kimling, L., Cornblatt, B. A. (1992). A summary of attentional findings in the New York High-risk Project. *J Psychiatr Res* **26**: 405–426.

Erlenmeyer-Kimling, L., Squires-Wheeler, E., Hilldoff-Adamo, U. H., *et al.* (1995). The New York High-risk Project. Psychoses and cluster A personality disorders in offspring of schizophrenic parents at 23 years of follow-up. *Arch Gen Psychiatry* **52**: 857–865.

Feinberg, I. (1982–83). Schizophrenia: caused by a fault in programmed synaptic elimination during adolescence? *J Psychiatr Res* **17**: 319–334.

(1990). Cortical pruning and the development of schizophrenia. *Schizophr Bull* **16**: 567–570.

Fenton, W. S., McGlashan, T. H. (1994). Antecedents, symptom progression, and long-term outcome of the deficit syndrome in schizophrenia. *Am J Psychiatry* **151**: 351–356.

Fish, B. (1987). Infant predictors of the longitudinal course of schizophrenic development. *Schizophr Bull* **13**: 395–409.

Garey, L. J., Ong, W. Y., Patel, T. S., *et al.* (1998). Reduced dendritic spines density on cerebral cortical pyramidal cells in schizophrenia. *J Neurol Neurosurg Psychiatry* **65**: 446–453.

Glantz, L. A., Lewis, D. A. (1997). Reduction of synaptophysin immunoreactivity in the prefrontal cortex of subjects with schizophrenia: Regional and diagnostic specificity. *Arch Gen Psychiatry* **54**: 943–952.

Goff, D. C., Coyle, J. T. (2001). The emerging role of glutamate in the pathophysiology and treatment of schizophrenia. *Am J Psychiatry* **158**: 1367–1377.

Grace, A. (1993). Cortical regulation of subcortical dopamine systems and its possible relevance to schizophrenia. *J Neur Transm (Gen Sect)* **91**: 111–134.

Haas, G., Sweeney, J. (1992). Premorbid and onset features of first-episode schizophrenia. *Schizophr Bull* **18**: 373–386.

Hafner, H., Maurer, K., Loffler, W., Riecher-Rossler, A. (1993). The influence of age and sex on the early course of schizophrenia. *Br J Psychiatry* **162**: 80–86.

Heresco-Levy, U., Javitt, D. (1998). The role of N-methyl-D-aspartate (NMDA) receptor-mediated neurotransmission in the pathophysiology and therapeutics of psychiatric syndromes. *Eur Neuropsychopharmacol* **8**: 141–152.

Hoffman, R., McGlashan, T. (1997). Synaptic elimination, neurodevelopment, and the mechanism of hallucinated "voices" in schizophrenia. *Am J Psychiatry* **154**: 1683–1689.

Jaskiw, G. E., Juliano, D. M., Goldberg, T. E., *et al.* (1994). Cerebral ventricular enlargement in schizophreniform disorder does not progress. A seven year follow-up study. *Schizophr Res* **14**: 23–28.

Javitt, D., Zukin, S. (1991). Recent advances in the phencyclidine model of schizophrenia. *Am J Psychiatry* **148**: 1301–1308.

Jernigan, T. L., Tallal, P. (1990). Late childhood changes in brain morphology observable with MRI. *Dev Med Child Neurol* **32**: 379–385.

Johnstone, E. C., Russell, K. D., Harrison, L. K., Lawrie, S. M. J. (2003). The Edinburgh High Risk Study: current status and future prospects. *World Psychiatry* **2**: 45–49.

Jones, P., Cannon, M. (1998). The new epidemiology of schizophrenia. *Psychiatr Clin North Am* **21**: 1–25.

Keshavan, M., Anderson, S., Pettegrew, J. (1994). Is schizophrenia due to excesive synaptic pruning in the prefrontal cortex? The Feinberg hypothesis revisited. *J Psychiatr Res* **28**: 239–265.

Keshavan, M. S. Development, disease and degeneration in schizophrenia: a unitary pathophysiological model. (1999). *J Psychiatr Res* **33**: 513–521.

Keshavan, M. S., Hogarty, G. E. (1999). Brain maturational processes and delayed onset in schizophrenia. *Dev Psychopathol* **11**: 525–543.

Keshavan, M. S., Reynolds, C. F., Miewald, M. J., *et al.* (1998a). Delta sleep deficit in schizophrenia: evidence from automated analyses of sleep data. *Arch Gen Psychiatry* **55**: 443–448.

Keshavan, M., Haas, G., Kahn, C., *et al.* (1998b). Superior temporal gyrus and the course of early schizophrenia: progressive, static, or reversible? *J Psychiatr Res* **32**: 60–65.

Keshavan, M. S., Stanley, J. A., Montrose, D. M., Minshew, N. J., Pettegrew, J. W. (2003). Prefrontal membrane phospholipid metabolism of child and adolescent offspring at risk for schizophrenia or schizoaffective disorder: an in vivo (31)P MRS study. *Mol Psychiatry* **8**: 316–323.

Kim, J., Kornhuber, H., Schmid-Burgk, W., Holzmuller, B. (1980). Low cerebrospinal fluid glutamate in schizophrenic patients and a new hypothesis on schizophrenia. *Neurosci Lett* **20**: 379–382.

Kovelman, J., Scheibel, A. (1984). A neurohistological correlate of schizophrenia. *Biol Psychiatry* **19**: 1601–1621.

Kraepelin, E. (1919). *Dementia Praecox and Paraphrenia*. Edinburgh: E. and S. Livingstone.

Lieberman, J. (1993). Prediction of outcome in first-episode schizophrenia. *J Clin Psychiatry* **54**(Suppl.): 13–17.

Lieberman, J., Koreen, A., Chakos, M., *et al.* (1996). Factors influencing treatment response and outcome of first-episode schizophrenia: implications for understanding the pathophysiology of schizophrenia. *J Clin Psychiatry* **9**: 5–9.

Lieberman, J., Sheitman, B., Kinon, B. (1997). Neurochemical sensitization in the pathophysiology of schiozphrenia: deficits and dysfunction in neuronal regulation and plasticity. *Neuropsychopharmacology* **17**: 205–229.

Lieberman, J., Chakos, M., Wu, H., *et al.* (2001). Longitudinal study of brain morphology in first episode schizophrenia. *Biol Psychiatry* **49**: 487–499.

Loebel, A. D., Liberman, J. A., Alvir, J. M. J. (1992). Duration of psychosis and outcome in first-episode schiozphrenia. *Am J Psychiatry* **149**: 1183–1188.

Mathalon, D. H., Ford, J. M., Rosenbloom, M., Pfefferbaum, A. (2000). P300 reduction and prolongation with illness duration in schizophrenia. *Biol Psychiatry* **47**: 413–427.

McGlashan, T., Fenton, W. (1993). Subtype progression and pathophysiologic deterioration in early schizophrenia. *Schizophr Bull* **19**: 71–84.

McGlashan, T. H., Hoffman, R. E. (2000). Schizophrenia as a disorder of developmentally reduced synaptic connectivity. *Arch Gen Psychiatry* **57**: 637–648.

McGlashan, T. H., Zipursky R. B., Perkins, D., *et al.* (2003a). The PRIME North America randomized double-blind clinical trial of olanzapine versus placebo in patients at risk of being prodromally symptomatic for psychosis. I. Study rationale and design. *Schizophr Res* **61**: 7–18.

(2003b). Olanzapine versus placebo treatment of the schizophrenia prodrome: one year results. *Schizophr Res* **60**(Suppl.): 295.

McGorry, P. D., Yung, A. R., Phillips, L. J., *et al.* (2002). Randomized controlled trial of interventions designed to reduce the risk of progression to first-episode psychosis in a clinical sample with subthreshold symptoms. *Arch Gen Psychiatry* **59**: 921–928.

McGrath, J. (2000). Universal interventions for the primary prevention of schizophrenia. *Aust N Z J Psychiatry* **34**(Suppl.): S58–S64.

Meltzer, H. (1994). An overview of the mechanism of action of clozapine. *J Clin Psychiatry* **55**: 47–52.

Mednick, S. A., Machon, R. A., Huttunen, M. O. (1988). Adult schizophrenia following prenatal exposure to an influenza epidemic. *Arch Gen Psychiatry* **45**: 171–176.

Moghaddam, B. (2002). Stress activation of glutamate neurotransmission in the prefrontal cortex: implications for dopamine-associated psychiatric disorders. *Biol Psychiatry* **51**: 775–787.

Morrison, A. P., Bentall, R. P., French, P., *et al.* (2002). Randomised controlled trial of early detection and cognitive therapy for preventing transition to psychosis in high-risk individuals. Study design and interim analysis of transition rate and psychological risk factors. *Br J Psychiatry Suppl* **43**: S78–S84.

Mrazek, P. J., Haggerty R. J. (1994). *Reducing Risks for Mental Disorders: Frontiers for Preventive Intervention Research*. Washington, DC: National Academy Press.

Murray, R. M., Lewis, S. W. (1987). Is schizophrenia a neurodevelopmental disorder? [Editorial] *Br Med J (Clin Res Ed)* **295**: 681–682.

Olney, J., Farber, N. (1995). Glutamate receptor dysfunction and schizophrenia. *Arch Gen Psychiatry* **52**: 998–1007.

Pettegrew, J. W., Keshavan, M. S., Panchalingam, K., *et al.* (1991). Alterations in brain high-energy phosphate and membrane phospholipid metabolism in first-episode, drug-naive schizophrenics. *Arch Gen Psychiatry* **48**: 563–568.

Pettegrew, J. W., McClure, R., Keshavan, M., *et al.* (1997). ^{31}P magnetic resonance spectroscopy studies of developing brain. In *Neurodevelopment and Adult Psychopathology*, ed. M. Keshavan, R. Murray. New York: Cambridge University Press, pp. 71–92.

Ruhrmann, S., Wagner, M., Wieneke, A., *et al.* (2002). Intervention in the initial phase of psychosis. *Acta Psychiatr Scand* **106**(S413): 19.

Scott, L., Kruse, M. S., Forssberg, H., *et al.* (2002). Selective up-regulation of dopamine D1 receptors in dendritic spines by NMDA receptor activation. *Proc Natl Acad Sci USA* **99**: 1661–1664.

Selemon, J., Rajkowska, G., Goldman-Rakic, P. (1995). Abnormally high neuronal density in the schizophrenic cortex. *Arch Gen Psychiatry*, **52**: 805–818.

Susser, E. S., Lin, S. P. (1992). Schizophrenia after prenatal exposure to the Dutch Hunger Winter of 1944–1945. *Arch Gen Psychiatry* **49**: 983–988.

Tamminga, C. A. (1998). Schizophrenia and glutamatergic transmission. *Crit Rev Neurobiol* **12**: 21–36.

Thompson, P. M., Vidal, C., Giedd, J. N., *et al.* (2001). Mapping adolescent brain change reveals dynamic wave of accelerated gray matter loss in very early-onset schizophrenia. *Proc Natl Acad Sci USA* **98**: 11650–11655.

Tsai, G., Passani, L., Slusher, B., *et al.* (1995). Abnormal excitatory neurotransmitter metabolism in schizophrenia brains. *Arch Gen Psychiatry* **52**: 829–836.

Weinberger, D. R. (1987). Implications of normal brain development for the pathogenesis of schizophrenia. *Arch Gen Psychiatry* **44**: 660–669.

(1995). From neuropathology to neurodevelopment. *Lancet* **346**: 552–557.

Weinberger, D. R., McClure, R. K. (2002). Neurotoxicity, neuroplasticity, and magnetic resonance imaging morphometry: what is happening in the schizophrenic brain? *Arch Gen Psychiatry* **59**: 553–558.

Woods, S. W., D'Souza, D. C., Wexler, B. E., Hoffman, R. E., McGlashan, T. H. (2002). Novel early interventions for prodromal states. *Acta Psychiatr Scand* **106**(S413): 12.

Woods, S. W., Breier, A., Zipursky, R. B., *et al.* (2003). Randomized trial of olanzapine versus placebo in the symptomatic acute treatment of the schizophrenic prodrome. *Biol Psychiatry* **54**: 453–464.

Wyatt, R. (1991). Neuroleptics and the natural course of schizophrenia. *Schizophr Bull* **17**: 325–351.

Zipursky, R. O. (1992). Widespread cerebral gray matter volume deficits in schizophrenia. *Arch Gen Psychiatry* **49**: 195–205.

Index